IYENGAR YOGA FOR MOTHERHOOD

Safe Practice for Expectant & New Mothers

IYENGAR YOGA FOR MOTHERHOOD

Safe Practice for Expectant & New Mothers

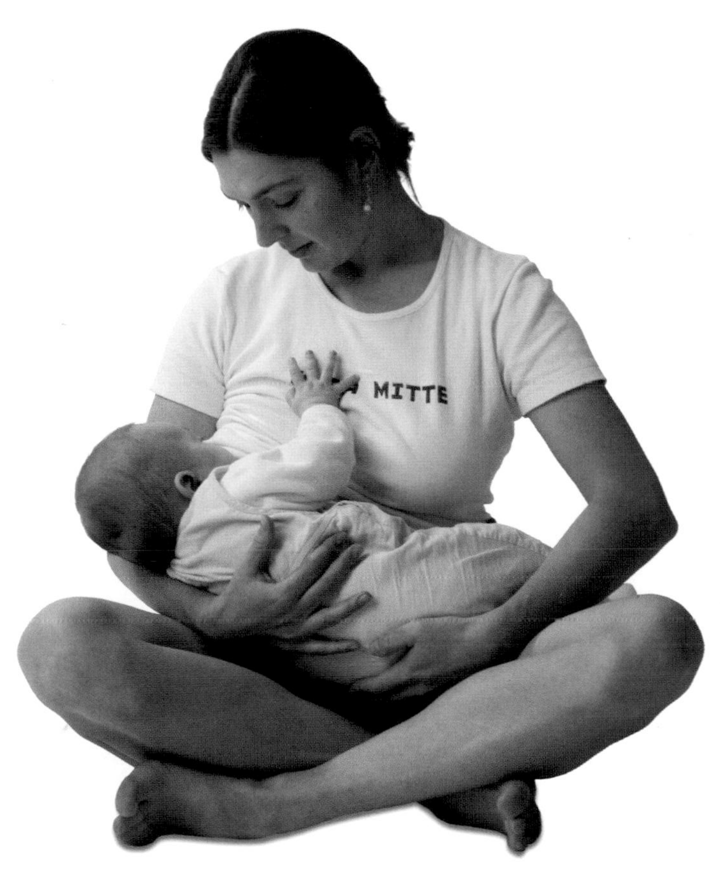

Geeta S. Iyengar, Rita Keller, & Kerstin Khattab

Photography by Dominik Ketz

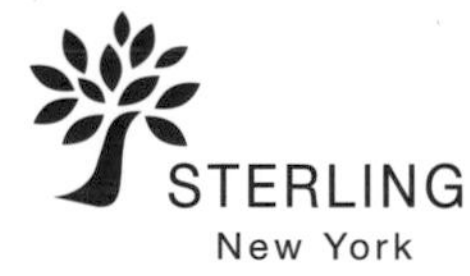

STERLING
New York

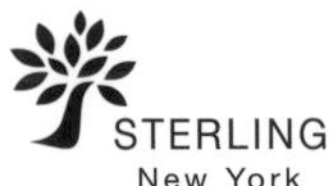
STERLING
New York

An Imprint of Sterling Publishing Co., Inc.
1166 Avenue of the Americas
New York, NY 10036

STERLING and the distinctive Sterling logo are registered trademarks of Sterling Publishing Co., Inc.

Penn Publishing Ltd.
1 Yehuda Halevi Street, Tel Aviv, Israel

ISBN 978-1-4027-2689-7

Distributed in Canada by Sterling Publishing Co., Inc.
c/o Canadian Manda Group, 664 Annette Street
Toronto, Ontario M6S 2C8, Canada
Distributed in the United Kingdom by GMC Distribution Services
Castle Place, 166 High Street, Lewes, East Sussex BN7 1XU, England
Distributed in Australia by NewSouth Books
45 Beach Street, Coogee NSW 2034, Australia

For information about custom editions, special sales, and premium and corporate purchases, please contact Sterling Special Sales at 800-805-5489 or specialsales@sterlingpublishing.com.

Manufactured in China

Lot #:
8 10 9 7

sterlingpublishing.com

Project Editors: Rachel Penn and Steve Magnuson
Design and Layout: Ariane Rybski
Editors: Jennifer Balick, Nina Davis, Jennifer Sigler

CONTENTS

Chapter 4: Sequences of Asanas for Beginners

Chapter 5: Sequences of Asanas for Advanced Students

PART IV: Miscellaneous

INVOCATION TO PATANJALI

Yogena chittasya padena vacam
Malam sharirasyacha vaidyakena
Yopakarottam pravaram muninam
Patanjalim pranjaliranato'smi

Abahu purushakaram
Shankha chakrasi dharinam
Sahasra shirasam shvetam
Pranamami Patanjalim

I bow before the noblest of sages Patanjali,
Who gave Yoga for serenity and sanctity of mind,
Grammar for clarity and purity of speech, and medicine for perfect health.

I prostrate before Patanjali who is crowned with a thousand-headed cobra,
An incarnation of Adishesha
Whose upper body has a human form, holding the conch in one arm,
Disk in the second, a sword of wisdom to vanquish nescience
In the third, and blessing humanity from the fourth arm,
While his lower body is like a coiled snake.

Where there is Yoga there is prosperity and bliss with freedom.

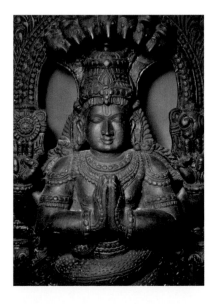

Prologue by B. K. S. Iyengar

I congratulate Geeta S. Iyengar, Rita Keller, and Kerstin Khattab on bringing out a book that is both beautiful and useful.

This holistic way to motherhood contains a fountain of wisdom showing ways for the mother-to-be to prepare herself, so that the child inside her—a gift of God—grows inside her body with devotion and protection through the proper nourishment of Yoga.

The practices of asana, pranayama, and *dhyana* (meditation), which are the progressive paths of Yoga, not only help keep your health in a perfect subjective state, but also keep the candle of inner light and life shining holistically.

Yoga also makes the Inner Light glow even after delivery, by bringing the child to live in harmony with the outer creation of beauty.

This book contains a fountain of information on anatomy, physiology, emotional confidence, and intellectual calmness, as well as on the five elements and the seven constituents (dhatus) of Ayurveda, which mold and blend the nectar of life through the five breaths (pranas), churning the energy or life force for physical and mental health.

Knowing well that physical and mental health are not the end, but the means, a philosophical touch has been added in this book. It will help you lead your life in the right direction through the rhythmic movement of the wheel of life and live in the conscientious divine state of holistic health, growing from the fetal stage to become a useful citizen of Mother Earth.

I am happy to share my thoughts on this work—a first of its kind for maintaining good health both during pregnancy and after delivery—and hope that it becomes a popular treatise for procreating healthy stars on Earth.

B. K. S. Iyengar

How to Use This Book

We decided to write this book in order to share the teaching that B. K. S. Iyengar and Geeta Iyengar have given throughout the last decades. We have crystallized their mountain of instruction into this one book, which introduces the subject even to beginners, so that they might benefit from the Yoga asanas (yogasanas), the pranayama, and the blessings of Ayurveda.

Beginning Students

- Please read everything carefully; don't practice just by looking at the photos.
- Always follow the "general rules" in Chapter 3.
- If you've never done Yoga before your pregnancy, confine yourself to the asanas (poses) and pranayama (breathing techniques) for beginners in Chapters 3 and 4. Chapter 6 deals with the delivery itself.
- If you don't feel well, or for any reason are not sure whether to practice the sequences given for the second trimester of pregnancy, follow the sequence that is given for throughout pregnancy.
- After delivery, you should follow the instructions given in Chapters 7 and 8. Omit the things you find difficult to follow, and practice the asanas that you can do with ease. When your period starts again, follow the instructions for during your period at the beginning of Chapter 8.

Advanced Students

- We ask advanced students not to try everything, not to experiment and take chances. Pregnancy and the time afterwards is a special stage in your life, when you have full responsibility for yourself and your baby. Always be aware of what and how you practice. Don't hesitate to skip asanas that you practiced before pregnancy.
- Be a daily beginner in your practice; always start with a fresh mind and be fully aware of the changes that are taking place in your body, breathing, and mind.
- Always follow the "general rules" in Chapter 3.
- When you're pregnant, work on Chapters 3 and 5. Chapter 6 describes the asanas for during your delivery. After your delivery, continue with Chapters 7 and 8. When your period starts again, follow the instructions for practicing during your menstrual cycle at the beginning of Chapter 8.
- Read the instructions carefully, because pregnancy and the time after delivery often involve a complete change in approach.

When to Practice What

- All the chapters mentioned above tell you what stage each exercise is intended for—a trimester either during your pregnancy or a term after your delivery. Always follow the indications that tell you what trimester, trimesters, or term you can practice any given asana.
- The asanas are classified in Chapter 3 (Sitting Asanas, Forward Bends, etc.).
- The classification gives you a quick and useful reference tool for finding all the asanas and in what trimesters they can be safely practiced; it does not, however, show the order in which they should be practiced.
- The asanas were taken from Chapter 3 and brought into practice sequences by the authors. **Sequencing is an art that takes experience and skill.**

B. K. S. Iyengar says: "When you practice with devotion and consciousness, you will find in one asana the depth and richness of the whole Yoga."

Props

In addition to the basic props that anyone practicing Yoga should have at home (such as a mat, bolster, blankets, etc.), we present on the next page and throughout the book some professional props that are generally to be found in professional Iyengar Yoga classes.

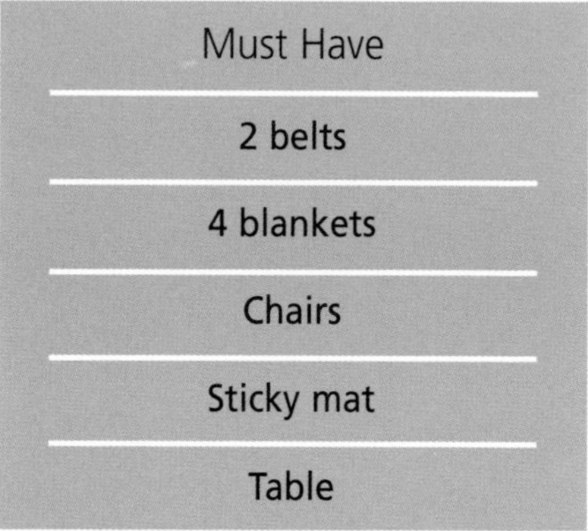

Must Have
2 belts
4 blankets
Chairs
Sticky mat
Table

Most of these professional props, however, can be substituted by simple home furniture: instead of a bench, you can use two chairs; instead of a trestle use a windowsill or a dining table. See examples in the table below, as well as in the relevant places throughout the book.

Optional / Professional
Bench or stool to give height
1 or 2 bolsters
Eye bandage
Foam blocks
Halasana table
Quarter-round block
Slanted blocks
Trestle, or windowsill
Wall ropes, installed as shown on page xv
Weight
2 wooden blocks

Props mentioned here can be bought at the addresses listed on the Useful Links and Addresses page 429. Please note: if you wish to install ropes at home, purchase them at one of the addresses listed in this book, and make sure to install them according to the instructions they come with, or the instructions given by the salesperson at the shop. **Do not, under any circumstances, use ropes that have not been properly and securely installed!**

These are the supplies you'll need to follow this book and practice on your own.

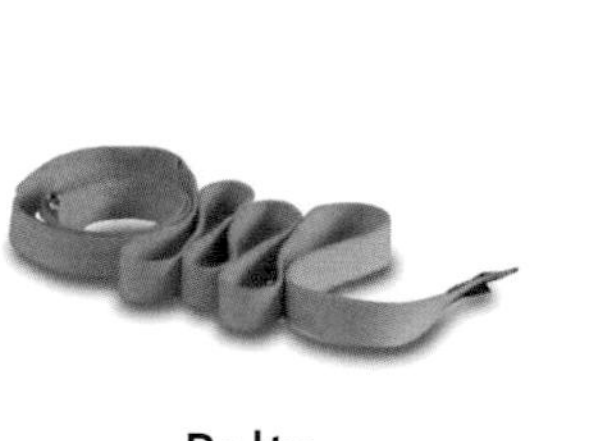

Belts

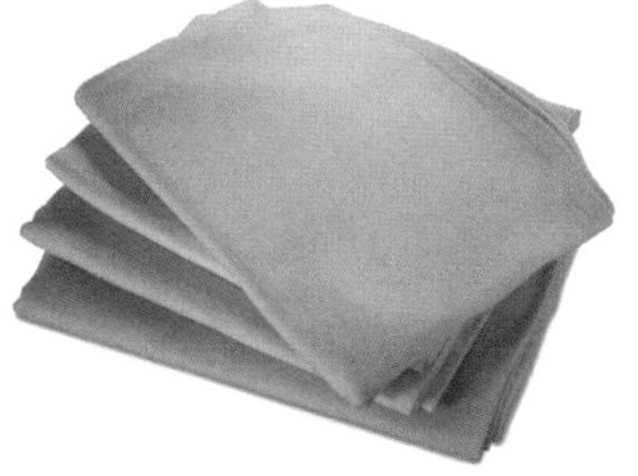

Blankets

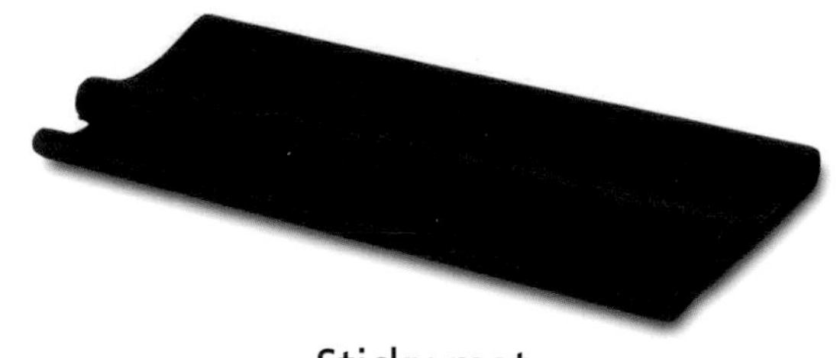

Sticky mat

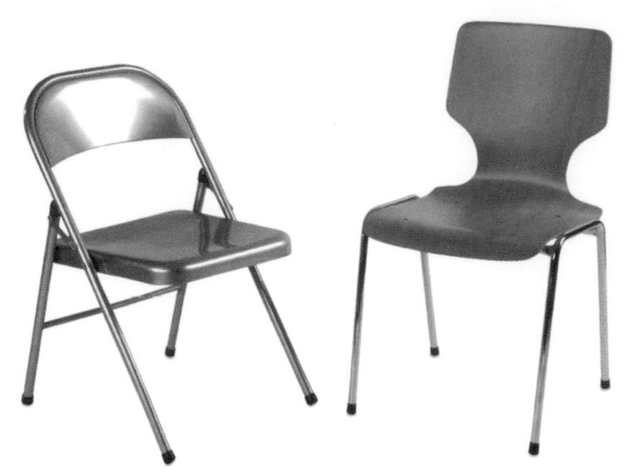

Chair (folding if possible)

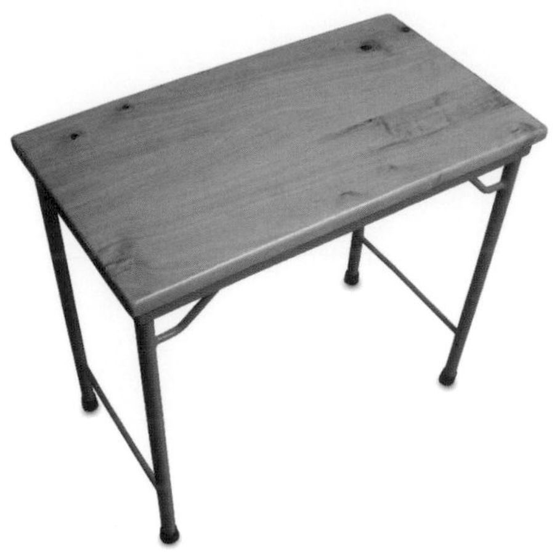

Halasana table

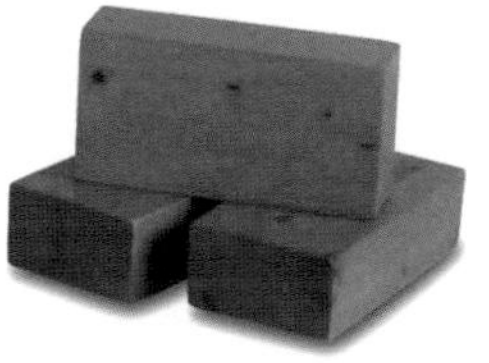

Wooden blocks

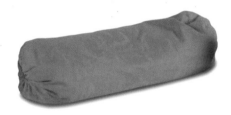

Bolsters

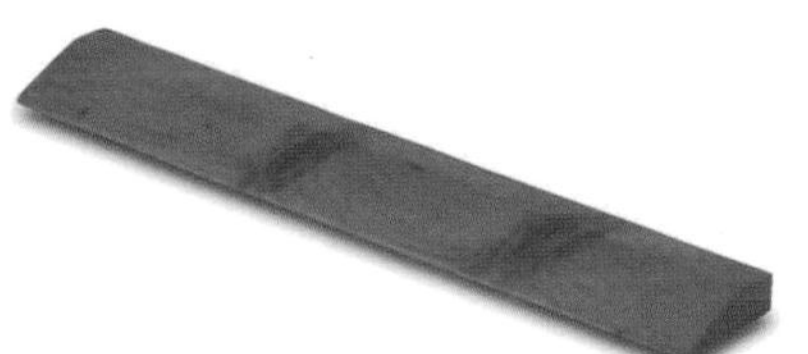

Slanted blocks

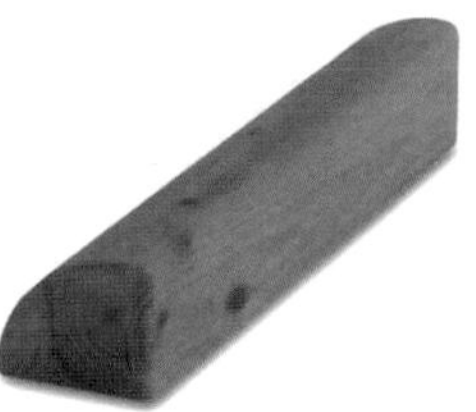

Quarter-round block (or you can use one of the blocks above)

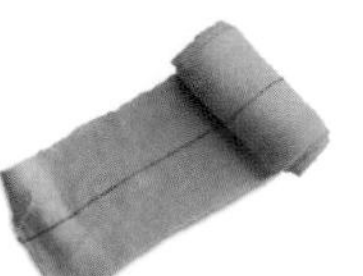

Eye bandage

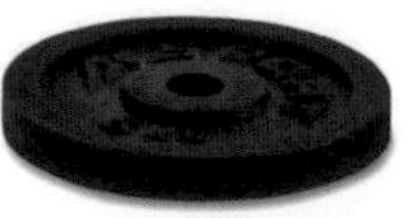

Weight

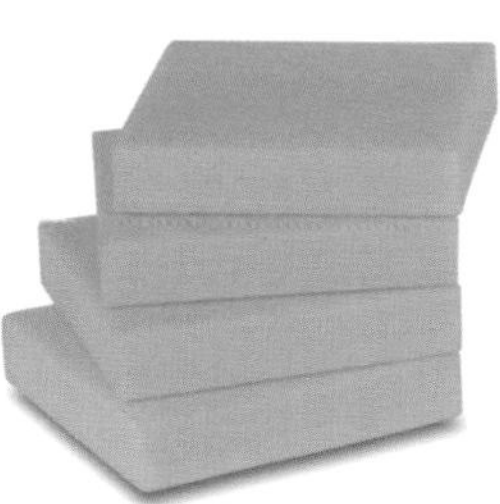

Foam blocks

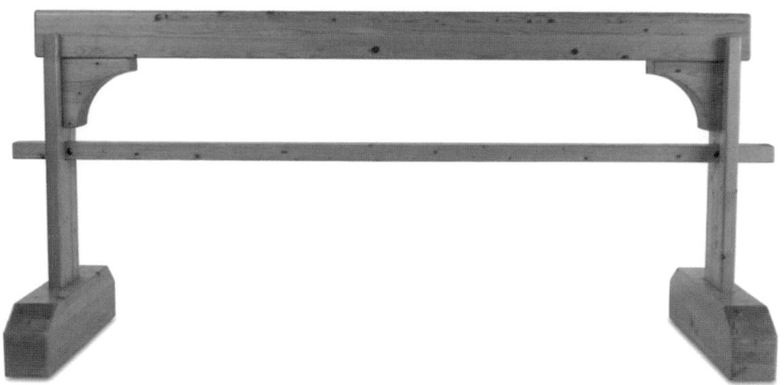

Trestle, table, or windowsill

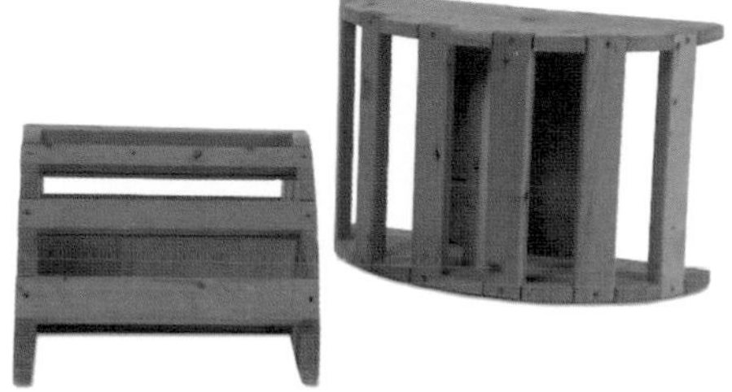

Viparita Dandasana bench

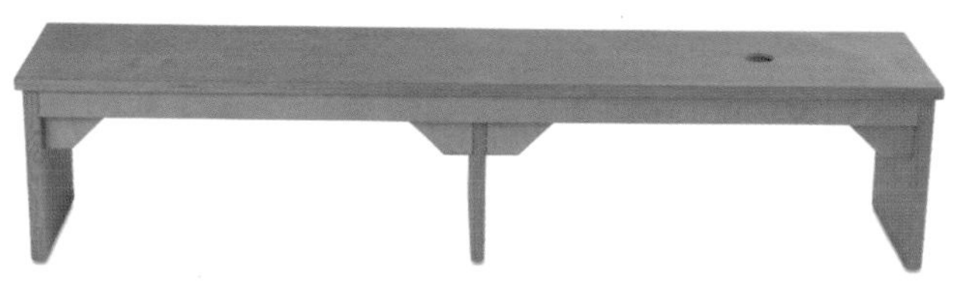

Bench

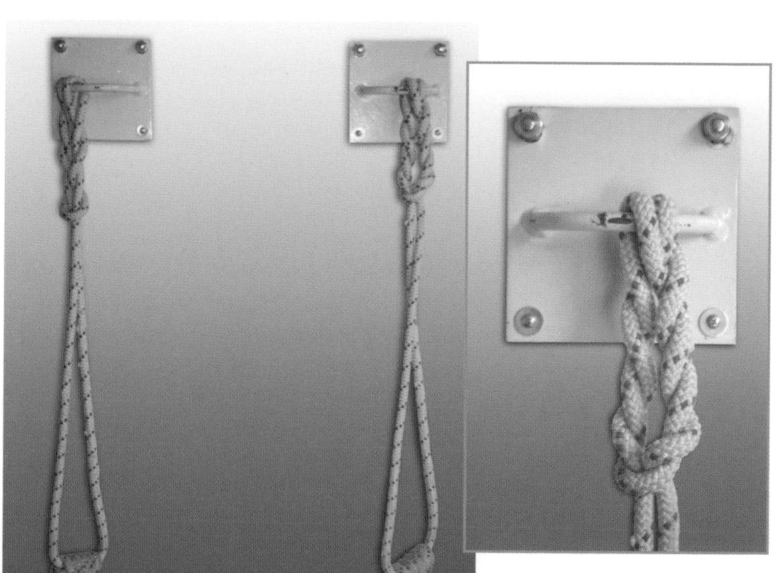

Ropes

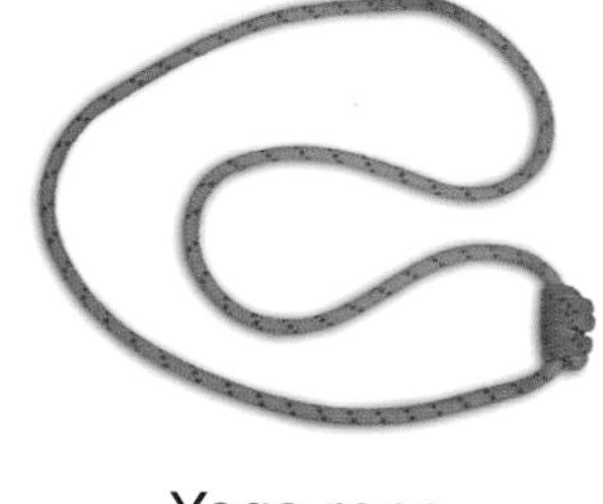

Yoga rope

IYENGAR YOGA FOR MOTHERHOOD

Safe Practice for Expectant & New Mothers

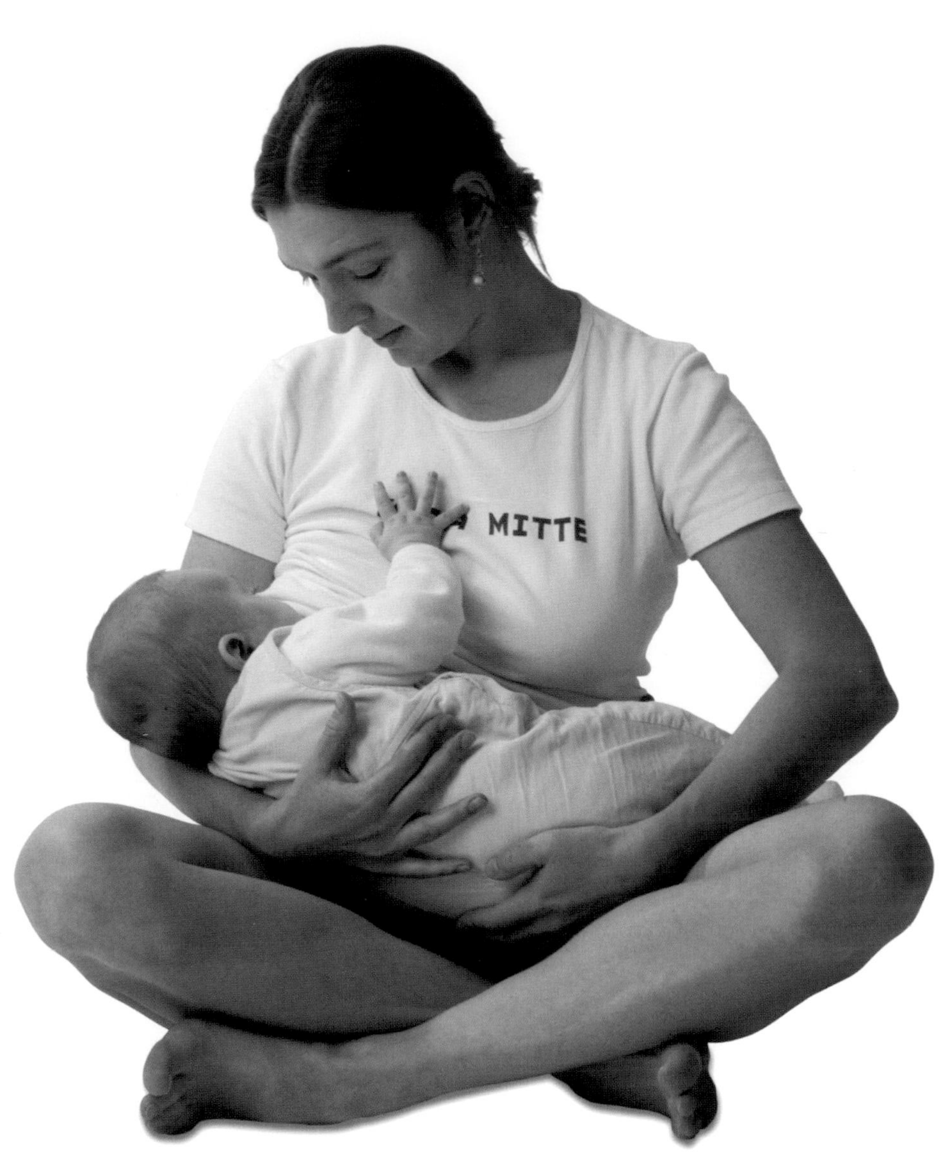
MITTE

PART I

An Introduction to Yoga, Motherhood, and Pregnancy

Chapter 1

Philosophical Background

Definition of Yoga

The word "Yoga" has its root in the Sanskrit word *yujir,* which means to merge, join, or unite. Yoga is the union of the soul with the eternal truth, a state of unalloyed bliss arising from conquests of dualities. The concept of Yoga is estimated to be thousands (8,000 to 10,000) of years old.

The study of Yoga discipline sharpens the power of discernment and leads to understanding the true nature of the soul, which cannot be fully comprehended by the senses or the intellect alone. The study of Yoga enables you to attain a pure state of consciousness and realize the inner self.

Yoga frees you from life's sorrows and from the diseases and fluctuations of the mind. It gives serenity, composure, and an inward unity amid the diverse struggles of life.

It is the art of knowing oneself and knowing the eternal truth. Yoga is the study of the functioning of the body, the mind, and the intellect in the process of attaining freedom. It is the experience of one's self-acquired knowledge and not the result of academic learning, of battling with logic, or of theoretical argumentation. Yoga is a philosophy and a way of life where art and science meet.

Patanjali's Definition

The great sage Patanjali has defined Yoga as *yogashchittavrttinirodhah*:

"The control of the fluctuations of the mind, the intellect, and the ego. Just as the moon is not reflected clearly in the turbid waters of a river, so also the soul is not properly reflected in an oscillating mind. A clear mind alone reflects the soul. For self-realization, the fluctuations of the mind have to be removed, enabling one to attain an unruffled mind." (1/1)

What Is Chitta?

The term *chitta* is used in the field of Yoga to indicate the mind in a comprehensive sense. Chitta is thus composed of mind, intellect, and ego. The mind is the bridge connecting the physical entity with the spiritual entity. When it is directed towards the physical, it gets lost in the pursuit of pleasure. When it is directed towards the spiritual, it is reaching its final goal. There is a perpetual tug-of-war between the two, with the mind being pulled in both directions according to the *guna*, or quality, that predominates, whether it be *sattva*, *rajas*, or *tamas*.

The *sattvic* state illumines the mind, giving calmness, composure, and serenity.

A *rajasic* state makes a person active, energetic, tense, and willful. The qualities of ambition, sternness, audacity, and pride will be profuse.

A *tamasic* state plunges a person into torpor, inertia, and ignorance.

As Lord Krishna explains to Arjuna in the Bhagavad Gita:

"Buddhiyukto jahatiha
Ubhe shukrtaduskrte
Tasmad yogaya yujyasva
Yogah karmasu kausalam."
(Bhagavad Gita 11:50, circa 500 BC)

"It is the knowledge of Yoga alone, that enables an intellectual whose mind is at peace to discriminate between good and evil and to steer the course of his life skillfully."

Yoga teaches one to do one's duty without thought of reward; to be involved in life's turmoil and yet to remain aloof; to act rightly and to liberate oneself from the sufferings of this life.

The Eight Branches of Ashtanga Yoga

The proper functioning of the body depends on the various limbs. The absence or sickness of any one limb affects the health of the whole body. The same principle applies to the study of Yoga and its branches. Any inadequacy in the study and the perfection of any of the eight steps of Yoga will hinder you from reaching self-realization.

The following are the eight branches as formulated by Patanjali:
Yama is conduct towards others or social discipline.
Niyama is conduct towards oneself or individual discipline.
Asana is practice of poses for physical discipline.
Pranayama is breath control for mental discipline.
Pratyahara is withdrawal or discipline of the senses.
Dharana is concentration.
Dhyana is meditation.
Samadhi is self-realization.

All eight branches are interlinked and interdependent. They appear to be different, but all lead to the same goal. As the rays of the sun are refracted to form the spectrum, so has Yoga been divided into eight components that are all interwoven.

Ordinary people—those who are not inclined towards the spiritual aspect—can practice Yoga for its physical benefits. The health of the body and mind is important to all, whether they wish to succeed in their worldly pursuits or in self-realization. Yoga gives equal fulfillment to the believer and to the atheist or agnostic alike.

Indeed, through Yoga, many an atheist or agnostic has become a believer; it is one of the beauties of Yoga that it keeps its doors open to all. Even *sanyasins*, who have renounced the world, can derive benefit from the practice of Yoga, because the health and the mental poise that it gives are necessary to all. On all those who seek physical well-being, mental peace, or concentration of mind, Yoga bestows whatever they demand and satisfies them all.

Lord Patanjali says:
"Yoganganusthanadasuddhiksaye
Jnanadiptiravivekakhyateh."
(Patanjali II, 28)

"The study of the eight limbs of Yoga leads to the purification of the body, the mind, and the intellect; the flame of knowledge is kept burning, and discrimination is aroused."

Chapter 1

Women and Yoga

In the Vedic period (circa 2,500–500 BC), women were held in high esteem. They enjoyed equal rights and opportunities.

Manu, one of the grandfathers of mankind according to Hindu philosophy, describes them as goddesses:
"Yatra naryastu pujyante ramante tatra devatah Yatretastu na pujyante sarvastatraphalah kriyah."
(Manu Smriti III, 55)

"Where women are respected, there gods dwell. Where they are disregarded, there all deeds go in vain."

There were also instances of women undergoing the sacred Brahman thread ceremony at that time. According to the Upanishads (holy texts circa 2,500 BC), *Brahman* or *Atman* is "breath, soul or seat of life, the 'universal one,' the Absolute, the Supreme Reality." Priests who dedicated their life to knowing Brahman and to practicing Yoga participated in an initiation ceremony. During the ritual, male initiates had their hair cut, and both females and males were given the holy thread that crosses the heart as a sign of their strength and zest to follow the ultimate life of a *Brahmacharin*. They studied the Vedas with their guru (teacher) and received training in various arts such as wrestling, archery, Yoga, music, and drama.

Gradually the woman's position became a subsidiary one and her freedom was curtailed, even though she was regarded as a mother and had to shoulder social responsibilities. She was considered the "weaker sex," and consequently held no social status. She lost the privileges she had enjoyed during the Vedic times. Studying with her guru and the thread ceremony were denied to her. In education she lagged far behind. The doors to the study of philosophy, science, arts, and Yoga were closed to her, with the result that her position deteriorated still further.

The status of women has considerably improved since the period after Vedic times. Today the path of Yoga is open to all, irrespective of race, caste, creed, and sex. Anyone can attain liberation through Yoga.

The many facets of woman shine in various fields; her intelligence, acumen, and creativity have a wider scope than men for fuller expression. On the stage of life she has to perform many roles—daughter, sister, wife, mother, and friend. She has to give her best in all these roles.

In *samkhyayoga*, a school of ancient Indian philosophy that was founded by Kapila, woman is compared to *prakriti* (nature). Like nature, she has to remain ever active. When she is, her life blossoms and her home is cheerful. That is why the playwright Kalidasa describes woman as the spark of life in a family. This very spark is what uplifts society.

Apart from the traditional roles mentioned above, a woman has an additional part to play in society. In this age of all-around competition, she has become doctor, lawyer, politician, and professor, and she has acquitted herself worthily. Yet, when the struggle exhausts even the upper limits of her patience, her body and mind get fatigued and her natural attention towards her family and children lessens. This results in negligence and frustration.

The Four Stages of Life

A woman's body is biologically created for certain specific functions. She has to undergo the four stages of life—childhood, adolescence, middle age, and old age. In each of these four stages, she undergoes physiological changes and has to face problems and internal conflicts. This affects her physical and physiological organs as well as her mind, and much of her energy is lost in coming to terms with life during the periods of change.

Motherhood is a woman's ordained duty. This is not merely a physical state, but a divine state. In giving birth, new responsibilities begin for her, and she has to prove herself. Motherhood adorns her with the sacred qualities of love, sacrifice, faith, tolerance, good will, and hard work. This is her highest religion, her *svadharma*.

These qualities are ingrained deep into her nature. They can make her feel somewhat servile when she is overwhelmed by the burdens of life, because she is not able to free herself from the plethora of duties that nature thrusts upon her. The endless struggle of being a woman and a mother, being tied to her work and her duty, trains her to face the world and its dualities with equanimity.

A woman has to pay a high price physically and psychologically in her multiple roles. The stabilization of physical and mental states is achieved by asanas and pranayama. Her salvation lies in practicing them.

Yoga is especially well suited for women, who although they have family responsibilities, can perform these Yogic asanas in the privacy and comfort of their own home.

Health According to Ayurveda

Ayurveda is the traditional Indian medicine. *Ayus* means "life" and *veda* means "science." Thus, Ayurveda is the science of life.

Western medicine, which defines health as the absence of disease, deals primarily with the symptoms of disease. The target of Ayurveda, however, is to maintain health—of body, mind, and soul—and to avoid disease. When illness does occur, Ayurvedic medicine uses a holistic process to find the reasons for the disease, in order to restore health completely.

The passage above sums up the philosophy of Ayurveda.

According to the philosophy of Ayurveda, ayus (life) is of four types: *hitayu*, *ahitayu*, *sukhayu*, and *duhkhayu*.

Hitayu is a saintly kind of life, in which the person is selfless, generous, thinks of all living beings, and has very good control over *kama* (desires).

Ahitayu is the opposite of this.

Sukhayu is a happy life, especially at an early age. The person is devoid of any diseases and enjoys the wealth and power to do any desired work. Whatever he does, he does in a rich manner.

Duhkhayu is the opposite of this.

Generally, a human life is a combination of these four types and one has to try hard to achieve hitayu and sukhayu.

Hita is a technical word that means maintaining or creating a balance of *doshas* (active principles of the body). It can refer to areas such as *ahara* (food), *vihara* (behavior), and psychological factors.

Ahita works against that; it means maintaining or generating an imbalance of doshas.

The Ayurvedic texts elaborate on hita and ahita for any kind of ayus (life), from conception till death. Then the *manam* (quantum) of the life can be decided on the basis of measuring the physical characteristics of newborn babies, which can denote the longevity or shortening of life.

The Nature of Physical and Mental Well-Being

No amount of wealth can equal health. Between the two, the choice is always with health, since wealth cannot be enjoyed without health, whereas wealth can be attained if one has health.

The Upanishads (Hindu scriptures, circa 2,500 BC) say:
"Health confers longevity, firmness, and strength; by this the entire terrestrial sphere will become affluent fully."

All virtuous acts and religious merits are attainable only if there is good health.

The *Charaka Samhita*, a text of Indian Ayurvedic medical science written by the ancient scientist Charaka, says:
"Dharmartha kama mokshanam Arogyam mulam uttamam."
(Charaka Samhita Vol. 1, 1:15) (1/2)

"The fundamental requirement of the body is good health in order to attain the four objectives of human existence, namely, acquisition of religious merits (*dharma*), wealth for living in comfort and generousness (*artha*), gratification of permissible pleasures and fulfillment of desires (*kama*), and lastly, the endeavor to obtain liberation from the shackles of the mundane cycles of births and deaths (*moksha*)."

Without health there is no strength. Strength is preserved only when health is maintained. Health of the body means both physical and mental health. It is a sign of a peaceful state of the body and the mind, when one is able to follow ethical codes, maintain moral standards, and fulfill social obligations.

Good health can neither be bought nor bartered. It cannot be acquired by force. It is a culture of external and internal cleanliness, dietary control, proper exercise of the limbs and the organs, physical and mental balance, and rest.

The Nature of Disease

Disease may be defined as a disturbance in the normal functioning of the body and the mind. Ayurveda describes health as the perfect harmony of bodily functions, a well-balanced metabolism, and the happy and poised state of the mind and the senses.

The science of Ayurveda has categorized the physiological functions of the body as falling under three headings: *chalana* (movement), *pachana* (digestion or assimilation), and *lepana* (respiration or illumination).

These correspond respectively to the three humors: *vata* (ether and wind), *pitta* (fire), and *kapha* (earth and water). These humors maintain a harmonious ratio of their own when the body is in a good state of health performing the above three functions.

Health is defined as equilibrium among the five factors:

1. The doshas (humors, or active principles of the body)
2. The dhatus (seven tissues of the body)
3. Agni (proper functioning of digestion and elimination of waste matter, which is called metabolism of the body)
4. Clarity or purity of the senses
5. Tranquility and peace of the mind

Any deficiency or excess in the normal quantity of the doshas or the dhatus, or any obstruction in their flow, brings about imbalance and results in indisposition causing disease.

Health According to Yoga

Like Ayurveda, Yoga recognizes the three afflictions, namely *adhyatmika*, *adhibhautika*, and *adhidaivika*.

Adhyatmika is concerned with both body and mind, that is, somatic and psychic diseases.

Adhibhautika afflictions are caused by nature's fury—epidemics, unnatural deaths at the hands of beasts, drowning, cyclones, tempests, sunstroke, and devastation by flood.

Daivika means destiny. Adhidaivika afflictions are caused by destiny: our own karmas are responsible for it. In adhidaivika you cannot trace the cause, but it happens. The child whose parents have AIDS may carry the disease although he or she is not responsible for it. Adhidaivika afflictions are hereditary diseases, which are passed on from parents to the child. Here, Yoga adds something more to the definition of health and makes it more comprehensive.

According to Yoga, any obstacle that prevents the realization of the self is an indication of physical indisposition causing a modification in the mental state, *chittavrtti*. The aim of Yoga is to restrain both physical disturbances and mental modifications.

The obstacles or impediments are: sickness, inaction, doubt, delusion, carelessness, non-abstention, inadvertent conception, non-attainment, instability in the *sadhana* (the practice of Yoga), sorrow, dejection, restlessness, and disturbed or arrhythmic breathing. These originate in the body or in the mind. Therefore, health means total freedom from physical and mental afflictions in order to achieve one's goal. Modern science is not at a variance with this definition; it agrees that the relationship between the body and the mind is intimate.

If life has to be protected, health must be maintained and the functioning of the various organs of the body, especially the central nervous system, should be well taken care of. Many diseases are due to mental depression, anger, grief, uninhibited sexual indulgence, anxiety, discontent, distrust, and other psycho-somatic disturbances. Many people given to mental weakness suffer from diseases of the imagination, which in many cases prove fatal. By developing such qualities as positive thinking, enthusiasm, courage, hope, and optimism, even weak bodies and minds can turn into strong, healthy ones.

The practice of Yoga brings a perfect balance in body and mind. It gives the body the health it needs to cooperate with the mind, so that steadiness, composure, and firmness are developed. Patanjali explains that the practice of Yoga enables one to avoid the pain that might be in store in the future.

So you can see that the practice of Yoga brings both physical health as well as mental health. It teaches how to conquer obstacles so that one can live peacefully and in perfect happiness to achieve the goal of life—self-realization.

Yoga Is Ideal for Women

"Nature meant woman to be her masterpiece."
John Ruskin

Her beauty and grace, as well as her gentle nature, bear witness to woman as the masterpiece of nature. She not only possesses external beauty, but her soft and graceful form belies her firmness of character and power of endurance. Woman is tender and flexible, and this makes her move with ease and grace, in contrast to man, whose body is rigid, rough, and robust. Yoga enhances elasticity, and it seems that the Creator has favored woman in making her body fit and suitable for Yoga.

A woman's muscles are soft and light compared to man's, which are large, coarse, and heavy. Her skeletal structure is less broad. She has the power to withstand physical strains and mental pressures to a far greater extent than man; this is not due to physical strength or power of endurance, but is nature's unique gift to her. Nature has also endowed her with the responsibility of perpetuating mankind. The wealth of a nation and the health of the future generation depend upon her physical and mental well-being.

From a careful study of the features distinguishing woman from man, meaning her physical body and her changing physiological functions and emotional states, it follows that, if she chooses to adopt yogasanas (Yoga + asanas = Yoga poses) and pranayama as part of her way of life, they will offer her added meaning and advantage.

72,000 *nadis* (fine energy channels and vessels) spring from the navel of the body. This indicates the importance of the navel region and of maintaining a soft, relaxed, lifted, and toned abdominal and navel structure. Good Yoga practice shows itself in a soft and relaxed abdomen, which reflects a soft and relaxed state of the throat and the thyroid.

This can only be achieved by practice that finds its balance starting from the feet. The exact rooting of the feet and aligned leg work enable you to balance your pelvis and lift your spine and entire torso. Good pose is instrumental in maintaining and ensuring the softness of abdomen, diaphragm, and throat. This in turn leads to soft, toned spinal and back muscles, which has positive effects on the internal organs and the organs of perception, the throat, the thyroid, and consequently the whole endocrinologic system.

The practice of yogasanas and pranayama helps the woman to align her anatomical and physiological structures, so that body-related stress is avoided. The tensions and upheavals of daily life can strongly affect the diaphragm and thus the breathing patterns, making her short of breath.

A woman has to learn that the muscles and anatomical structures are meant to structure the outer and inner body and to balance all bodily systems, in order to balance the breathing and the mind.

Yoga helps a woman fulfill her tasks and maintain her complexion's luster and femininity. She has no need of cosmetics, because good blood circulation makes her skin glow.

Yogic practices, without exaggeration, are ideally designed to help a woman in all the conditions and circumstances of her daily life. Yogasanas exercise the entire body and revitalize all the physiological systems, resulting in a sound mind in a sound body. Each asana cultivates the body and the mind evenly. Yogasanas and pranayama have withstood the test of time and are helpful for all the needs of men and women in their pursuit of perfect health and supreme happiness.

The Difference between Yoga and Other Physical Exercises

All types of exercises have two features: motion and action.

Asanas exercise the front, back, side, and interior portions of the body equally, as every pose is a complete entity in which each part of the body has a particular role to play. Motion is constant movement from position to position or from place to place. Asanas, though appearing static externally, are full of dynamic action within. A full range of movements and actions such as horizontal, vertical, diagonal, and circumferential extension and expansion are created while performing the poses. This requires skill, intelligence, and application. No portion of the body or the mind is left untouched when an asana is carefully and correctly performed.

Asanas are psycho-physiological, unlike physical exercises that are purely external. While asanas develop body consciousness, they also generate internal consciousness and stabilize the mind. Yoga is a culture of body, mind, and soul.

In other physical exercises, body movements may be done with precision alone, whereas in Yoga, a deeper awareness is cultivated, bringing balance and alignment of body and mind.

Like physical exercises, asanas develop muscles and remove stiffness so that the body movements become free. However, they are more concerned with the physiological body and the vital organs than with the physical body. They strengthen and revitalize organs such as the liver, spleen, intestines, lungs, and kidneys. Each asana works on the entire system. It is an organic exercise that removes toxins.

The health of the entire body depends on the digestive system. Its malfunctioning is the root of many diseases, and asanas help alleviate them.

The practice of asanas and pranayama makes the respiratory system work to its optimum, ensuring the proper supply of oxygen to the blood and improving circulation.

The endocrine glands are ductless glands that secrete hormones, which are circulated throughout the body and are essential for physical and mental health. Certain asanas stimulate these glands to ensure their proper functioning, while others normalize the over-functioning of the hormones and maintain a balance in the system.

Asanas and pranayama are a great help in the proper functioning of the brain, the nerves, and the spine. The brain is the seat of thinking, reasoning, memorizing, perceiving, and directing. It is the controller of voluntary and involuntary movements in our body. The body and the brain are constantly interacting. In facing the turmoil of life, they are under continual stress; a tired brain affects the entire system. This constant strain creates anxiety and worry, leading to psychoneurosis, neurasthenia, hysteria, and a host of psychoneurotic diseases.

Asanas such as Shirshasana, Sarvangasana, Halasana, and Setu Bandha Sarvangasana supply fresh blood to the brain and keep it alert and yet restful. Yoga thus has the unique quality of being able to soothe the nerves, quiet the brain, and refresh and pacify the mind.

Yoga practice is not limited to the young and strong. In fact, it is particularly beneficial to those over 40, when the recuperative power of the body is declining and resistance to illness is weakened. Yoga does not dissipate energy; it generates it, filling you with vitality. With a minimum of effort, you obtain great benefit.

Yoga is not only preventive, but also curative. Unlike other systems, its aim is to develop symmetry, coordination, and endurance in the body. It activates the internal organs and makes them function harmoniously.

A Naturopathic Treatment Process

Yoga is a naturopathic process of treatment, with slow but certain progress. It can complement the medicines provided by modern science by speeding recovery and helping to counteract harmful side effects.

Yoga strengthens the body's natural defenses that fight disease and can check the advance and intensity of chronic disease. It is advisable to practice Yoga before an operation, as this relaxes the nerves and the inner organs and quiets the mind. Practice is again necessary after the operation to help the wound heal quickly and to regain strength. In cases of accidents, when other forms of exercise are impossible, the door to Yoga is open.

Asanas are most helpful in eradicating fatigue, aches, and pains. They heal and also help the healthy to remain so.

Yoga has a special gift to offer those active in sports. The asanas can help correct the faulty muscle movements that cause strains and sprains. They create freedom from pressure and tension, increase range of movement, and give speed, elasticity, strength, endurance, and coordination to the entire system. When athletes suffer from exhaustion, they can easily recover their energy by practicing asanas.

The practice of Yoga has a tremendous effect on character and makes one morally and mentally strong. One's approach to life becomes more positive and tolerant. Pride and egoism are eradicated and humbleness and humility set in. One becomes more thoughtful and discriminating and acquires intellectual clarity. This leads one towards a contemplative state.

Thus the art of Yoga is unique in nature. It has everything to give according to one's need.

Milestones in a Woman's Life

The ideal age to begin Yoga is 12 to 14. This does not mean that Yoga should not be started earlier; on the contrary, it is good to start around the age of eight, but little ones should not be forced to be too serious. It is enough to introduce Yoga to the child in a playful manner with the purpose of creating interest so that a foundation is laid. Even if you didn't start at an early age, however, this should not prevent you from starting later; Yoga may be started at any time.

"The young, the aged, the diseased, and the weak—all may take to the practice of Yoga and derive its benefits without hindrance."
(Hatha Yoga Pradipika (1:64)
written by Svatmarama, 800 AD)

B. K. S. Iyengar began to teach Yoga to the Queen Mother of Belgium when she was 84 years old. She had never practiced it before. Her head and entire body had tremors. With perseverance, she did Shirshasana (headstand) for the next eight years.

Pregnancy - General

The saying "As you sow, so shall you reap" is apt in the case of pregnant women. A woman who has looked after her health will reap the reward by having a healthy pregnancy and delivery. It is absolutely essential for a pregnant woman to maintain her physical and mental well-being both for her own sake and for the sake of the child within.

There are mistaken notions about Yoga for pregnant women. Some women fear that it may lead to miscarriage. This is, however, nothing but an old wives' tale. In asanas, the uterus is exercised to become strong and to function more efficiently so that the delivery can be normal.

We recommend that a woman begin to practice Yoga before conception, to improve maternal health and ensure sound health for future generations.

Pregnant women are advised to be careful during the first trimester. Just as medical science does, Yoga recommends prenatal care. The mother needs blood rich in hemoglobin and normal blood pressure during pregnancy. Asanas are meant to avoid dangers such as high blood pressure, rapid weight gain, and albumins in the urine.

There is a chance of miscarriage during this period due to improper formation of the placenta, prolapse, or muscular weakness of the uterus. It is dangerous to lift heavy loads and be overly active. Yogasanas, however, are non-violent; they strengthen the pelvic muscles and improve blood circulation in the pelvic region. They strengthen the reproductive system, exercise the spine, and make the time of pregnancy bearable.

Your Pregnancy

In the first trimester, the asanas you should concentrate on are Parvatasana, Supta Virasana, Upavishtha Konasana, Baddha Konasana, Shirshasana, and Supta Padangushthasana 2. These expand the cavity of the pelvic region, creating space inside the uterus and ensuring proper blood circulation and adequate room for the movement of your unborn child.

In addition, if you practice pranayama, it calms your nerves, gives you confidence and courage, and conquers fatigue. Even inverted poses, performed correctly, are beneficial. Under the guidance of an experienced Iyengar Yoga teacher, you can practice these asanas up to the ninth month. When your breathing becomes heavy, however, they should be stopped. A woman in the state of advanced pregnancy is herself the best judge. She can assess that certain asanas are not possible due to heaviness in the pelvis and abdomen, and consequently the heart.

Very often, it's fear that makes you reluctant to practice. You might think of discontinuing Salamba Shirshasana, Salamba Sarvangasana, and Halasana. These inversions, however, are not harmful. With years of experience and observation, we have found that during advanced pregnancy, you will enjoy doing inversions.

As you approach the delivery, you'll find Halasana difficult, so it is the first asana to drop. The second is Salamba Sarvangasana, in which you'll find the abdomen becoming heavier.

Salamba Shirshasana, however, you'll probably feel like continuing until the end. You can also continue asanas such as the sitting ones with concave back and spine-strengthening ones until the end of pregnancy. You can do Ujjayi Pranayama 1 and Viloma Pranayama Stage 1 and 2 throughout pregnancy.

In the early stages of pregnancy, morning sickness, dullness, and weakness may appear. Sometimes there are discharges or pain in the pelvic region, swelling or numbness in the feet, swollen and varicose veins, backache, constipation, fluctuations in blood pressure, toxemia, headache, dizziness, blurred vision, and frequent urination. With these conditions, even though asanas can help you, you may find it difficult to practice Yoga.

In advanced pregnancy, surprisingly, you'll find it much easier to practice.

Miscarriage

A short time after a miscarriage, you can safely restart asanas and pranayama without straining the abdominal organs. As steadiness and progress are maintained, you can increase the duration as well as the number of asanas. Start with supine poses and inversions before going for back-bending, twisting, or forward-bending asanas.

Delivery

Labor pains are natural. They indicate that various muscles in the pelvic region, and mainly the muscles of the uterus, are contracting, to help expel the baby. However, anxiety and mental stress aggravate labor pains and delay the baby's emergence.

If you practice yogasanas during pregnancy, your strengthened uterine muscles will function more efficiently during delivery. Baddha Konasana and Upavishtha Konasana are extremely beneficial, as they help broaden the pelvic area and dilate the cervix.

Pranayama strengthens the nerves to enable you to breathe calmly in the periods between contractions, which is essential for easy delivery. It helps to relax the nerves and avoid mental tension.

If the delivery is normal, or even after a cesarian section, it is advisable to restart asanas and pranayama in order to regain your health and strengthen the abdominal organs.

Lactation

After delivery, you need mental and physical rest. The abdominal muscles become lax after delivery, so Shavasana and Ujjayi Pranayama 1 are helpful at this stage.

The child should have pure breast-feeding. According to medical science, every ounce of maternal milk requires 400 ounces of oxygen. In Shavasana, the abdomen and internal organs do not protrude, which allows them to relax completely. This in turn allows the diaphragm and lungs to expand fully in the deep breathing of Ujjayi Pranayama, which increases your oxygen intake and helps lactation.

After the first month, you can perform the asanas that are recommended for the first term after delivery. These asanas stimulate the pituitary gland, which secretes the hormone prolactin that controls lactation. They also relieve heaviness in the breasts and bring firmness to their muscle fibers.

After delivery, fat generally accumulates around the buttocks, hips, and breasts, and there is a tendency towards flabbiness. In the second term after delivery, you should perform asanas that help contract the abdominal and pelvic muscles to their former shape.

There is no harm in doing Yoga if you have undergone a surgical operation such as a tubectomy or hysterectomy. However, start carefully and gradually—only after resting completely for two months and avoiding strain and overstretching. (*see "After a Cesarian Section," page 251*).

Menopause

At around the age of 40 to 50, women experience changes in the menstrual cycle. Menstruation either stops suddenly, becomes irregular, or lessens in quantity. All these are natural signs that the reproductive functions are coming to an end.

Just as physical and psychological disturbances occur at the beginning of menstruation, you have to face them again during menopause. As the ovaries stop functioning, glands including the thyroids and the adrenals become hyperactive, causing an imbalance of hormones. As a result, you may suffer from hot flashes, high blood pressure, heaviness in the breasts, and a range of other changes. You may experience loss of balance and poise, and this can result in a short temper, depression, and anxiety.

This is a critical period of adjustment. You can learn to face these new challenges by improving your physical and mental stability. The practice of asanas is extremely beneficial, as it calms the nervous system and brings emotional balance.

Yoga is a gift for old age. If you take up Yoga when you're old, you gain not only health and happiness but also freshness of mind, since Yoga gives you a bright outlook on life. You'll be able to look forward to a happier future, rather than looking back into the past, which has already receded into darkness. The loneliness and nervousness that create sadness and sorrow are swept away by Yoga as a new life begins. So it is never too late to begin.

You can only experience the meaning of Yoga, however, by practicing it.

Yoga's Benefits

Beauty from the Inside

Yoga asanas strengthen your nerves, ligaments, and internal organs. They improve blood circulation, give inner poise, and balance the outer body. This has positive effects on the proportions of your body, providing you with a lovely figure and enhancing your beauty. Due to improved blood circulation, your skin becomes soft and silky. Your voice becomes melodious, your eyes shiny, and your breath fresh. Your entire personality gains charm and spiritual presence. If you practice Yoga on a regular basis, you won't need cosmetics and other beauty enhancements: your beauty comes from the inside.

Benefits during Pregnancy

The practice of Yoga helps in good digestion, healthy blood circulation, and light, easy breathing. Asanas and pranayama help to end tiredness and nervous tension, and to rid the body of toxins, enabling you to enjoy a state of mental and physical health and well-being.

The asanas in this book have been chosen to give maximum space inside the uterus for the child to move and grow freely. If regularly practiced, they also prepare you for a natural and easy birth.

Empirical tests have proven that not only the physical health of the expectant mother but also her emotional and mental state affect the future healthy development of the unborn child. Yogasanas and pranayama, as well as a healthy lifestyle, highly enhance the child's future health.

A Feeling of Radiant Health

Some pregnant women might not be able to follow all the asanas that are recommended in this book. If you feel exhausted after practicing Yoga, it means that something is wrong. It could be that your practice was either too intense or incorrect. Please turn to an experienced Iyengar Yoga teacher for guidance.

In some specific cases, lying on your back can cause pressure on the inferior vena cava (lower vein that leads to the heart). If you feel dizziness or nausea, always turn onto your left side.

Chapter 2

Preparing for Pregnancy

Before Conception

From the Yogic point of view, the time before a child is conceived is as important as the actual pregnancy. Once you have decided to become pregnant, you should prepare yourself through a balanced diet (*see "Ayurvedic Recipes and Health Tips," page 415*) and give up alcohol, drugs, nicotine, and caffeine.

This is not only recommended for the woman, but also for the man. The decision should be taken by both of you to get pregnant. The woman and the man alike have to prepare holistically for motherhood and fatherhood respectively. Although this chapter is addressed to women, it is also advisable for men to practice Yoga. What is good for the female pelvis and her reproductive organs is, of course, also good for the male pelvis and his reproductive organs.

Yoga practice will gently improve the blood circulation of the pelvis and the reproductive organs. It will strengthen the spine and consequently the uterus, and will enhance fertility. Mentally, Yoga creates equilibrium and emotional balance.

It is important to adjust the practice of asanas according to your menstrual cycle. Especially for a woman who wants to become pregnant, this adjustment for your menstrual cycle is a prerequisite for conception.

I. V. F. (In Vitro Fertilization):
The whole chapter is relevant also for those women who wish to conceive through I. V. F..

◇

Sequences for during Your Period

During the first hours of menstruation (48 to 72 hours), complete rest is advisable. You can practice the following, however, to alleviate fatigue and to reduce excessive menstrual discharge:

• Shavasana

(page 366)

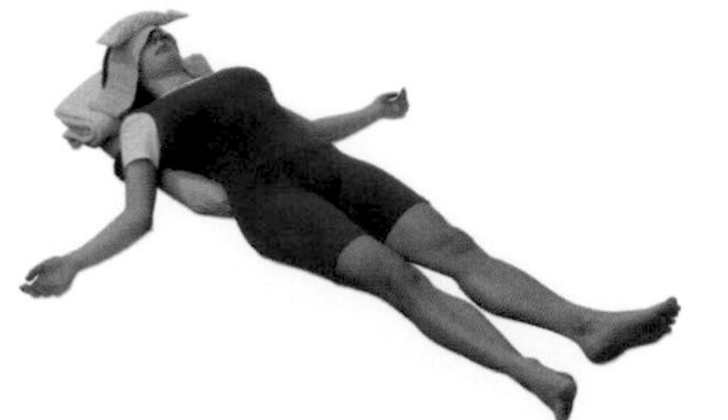

• Viloma Pranayama

(Stage 1 and 2 in Shavasana, page 151).

• Supta Baddha Konasana

(bolster crosswise, page 127)

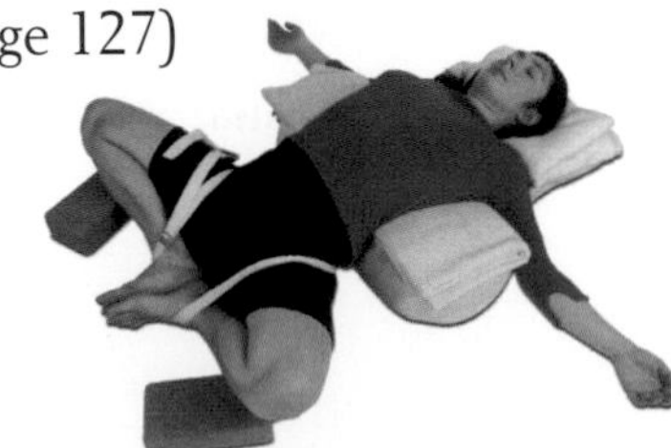

Depending on how you feel, you can start the following sequence on the third, fourth, or fifth day of your period:

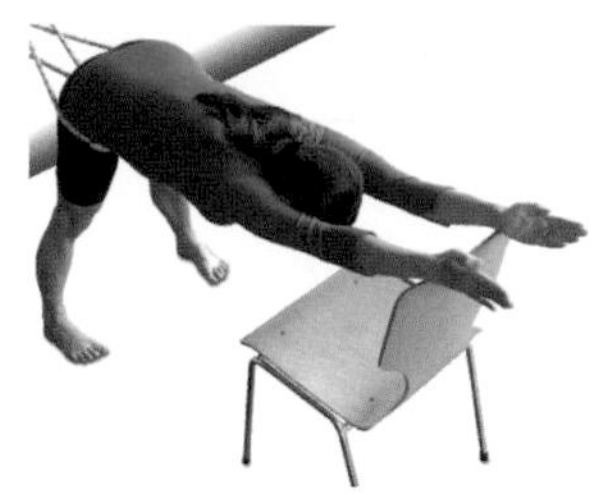

1 Ardha Uttanasana, *page 61*

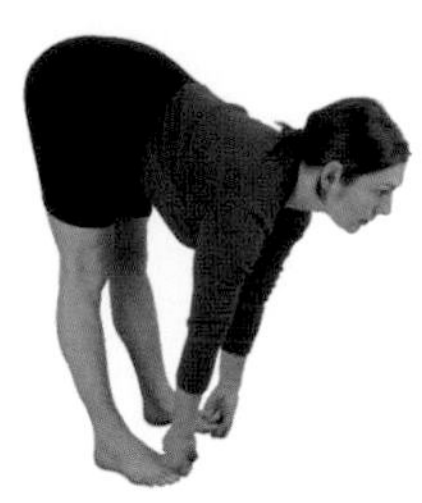

2 Padangushthasana (concave back), *page 297*

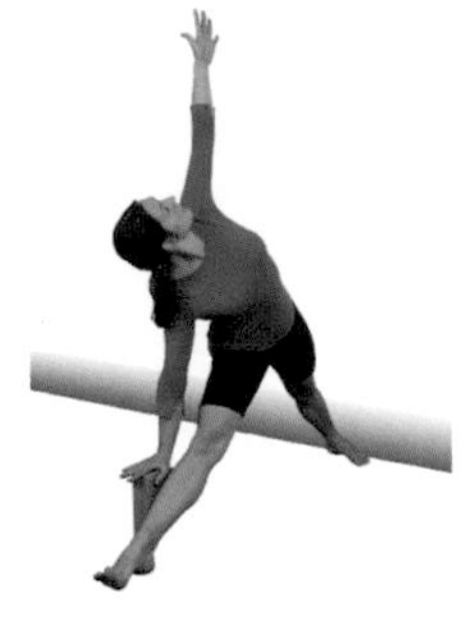

3 Utthita Trikonasana (back foot against wall), *page 281*

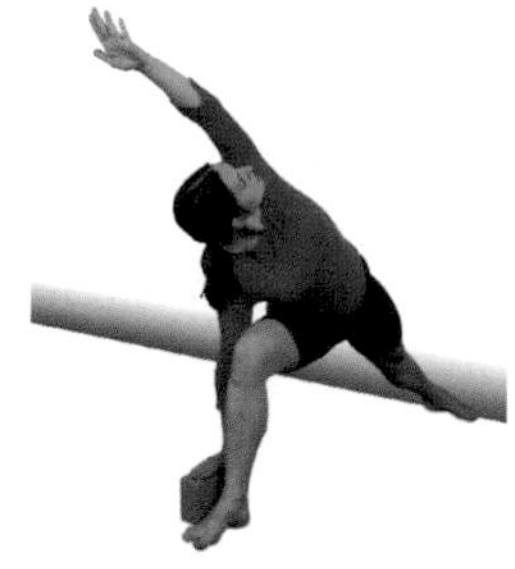

4 Utthita Parshvakonasana (back foot against wall), *page 282*

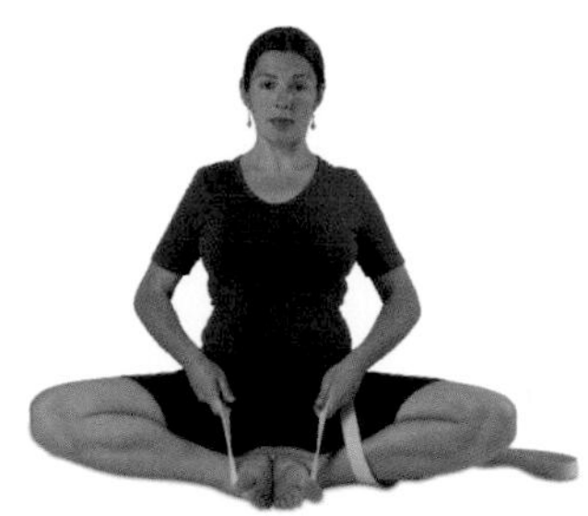

5 Baddha Konasana (bolster/s), *page 67*

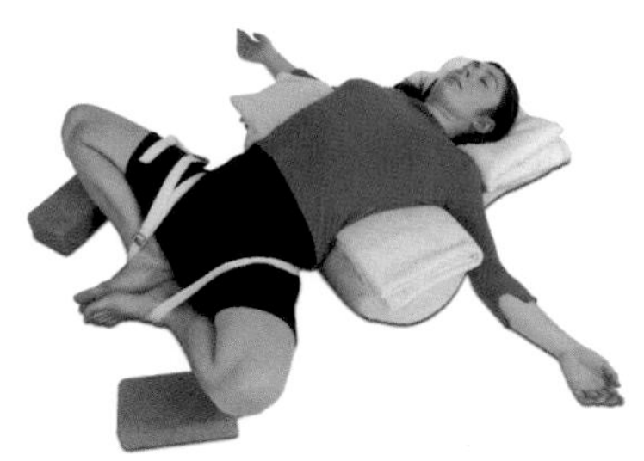

6 Supta Baddha Konasana (bolster crosswise), *page 127*

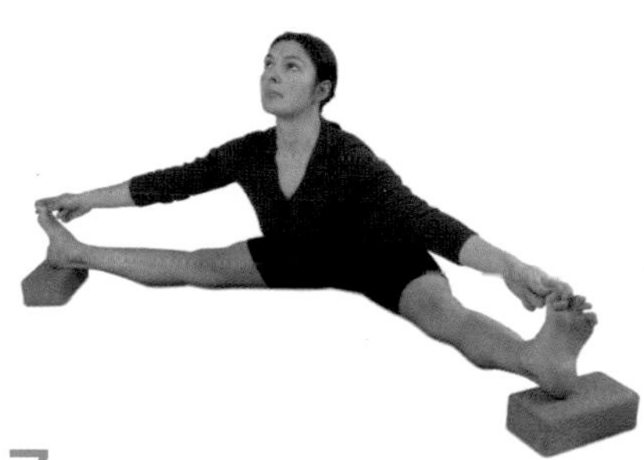

7 Upavishtha Konasana (concave back), *page 316*

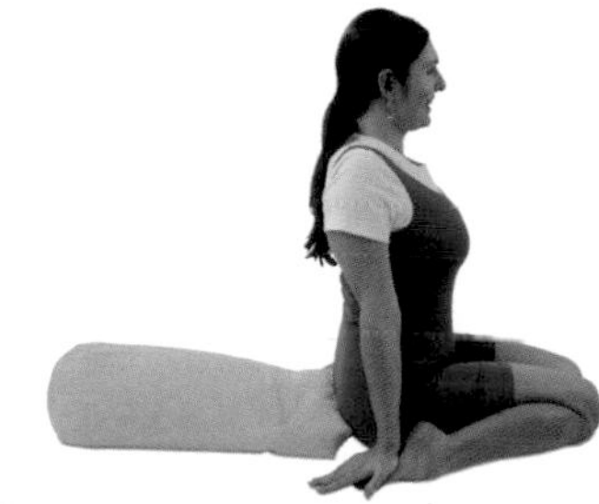

8 Virasana, *page 302*

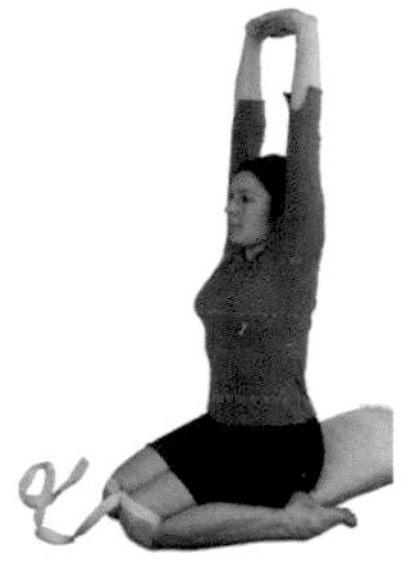

9 Parvatasana in Virasana, *page 74*

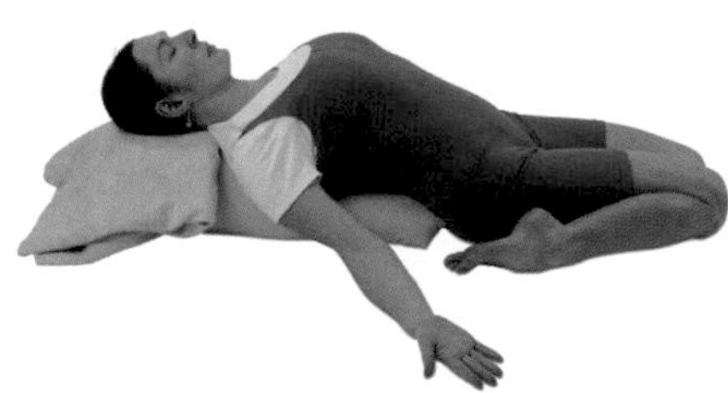

10 Supta Virasana (bolster/s), *page 367*

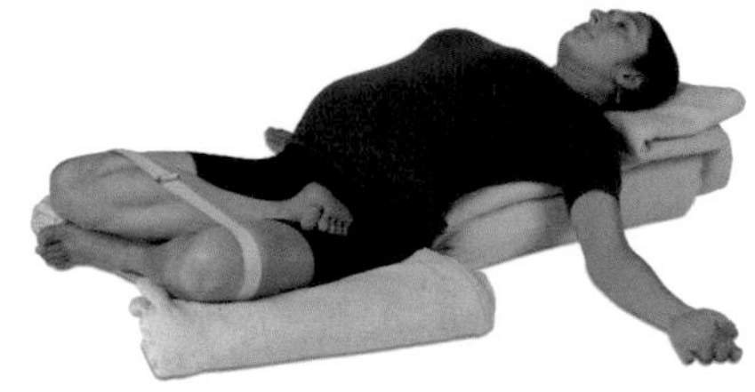

11 Matsyasana (bolster/s), *page 131*

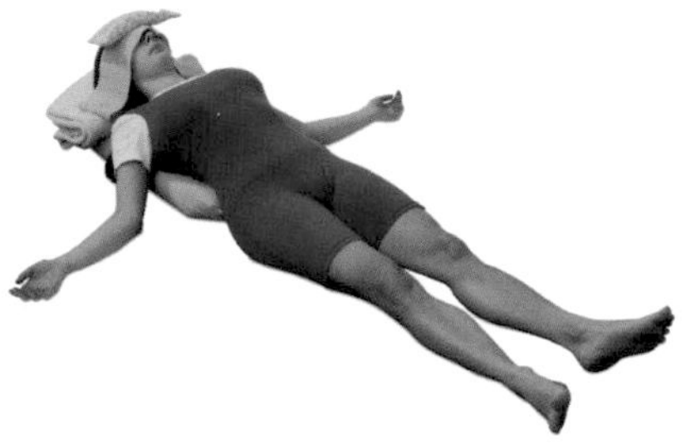

12 Shavasana, *page 366*

You can practice forward bends when the flow is at its heaviest. Towards the end of your period, you can practice the following supine and supported positions:

- **Dvi Pada Viparita Dandasana**

- **Setu Bandha Sarvangasana, Baddha Konasana,** and **Upavishtha Konasana**

This program is also helpful when you suffer from pain, profuse bleeding, and cramps. You should resume inverted poses like Salamba Shirshasana and Salamba Sarvangasana only after your period has ended.

On the first day after your period, you can resume normal practice; you should, however, practice as recommended for the second term after delivery.

After Your Period Has Stopped: Phase before Ovulation

Concentrate on inverted poses like Salamba Shirshasana, working with blocks and belts; Dvi Pada Viparita Dandasana; full arm balance (Adho Mukha Vrikshasana); forearm balance (Pichcha Mayurasana); and Salamba Sarvangasana, Halasana, Setu Bandha Sarvangasana, and Viparita Karani.

It is absolutely necessary to clean the uterus completely after your period. For this, we recommend concave positions and working with blocks, the wall, and wall ropes. These help to straighten and align the pelvis and inner organs.

Fertility Issues

There can be many reasons why a couple is not able to become parents. Disturbances in the female cycle are but one possibility. If a couple is experiencing fertility problems, it is best to consult a specialist and obtain an exact diagnosis.

Mental stress, malnutrition, rapid weight loss, and anorexia nervosa are among the factors that disturb the excretion of the hormone GnRH (gonadotropin releasing hormone) into the hypothalamus region of the brain. This, in turn, negatively affects the secretion of the hormones FSH (follicle stimulating hormone) and LH (luteinizing hormone), which regulate the menstrual cycle and ovulation Disturbances of the hypothalamus can even lead to complete amenorrhea (absence of periods).

Sometimes the urge to conceive a child is so strong that a hormonal imbalance can result. This is why yogasanas like resting or restorative poses and pranayama are recommended for mental stress.

Mental Stability

We recommend the following sequence for mental stability:

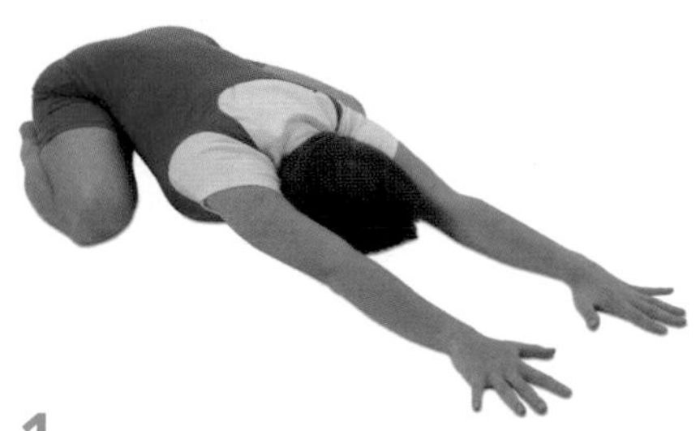

1 Adho Mukha Virasana, *page 317*

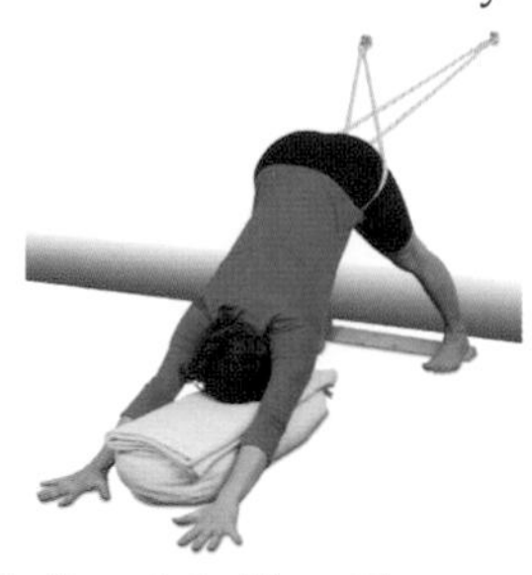

2 Adho Mukha Shvanasana (wall ropes or hands on wall, head supported), *page 299*

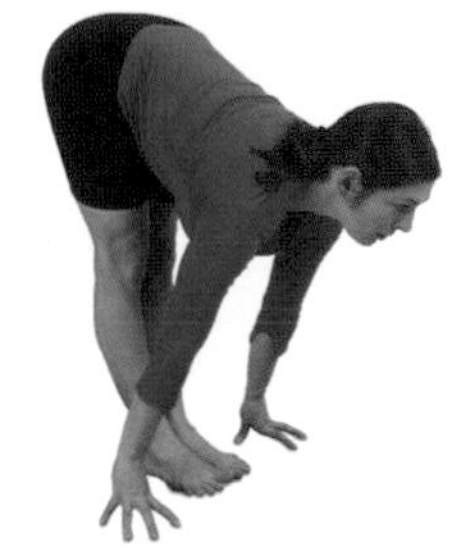

3 Uttanasana (concave back), *page 213*

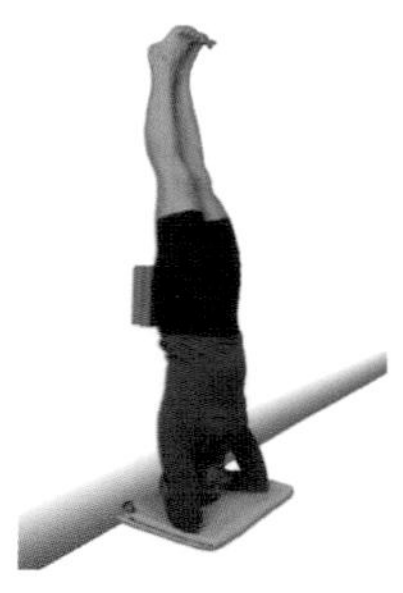

4 Salamba Shirshasana, *page 100*

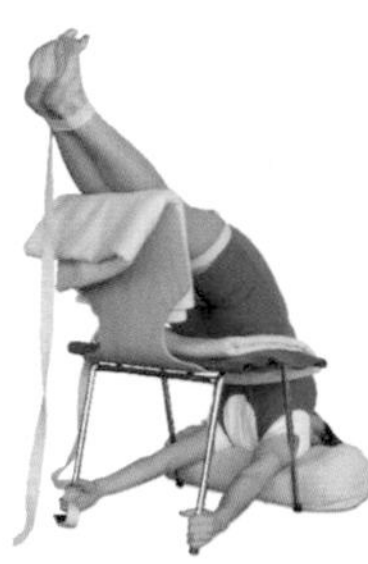

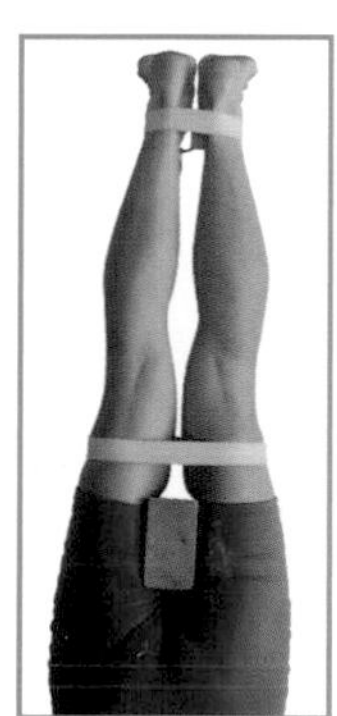

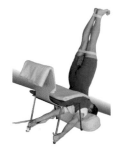

5 Salamba Sarvangasana and Niralamba Sarvangasana (with and without block and belt), *page 330*

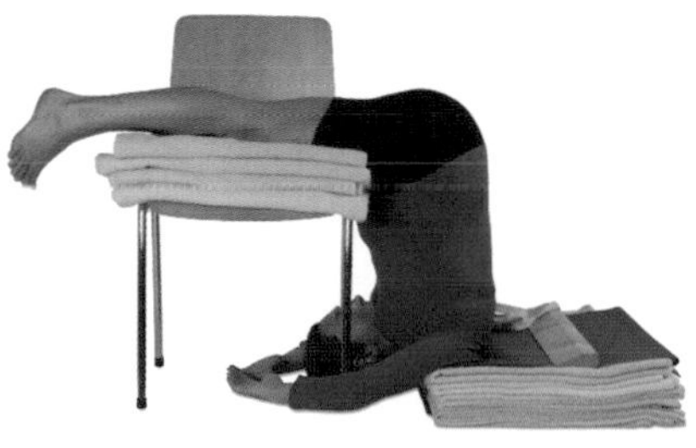

6 Ardha Halasana, *page 105*

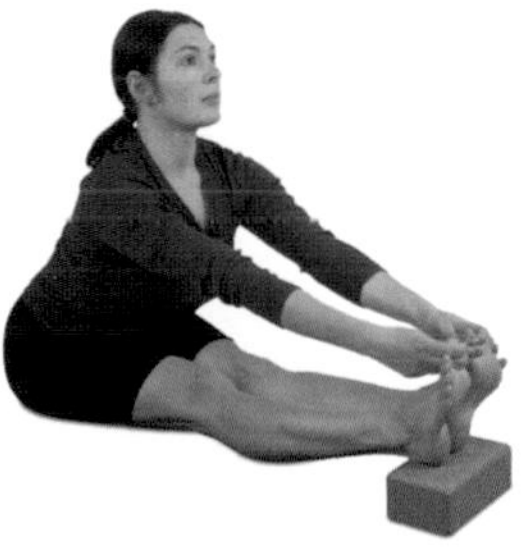

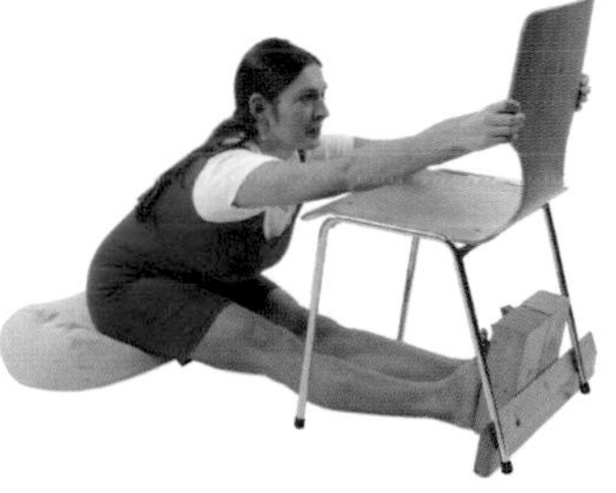

7 Pashchimottanasana (concave back), *pages 308–309*

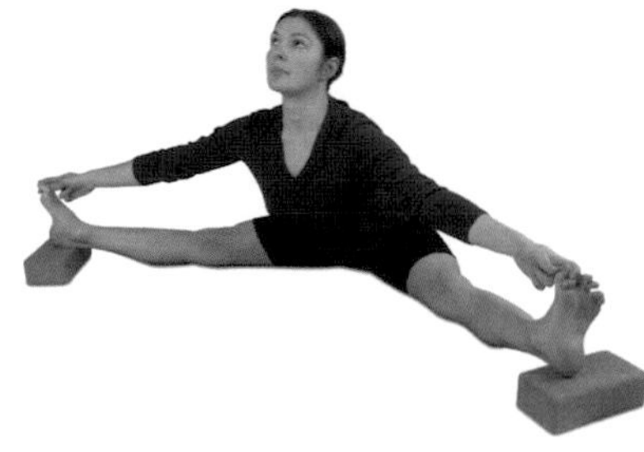

8 Upavishtha Konasana (concave back), *page 316*

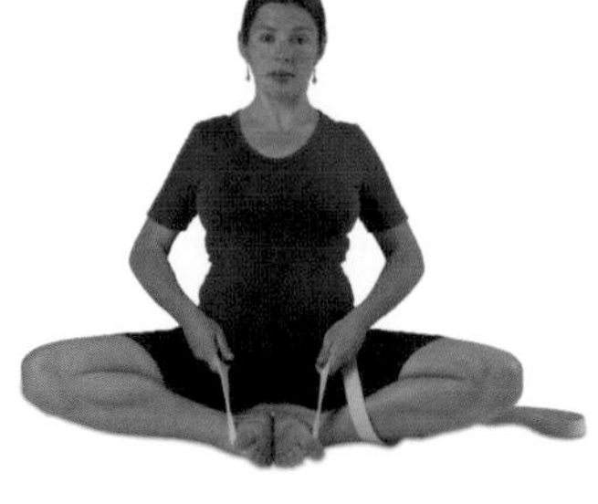

9 Baddha Konasana, *page 67*

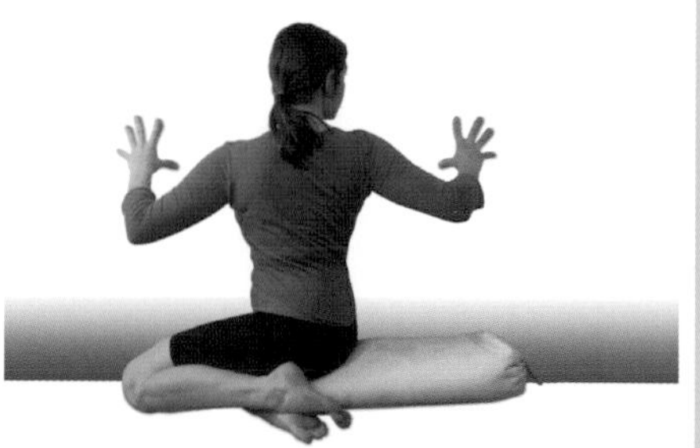

10 Bharadvajasana 1, *page 319*

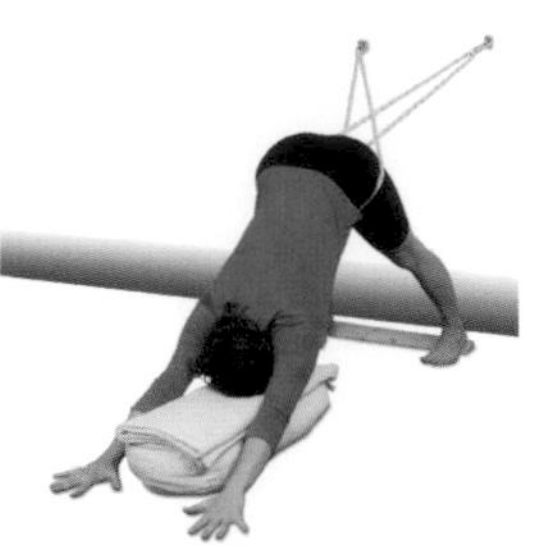

11 Adho Mukha Shvanasana (wall ropes or hands on wall, head supported), *page 125*

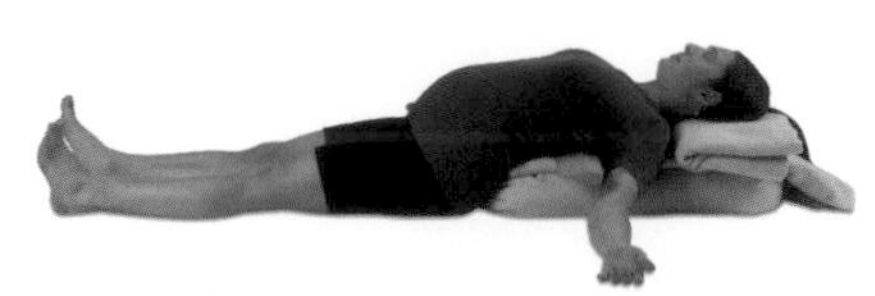

12 Shavasana, *page 134*

13 Ujjayi Pranayama 1, Viloma Pranayama Stage 1 and 2, and Pratyahara, *page 151*

◇

There are many possible organic reasons for reduced fertility; it can originate in the anatomy itself, or in hormonal deficiencies at the level of the hypothalamus (a part of the brain that secretes substances that control metabolism), the pituitary gland, the reproductive organs, or the reproductive cells. We recommend the following sequence to improve the physical and physiological stability of the body and the reproductive organs:

Physical and Physiological Stability: Preparing the Ground

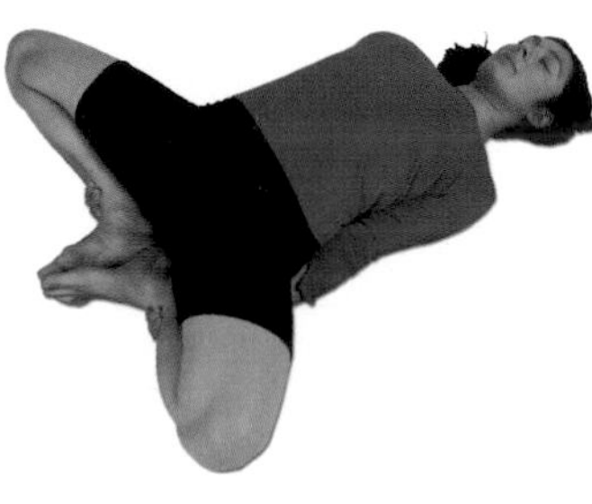

1 Supta Baddha Konasana (active, arms extended), *page 126*

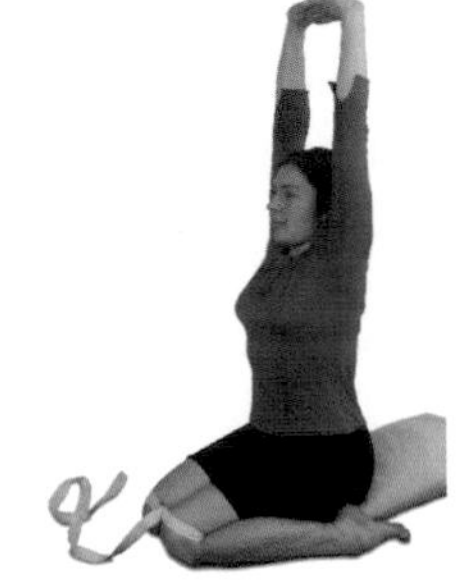

2 Parvatasana from Virasana, *page 74*

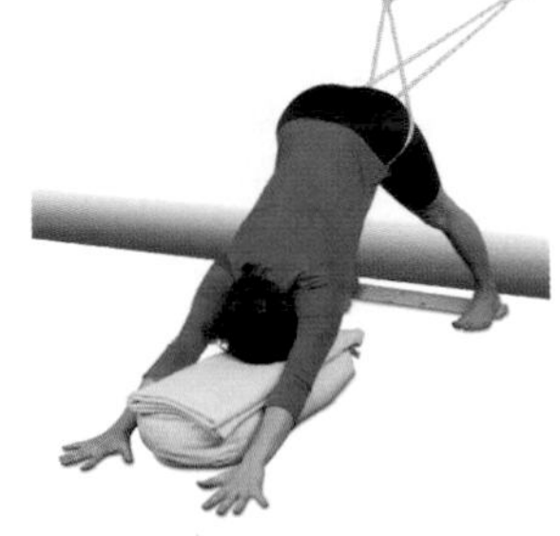

3 Adho Mukha Shvanasana, (wall ropes), *page 125*

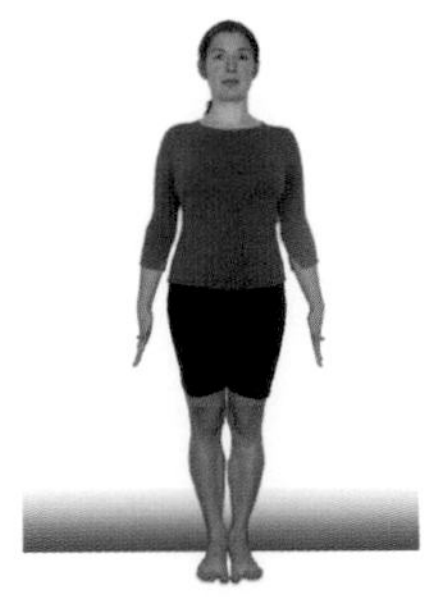

4 Tadasana, *page 32*

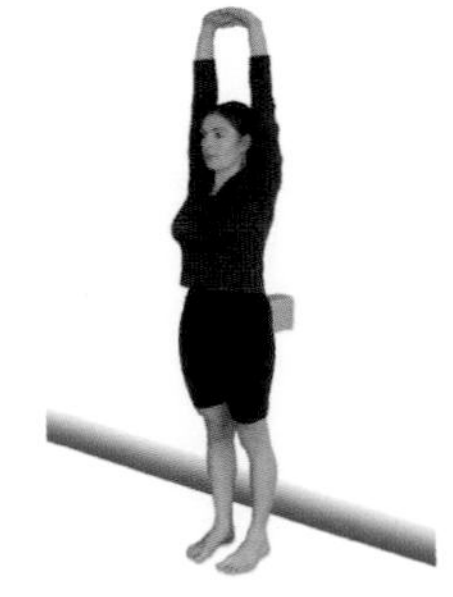

5 Urdhva Baddhanguliyasana in Tadasana (with a brick), *page 275*

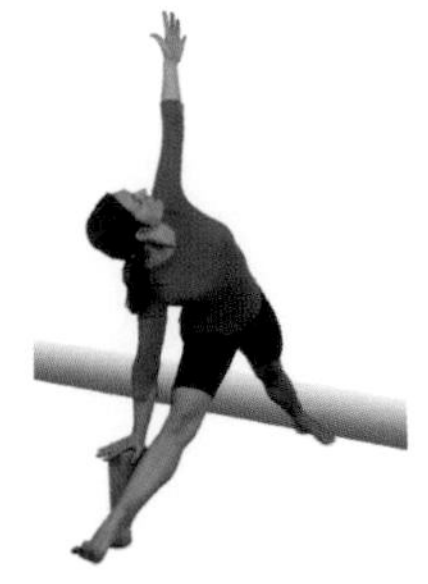

6 Utthita Trikonasana (back foot against wall), *page 281*

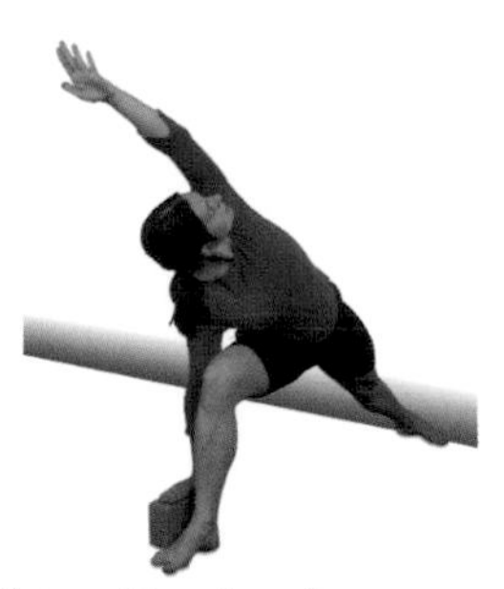

7 Utthita Parshvakonasana (back foot against wall), *page 282*

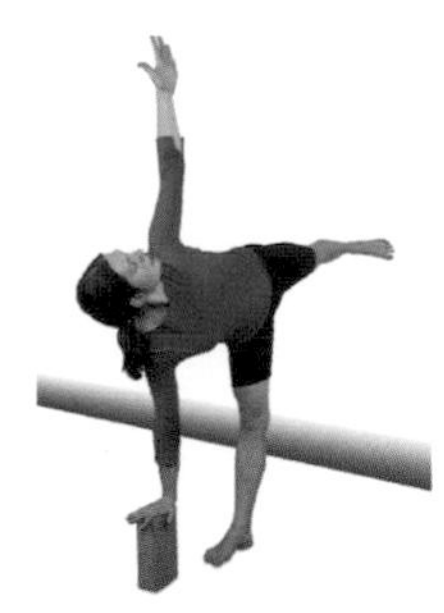

8 Ardha Chandrasana (back foot against wall), *page 283*

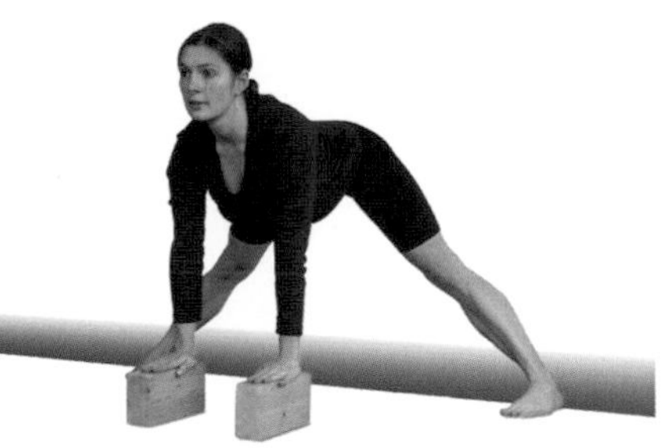

9 Prasarita Padottanasana (heels and buttock bones against wall), *page 296*

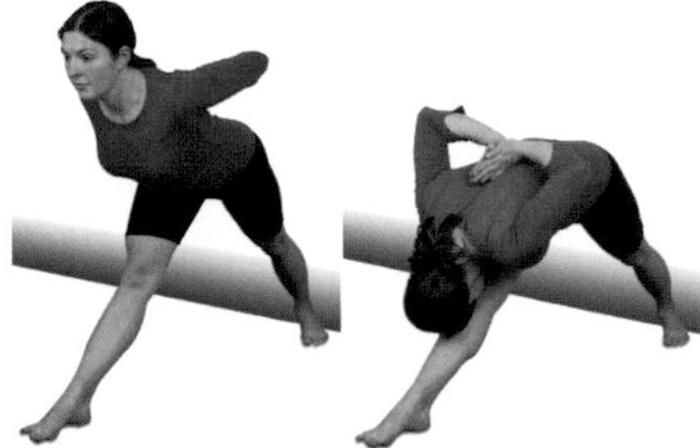

10 Parshvottanasana (back foot against wall), *page 287*

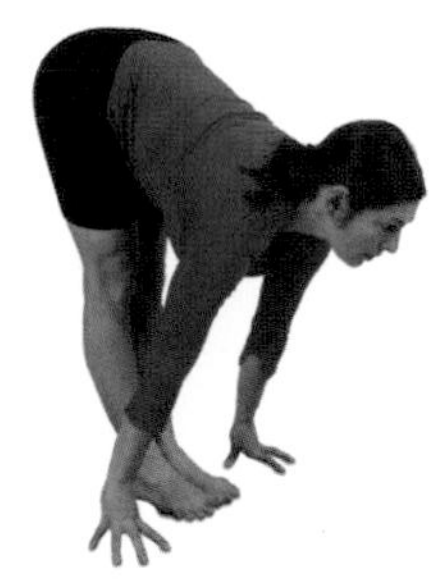

11 Uttanasana (concave back), *page 294*

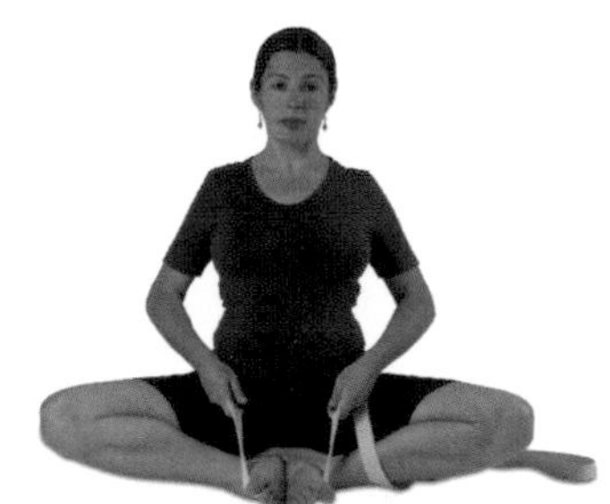

12 Baddha Konasana (straight back), *page 67*

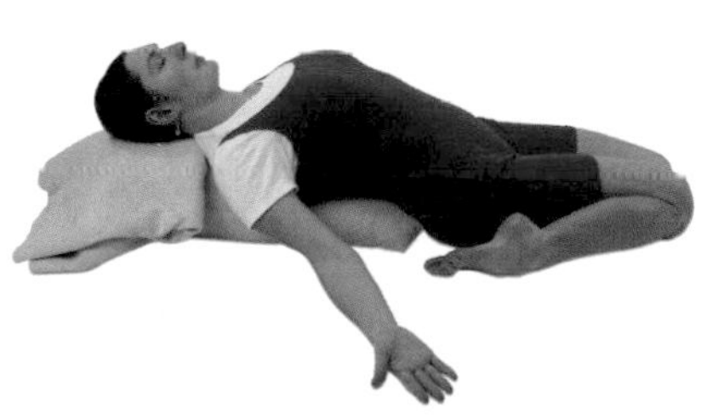

13 Supta Virasana (bolster), *page 367*

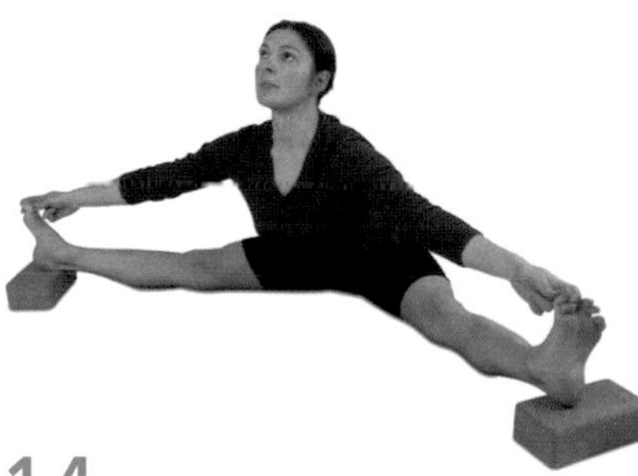

14 Upavishtha Konasana (concave back), *page 316*

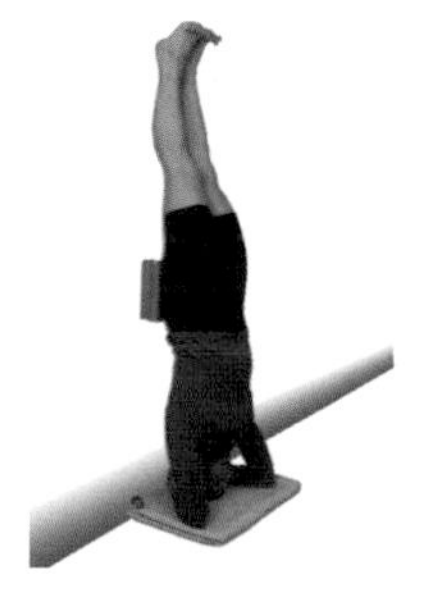

15 Salamba Shirshasana (align the pelvis), *page 100*

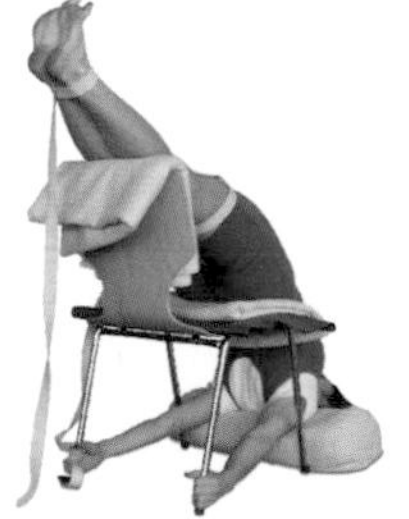

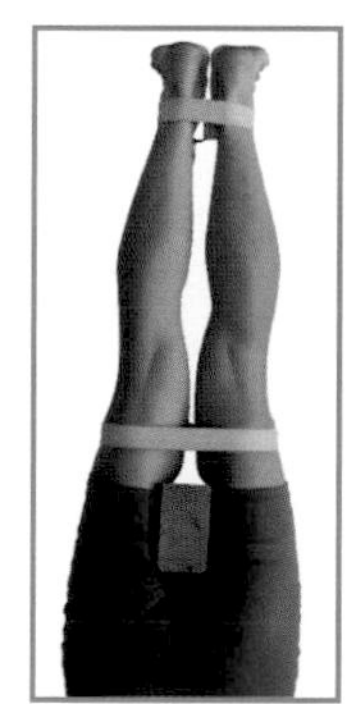

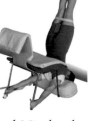

16 Salamba Sarvangasana and Niralamba Sarvangasana (align the pelvis, with and without belt), *page 330*

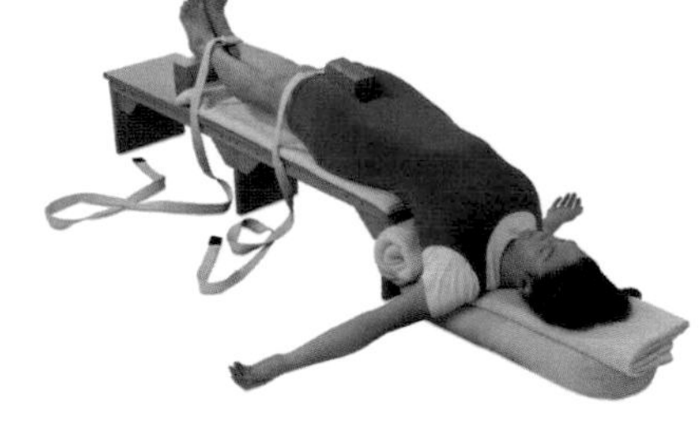

17 Setu Bandha Sarvangasana, *pages 107 and 334*

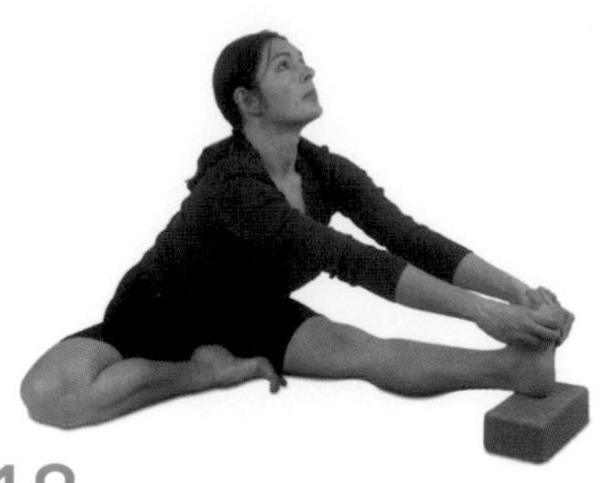

18 Janu Shirshasana (concave back), *page 306*

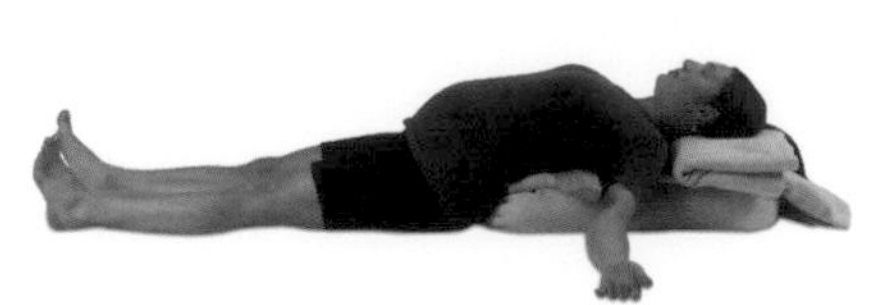

19 Shavasana, *page 134*

20 Ujjayi Pranayama 1, Viloma Pranayama Stage 1 and 2, and Pratyahara, *page 141*

If possible, alternate between the two sequences above every day. If you practice the pranayama before the asanas, you should take a break of at least 30 minutes. If you practice the pranayama after the asanas, take a rest of at least 15 minutes in Shavasana.

After Your Period Has Stopped: Phase after Ovulation

If you want to get pregnant but have problems conceiving, you should be careful with yogasanas in this phase of your cycle.

At this stage, the fertilized egg embeds itself in the endometrium, so you should not practice

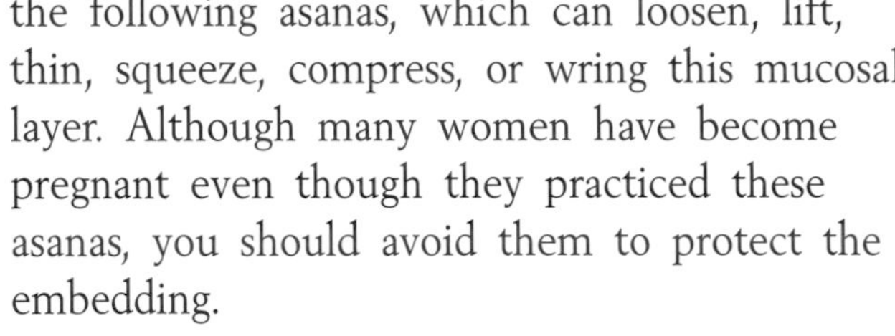

the following asanas, which can loosen, lift, thin, squeeze, compress, or wring this mucosal layer. Although many women have become pregnant even though they practiced these asanas, you should avoid them to protect the embedding.

Asanas to avoid are the following:

- Asanas like Parivritta Trikonasana, which have a lifting and wringing action; this holds true for all twists.
- Asanas with full forward extension like full Pashchimottanasana (head down), which compress the uterus.

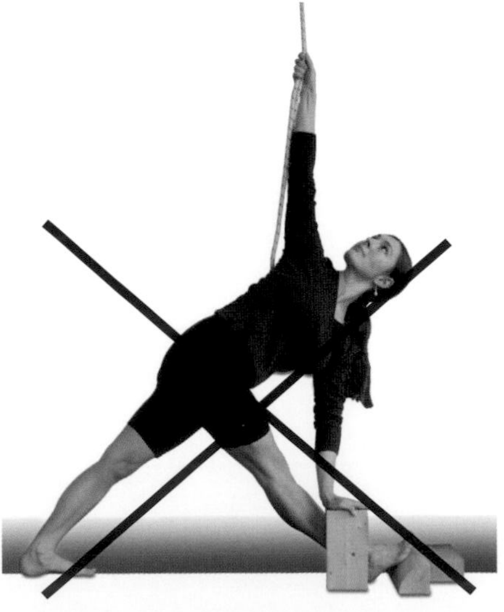

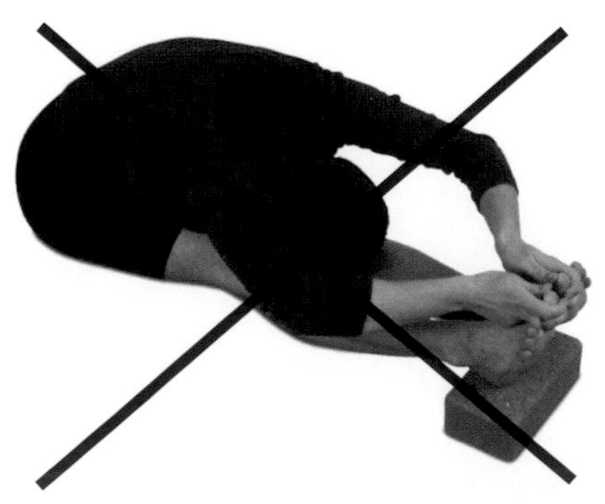

- Twisting asanas against a bent leg like Marichyasana 3 or Parivritta (twist in) Parshvakonasana, which combine the two previous actions.

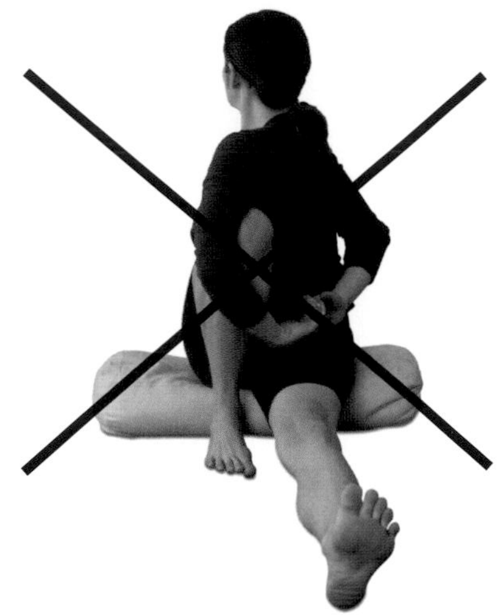

- Back bends like Dhanurasana and Urdhva Dhanurasana, which have a stretching and thinning action.

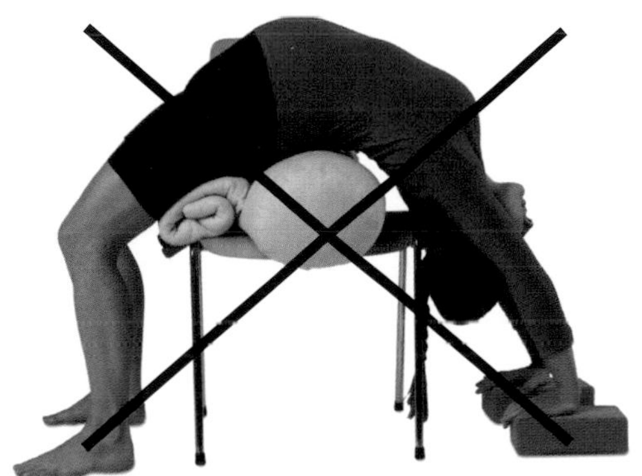

- Asanas like Urdhva Prasarita Padasana, which put too much pressure on the pelvic floor. This can also happen in all balancing, sit-up, and drop-back asanas, where the abdominal muscles create pressure down on the uterus.

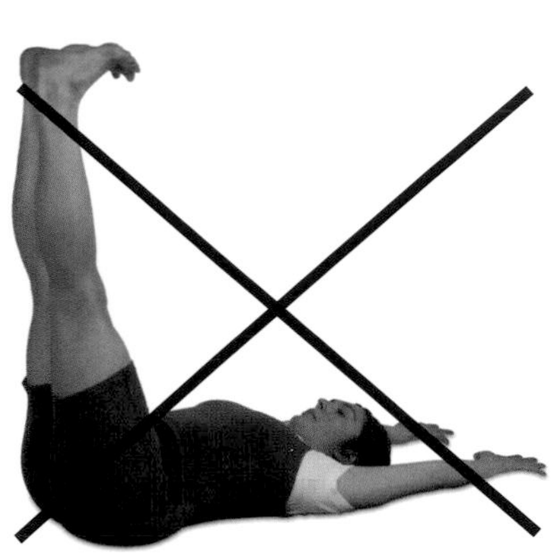

In general, you should not exaggerate with Yoga practice or other sports activities. This recommendation is especially true for women who suffer from a weakness of the corpus luteum, when the secretion of progesterone is not sufficient for the fertilized egg to become embedded. With this special condition, you should not practice the above-mentioned asanas at all, but rather stick to the two sequences for mental, physical, and physiological stability.

The Importance of Proper Body Alignment

Proper alignment of the body is important in avoiding physical, physiological including hormonal, and mental stress. To achieve it, you should practice asanas that provide proper alignment of the pelvis and the spine, so that the awareness and consciousness of this will influence your daily life. Tilting the pelvis in either direction also tilts and applies pressure to the uterus and its inner lining.

Proper alignment for pregnancy is also the proper alignment for delivery. For advice, contact an experienced Iyengar Yoga teacher.

Preventing Miscarriages

Sequence to Balance the Thyroid Gland

The importance to your pregnancy of a healthy thyroid gland cannot be overstated. That's why it is so highly recommended for you to practice Yoga, which balances the thyroid, before you conceive.

A deficiency in the secretions of the thyroid gland can result in miscarriage; asanas that help in this area are listed below. If possible, practice these under the guidance of an experienced Iyengar Yoga teacher.

• Salamba Shirshasana

(with precise alignment, page 100)

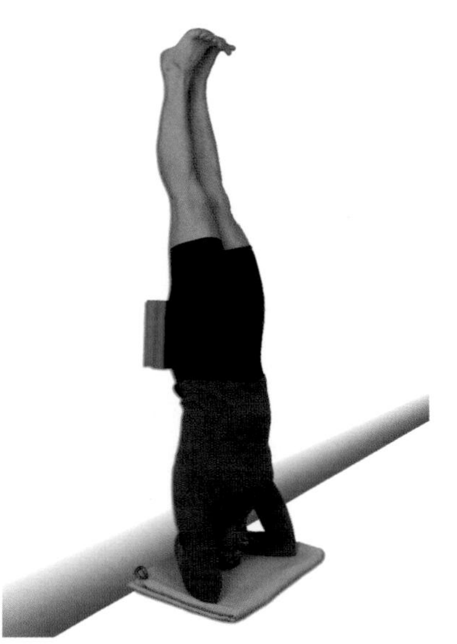

• Salamba Sarvangasana and Niralamba Sarvangasana

(with precise alignment, alternatively with and without block and belts, page 330)

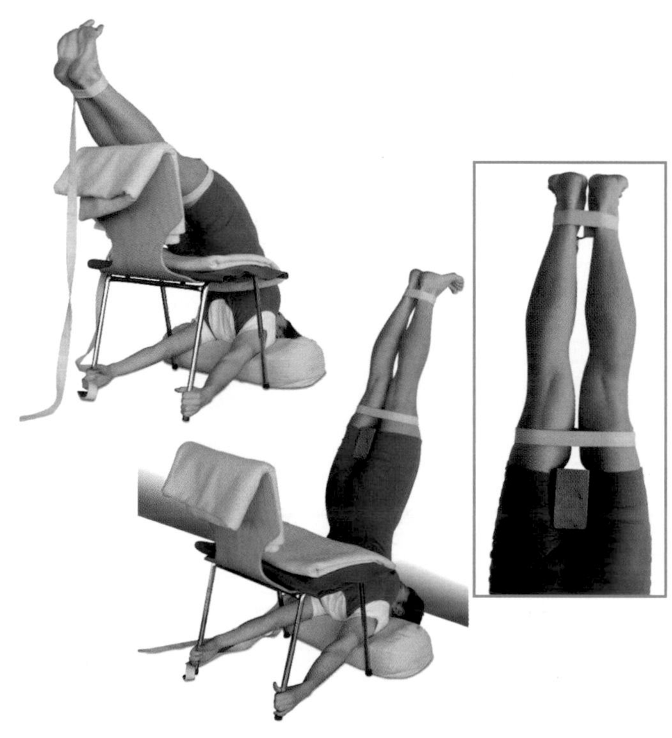

• Setu Bandha Sarvangasana

(supported, page 107)

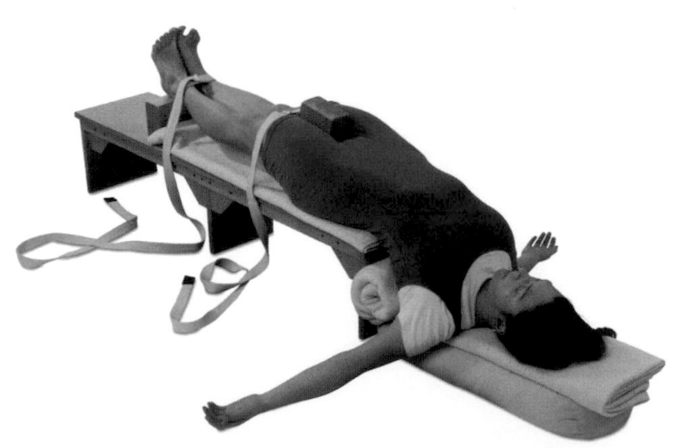

• Janu Shirshasana

(concave back, page 306)

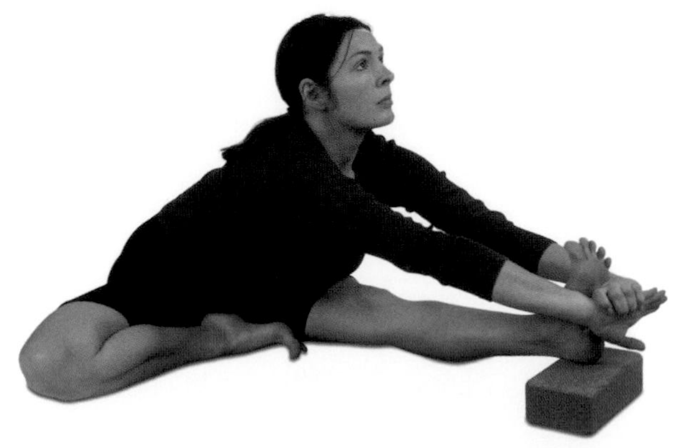

Helpful Asanas for a Tendency to Miscarry

Miscarriages that take place in the first three months of pregnancy are often the result of insufficient development of the placenta, prolapse (slipping) of the uterus, muscular weakness, or a hormonal imbalance.

If you have a disposition toward miscarriage, you should not practice standing poses, but rather should concentrate on forward bends done with a concave back, including:

• Janu Shirshasana:

(Urdhva Hasta, page 82) (concave back, lower chest lifted, pages 83 and *306*)

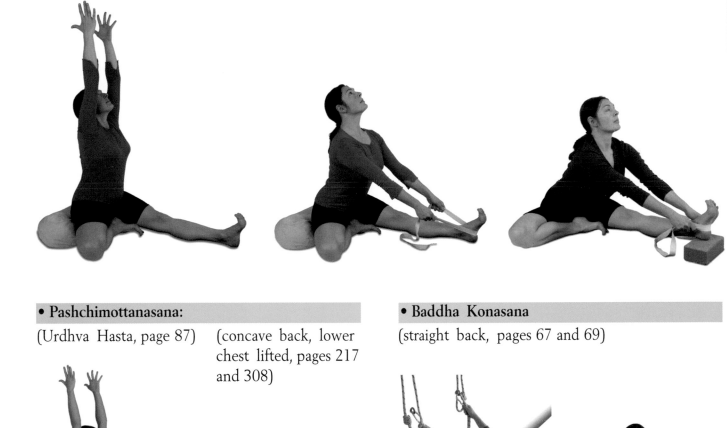

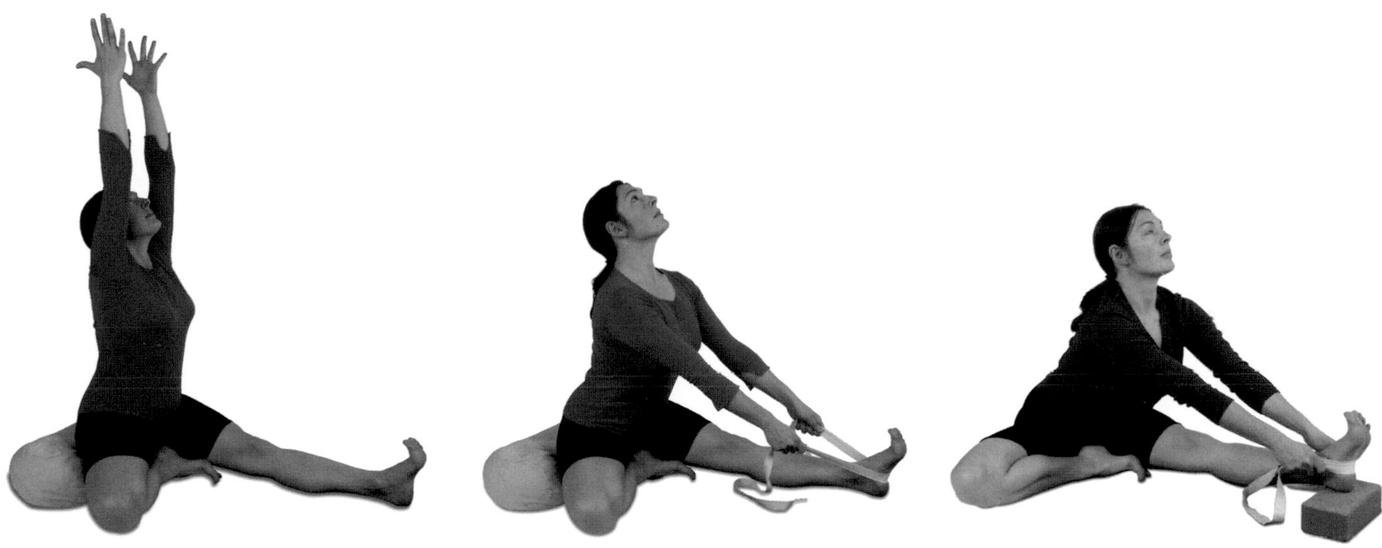

• Pashchimottanasana:

(Urdhva Hasta, page 87) (concave back, lower chest lifted, pages 217 and 308)

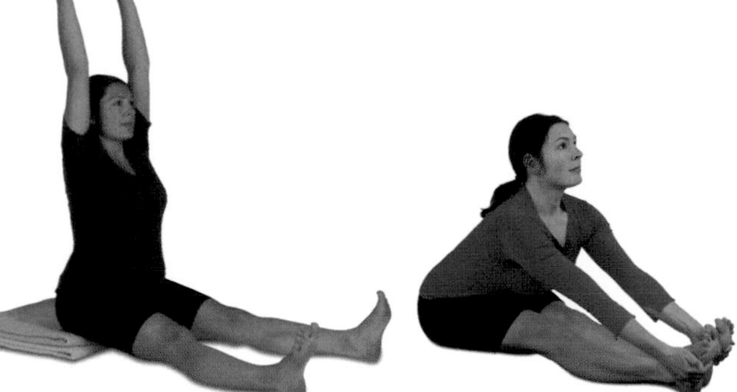

• Baddha Konasana

(straight back, pages 67 and 69)

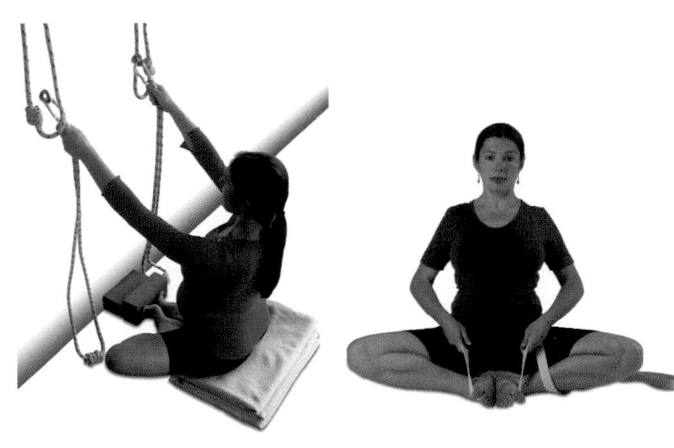

• Salamba Shirshasana

(page 99)

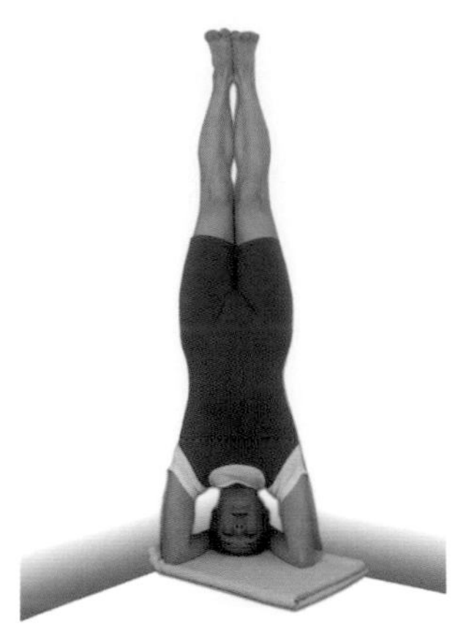

• Salamba Sarvangasana

(page 331)

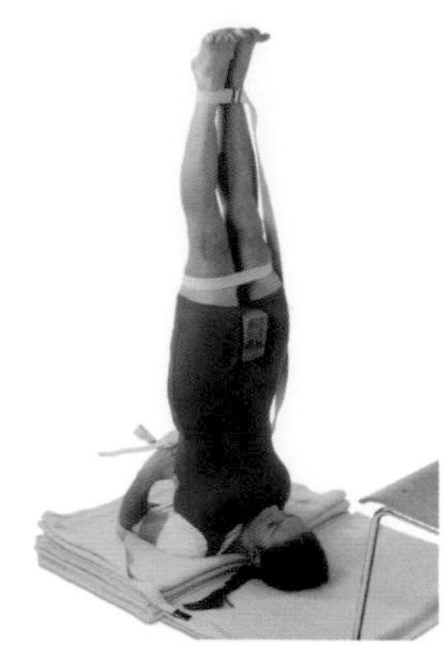

• Shavasana

(page 134)

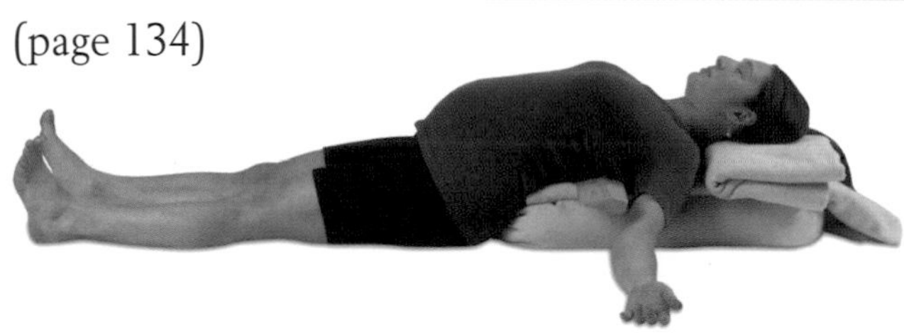

> Twice a day, in the morning and the evening, for 10 to 15 minutes.

> Whenever you feel like taking a rest, practice Shavasana with a support for the spine. Make sure that your elbows are resting on the floor, your eyes are closed, and your breath flows softly in and out.

• Ujjayi Pranayama 1

(on a regular basis and after a miscarriage, page 148).

If you have already had a miscarriage due to a malfunctioning of the endocrinologic system or any other reason, you should consult an experienced Iyengar Yoga teacher. In these cases, precise work in Salamba Shirshasana and Salamba Sarvangasana is a great help.

Other suggestions include a balanced diet and renouncing toxins like alcohol, drugs, and caffeine.

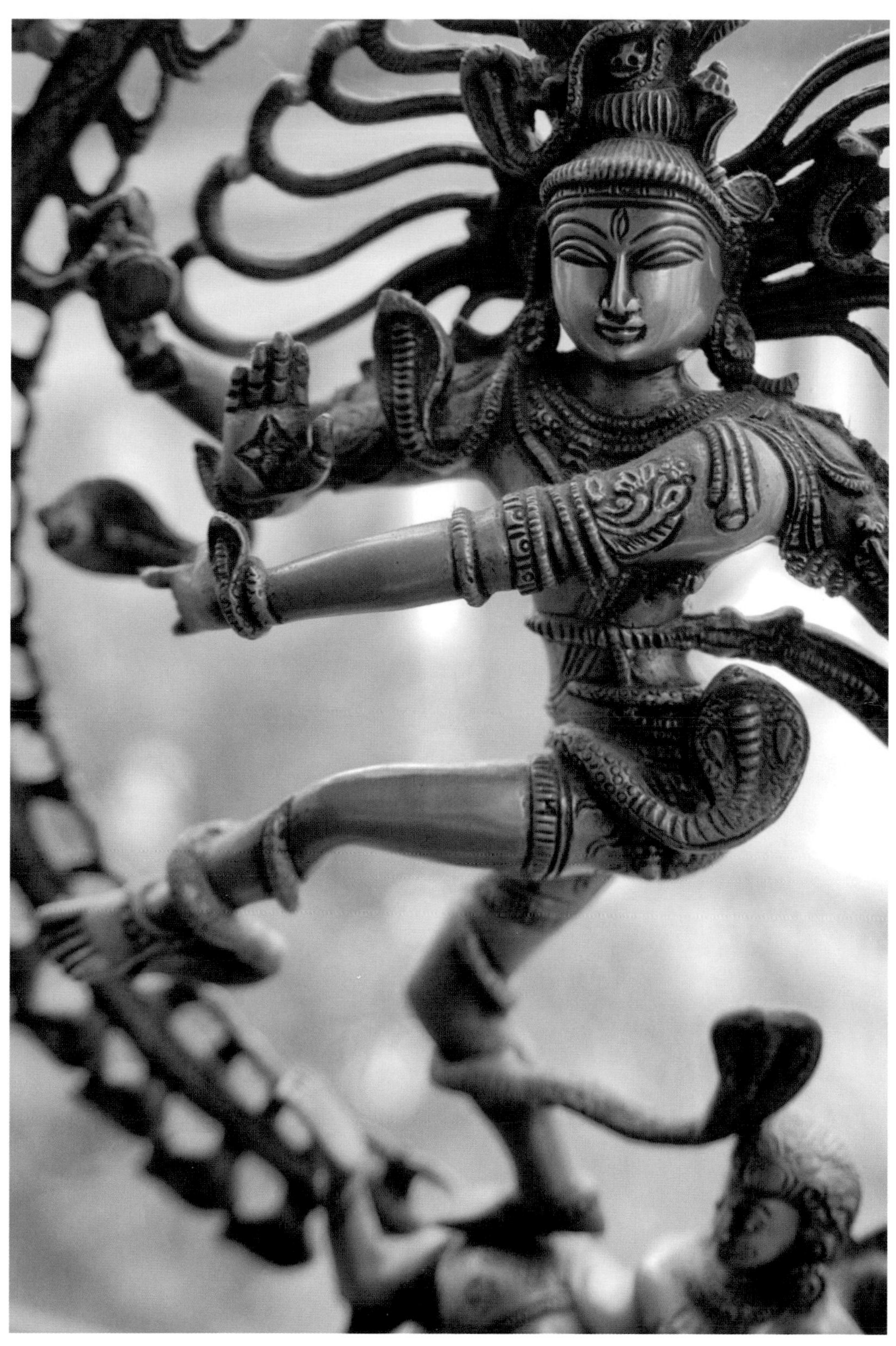

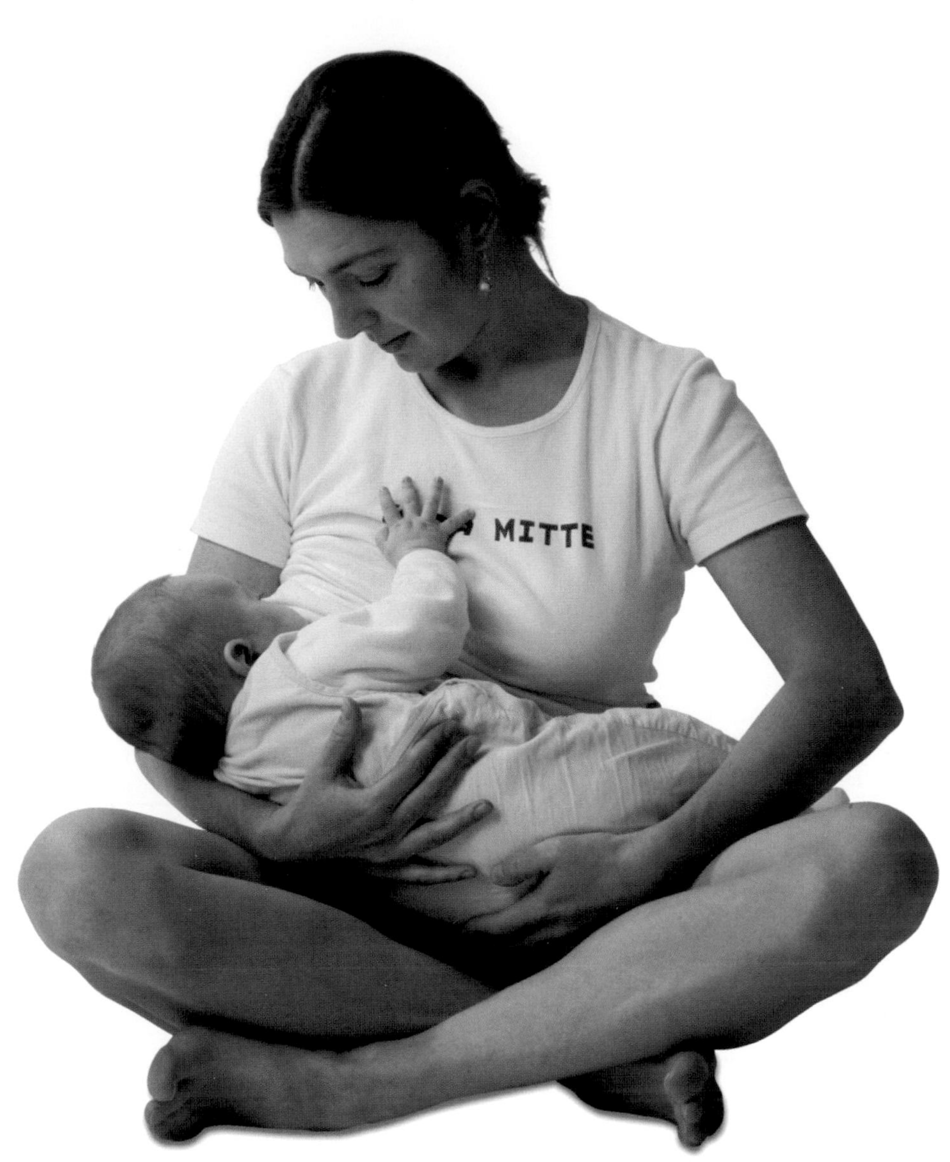
MITTE

PART II

Yoga During Pregnancy

CHAPTER 3
DETAILED DESCRIPTIONS OF ASANAS FOR ALL STUDENTS

CHAPTER 4
SEQUENCES OF ASANAS FOR BEGINNERS

CHAPTER 5
SEQUENCES OF ASANAS FOR ADVANCED STUDENTS

CHAPTER 6
DELIVERY

Chapter 3

Detailed Descriptions of Asanas for All Students

Practicing asanas and pranayama during pregnancy will maintain and secure the new life and create space for it to develop freely.

We recommended that you use the suggested props; this not only makes the poses easier and more comfortable, but also increases your sensitivity.

The asanas in this chapter are for both beginners and advanced students. We offer special guidance for beginners where needed. We specify which asanas are suitable for beginners and which for advanced students, as well as which asanas are appropriate for which trimester of pregnancy.

IMPORTANT:
If yours is considered a high risk pregnancy, do not attempt to use this book on your own. Seek the personal assistance of a certified Senior Iyengar Yoga teacher.

General Rules

As you perform the asanas, remember that you're practicing in order to protect yourself and the baby in your womb. Simply keeping this thought in mind goes a long way. You'll find that you enjoy doing the asanas more, because they develop a kind of sensitivity that makes you feel the freedom and atmosphere for growth that you are creating for your baby.

- Avoid pressure on your abdomen and pelvis.
- Avoid squeezing movements or those that put pressure on the pelvic floor.
- Practice quietly and gently, without creating body stress and tension.
- Observe your breathing; it is an indicator of whether you're using too much force and thus creating too much tension. Your breathing should be gentle, quiet, rhythmic, and natural.
- Be aware that you're practicing for yourself and the healthy growth of your baby.

Coming out of a pose:

In performing the asanas, you create space. When you come back from an asana, maintain that space. Don't collapse and shrink the space you have acquired; stay open and maintain the expansion, extension, and state of mind.

Cautions

1. The asanas we recommend for pregnancy are safe, and they maintain good health and strengthen and tone the muscles. However:

As soon as you have conceived, stop practicing the following asanas:

- Parivritta Trikonasana (page 290) and Parivritta Parshvakonasana (page 155)
- Marichyasana (pages 314 and 320) and Ardha Matsyendrasana (page 324)
- Urdhva Prasarita Padasana (page 350)
- Dhanurasana (page 239)
- Pashchimottanasana (pages 87 and 308)

These squeeze and compress the fetus and could lead to miscarriage.

2. As you do the standing poses, avoid jumping to spread your legs. Instead, merely spread your legs and adjust the distance. Always practice on a sticky mat to avoid slipping.

3. Avoid rapid movements, jerking or jolting your body, and hurrying to finish your practice. Go slowly and do each asana with awareness and understanding.

4. Don't hold your breath. Your breathing, though not deep, should be smooth and soft, without restriction or interruption. Your diaphragm region should not be tensed, tightened, or compressed.

5. Coming out of a pose, don't collapse, but rather maintain the lift, the extension, the expansion, and the state of mind you have created in an asana.

6. The standing asanas like Utthita Trikonasana, Utthita Parshvakonasana, and Ardha Chandrasana help to strengthen the spine and broaden the pelvis. Therefore, while performing these asanas, be very careful to stretch the spine and avoid compression of the uterus. **If you have a tendency to miscarry, you should avoid the standing asanas completely.**

7. **If you have a tendency toward repeated miscarriages due to a problem in glandular function, you should seek the advice of an experienced, trained Iyengar Yoga teacher**. The inverted asanas such as Salamba Shirshasana and Salamba Sarvangasana are very helpful. The causes of miscarriage can include muscular weakness and a weak constitution. You should concentrate more on forward-extending asanas like Janu Shirshasana, Pashchimottanasana, and Baddha Konasana done with a concave back and the lower chest lifted.

8. In the forward-extending asanas, you should not bend forward, which compresses the fetus. However, making the spine concave and lifting the lower chest helps tremendously, as the fetus gets space to move freely within. The uterine system should not get compressed or constricted, as downward pressure may cause miscarriage. *Actions that involve bending far forward are meant for nonpregnant women only.* At the beginning of the second trimester, you might still practice at a 45° angle, but with the growth of the fetus, you should take care that it is not compressed. At the end of your pregnancy, you might end up practicing at an angle of 80° to 90°.

9. You should practice pranayama regularly throughout the pregnancy and afterwards, even if you have had a miscarriage.

10. Practice Shavasana regularly as well, preferably twice a day, in the morning and in the evening. In fact, it can be done whenever you feel like you need a rest.

11. You should feel comfortable doing the asanas; understand your capacity and use discretion. A faulty pose, hurrying, overenthusiasm, strain, and force can cause injuries. Pay special attention to careful spinal extension, avoiding compression, and to proper breathing.

12. Be sure to get regular medical checkups. If the fetus is found in an abnormal position (e.g., sideways) seek appropriate medical care. In such cases, a capable Yoga teacher's advice is also essential. If the fetus is in breech position, you can still practice asanas.

13. Practicing asanas and pranayama should make you feel mentally well and secure. A sound and healthy practice reduces fatigue and depression and gives you a feeling of strength and inner balance.

Frequently Asked Questions

Q: What is the ideal time to practice?

For any study or practice, early morning is the ideal time because your mind and body are fresh and relaxed. Beginners, however, may have stiff muscles, so they can practice in the afternoon or evening, when the muscles are more elastic. Of course, if your schedule doesn't allow for morning practice, then you can practice in the evening.

Q: Should I take a bath or a shower before practice?

Yes, with an oiling of the body first, 20 to 30 minutes before you start, which softens the muscles. You can also bathe 20 to 30 minutes afterwards.

Q: Should I practice on an empty stomach?

Yes, if possible, but a cup of tea won't hurt. After a light meal, such as soup, you should wait for one hour. After a full meal, you should wait four hours. After practicing, you can drink, but should wait one hour before you have a full meal. If you feel very weak in the morning and need to have breakfast, then do so and practice after an hour. You can practice head and shoulder balance before the evening meal.

Q: Are there asanas that I can do directly after a meal?

Yes. Some asanas enhance digestion, including:
- Virasana
- Supta Virasana
- Baddha Konasana
- Supta Baddha Konasana
- Svastikasana
- Supta Svastikasana
- Matsyasana

Q: Can I practice immediately after sunbathing?

No. You should wait 30 minutes, so the body can cool down.

Q: Shall I use props like a mat, bolster, and blankets?

Yes. Make use of all the props that are recommended, so that you can adjust your body more easily to the pose and give freedom to the life in your womb.

Q: What shall I wear for practice?

Wear comfortable clothes that you can freely move in, preferably made of cotton. When it is cold, dress warmly.

A Word to Teachers

The asanas you teach should be easily performed. They should reduce common pregnancy problems and warning signals like nausea, morning sickness, constipation, water retention, headache, and toxemia. The asanas should balance the digestive and urinary systems and blood circulation. They should ensure free breathing.

In teaching pranayama, try to reduce symptoms like fatigue and nervous tension, and enable the expectant mother to enjoy mental and physical health during the different stages of her pregnancy.

For questions, seek the advice of an experienced senior teacher.

Instructions and Benefits

The three trimesters of pregancy refer to the following weeks:

1st trimester: weeks 1 to 16
2nd trimester: weeks 17 to 29
3rd trimester: weeks 30 to 40

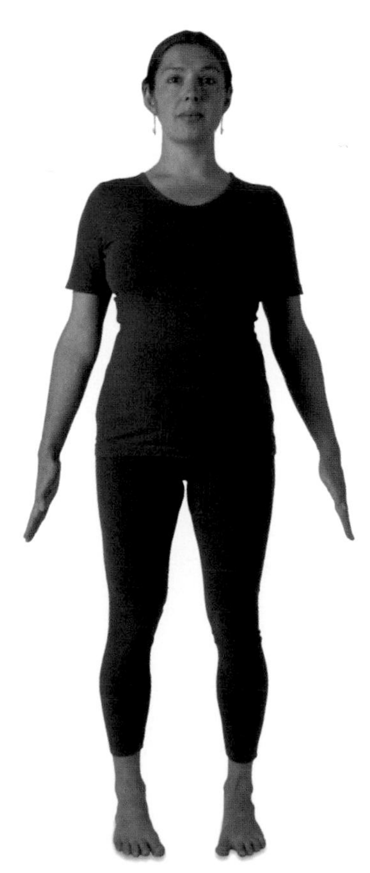

Standing Asanas
Uttishtha Sthiti

Tadasana or Samasthiti
Mountain pose

Tadasana means "erect and steady like a mountain." This pose is called the mountain pose. It promotes an alert body, mind, and brain.

Tadasana is one of the basic poses of the standing asanas. From here, you explore the other standing asanas. In Tadasana, you learn how to balance your weight on both feet and on each sole. You learn to ground your feet and how this grounding helps to stretch your legs, straighten your pelvis, and lift your entire spine, including your head.

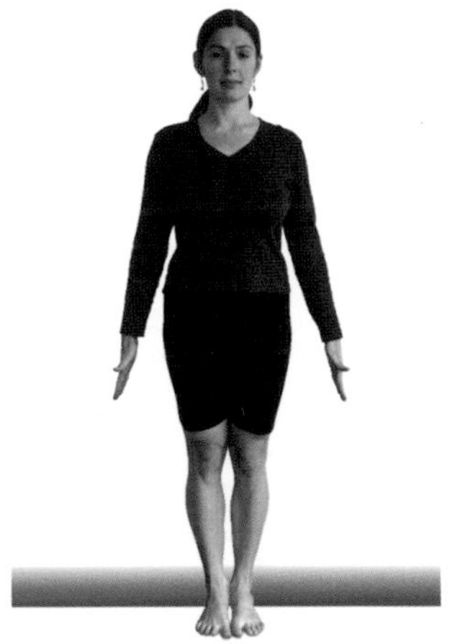

1st trimester

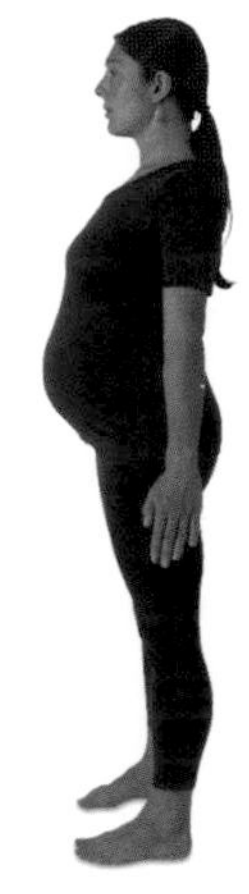

2nd trimester

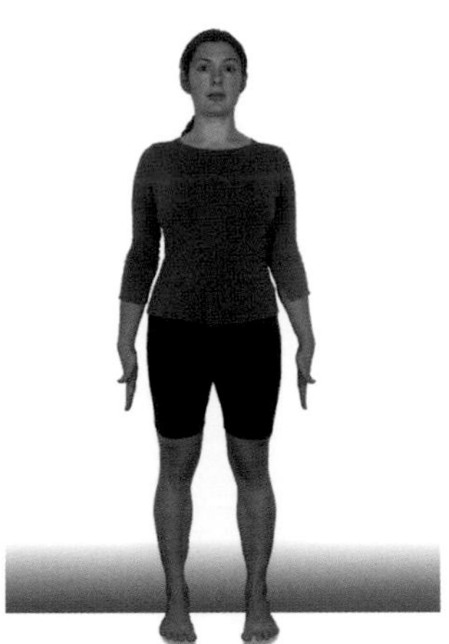

3rd trimester

Advanced pregnancy: In the third trimester, to draw the internal organs up away from the pelvic floor, turn your toes in.

1 Stand erect with your feet together (during the first trimester) and your big toes and heels touching. The weight of your body is neither on the heels nor on the toes, but in the center of the arches.

2 Don't tighten your toes; stretch them from the bottom and keep them relaxed. (This is the position of the toes in all standing poses.)

3 Keep your ankles in line with each other.

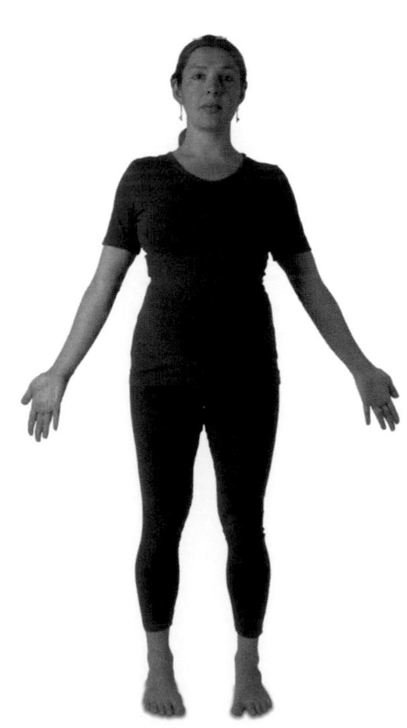

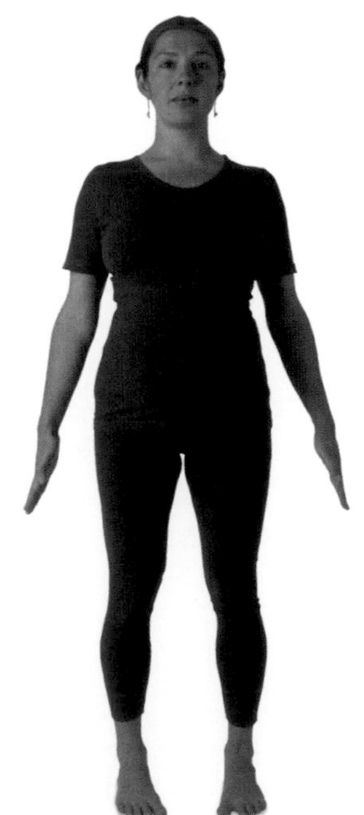

4 Tighten your kneecaps upward and tighten your front thigh muscles.

5 Keep your spine erect, raise your breastbone, and expand your chest. Don't let your abdomen protrude, but lift it upward.

6 Keep your neck erect and your head straight; don't tilt your head forward or backward.

7 Look straight ahead.

8 Keep your arms by your sides, and extending downward; turn your hands and arms out. Then, maintaining the lift of your chest and its sides, turn your hands in and extend them downward.

9 Remain in the pose for 20 to 30 seconds.

1st trimester: Keep your feet together.
2nd trimester: Place your feet hip-width apart, to avoid pressure on the pubic plate. Keep the outer sides of your feet parallel.
3rd trimester: For better alignment, make use of the wall.

Benefits

Counteracts cramps in the calf muscles during the night

Counteracts curvature of the spine and pain in the hip

Tadasana with Wall and Quarter-round Block

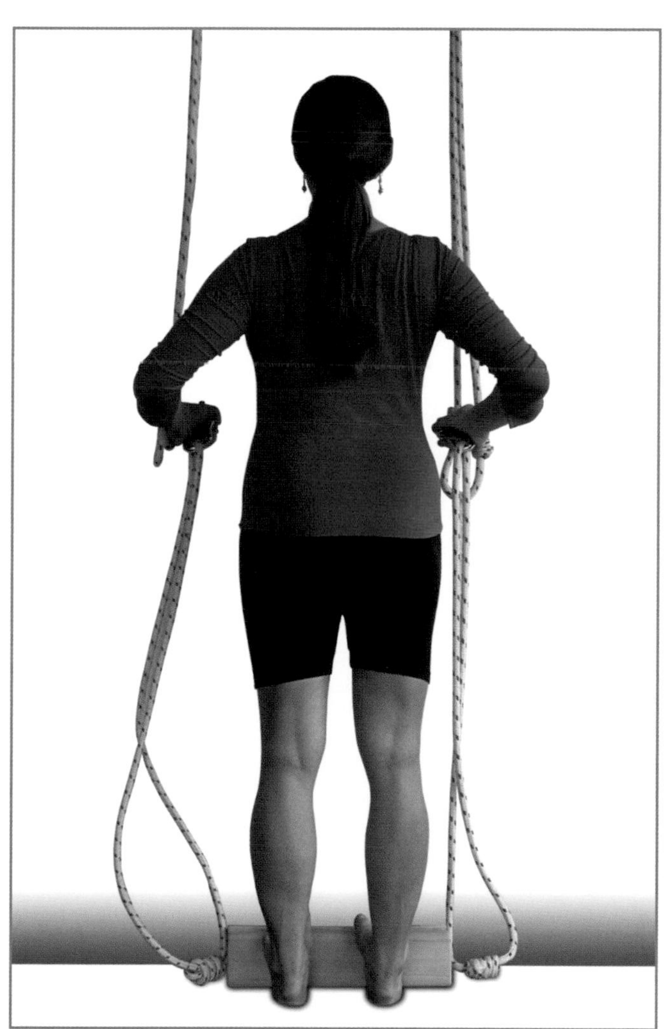

Using ropes is optional

1 Place your heel down on the floor and the balls of your feet on the block.

2 Stretch the bottoms of your toes away from your soles.

3 Tuck your tailbone down and inward; don't project it backward.

Urdhva Baddhanguliyasana in Tadasana
Mountain pose with bound hands

In this pose, the whole body extends upward like a tree.

1 Stand erect in Tadasana (page 32).

2 Interlock your fingers, turn your wrists and palms outward, and stretch your arms forward in line with your shoulders.

3 Move your extended arms upward by the sides of your ears. Your palms should face the ceiling.

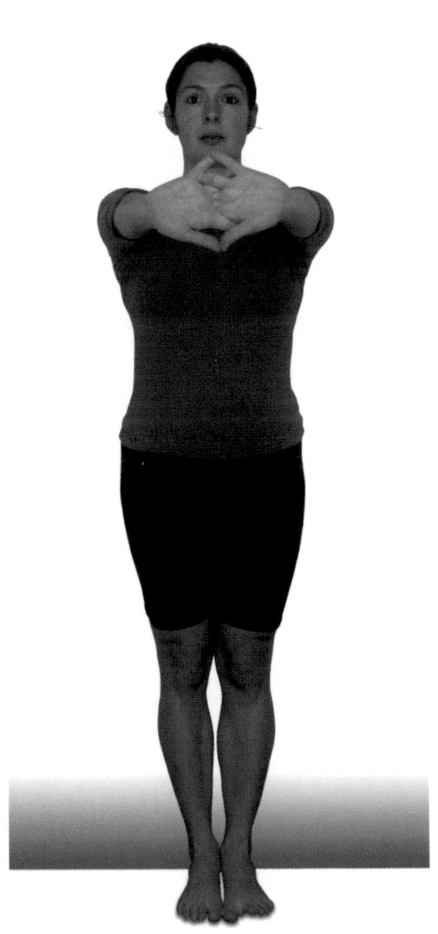

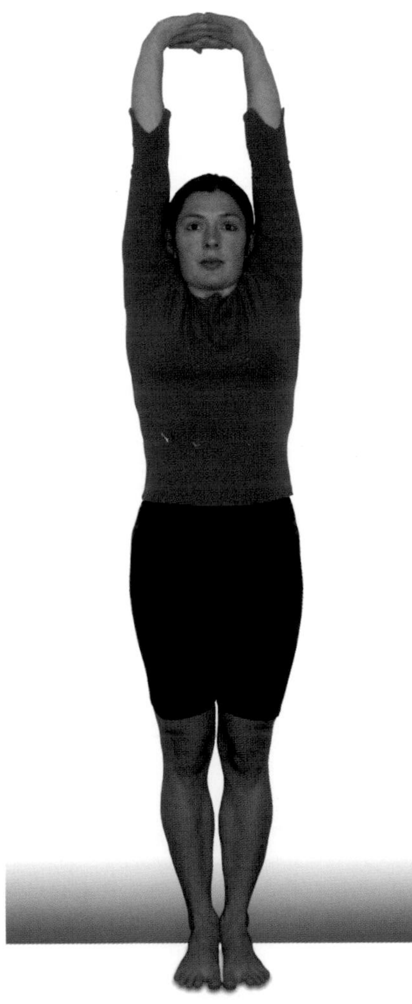

1st trimester: no
2nd trimester: yes
3rd trimester: yes

Benefits

Tones the shoulder muscles
Lifts the spine

Gives poise and balance
Revitalizes body and mind

Contraindications

Symptoms of toxemia

Feelings of exhaustion or tiredness

4 Move your back ribs forward. Lift your chest and tuck your shoulder blades in deep.

5 Keep your head erect and look straight ahead.

6 Breathing normally, maintain this pose for 10 to 15 seconds.

7 Maintaining the space you have created in the spine and the chest, lower your arms, come back, change the interlocking of your fingers, and repeat.

Coming out of the pose

Maintain the space you have created in the spine and the chest while coming back.

Urdhva Hastasana

Mountain pose with arms stretched upward

1st trimester: no
2nd trimester: yes
3rd trimester: yes

Benefits

- Tones the shoulder muscles
- Lifts the spine
- Revitalizes body and mind

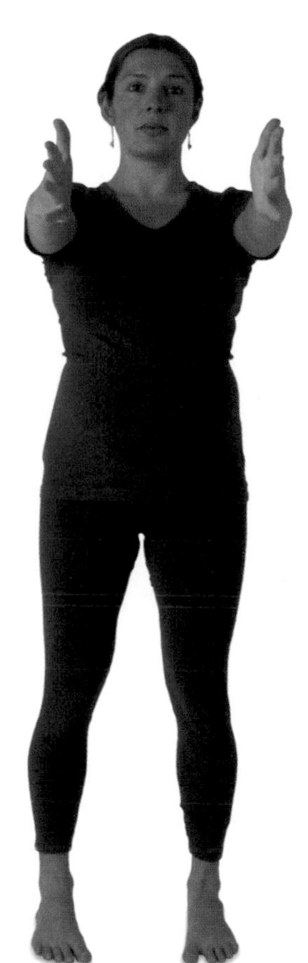

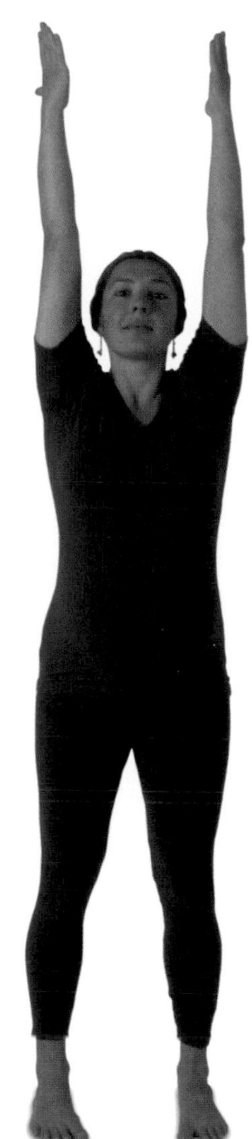

1 Stand erect in Tadasana (page 32).

2 Stretch your hands downward, palms facing your outer thighs.

3 Elongating your fingers, stretch your arms forward in line with your shoulders.

4 Inhale and stretch your arms upward to the ceiling alongside your ears.

5 Breathing normally, maintain the pose for 10 to 15 seconds.

6 Maintaining the space you have created, lower your arms with the same stretch.

Variation

Urdhva Hastasana, with ropes

Grip the ropes firmly and lift your torso upward.

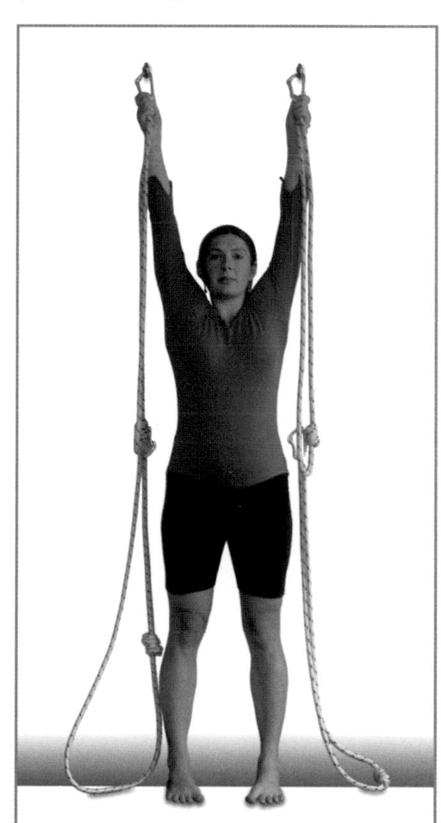

NOTE

You can do Tadasana, Urdhva Baddhanguliyasana and Urdhva Hastasana also in a lying down position.

Pashchima Namaskarasana in Tadasana

1st trimester: no
2nd trimester: yes
3rd trimester: yes

Benefits

See Gomukhasana in Tadasana, page 37

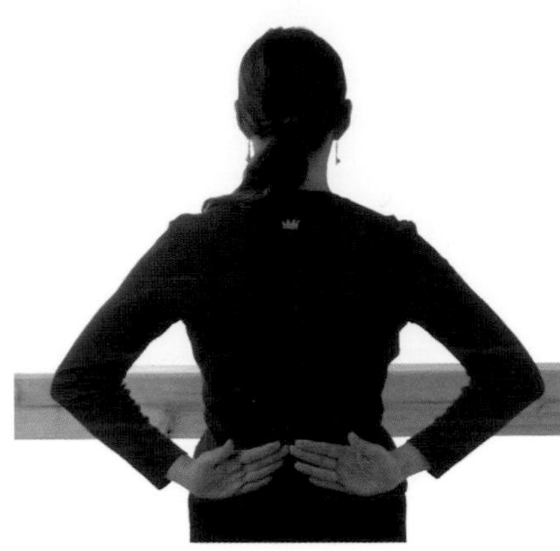

1 Stand erect in Tadasana (page 32).

2 Join your palms behind your back, fingers pointing towards your waist. Turn your wrists and palms inward and bring both palms up above the middle of your back.

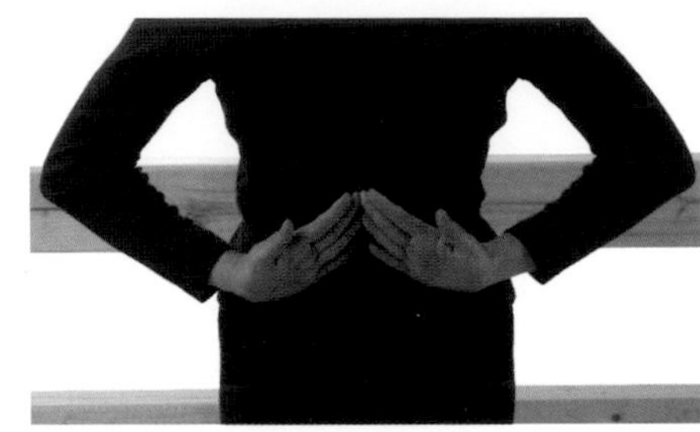

3 Keep your fingers in line with your shoulder blades and pointing upward.

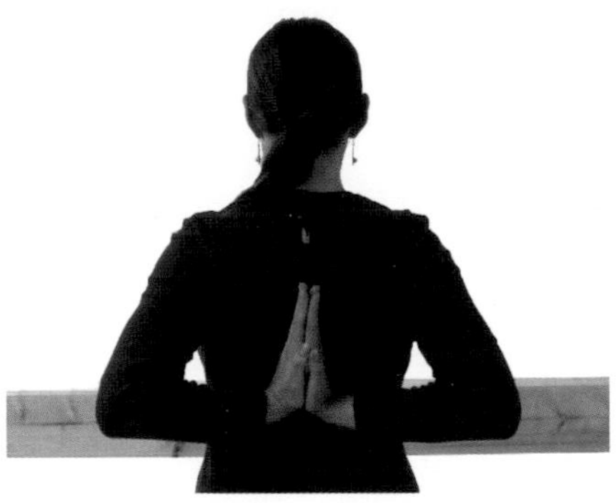

4 Press your palms against each other and move your elbows backward, so that your chest is not constricted. Expand your chest and raise your breastbone.

5 Keep your thighs back, your pelvis erect, and your abdomen lifted.

6 Breathing normally, remain in the pose for 15 – 30 seconds.

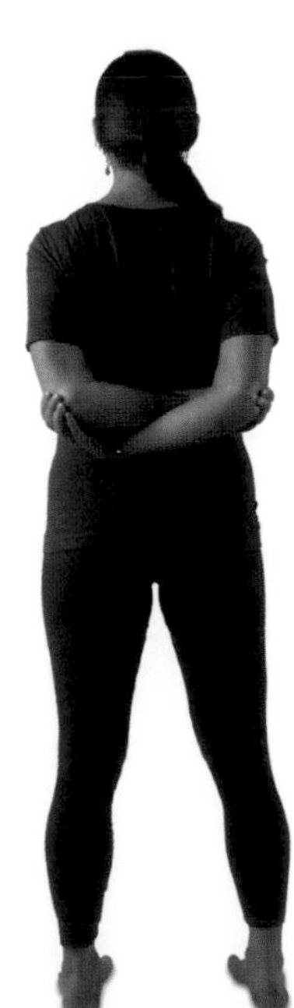

Help

If you can't bring your hands together, grip your elbows in Pashchima Baddha Hastasana.

Remember to reverse your grip and repeat accordingly.

Coming out of the pose

Maintain the lift and broadness of the chest and relax your hands.

Gomukhasana in Tadasana
Cow face in mountain pose

1st trimester: no
2nd trimester: yes
3rd trimester: yes

1 Stretch your left arm down and your right arm up.

2 Bend your left arm backwards and bring your left hand between your shoulder blades. Extend the fingers of your left hand upward.

3 Bend your right arm. Extend your right hand down to the left hand and grip.

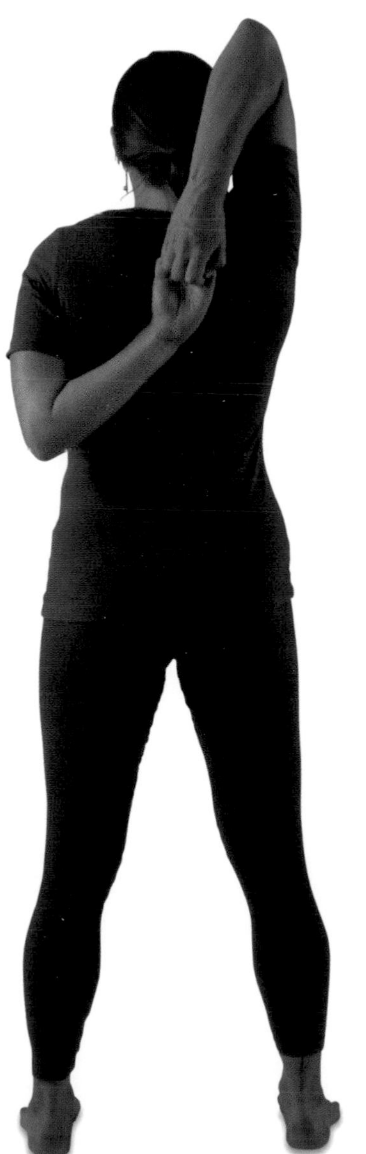

4 Extend both elbows away from each other and move them farther back, without pushing your head.

5 Keep your head in line with your spine.

6 Loosen your grip, extend your arms once more, and change sides.

Coming out of the pose
Maintain thc lift and broadness of your chest and relax your hands.

Benefits
Pashchima Namaskarasana and Gomukhasana (*below*) are especially good for: arthritis, stiffness in the neck, shoulders, elbows, and wrist

Contraindications
Feelings of exhaustion or tiredness

Symptoms of toxemia

Help
If you can't grip your fingers, use a belt.

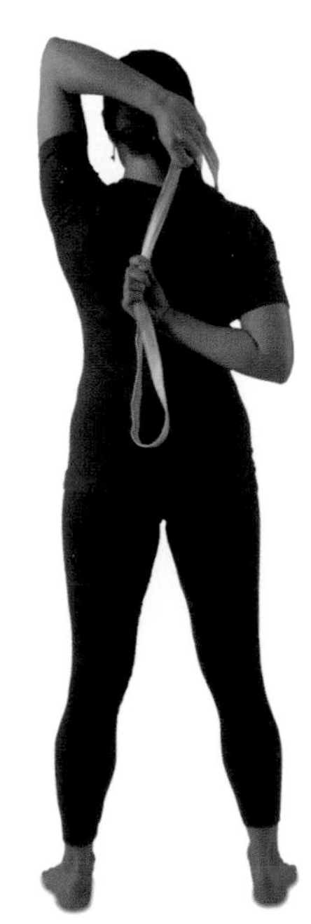

Utthita Trikonasana
Extended triangle pose

Utthita means "extended," and *trikona* means "triangle." This is an extended triangle pose, aimed at broadening the pelvis and chest.

1 Stand next to a wall.

2 Stand erect in Tadasana (feet hip-width apart, page 32), outer feet parallel.

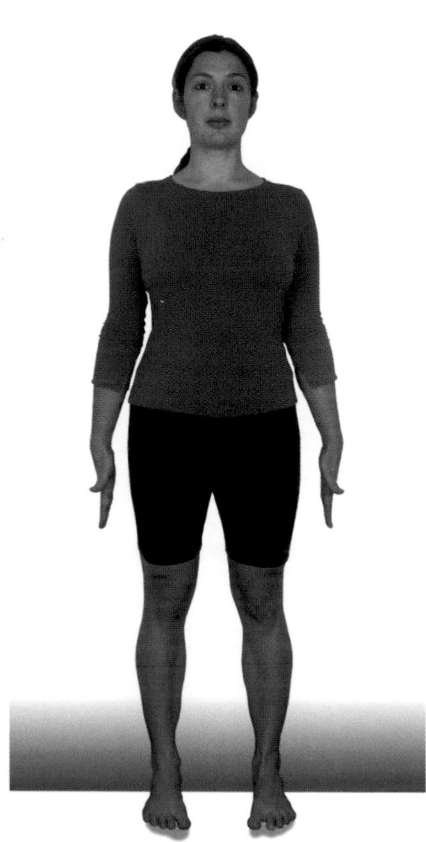

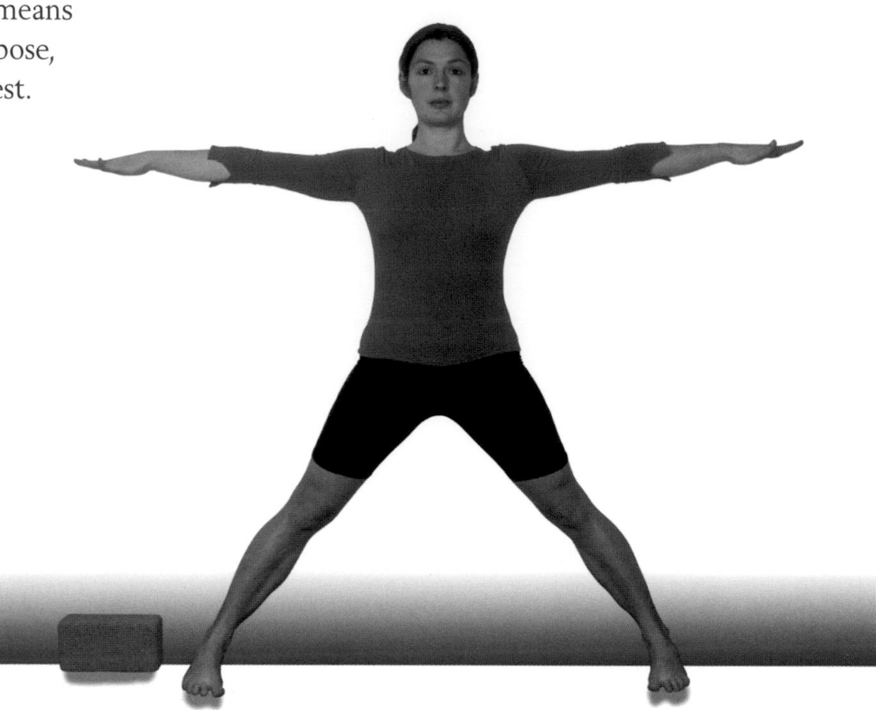

3 While inhaling, spread your legs 3 feet apart and stretch your arms sideways in line with your shoulders. Keep your palms facing the floor.

4 Turn your right leg 90° to the right. Turn your left foot slightly inward. Tighten your knees and thighs. Your mid foot, mid knee, and mid thigh should be all in one line. Take one or two breaths.

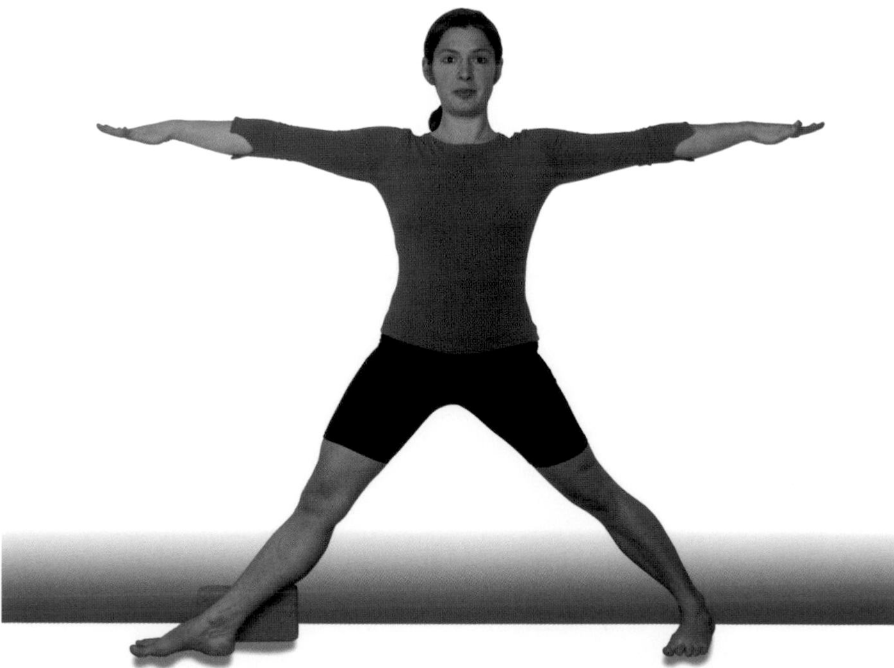

5 While exhaling, bend your torso sideways to the right. Hold your right ankle with your right hand, or place your right hand on a block.

6 If you are new to Yoga and your palm cannot reach your ankle, or if the side of your pelvis gets compressed, then keep your palm in the middle of your shinbone.

7 Raise your left arm in line with your shoulders and your right arm. Keep your left palm facing forward. Stretch both arms, keeping your elbows tight.

8 Turn your neck and look at your left thumb. If turning your head causes pain or strain, then keep your head in line with your spine.

9 This is the final position of the asana. Breathe normally and remain steady for 20 to 30 seconds, observing the following points in "Check Yourself" below.

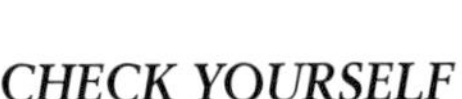

1st trimester: yes (with support)
2nd trimester: yes
3rd trimester: yes

Benefits

- Gives proper alignment of the legs
- Relieves backache and neck pain
- Strengthens the lower spine
- Frees space for the diaphragm

Contraindications

- Nausea (at the time of your practice, not in general)
- High blood pressure

HINT: To lessen fatigue, you can come back to Tadasana after you have done the asana on one side and then restart it on the other side.

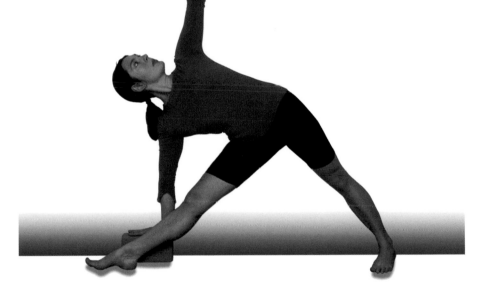

CHECK YOURSELF

- *Keep your thigh muscles tight and your kneecaps pulled in and up.*
- *The back of your left leg, your hips, and the back of your chest should all be in one line.*
- *Expand your chest by tucking in your shoulder blades.*
- *Extend the front of your torso from pelvis to chest in the direction of your head. Keep the sides of your torso parallel.*
- *Don't hold your breath while you're in the pose.*
- *While staying in the pose, elongate your lower chest, creating space between your chest and abdomen.*
- *As you come out of the pose, maintain the expansion of your body, inhale, lift your right hand away from your ankle, raise your torso, and come back.*
- *Turn your legs and feet to the left and repeat to the left side.*
- *You may also close your feet in Tadasana and then repeat to the left side.*

Utthita Parshvakonasana

Extended lateral angle pose

Utthita means "extended," *parshva* means "side," and *kona* indicates an "angle." This asana aims at broadening the pelvis and chest.

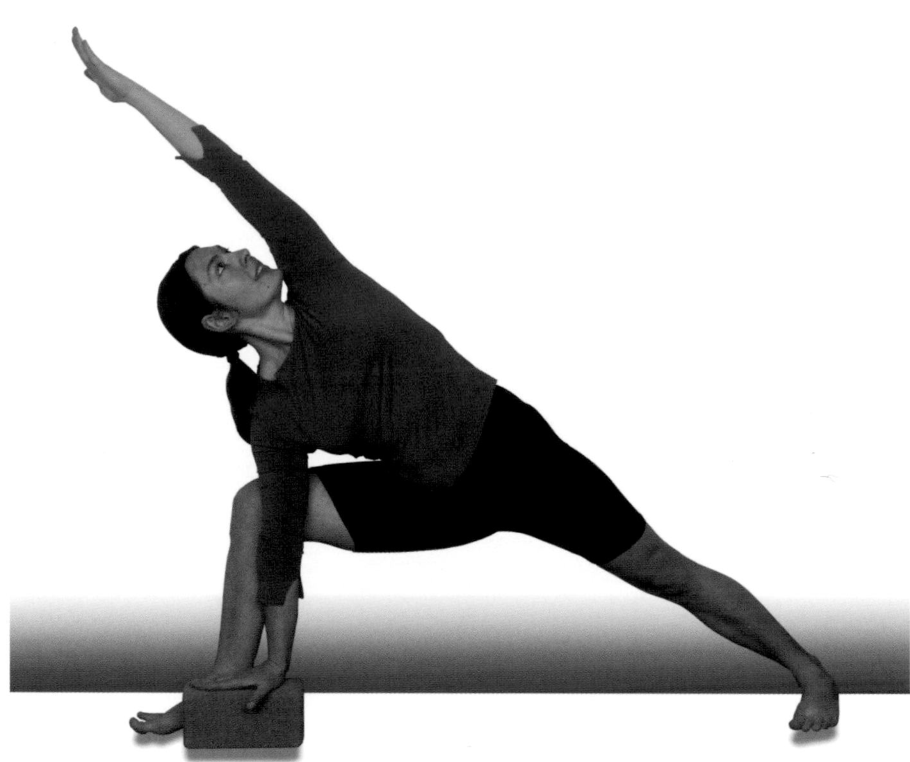

1 Stand next to a wall in Tadasana (page 32).

2 While exhaling, spread your feet 4 to 4½ feet apart. Extend your arms sideways.

3 Turn your right leg to 90° and your left foot slightly in. Tighten your knees and thighs. Place a wooden block by the inner edge of your foot. When you are practicing against a trestle or table, you can also place a block by the outer edge of your foot.

4 Bend your right leg at the knee until your thigh and calf form a right angle. Your right thigh is parallel to the floor, and your shin is perpendicular to it. Take one or two deep breaths. If the distance is not right and you have to adjust, then always adjust from the back leg, in order not to disturb your bent front leg.

5 Exhale and move your torso sideways to your right foot. Place your right palm or your fingertips on the block, creating space between your right thigh and the right side of your torso. Make sure that your abdomen does not press against your thigh. Your chest should also remain free so you can breathe easily.

6 Stretch your left arm straight up, turn it so that your palm is facing your head, move the arm over your head, turn your neck, and look up.

7 If it's difficult to turn your head, then keep your left arm straight up as in Utthita Trikonasana, with your head facing forward or up.

8 This is the final position. Breathe normally and stay in the pose for 20 – 30 seconds.

9 While inhaling, lift your right hand from the floor, lift your torso, and keep your right leg at the right angle. Then, straighten your right leg and turn your legs and feet to the left side to repeat.

10 From the left side, come back to Tadasana.

1st trimester: yes (with support)
2nd trimester: yes
3rd trimester: yes

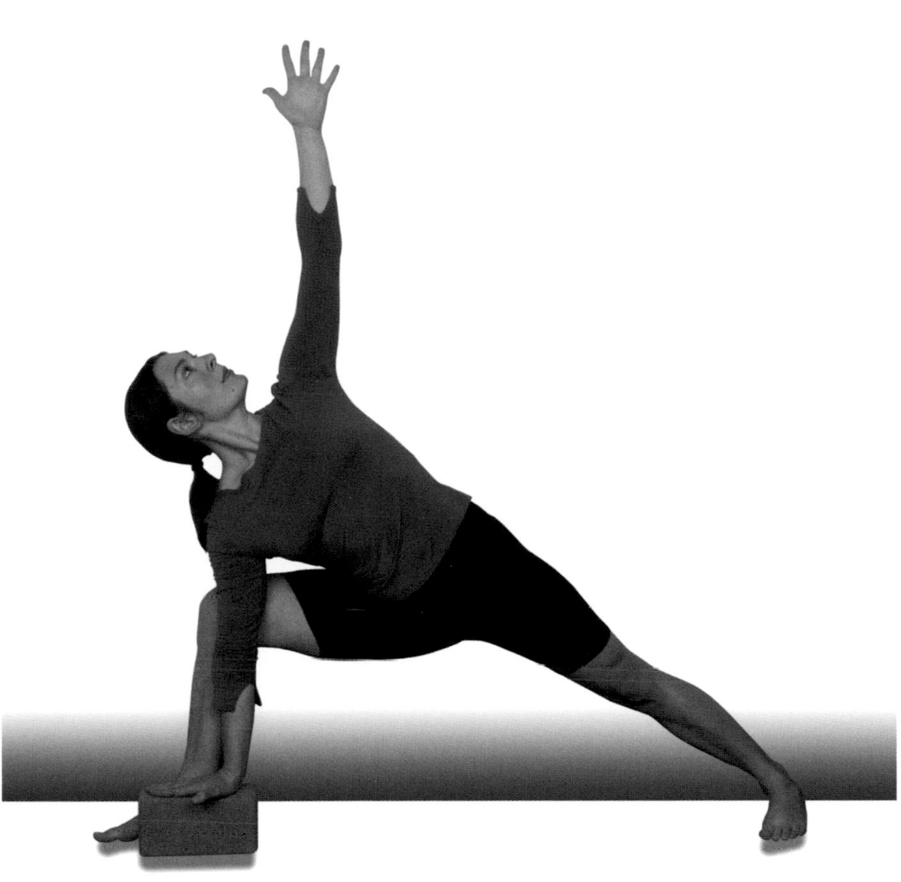

Benefits

- Relieves hip and arthritic pains
- Corrects digestion, flatulence, and elimination problems
- Removes backache and lower back pain
- Helps breathing
- Creates lightness
- Prevents urine retention

Contraindications

See Virabhadrasana 2, page 42

HINT: To lessen fatigue, you can come back to Tadasana after you have done the asana on one side and then restart it on the other side.

CHECK YOURSELF

> *Tuck your right buttock in so that it remains in line with your outer knee.*

> *Tighten your front thigh muscle and stretch the hamstrings (muscles behind the knee) of your left leg.*

> *Extend your left armpit, biceps (front upper arm muscle), wrist, palm, and elbow. From your left ankle to left wrist there should be one stretch, so that your body does not sway.*

> *Tuck your shoulder blades in. Turn the left side of your torso upward and backward, so that your chest is expanded and the back of your body remains in one line.*

> *If your right side feels short and tight, place your lower arm on your upper thigh, move the knee farther out and your right buttock farther in, and lift your right side and right chest farther using the resistance in your feet, legs, and pelvis. Practice the same way on the other side.*

Virabhadrasana 2
Warrior 2 pose

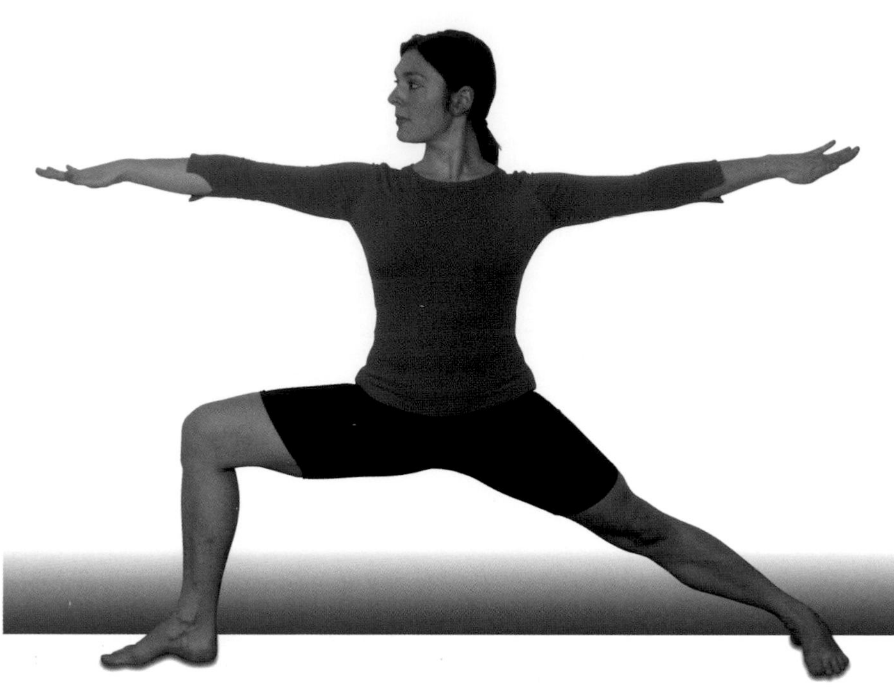

This pose is named after Virabhadra, a warrior; it gives balance and brings firmness.

Although this asana, like Virabhadrasana 1, is very beneficial for morning sickness, you shouldn't perform it when you are actually nauseated.

1 Stand next to a wall in Tadasana (page 32).

2 While inhaling, spread your legs 4 to $4\frac{1}{2}$ feet apart and stretch your arms sideways in line with your shoulders, palms facing down.

3 Turn your right leg 90° to the right and your left foot slightly in. Keep your legs straight. Take a deep breath.

4 While exhaling, bend your right leg.

5 Turn your head to the right and keep your left eye focused on your right hand.

6 Breathe normally, remain steady for 10 to 15 seconds, and observe the points in "Check Yourself."

CHECK YOURSELF

> Expand your chest.

> Stretch both arms sideways as though they were being pulled apart.

> Keep your anus and the crown of your head in line.

> Widen your pelvic region sideways, to give the fetus more room to move.

> Maintaining the space, come back with an inhalation, and repeat on the left side. From there, close your feet in Tadasana.

> Don't allow your torso to lean towards your bent leg as you bend the knee.

> Keep the sides of your torso parallel.

> While turning your head to the right, don't also turn your torso to the right, but stretch your left arm back in line with your left leg towards your left foot.

> Create resistance in your left leg (the back leg).

Coming out of the pose

Maintain the space you have created, feel both feet, inhale, and come up.

Guidance for All Three Asanas

- Beginners can practice the asanas in the second and third trimesters, and advanced students in all three trimesters of pregnancy (*see also Chapter 4, "Classification of Asanas," pages 169 – 170*).

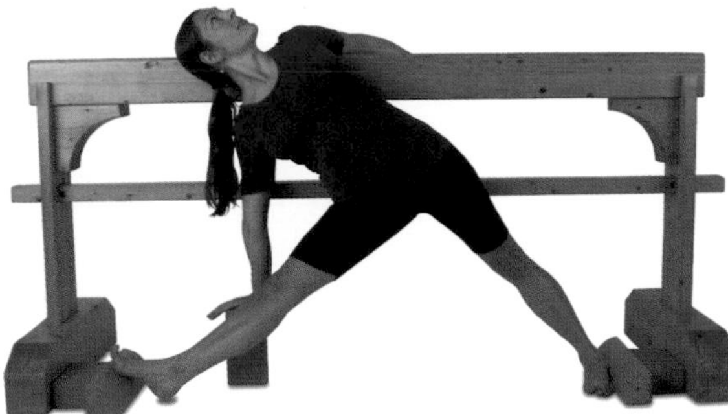

- For more balance, practice with your back, back of the heel, hips, and back of your head touching the wall. This will allow you to extend your spine upward easily, and exert less effort while enjoying the maximum advantage from the asana. You also won't feel heaviness in your abdomen, because your weight is properly distributed between the front and back of your torso.

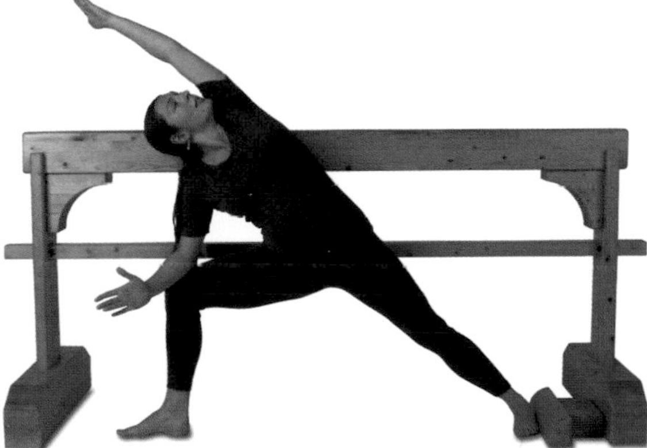

- Practice against a trestle (or a table), especially in the third trimester, when your abdomen is so heavy that alignment and balance are difficult. Keep your back foot against a block under the trestle (or leg of table).

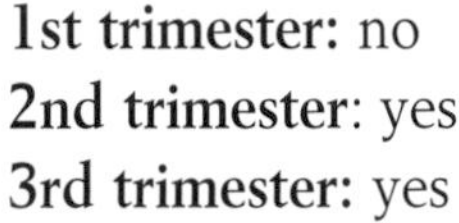

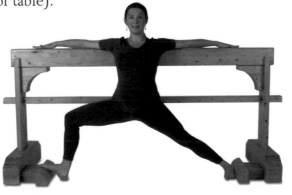

1st trimester: no
2nd trimester: yes
3rd trimester: yes

Benefits

- Brings lightness to the abdominal area
- Prevents urine retention
- Reduces morning sickness
- Massages the liver and spleen, improving digestion
- Strengthens the pelvic region
- Lubricates the spinal vertebrae

Contraindications

- High blood pressure
- Heart problems
- Toxemia
- Dizziness

HINT: To lessen fatigue, you can come back to Tadasana after you have done the asana on one side and then restart it on the other side.

DETAILED DESCRIPTIONS OF ASANAS FOR ALL STUDENTS

Parighasana
Gate pose

Parighasana is an assisting asana; it improves Utthita Trikonasana and Utthita Parshvakonasana.

1st trimester: no
2nd trimester: yes
3rd trimester: as long as you feel comfortable

Benefits
Extends the sides of the torso
Lengthens and softens the abdominal wall

Step 1

1 Kneel on a blanket, keeping your hands on your waist.

2 Your shinbones should press into the blanket, and your feet and toes should point straight back.

3 Lift your right leg, turn your right foot to the side, and keep it bent at 90°, as in Virabhadrasana 2.

4 Keep your knee turned out.

5 Come back to the center and repeat on the left.

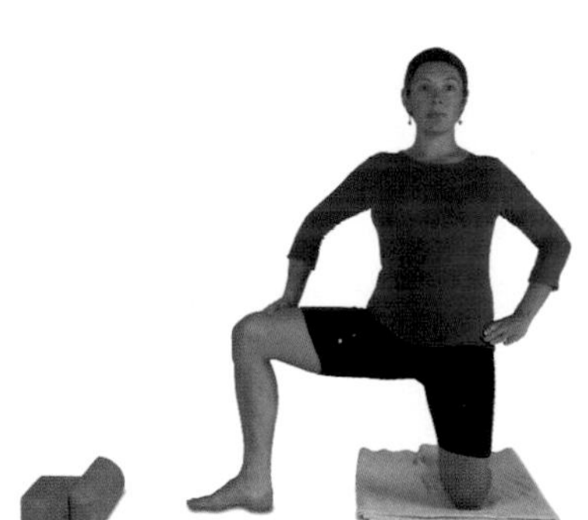

Step 2

1 Without changing the level of your buttocks, extend your right leg straight out to the side in line with your right hip, extend your heel, place the balls of your feet on a block or against the wall, and keep your leg straight and the kneecap tight.

2 Keep your shinbone, ankle, and metatarsals of the bent knee pressed on the floor.

3 Extend your arms straight out to the sides at shoulder level.

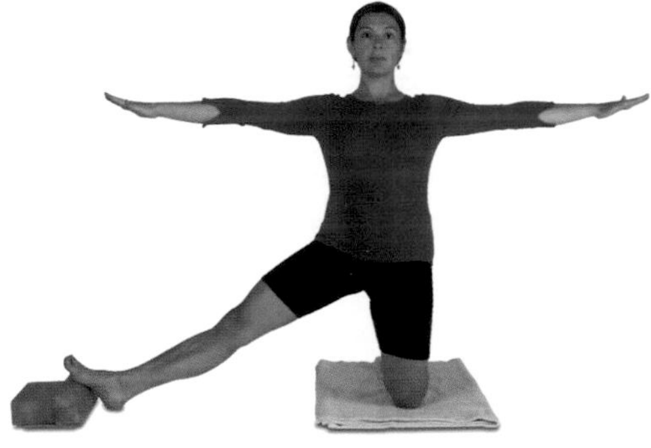

Step 3

1 Exhale, and with your chest and abdomen facing forward, bend your torso to the side of your right leg.

2 Place your right hand on your right shinbone.

3 Exhale and extend your left arm over your head in line with your left ear.

4 Breathe normally.

5 Develop your ability to rotate your torso towards thc ceiling as in Utthita Parshvakonasana.

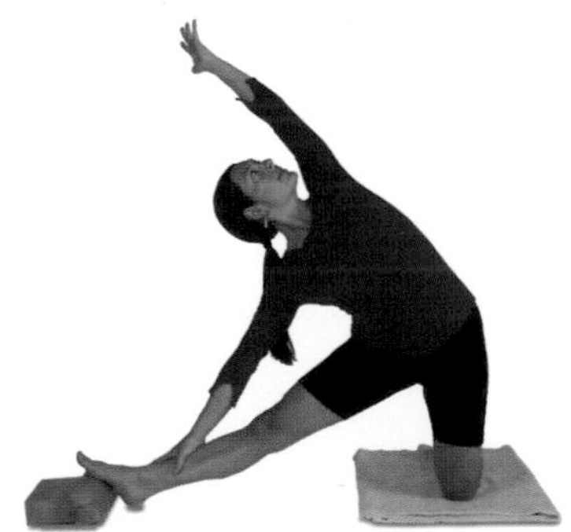

Coming out of the pose

Put your left hand on your waist, lift your torso, and come up. Come back to the center and repeat on the other side.

Ardha Chandrasana, Elevation

Half moon pose

Ardha means "half," and *chandra* means "moon." This pose resembles the half moon.

This pose is a great gift to the pregnant woman. It brings lightness to her body, and with the extension and expansion inherent in the asana, a feeling of freedom and abandon. Some standing asanas can increase the feeling of nausea that is common among pregnant women, which is why they should be omitted. This asana, however, is a great help.

Ardha Chandrasana, Upavishtha Konasana, and Baddha Konasana are relief-giving poses. They help you to breathe freely, calmly, quietly, and confidently.

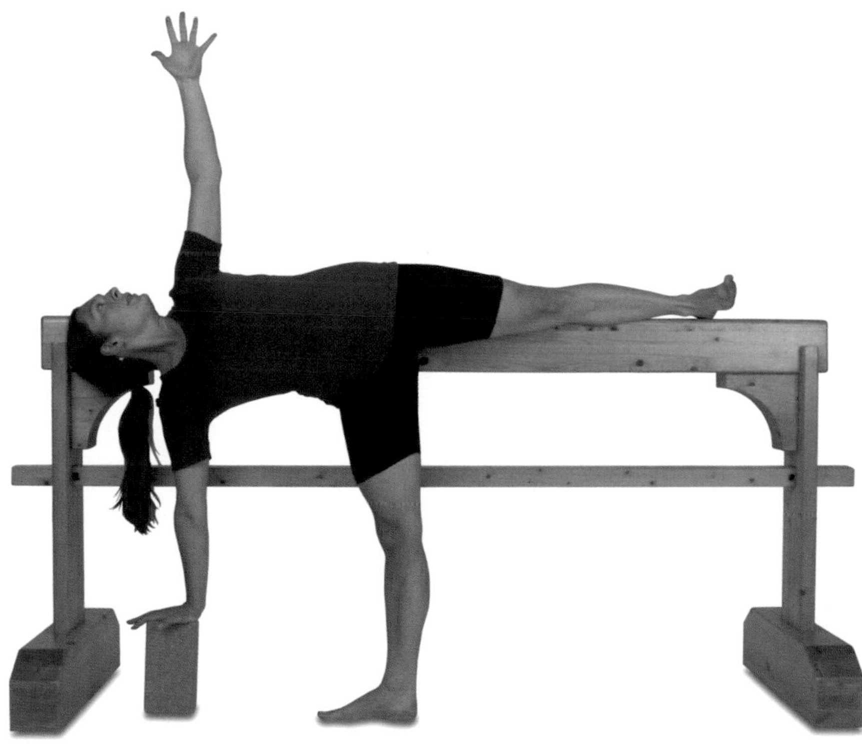

1st trimester: yes (with support)
2nd trimester: yes
3rd trimester: yes

Benefits

- Makes you feel light and elated
- Eliminates mental and physical dullness and fatigue
- Reduces anxiety, nervous tension, and occasional depression due to fatigue
- Checks bleeding during pregnancy
- Eliminates discomfort, heaviness, and throbbing in the breasts
- Strengthens and firms the breast
- Strengthens the spine and pelvic muscles
- Expands the lower abdominal region, allowing the fetus to float freely
- Strengthens the placenta
- Reduces itching
- Relieves upward pressure from the fetus resulting in heavy breathing and tiredness, especially in mid-pregnancy. The torso gets organically spread out from inside, creating space between the thorax, abdomen, and diaphragm.
- Reduces nausea and vomiting
- Loosens heavy, knotted feelings and tones the abdomen
- Prevents cramps caused by the uterus, creating pressure on the pelvic nerve. The torso and spine get extended and expanded, lessening the pressure.

1 Stand in Tadasansa (page 32) with your back against the wall. Have a block on your right side.

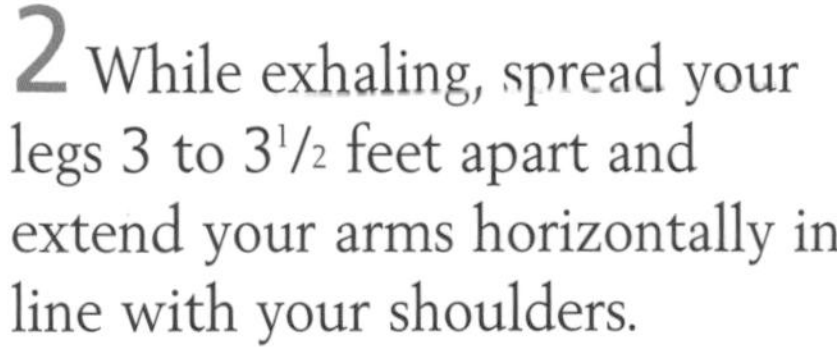

2 While exhaling, spread your legs 3 to 3½ feet apart and extend your arms horizontally in line with your shoulders.

3 Do Utthita Trikonasana on the right side. Take one or two deep breaths.

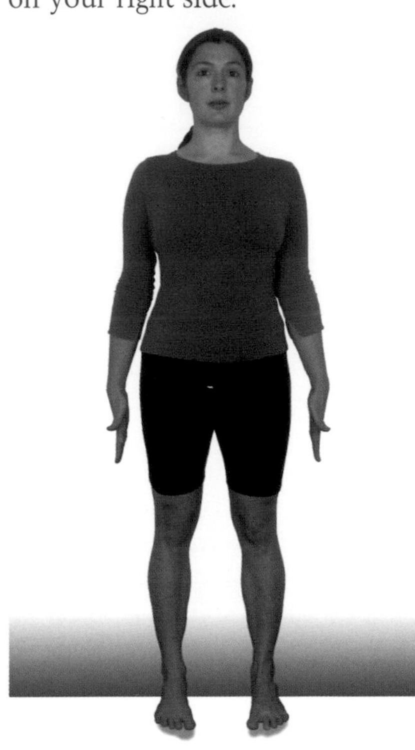

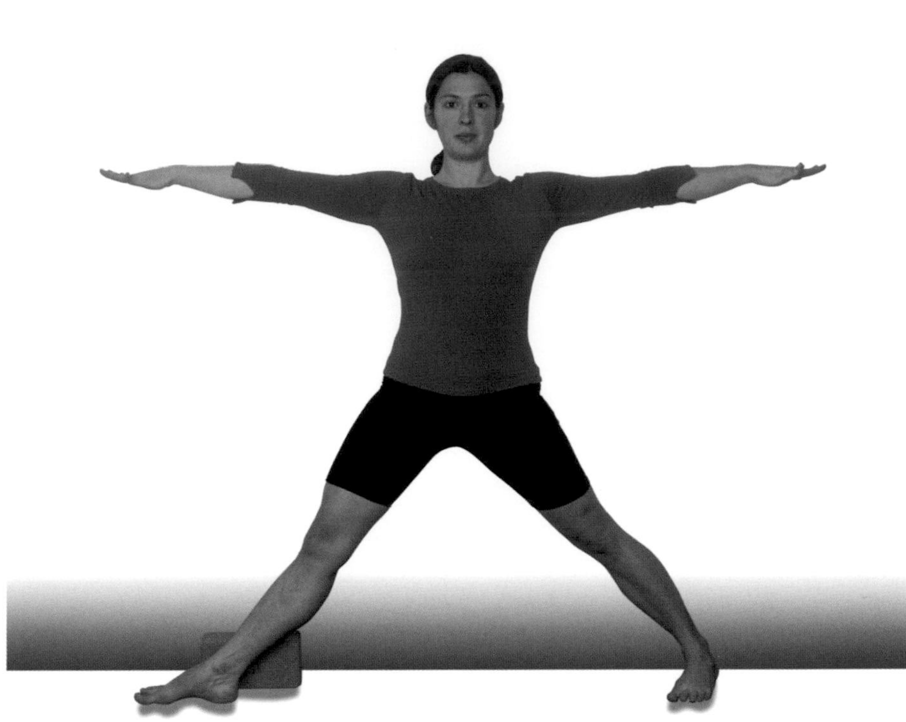

4 Exhale and bend your leg slightly. Rest the palm of your right hand on the block or a raised surface, about one foot in front of your leg, so that your spine does not slant downward.

If you keep your palm on the floor (as a nonpregnant woman might do), your spine will slant downward and the sides of the pelvis will narrow, which is harmful to the fetus.

5 While lowering your arm, move your torso and raise your left heel so that it comes up with no extra effort. Your heel and leg should rise like a seesaw.

6 Exhale, extend your torso towards your head, and raise your left leg. Straighten your right leg and keep it firm.

7 Raise your left arm in line with your shoulders.

8 This is the final position. Breathing normally, remain steady for 10 – 15 seconds.

Coming out of the pose

• Maintain the space in your chest and the firmness of your back leg.

• Exhale, bend your right leg, lower the left leg to the floor, and come back to Utthita Trikonasana.

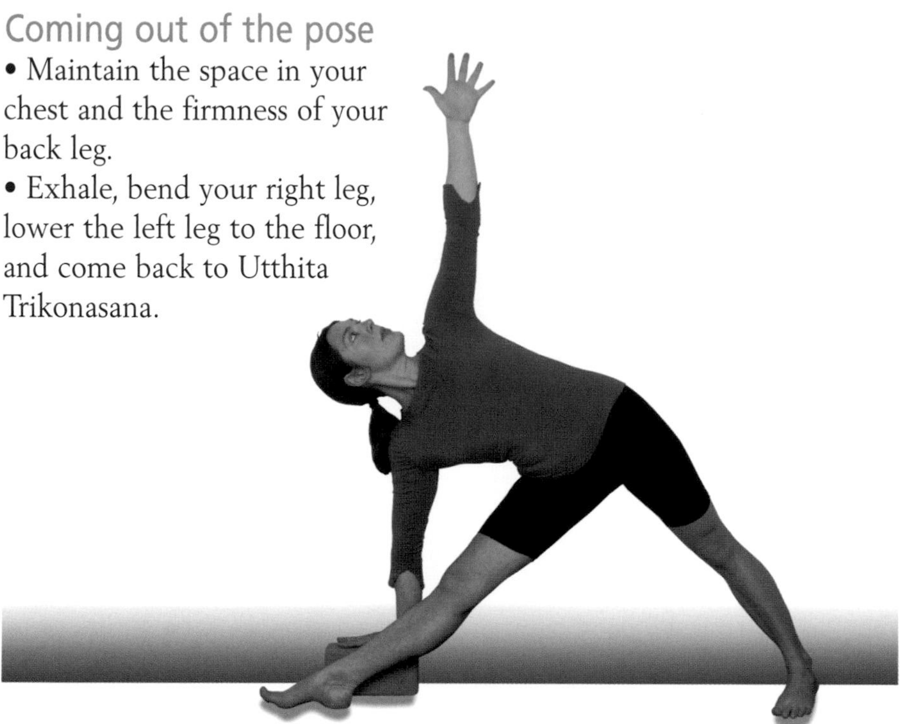

Benefits

Provides space in the uterus and freedom to breathe through vertical and horizontal expansion and extension

Regulates blood pressure

Maintains proper kidney function, thus preventing water retention, kidney inflammation, and back pain

Tucks the tailbone in, distributing your weight evenly. This gives relief to the lowered uterus during the latter stage of pregnancy, bringing freedom to the uterine and vaginal opening and easing delivery. (To avoid pain, women often stand with the tailbone protruding, which actually increases pain and other problems.)

Contraindications

Toxemia

CHECK YOURSELF

> *Keep your right leg perpendicular and your left leg slightly raised, extend the toes of your left foot, and synchronize the action of raising the left leg and straightening the right leg.*

> *Tuck your shoulder blades in and expand your chest.*

> *The back of your left leg, the back of your torso, and the back of your head should be in line.*

> *The weight of your body remains on your right thigh and hip.*

> *The left side of your torso should face the ceiling.*

> *Widen your pelvis by turning your left pelvic bone up.*

> *Tuck in your tailbone.*

> *Create a good space between your right thigh and right arm for the right side of your pelvis to open; it should not be compressed.*

> *Tuck your buttock bones in.*

> *Keep your left leg in line with the pelvic bone or even slightly higher, so that the uterus does not get compressed. If the leg is lower than pelvic level, the abdomen gets pulled, causing pain. Extend the lifted leg and elongate it towards the foot. It should not gravitate downward.*

> *Your spine should not be in a slanted position or gravitate downward.*

> *Your armpit and groin should be in line.*

> *Straighten up your top hand in order to lessen the heaviness in your chest and breast. Better yet, hold on to a trestle, as shown here, or something similar, with the raised hand.*

Help and Variations

- To lessen fatigue, you can come back to Tadasana after you have done the asana on one side, and then restart it on the other side.
- For safe balance, always use the support of a wall or a trestle.

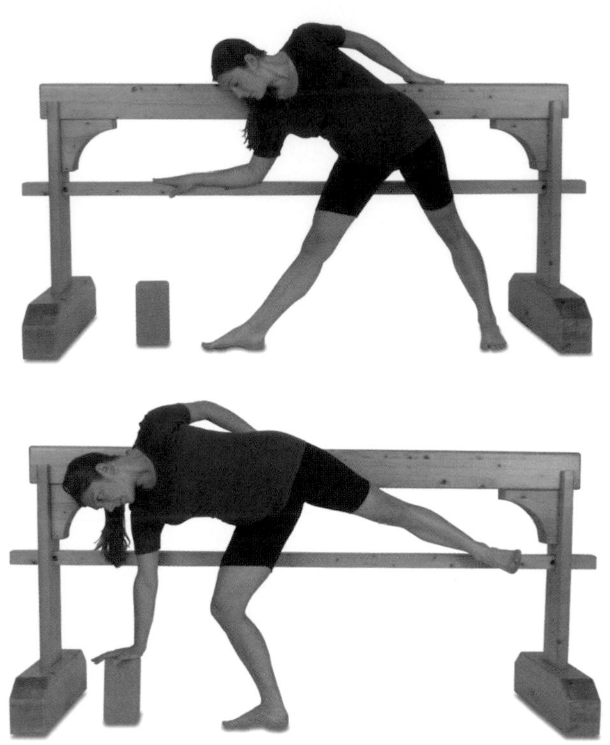

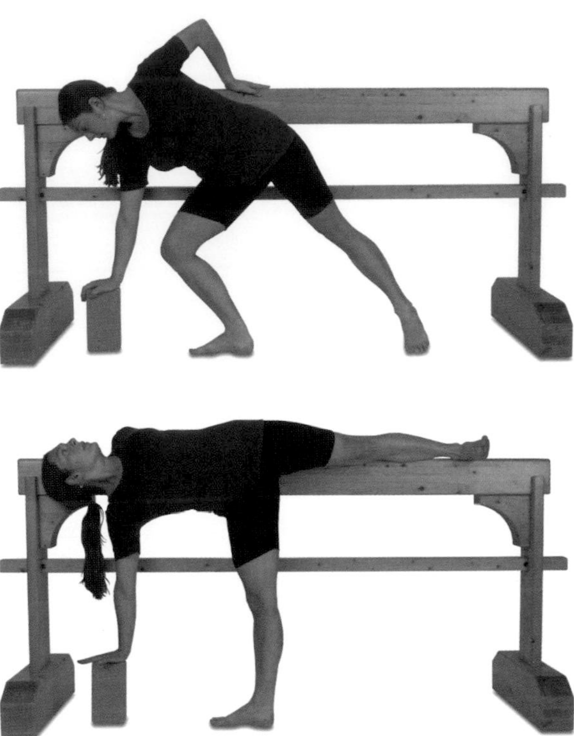

- You can also use the wall and a chair as shown in the photos.
- If you are overweight or find it difficult to do Utthita Trikonasana, you can synchronize the placing of the hand and the lifting of the leg only.

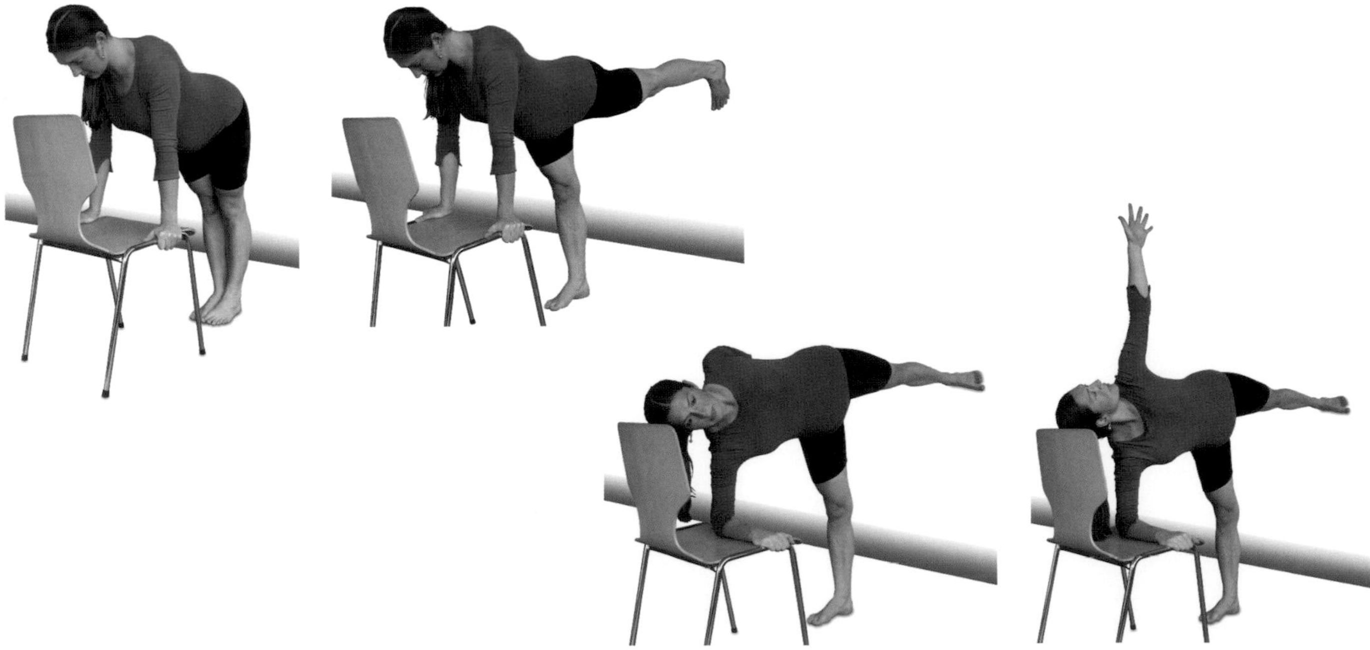

Parshvottanasana

Intense chest stretch pose

It is essential for a pregnant woman to keep the pelvis joints free and moving. A broadened pelvis and free hip joint help you have an easier delivery. This asana broadens and expands the pelvic and abdominal regions, to give you lightness and freedom.

Parshva means "side" or "flank," and *uttana* means "an intense stretch." This pose stretches the sides of the chest.

1 Stand in Tadasana (page 32).

2 Start with Pashchima Namaskarasana: join your palms behind your back, fingers pointing down towards your waist. Turn your wrists and palms inward and bring both the palms up above the middle of your back.

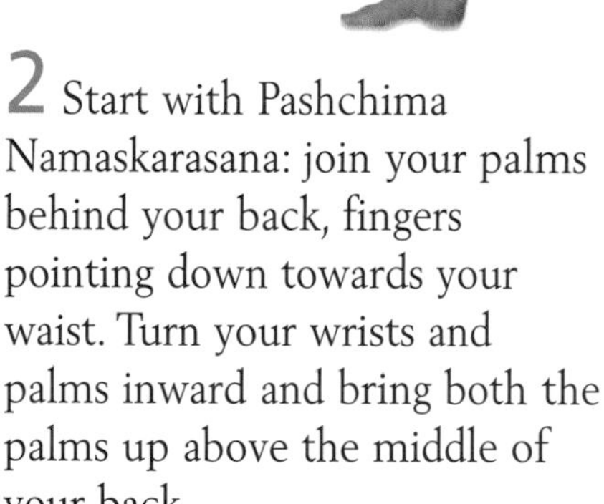

3 Keep your fingers in line with your shoulder blades and pointing upward.

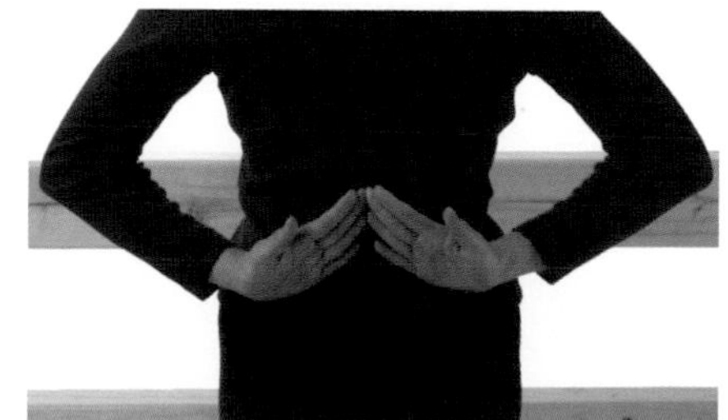

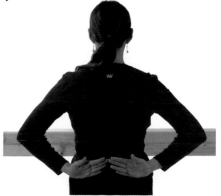

1st trimester: yes (with support)
2nd trimester: yes
3rd trimester: yes

Benefits

- Strengthens the abdominal muscles
- Eliminates lower back pain
- Softens the diaphragm and expands the chest cavity
- Removes body stiffness
- Frees the abdomen from heaviness
- Eases morning sickness
- Keeps the pelvic joints free and moving
- Broadens the pelvic and abdominal regions
- Gives lightness and freedom
- Makes delivery easier
- Brings down high blood pressure
- Can be practiced throughout pregnancy

Contraindications

See "Help and Variations" on page 51

Hint: To lessen fatigue, you can come back to Tadasana after you have done the asana on one side and then restart it on the other side.

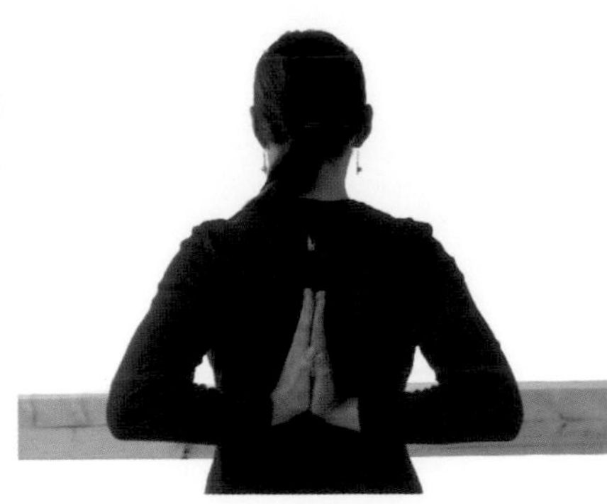

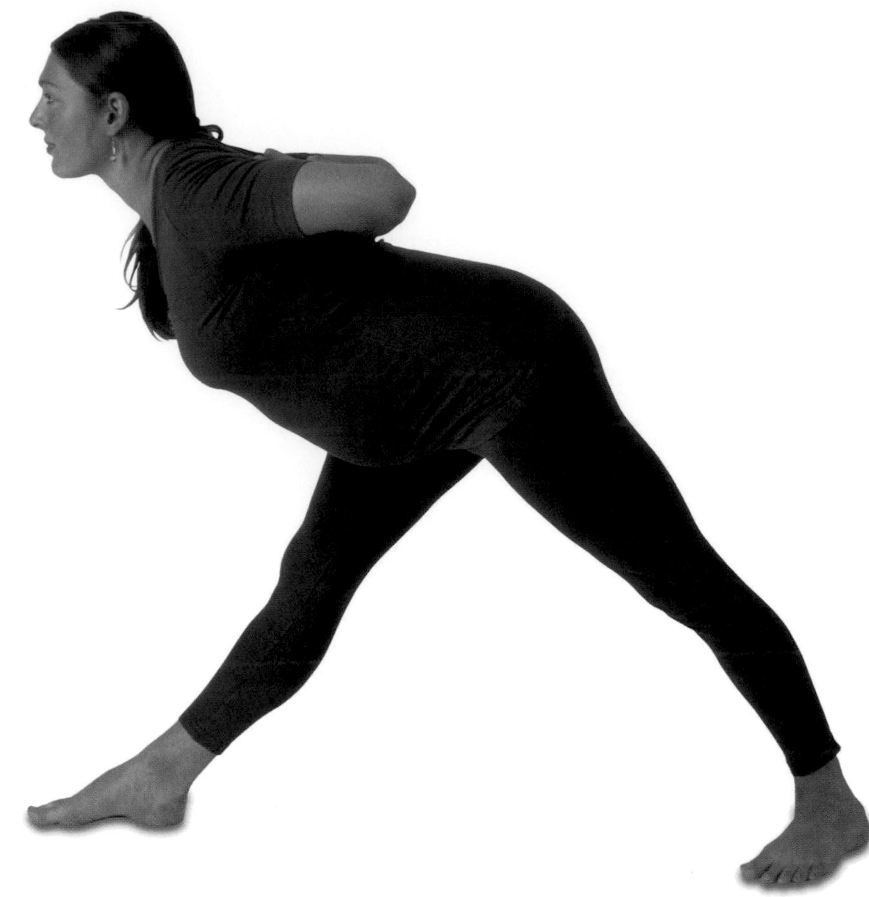

4 Press your palms against each other and move your elbows backward so that your chest is not constricted. Expand your chest and raise your breastbone.

5 While inhaling, spread your legs 3 to 3½ feet apart. Remain in this position for a while, breathing normally.

6 Turn your right leg 90° out to the right and the left leg inward. Simultaneously, turn your torso to the right.

7 Don't extend your head backward (like a nonpregnant woman would do).

8 Instead, raise your pelvis and extend and expand your chest. Stay in this position for 10 to 15 seconds.

9 When you bend your torso to your right leg, your torso should remain parallel to the floor so that there is no pressure on the abdomen.

10 Your spine, from the tailbone towards the cervical area, should extend towards your head. Don't attempt to touch your knee.

11 Stay in this final position for 20 to 30 seconds, breathing normally.

12 Maintaining the broadness of your pelvis and chest, come up, repeat to the left side, and come back to Tadasana.

CHECK YOURSELF

> *Keep the center of your torso over the center of your thigh.*

> *Tighten your legs and extend your spine towards your head.*

> *Keep both pelvic bones parallel.*

> *Keep your chest expanded; don't cave it in.*

> *Rotate the left side of your abdomen to the right so that it is parallel to the floor.*

> *Make sure that your abdomen is not compressed against your thigh. As your pregnancy progresses, it will limit how far you can lower your torso.*

Help and Variations

- You can split the asana into two parts, as follows:
  - First part: hands and arms only
  - Second part: hands, arms, and legs

- If you can't perform this asana with your hands folded behind your back, you can grip your elbows instead.

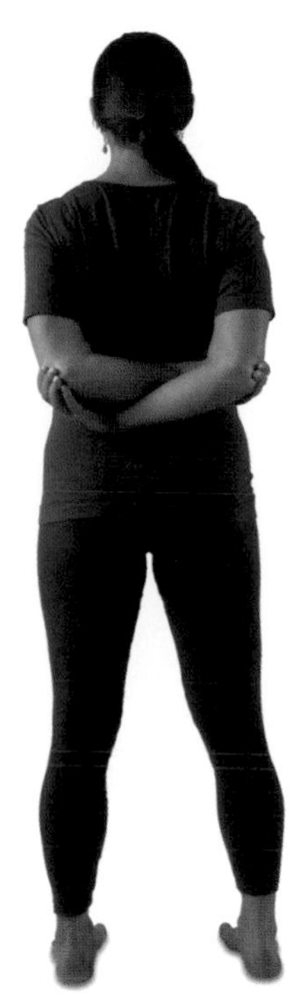
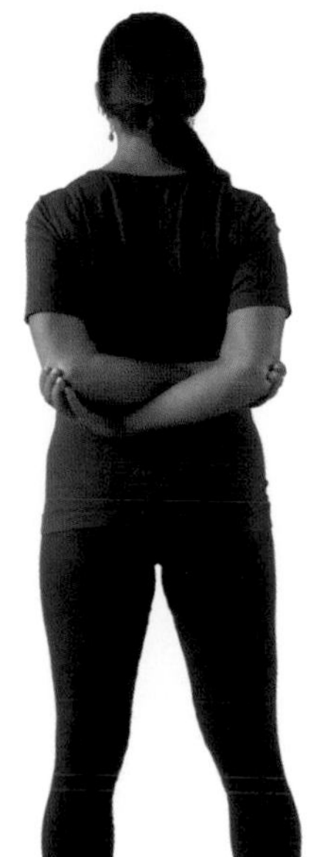

- If you're having trouble balancing, you can rest your palms or your fingers on either side of your foot at the height of two blocks.

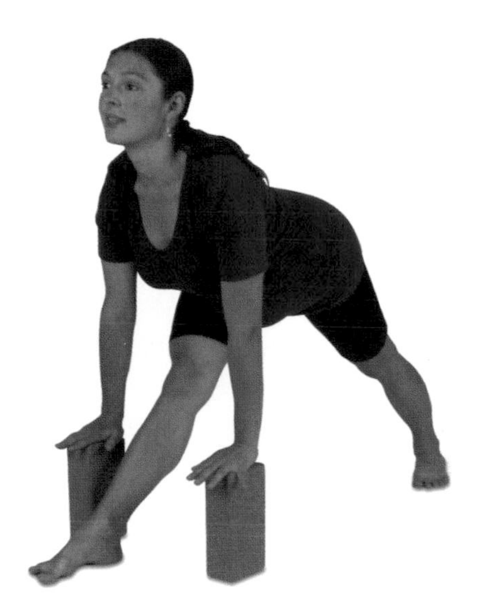

- For more weight on the back foot, you can put the sole of your front foot on a quarter-round block.

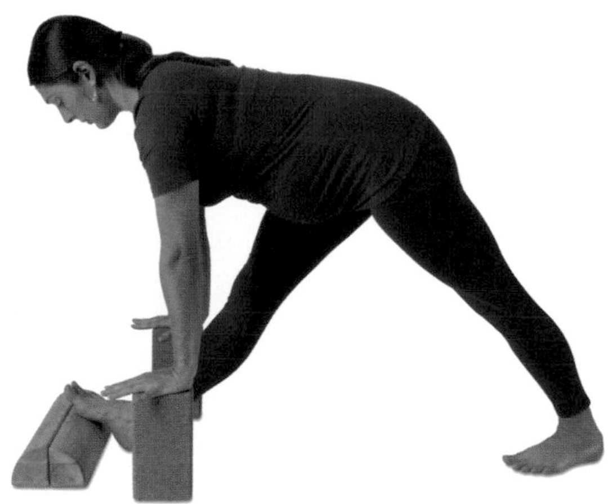

- For a good elongation of your sides, stretch your arms over the back of a chair.

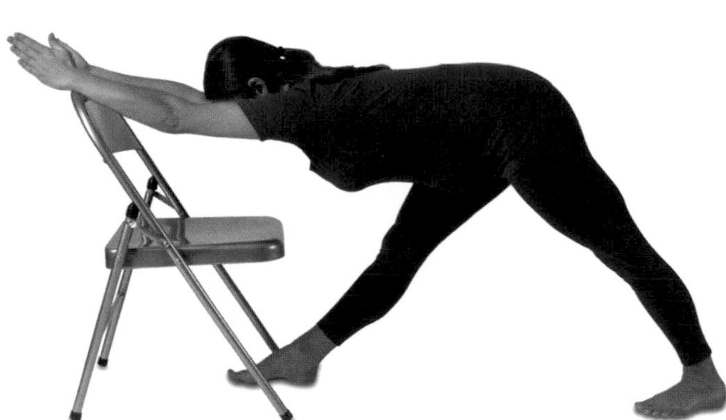

Virabhadrasana 1 and 3: Strength and Balance

Virabhadrasana 1
Warrior pose 1

This pose is named after Virabhadra, a warrior; the asanas give a sense of balance and bring firmness.

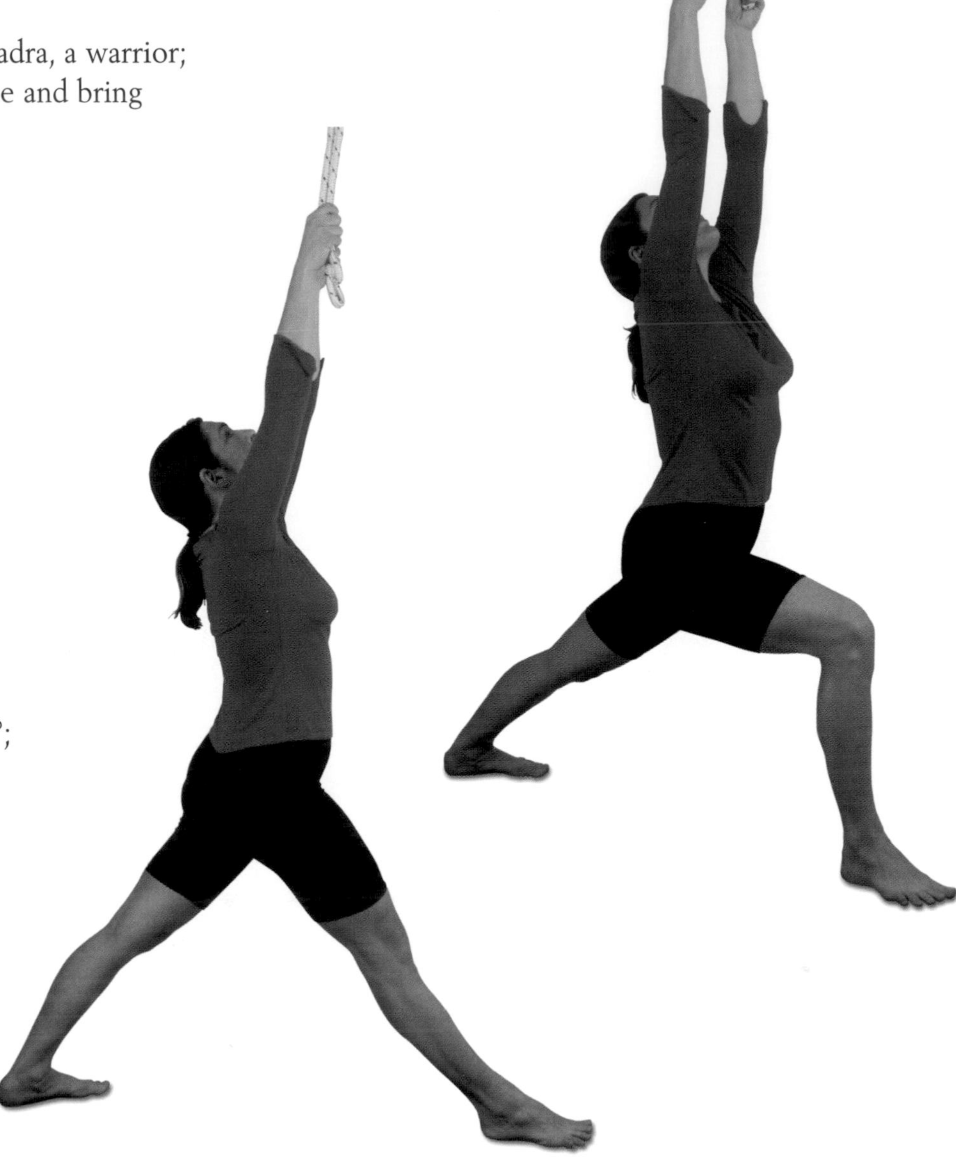

1 Stand in Tadasana (page 32) and grip the ceiling ropes or the doorframe above you.

2 Exhale and put your right foot forward and your left leg back.

3 Grip the rope or the doorframe firmly, exhale, and bend your right leg.

4 As a pregnant woman, don't try to bend your front leg to 90°; it's better to keep the thigh slightly up. This ensures that your abdomen is not pressed against your thigh.

5 Extend your back leg backward.

6 Instead of looking up, you may keep your head straight.

7 Stretch your spine upward towards your head to avoid pressure on the uterus.

CHECK YOURSELF

> *Keep your left leg firm and straight while bending your right leg.*
> *Grip the ceiling ropes and stretch your arms. When you're pregnant and you stretch your arms up, your floating ribs (two lower ribs on either side) unlock and lift, which prevents pressure on the abdomen.*
> *Keep your hands, head, and anus in line with each other.*
> *It is important to keep your spine in a healthy state throughout the pregnancy. To firm up the spine, both pelvic bones should be balanced: parallel, facing forward, and not tilting to the side.*

8 This is the final position. Breathe normally and stay for 10 seconds.

9 Maintaining the space in your spine and torso, inhale, come back, close your feet, and repeat to the left side.

10 Come back to Tadasana.

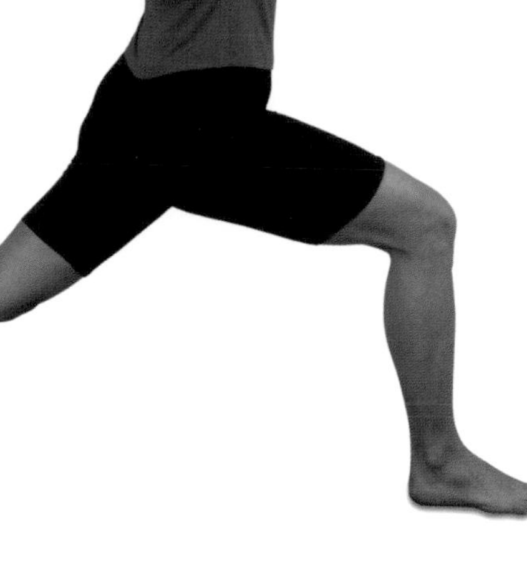

1st trimester: no
2nd trimester: yes
3rd trimester: yes

Benefits

- Gives a sense of balance and firmness
- Reduces the intensity of morning sickness (should not be performed, however, while you have morning sickness)
- Helps massage the liver and the spleen, which improves digestion
- Relieves heaviness in the abdomen
- Alleviates tailbone pain
- Relieves flatulence
- Flushes the kidneys; in the later stages of pregnancy, helps relieve the feeling of being knotted up inside

Help

For stability and balance:

- Practice the asanas with your fingers against the wall and the sole of your front foot supported.
- Practice with the trestle, or a table, for total lift and stability.

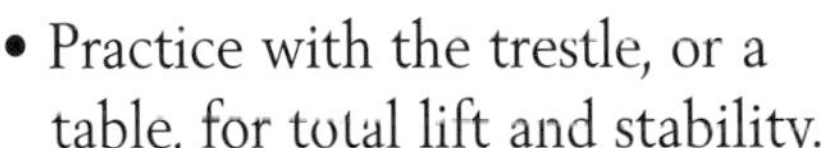

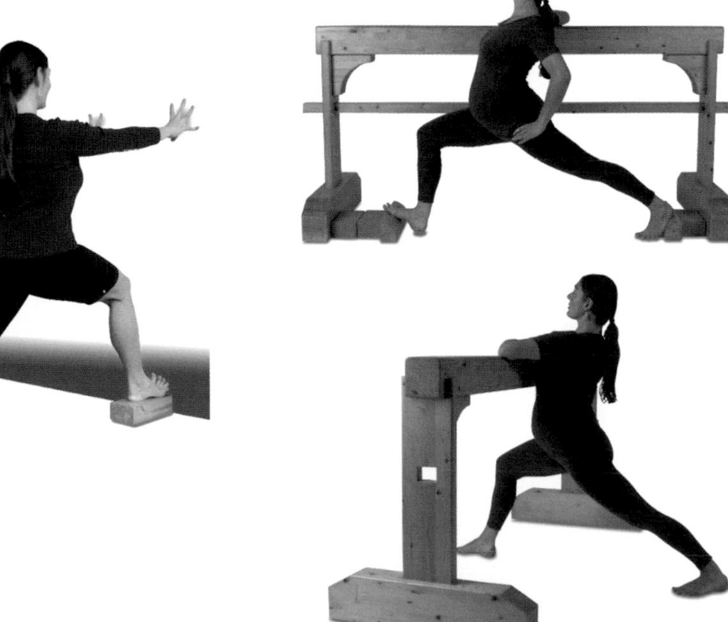

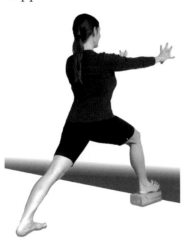

Contraindications

- High blood pressure
- Swelling in the legs
- Tendency to miscarriage
- Vaginal discharge
- Persistent vomiting
- Avoid the asanas in the last two months if your abdomen is getting too heavy and you feel discomfort.

Virabhadrasana 3
Warrior pose 3

1st trimester: no
2nd trimester: yes
3rd trimester: yes

With full support for arms and lifted leg, this asana develops poise and balance, strengthens the legs, and tones the abdominal organs.

Benefits
Tones the spine
Relieves backache and hip problems
Tones the muscles around the tailbone
Rests the heart

Preparation:
Have a table or other raised surface where you can stretch your arms, and the back of a chair or something similar for the lifted foot.

1 Stand in Tadasana (page 32) and lift your arms to Urdhva Hastasana (page 35).

2 Bend forward to Ardha Uttanasana (page 60).

3 Put your arms on a trestle or table and stretch them forward.

4 Bend your legs and stretch your left leg backward, rest your foot or shin on the support behind you, and straighten your front leg.

5 Keep your right leg firm and steady and pull in the kneecap.

6 Stretch your left leg backward and your torso forward.

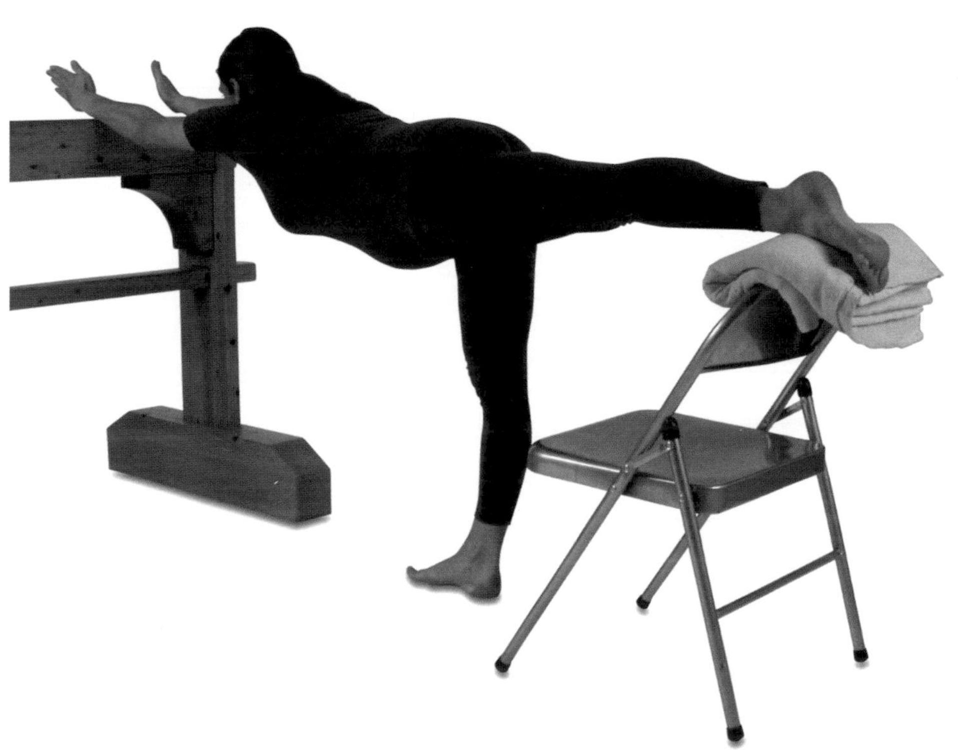

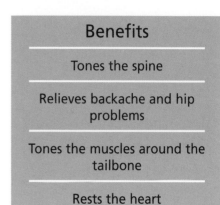

7 The center of gravity is in your right leg; extend the sides of your torso forward towards your arms.

8 Keep your pelvis bones parallel to the floor.

9 Breathing normally, maintain 10 – 15 seconds, put your left leg down, and repeat on the left side.

10 Maintaining the firmness and extensions of the sides of the torso, come back with an inhalation. Stand in Tadasana or rest in Ardha Uttanasana.

Prasarita Padottanasana
Expanded leg intense stretch pose

Many pregnant women complain of back pain and a feeling of "tightness" causing discomfort and heaviness. Their joints feel heavy and inflexible. Prasarita Padottanasana, which answers these complaints, is an ideal asana for both pregnancy and menstruation.

Prasarita means "extended" or "expanded," and *pada* means "foot" or "leg." This pose provides an intense stretch of the legs and spine, and prepares the body and mind for the leg work in the standing asanas. It teaches grounding and the coordination of different stretching directions.

It also teaches the opening of the inner space, and the surrender to wideness, deep breathing, and relaxation of the senses and the brain. As you can imagine, its positive effects are equally comprehensive.

Step 1

1 Start in Tadasana, the mountain pose, feet hip-width apart.

2 Turn your inner arms and your hands out to lift and widen the chest.

3 Keeping your chest lifted, turn your hands in.

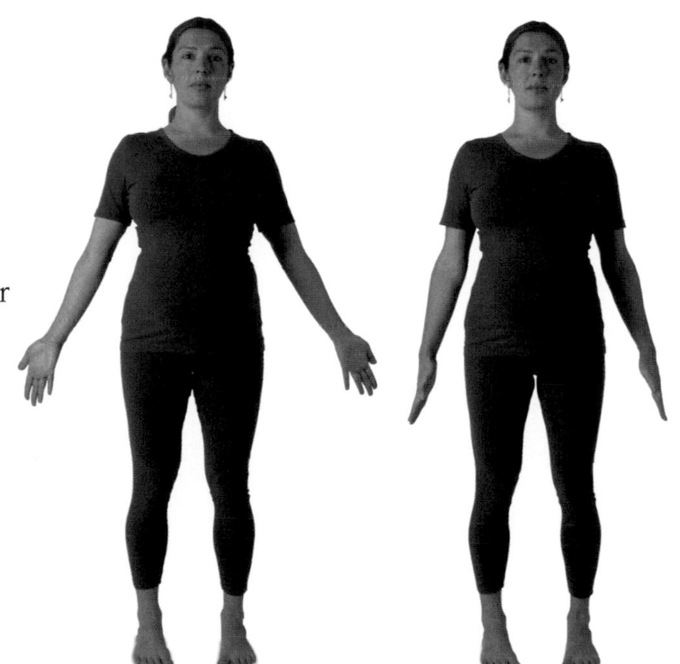

1st trimester: yes, with concave back
2nd trimester: yes
3rd trimester: yes

Benefits

- Develops and strengthens the ligaments and muscles of the feet, knees, legs, and hips
- Stretches and widens the pelvic region
- Lifts all the organs of the torso and keeps them in place
- Improves breathing and rests the heart
- Reduces high blood pressure
- Increases blood circulation and improves digestion
- Reduces pressure and heaviness in the pelvic and abdominal regions caused by prolonged standing or sitting
- Gives more flexibility to the lower spine
- Soothes the nervous system
- Relieves morning sickness and nausea
- Especially when your forehead is resting on the seat of a chair, lessens nausea, relaxes the head, and eases breathing

Contraindications

- Symptoms of toxemia
- Exhaustion

4 Spread your legs 4 to 4½ feet apart. Don't jump!

5 Keep the outer sides of your feet parallel, spread your soles well, and spread your toes and stretch them forward.

6 Be firm in the outer part of your feet and your entire heel with its inner and outer rim. Broaden the balls of your big and little toes and place them on the floor.

7 Lift your kneecaps and pull their center deep into your knees.

8 Bring your shinbones and upper thighs back.

9 Move your tailbone down and in.

10 Lift the skin of your abdomen, navel, and breastbone.

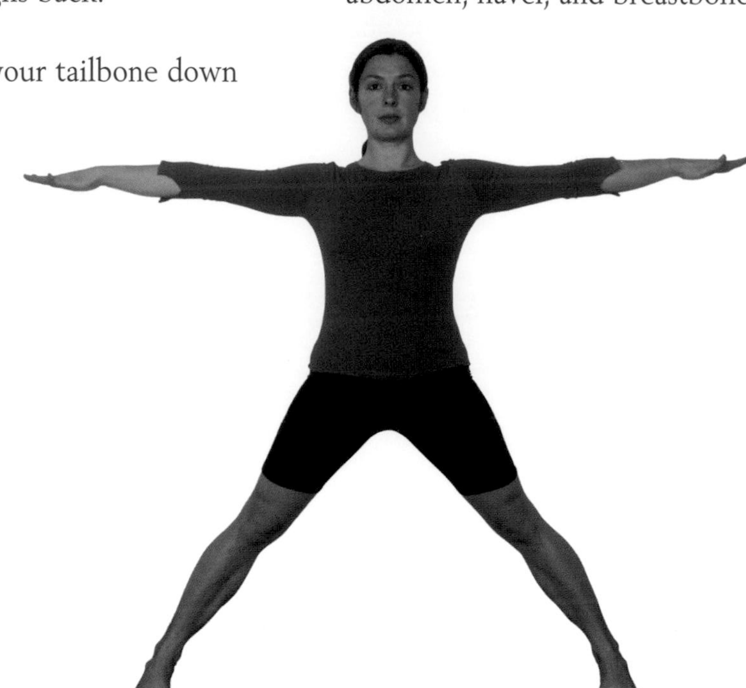

◇

Step 2

1 Bend forward and stretch your shins, knees, and upper thighs backward. From the resistance of your legs, stretch your whole spine forward and place your hands on blocks on the floor below your shoulders.

2 Keep your buttock bones and heels in line. Continue to stretch your whole spine forward together with your navel, chest, and armpits.

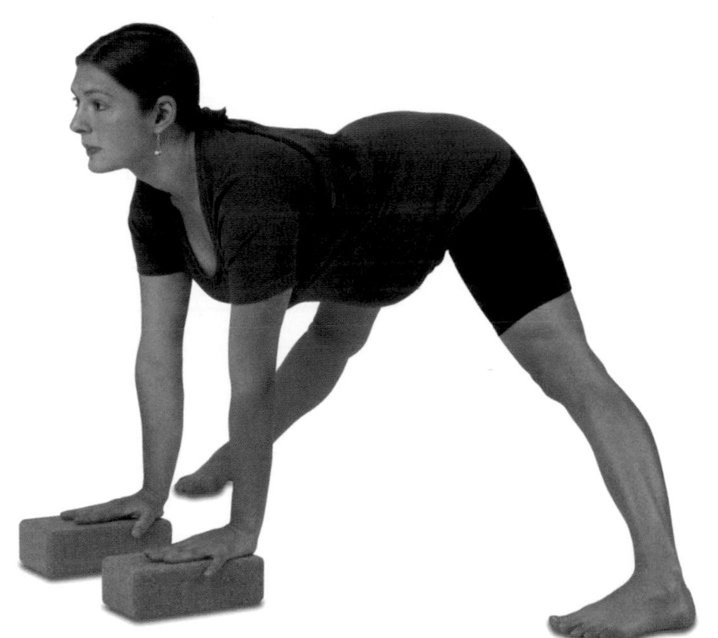

3 Widen your collarbone, move your shoulders away from your ears, elongate your neck and its sides, and lift your chin away from your chest.

4 Move your buttock bones up and away from each other as much as possible, so as to pull in the sacrum (bone plate between spine and tailbone). Maintain the length of the sides of your torso and abdominal wall.

5 Stay in the pose for 30 to 60 seconds; if you feel comfortable, you can keep up the good work even longer. If your concentration is lessening, then come out earlier.

Help

- You can practice Prasarita Padottanasana as a substitute for Salamba Shirshasana (page 97) if you feel too exhausted or have problems with your cervical (upper) spine or eyes.
- If the fetus is causing pressure on the pelvic floor and it's difficult to lift your abdomen, you should practice with your outer feet against blocks and your hands on blocks or a chair.

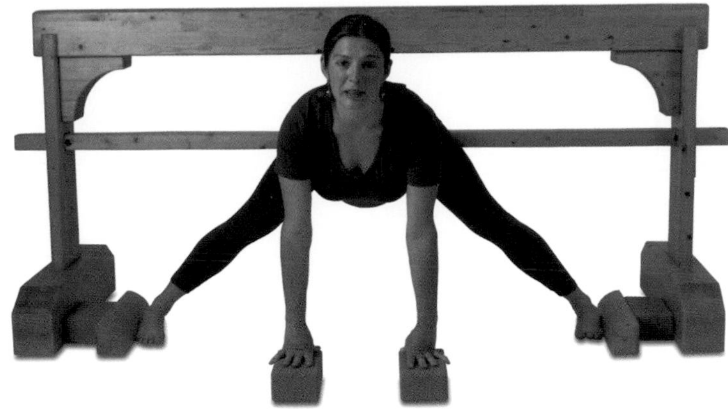

Use a trestle or a table

CHECK YOURSELF

> *Maintain the rooting of the balls of your thumbs, your index fingers, and your feet.*
>
> *Intensify the work in your legs by stretching your front thighs back and lifting your inner legs. This lifts the groin and the buttock bones away from your inner legs and allows your entire spine to stretch away from the pelvis, parallel to the floor.*
>
> *Breathe evenly.*

Coming out of the pose

1 Don't jump out of the pose; walk your feet together.

2 Inhale and lift your torso.

3 Close your feet to hip-width in Tadasana.

4 Feel the wideness of your pelvis, the grounding of your feet, and the vitality and length of your inner legs. Enjoy the deeper breathing and the peace of mind.

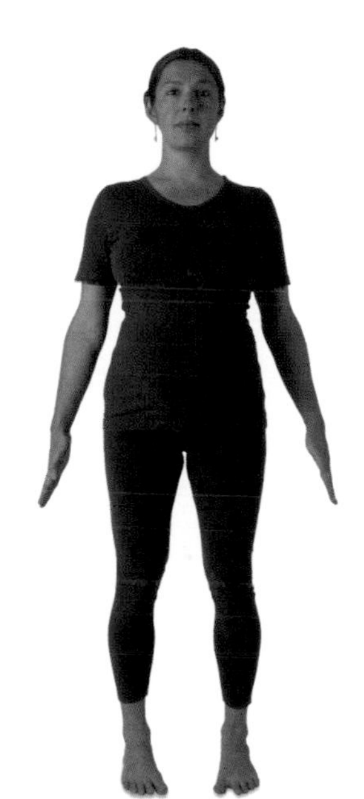

Special Instructions

Horizontal Stretch

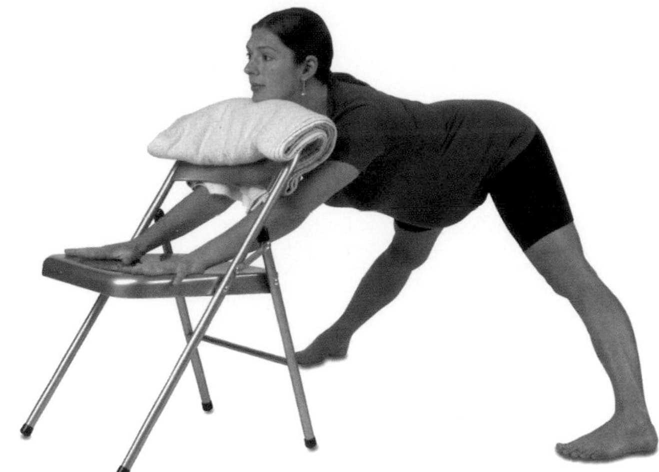

- During pregnancy, you should stretch your spine with a concave back. This helps to loosen stiff elbow and knee joints.
- Stretch your spine parallel to the floor to relieve back pain and joint pain.
- The horizontal stretch allows your heart to rest.
- In the original asana, the spine and head are stretched vertically down to the floor. While pregnant, you should stretch your spine only horizontally, that is, with a concave back, so that your torso is concave from the hips to the neck. Your abdominal area and waistline stretch towards your head. This gives good support for the baby.

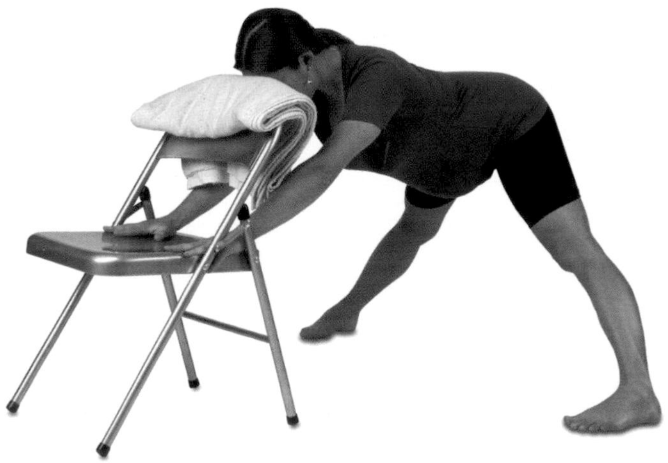

Using a Chair

- If your back is stiff, using a chair gets you deeper into the pose and allows you to stay in it longer. It also helps you stretch your spine parallel to the floor.
- Step 1 with concave back and chin on the back of the chair.
- Step 2 with forehead resting on the backrest or seat of the chair.
  Especially when your head is resting on the seat of a chair, this asana lessens nausea, relaxes the head, and eases breathing.

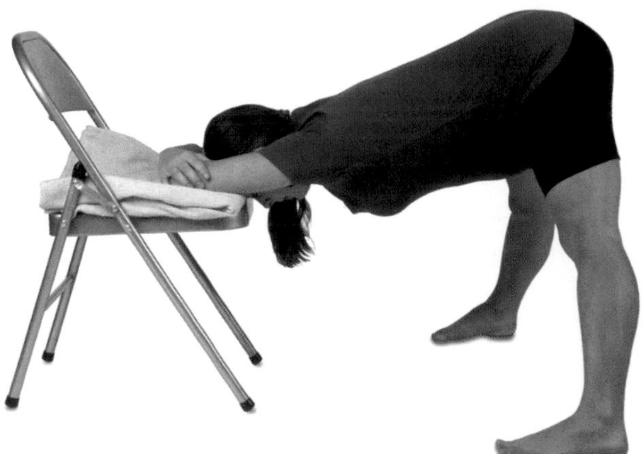

Practice with a chair as described above if you have:

- High blood pressure
- Stiffness in the 2nd and 3rd trimesters of pregnancy
- Heavy menstrual bleeding
- Exhaustion
- Severe headache

Ardha Uttanasana
Half intense forward stretch pose

1st trimester: yes
2nd trimester: yes
3rd trimester: yes

Ardha (half) Uttanasana is the last of the asanas in the chain to be performed before Salamba Shirshasana, and the first asana to be performed after it.

In the original asana, the body is doubled up. But when you're pregnant and have to be careful not to compress your abdomen, you'll perform it only up to the intermediate stage of your pregnancy, and afterwards in a modified form.

In advanced pregnancy, it is difficult to keep your feet together, since your abdomen is pressing on the pubic plate. In addition, bending down too much and pressing your uterus against your thighs pushes the baby up. This might cause a turning of the baby, which is certainly to be avoided.

For these reasons, the asana should be performed with your legs apart and your hands on a raised support, ensuring that there is no pressure on the abdomen.

Benefits

The benefits below refer to all the variations of Ardha Uttanasana

- Alleviates depression
- Calms the mind
- Relieves stomach pain
- Strengthens the abdominal organs
- Helps the free flow of digestive juices
- Creates space for the fetus to grow and extend its limbs
- Lengthens and straightens the back of the cervix and the vagina, increasing blood circulation in that area
- Restores normal blood pressure
- Soothes lower back pain

◇

Modified Technique

1 Stand in Tadasana (page 32) and spread your legs 1 to 1½ feet apart, with the outer sides of your feet parallel.

2 Inhale, stretch your arms to Urdhva Baddanguliyasana in Tadasana (page 34) and then to Urdhva Hastasana (page 35).

3 Exhale, extend your spine, and bend your torso forward.

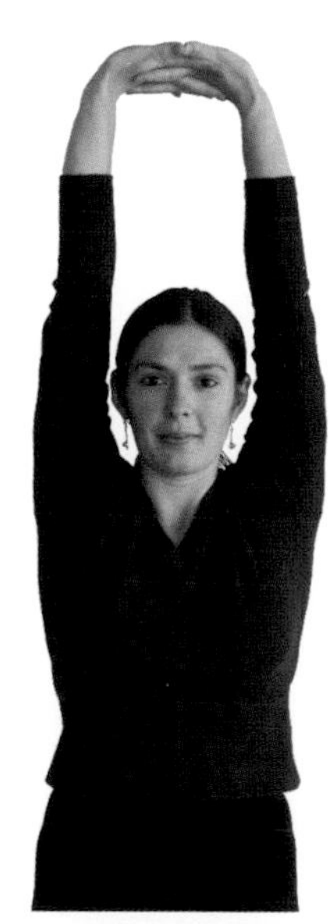

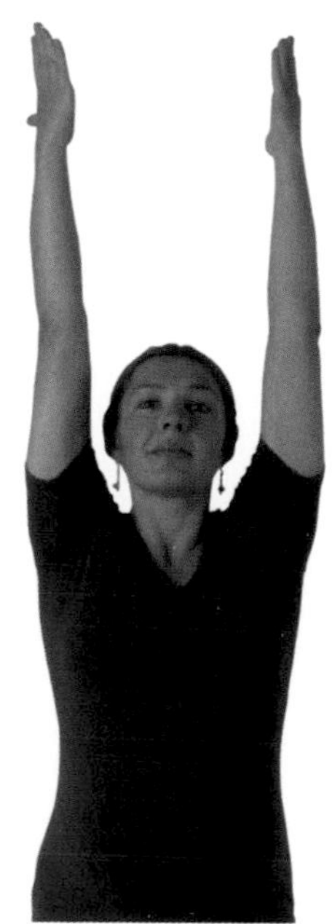

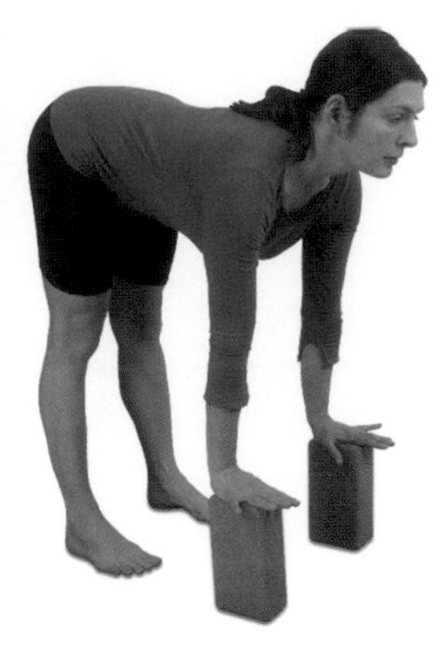

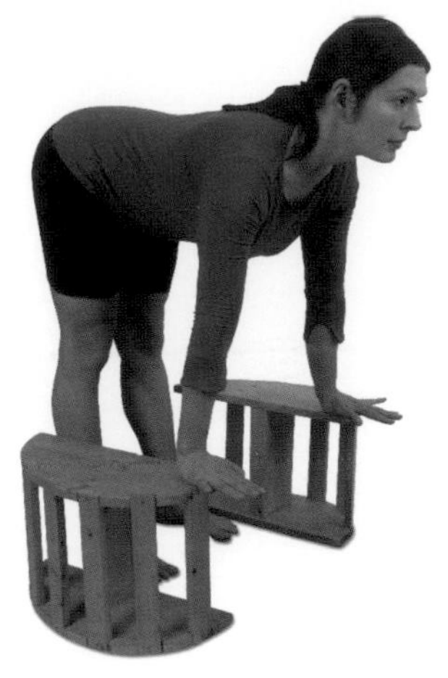

4 From the 3rd to 5th month: Rest your palms on a raised surface, such as two blocks.

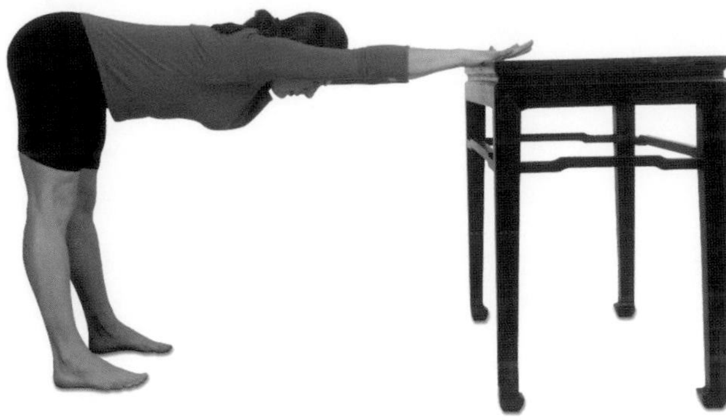

5 From 5th to 7th month: Extend your arms against a table or trestle.

6 In the 7th and 8th months: Keep your folded arms supported by a raised surface like a stool, table, or trestle.

a back concave

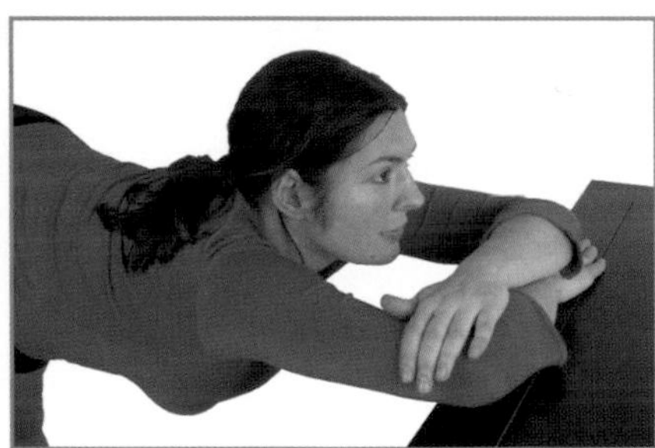

b head in line with the spine

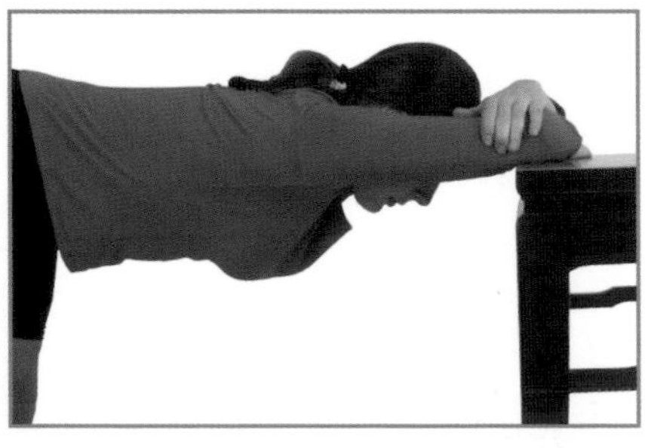

7 Up to the last month: Bend your elbows, extend your lower arms, and bring the crown of your head against the support. When your arms are anchored on the stool, table, or platform, your torso gets extended from the legs to the arms, which should bring you tremendous relief. Put a belt around your elbows to keep them in.

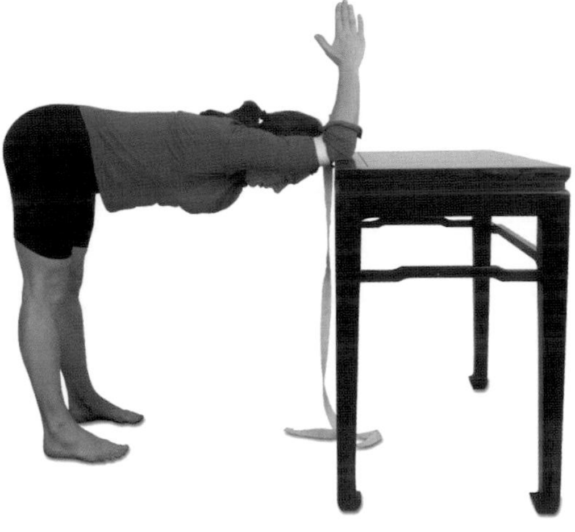

8 Stay in this pose for 30 to 60 seconds, breathing normally.

9 Maintaining the space you've created, place your hands properly so they can give support, walk in, inhale, and come up.

Ardha Uttanasana, with Ropes and Chair

For working in the concave position, hands on a chair.

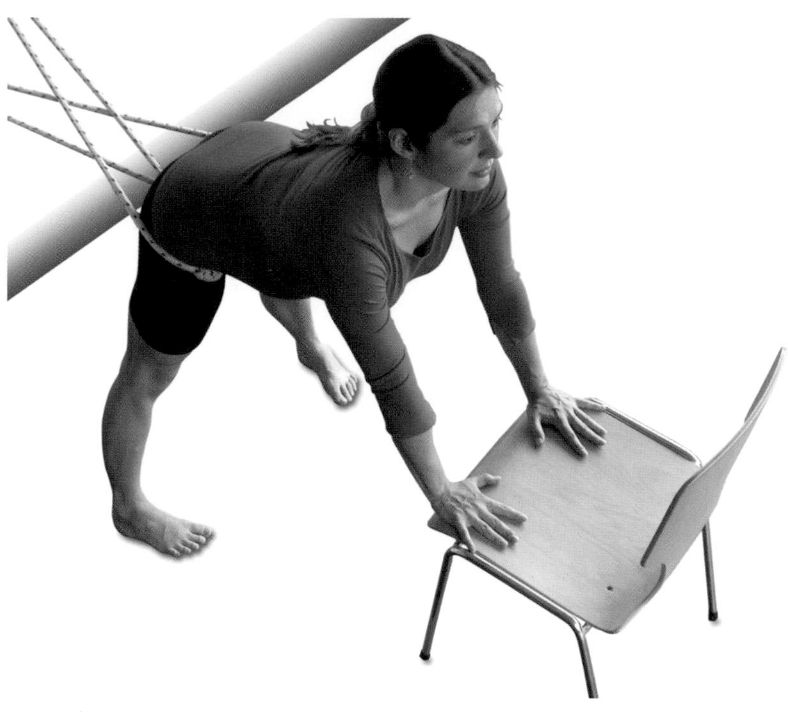

For more extension: stretch your hands over the back of the chair.

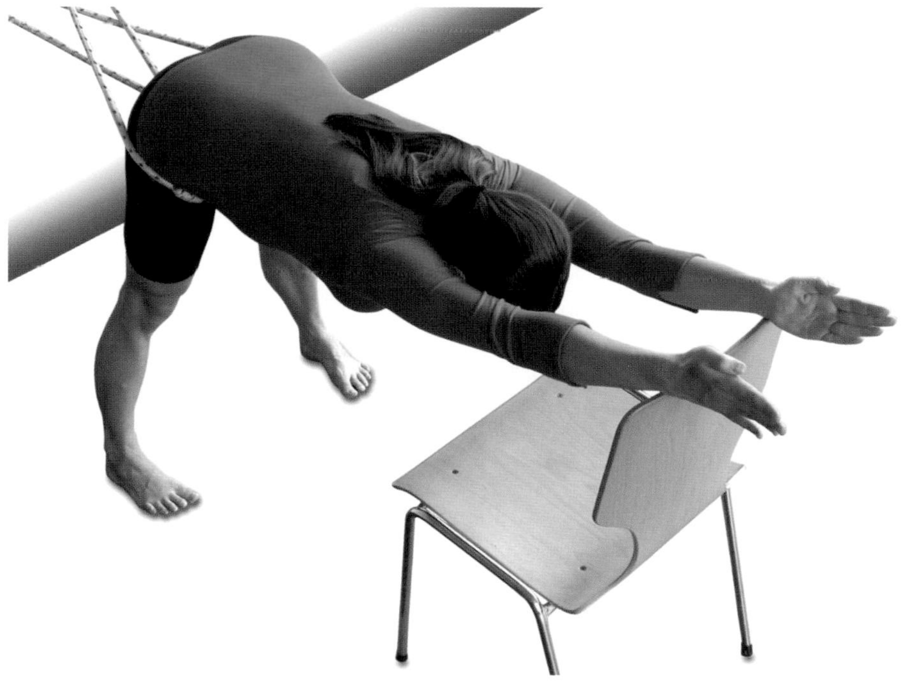

CHECK YOURSELF

- > *Extend your dorsal and lumbar (mid and lower) spine.*
- > *Open your chest.*
- > *Turn your toes in and heels out to reduce abdominal pressure.*
- > *Extend your lower ribs.*
- > *Don't bend your knees; pull your kneecaps and front thigh muscles up.*

Adho Mukha Shvanasana

Downward-facing dog pose

This asana is the second in the chain of asanas to be performed before Salamba Shirshasana, coming after Maha Mudra. It is important in the chain because it is designed to do away with fatigue.

Adho means "downward," *mukha* means "face," and *shvana* means "dog." This asana resembles a dog stretching with its head down.

1 Stand in Tadasana (page 32).

2 Exhale and come down to Uttanasana (page 213).

3 Place your palms on the blocks for support.

4 Bend your knees and place your legs 4 to 4½ feet back, one by one; you can do so by walking a few steps back. Spread your palms and extend your fingers. Keep your feet parallel and extend your toes.

As your pregnancy advances, keep your feet farther apart. Here they are kept mat-width apart, with the side of the little toe touching the edges of the mat.

5 Stretch your thighs backward and pull your kneecaps in, place your heels on the floor, and take one or two breaths.

6 Exhale, stretch your arms and legs, and push your thighs back. Move your torso towards your legs.

7 Press your heels into the floor and place your forehead on the bolster. (Do not force your head to reach the bolster; rather, increase the height of the bolster until your head reaches it easily.)

8 Remain in this final position for 15 to 20 seconds, breathing normally.

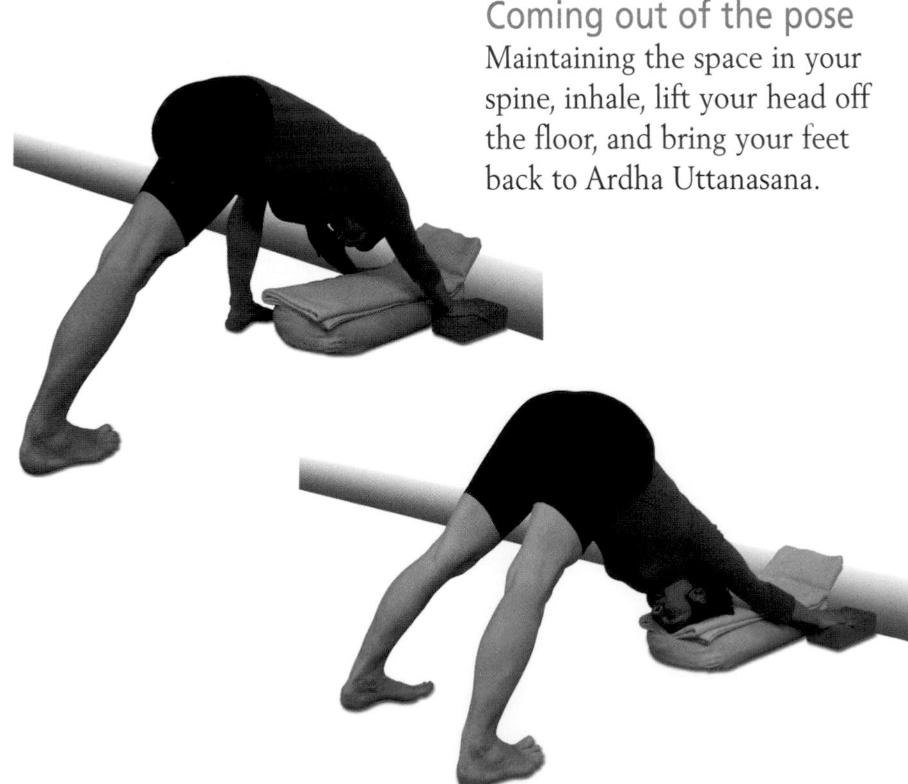

CHECK YOURSELF

> *Don't bend your knees.*
> *Tuck your shoulder blades in and broaden your chest.*
> *Lock your elbows.*
> *Creating resistance, extend your index fingers and thumbs.*
> *Keep your outer feet parallel.*
> *Keep your inner ankles lifted.*
> *Stretch your inner thighs and knees back.*
> *Relax your diaphragm and throat.*

Coming out of the pose

Maintaining the space in your spine, inhale, lift your head off the floor, and bring your feet back to Ardha Uttanasana.

Using other Props

1 Take an even higher support for your hands, like a chair or bench.

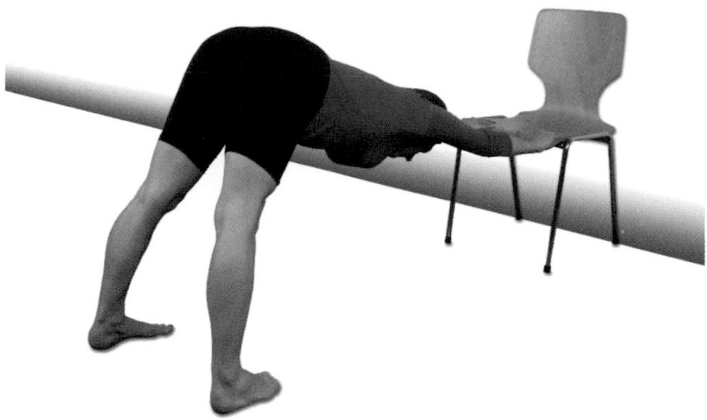

- Put your hands on the support and walk back.
- Come back to Uttanasana.

2 Practice Adho Mukha Shvanasana with wall ropes, support for your head, and a slanted plank for your heels.

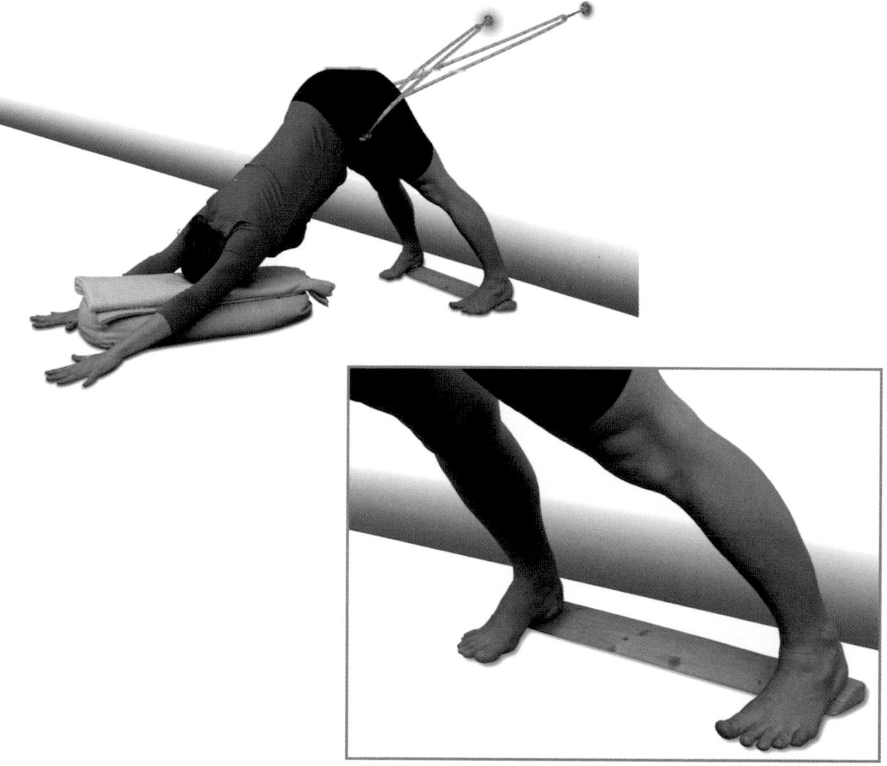

1st trimester: yes
2nd trimester: yes
3rd trimester: yes

Benefits

With your head resting on a support, brings a calm feeling, lowers blood pressure, and relieves headaches

Brings about a feeling of exhilaration

Increases blood supply to the brain

Eliminates shortness of breath, extreme fatigue, and palpitations

Restores normal blood pressure and heartbeat

Lightens and softens the diaphragm, and enlarges the chest cavity

Tones the nervous system and counteracts forgetfulness, moodiness, and depression

Strengthens the spinal muscles and extends the spine

Removes pain from the lower back at the tailbone

Brings freedom of the floating ribs (two lower ribs on either side) and opens intercostal muscles

Lessens swelling in the legs and ankles

Prepares you for Shirshasana by relieving heaviness of the head and stopping the onrush of blood to it

Sitting Asanas
Upavishtha Sthiti

Dandasana
Staff pose

Danda means "stick." This asana resembles a stick or a staff. Just as Tadasana is the basic pose for the standing asanas, Dandasana is the basic pose for all the sitting asanas.

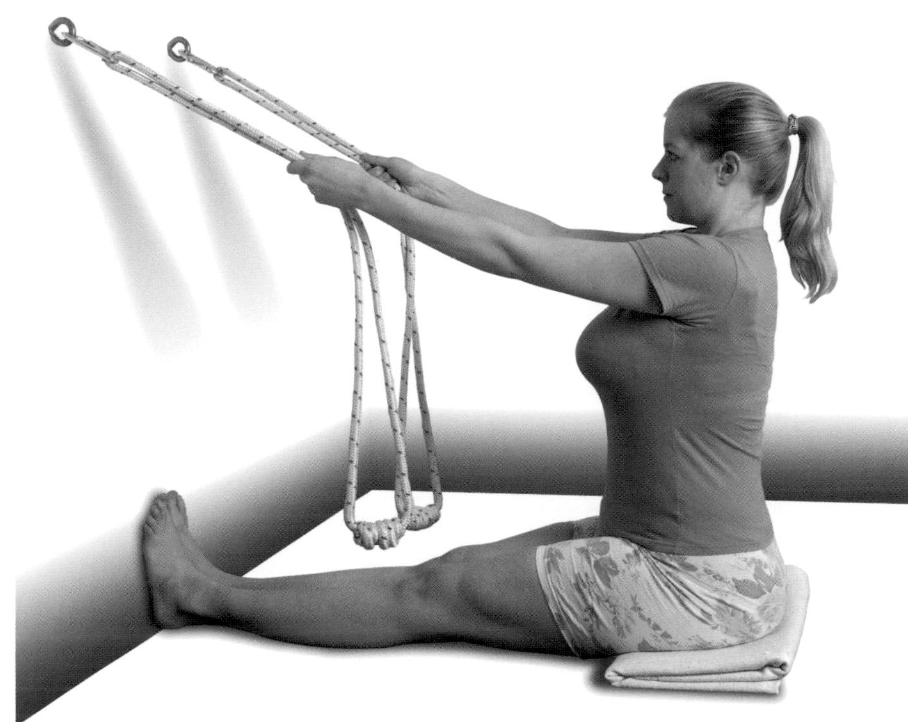

1 Sit on a folded blanket 3 to 4 inches thick (or a bolster), with your buttocks higher than your feet.

2 Sit up straight with your legs extended forward.

1st trimester: Keep your thighs, knees, ankles, and toes together.

2nd and 3rd trimesters: Place your feet 1 to 1½ feet apart to allow space for your abdomen and lessen pressure on the pubic bone.

3 Extend your toes towards the ceiling.

4 Keep your palms on the floor by the sides of your hips, with your fingers pointing forward.

5 Keep your chest up and your head and neck erect and look straight ahead.

Contraindications and Help

- If you have weak back muscles or heart problems, you should sit with your back against the wall or as shown here, with your feet against the wall, using the wall ropes for support.

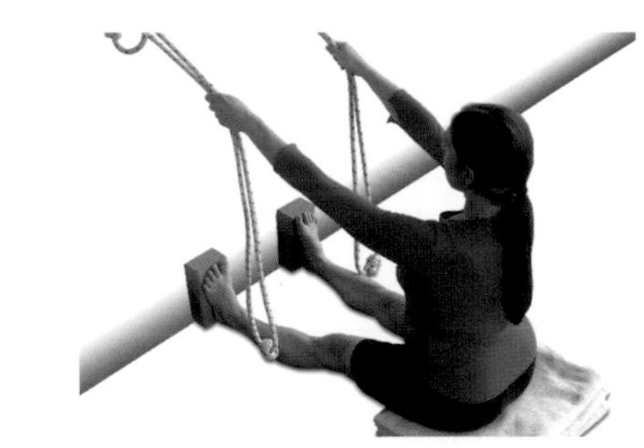

with wall and ropes, feet against wall

- If you have the help of a teacher, you could also practice as shown here.

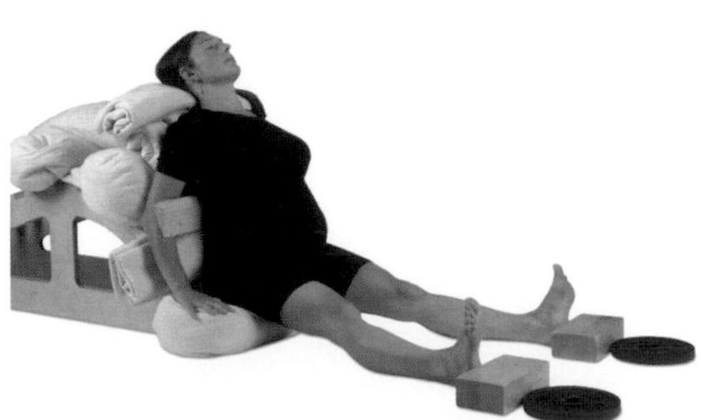

(for Dandasana and Urdhva Hasta Dandasana)

2nd and 3rd trimester: feet apart

1st trimester: yes, holding for no longer than 5 seconds
2nd trimester: yes, with feet apart
3rd trimester: yes, with feet apart

Benefits

- Stretches the leg muscles
- Massages the abdominal organs
- Strengthens the waist muscles
- Tones the kidneys
- Trains you to sit with your spine erect

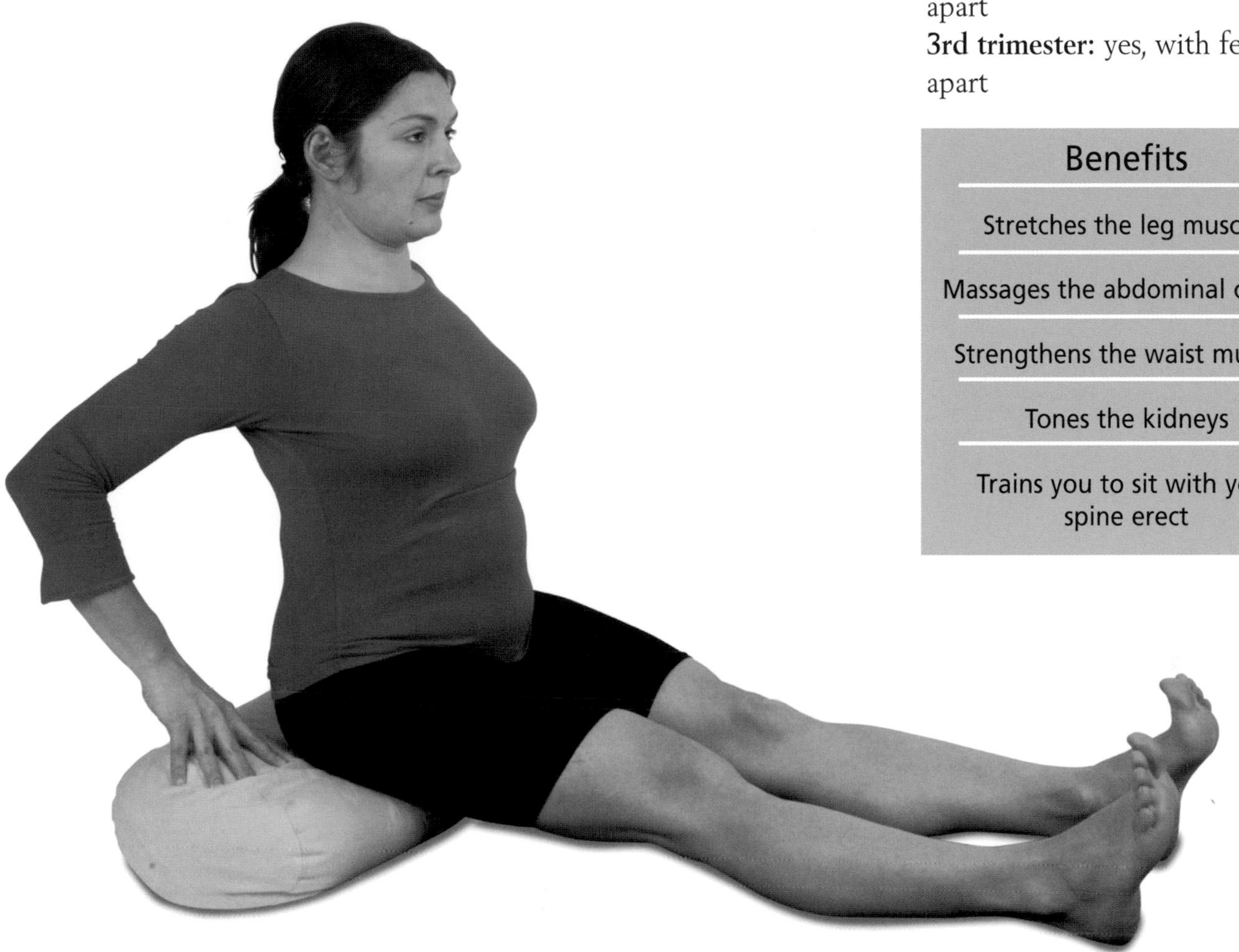

6 This is the final position. Remain for 5 seconds, breathing normally and observing the points in "Check Yourself."

Coming out of the pose

Maintain the length and firmness of your spinal column, inhale, and bend your legs.

CHECK YOURSELF

> *Press your knees and thighbones towards the floor and raise your waist.*

> *Keep your buttocks, back, and head in one line, perpendicular to the floor.*

> *Firm up your spinal column and expand your ribs and chest.*

> *Lift your abdominal organs upward.*

> *Stay for 30 to 60 seconds, maintaining the length and firmness of the spinal column. Inhale and bend your legs while coming back.*

Urdhva Hasta Dandasana

Staff with arms stretching upward pose

1 Elongating your fingers, stretch your arms forward in line with your shoulders.

2 Inhale and stretch your arms upward towards the ceiling alongside your ears.

3 Maintaining the lift and pressing your knees and thigh-bones towards the floor, raise your waist and the sides of your chest.

4 Tuck your shoulder blades in.

5 Stay for 10 to 15 seconds, maintaining the lift of your chest and its sides and lowering down your stretched arms.

Contraindications and Help

- If you have heart problems such as palpitations or high blood pressure, you should practice this asana with wall ropes, sitting on a support with your back against the wall.

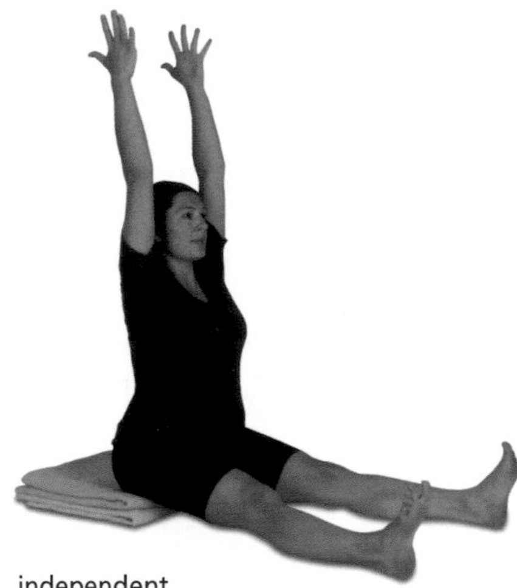

independent

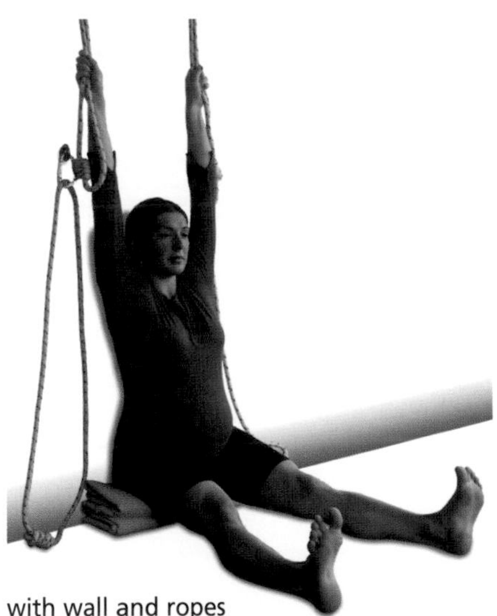

with wall and ropes

1st trimester: yes, holding for no longer than 5 seconds
2nd trimester: yes, with feet apart
3rd trimester: yes, with feet apart

Benefits

- Strengthens and stretches the leg muscles
- Lifts the abdominial organs
- Lifts the sides of the trunk
- Lifts the abdominal skin
- Strengthens the waist muscles
- Tones the kidneys
- Trains you to sit with your spine erect
- Prepares for all sitting forward-bending actions

Baddha Konasana

Bound angle pose

1st trimester: yes
2nd trimester: yes
3rd trimester: yes

Among the asanas recommended for pregnant women, Baddha Konasana tops the list. It tones the kidneys and pelvic region, and frees the respiratory system. This asana is always performed with a straight back, so that you can extend the spine without overworking the lumbar region (lower back).

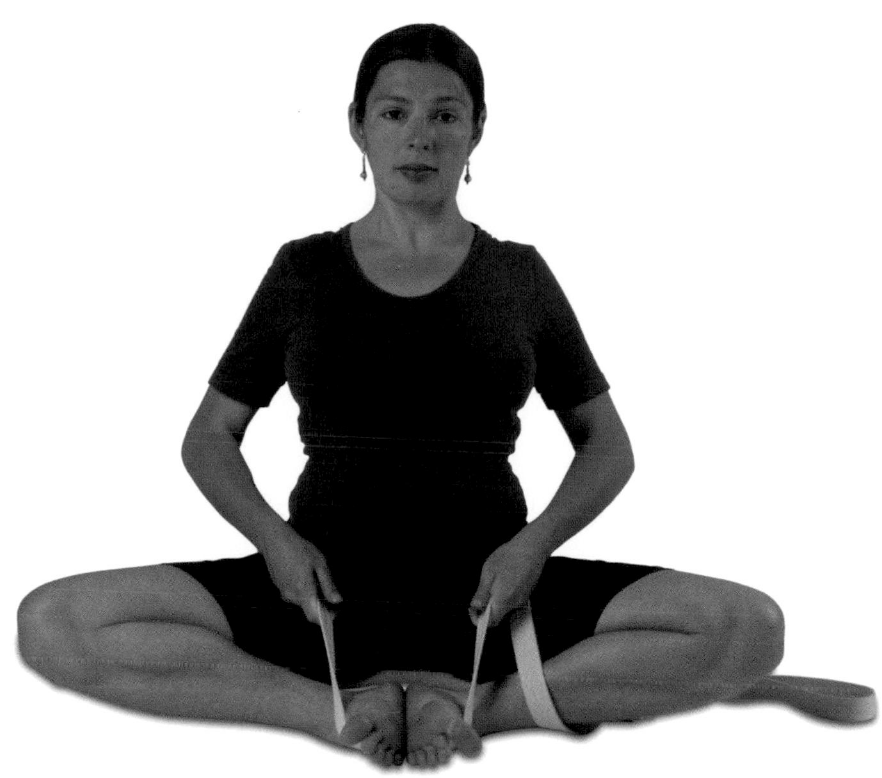

1 Sit in Dandasana (page 64) on a folded blanket 3 to 4 inches thick (or a bolster) under your buttocks, so that your buttocks are higher than your feet.

2 Bend both legs at the knees and bring your feet towards your groin.

3 Bring your soles and heels together as in Namaste (the Indian way of salutation).

4 Hold both feet with your hands or a belt and bring your heels towards your perineum. The outer edges of your feet should touch the floor. Breathe normally.

5 Widen your thighs and touch the floor with your knees.

6 Extend your groin and rest your knees on the floor in line with your thighs.

Benefits

- Soothes back pain
- Strengthens the muscles of the pelvic region and lower back
- Tones up the kidneys and helps alleviate urinary and uterine disorders
- Lessens the frequent passing of urine and the associated burning sensation
- Helps eliminate vaginal discharge and the resulting discomfort and irritation
- Reduces tension of the skin and abdominal muscles, which causes a stretching and itching sensation
- Corrects pressure of the uterus on the large veins in the pelvis, which can cause obstruction in the circulation resulting in fluid retention.
- Gives freedom to pelvic floor muscles because of the positioning of the legs, which open out like petals of the lotus flower
- Sitting with your back supported against the wall helps the respiratory system, not requiring any extra effort to keep your spine lifted, especially in the advanced stages of pregnancy.
- Alleviates heaviness in the lower abdomen and eases breathing
- Relieves compression of the vagina, anus, and lower part of the spine

7 Pull your heels closer towards the perineum, keeping your calf muscles alongside your inner thighs.

8 Hold your feet with your hands, press your knees, ankles, and thighs towards the floor, and stretch your torso upward. Be careful of the abdominal region and keep your neck straight.

9 Stay in this final position for 30 to 60 seconds, breathing normally. Later, increase the time as much as possible.

10 Maintaining the lift and the length in your inner legs, inhale and come back to Dandasana.

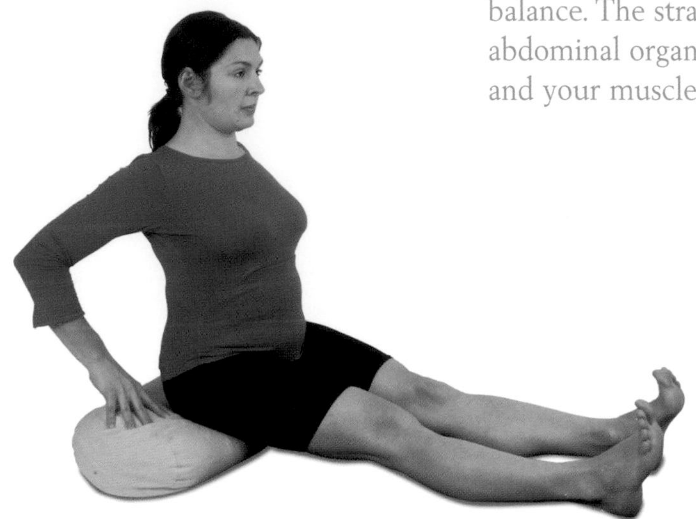

11 To sit longer in this position, keep your back against a wall so that it is supported throughout and you feel no back strain.

Hint: If you can sit quietly in the asana for 5 to 10 minutes with normal breathing, you will experience an inner peace and balance. The strain on your abdominal organs is lessened, and your muscles are relaxed.

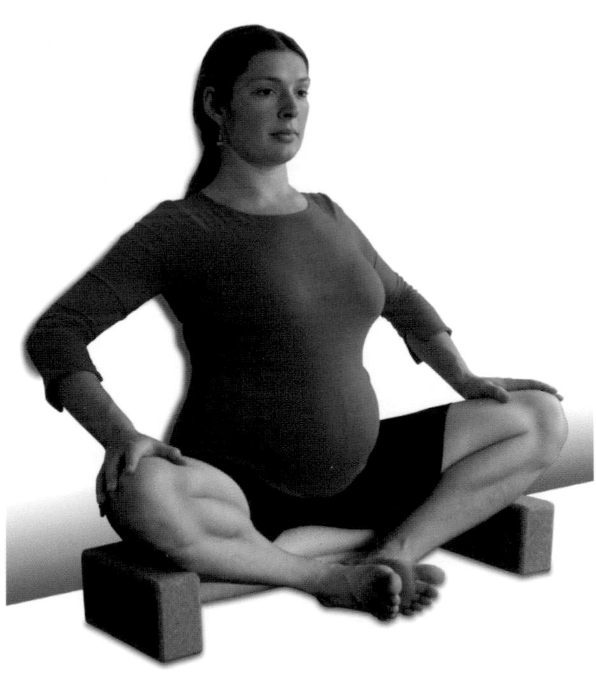

This asana is also recommended for the practice of pranayama (page 143)

CHECK YOURSELF

> *Press the sides of your shinbones down.*
> *Extend your torso from the navel upward; the firmer the grip of your hands on your feet, the better the lift of the torso.*
> *Keep your shoulder blades broad and tucked in.*
> *With your buttocks higher than your feet, your heels will not come close to the perineum.*

Help

- If you're less flexible, you may not be able to rest your knees on the floor. Don't force your knees down, but extend your groin towards your knees. If you can't do this, and your knees remain higher than the pelvic region, allow your legs to gravitate naturally, without applying any force.

- To practice opening the groin, you can place a rolled blanket under your outer ankles. Spread the ball of your big toes apart and rest your feet on their outer edges, so that your inner legs can easily open to the sides.

- In the last weeks of the pregnancy, for more lightness of the spine and the abdomen, ask someone to place a block and a 10 kg/20 lb. weight against the bottom of your toes, or practice with a block, a support, and wall ropes.

- Place a block or rolled blanket under each shin and let them rest on it. This will ease the pressure on the groin and make you more comfortable. This kind of support is particularly recommended if you have arthritis in the knees and ankles. (*See also Upavishtha Konasana, page 70.*)

- To sit longer in this position, keep your back against a wall so that it is supported throughout and you feel no back strain.

- You can rest the sides of your palms by the sides of your buttocks as in Dandasana, instead of holding your feet.

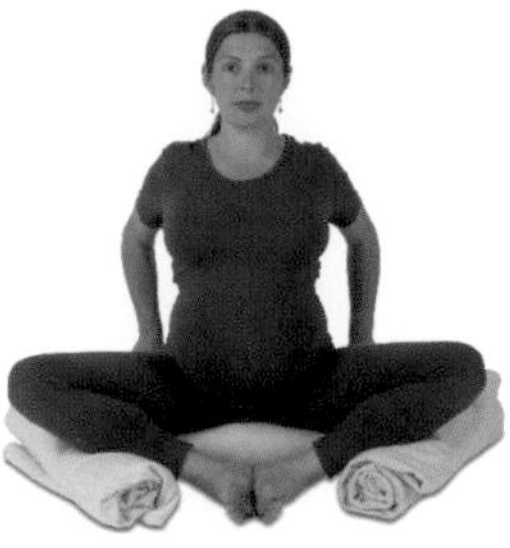
knee support

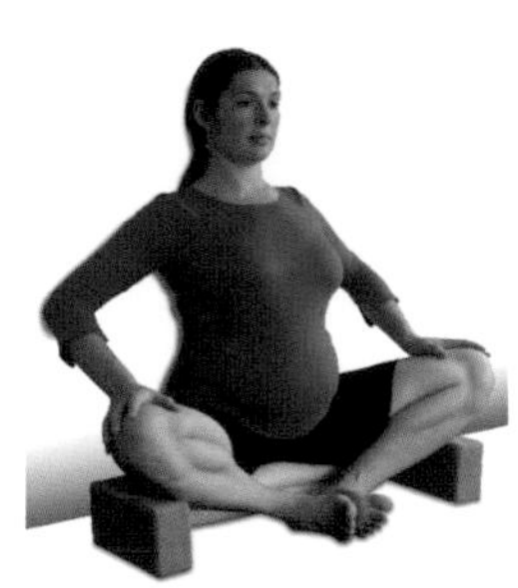
wall support

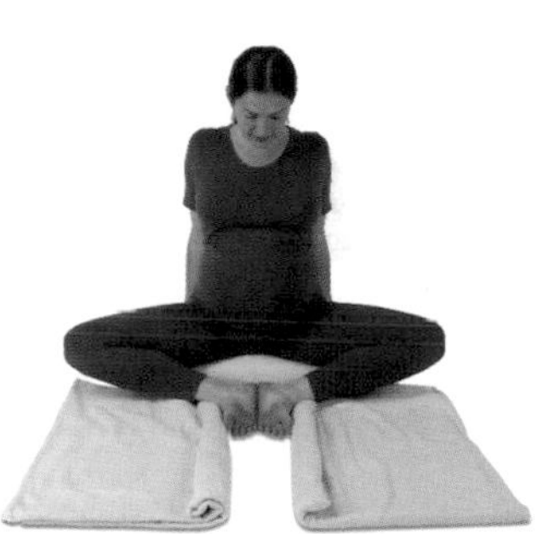
ankle support

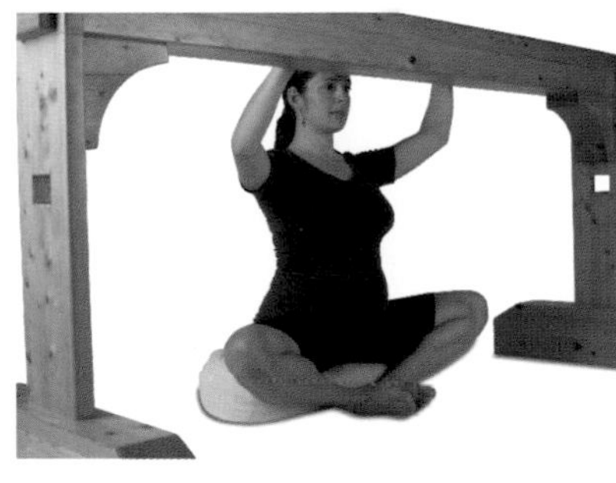

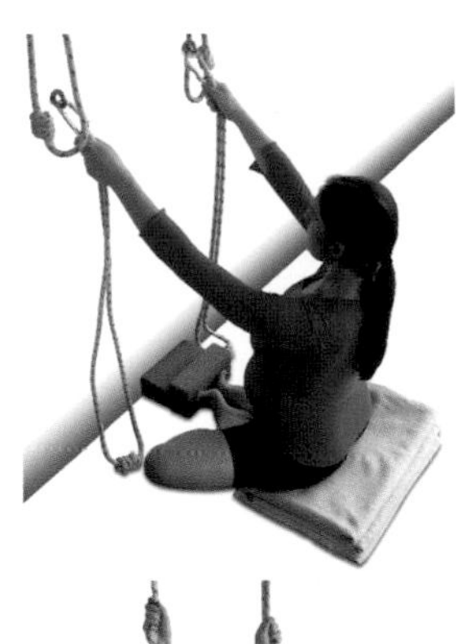

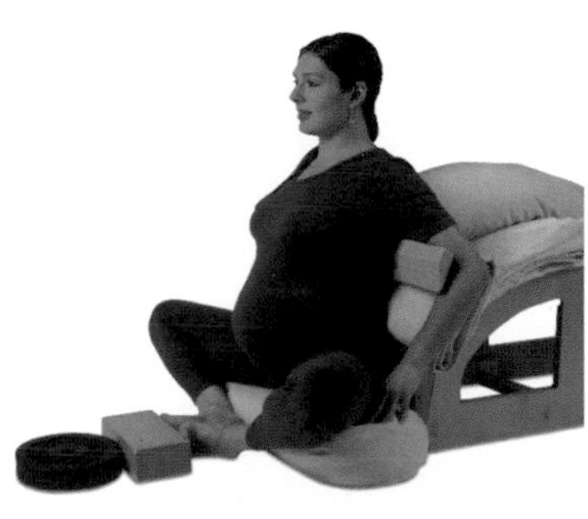
foot support and vesting

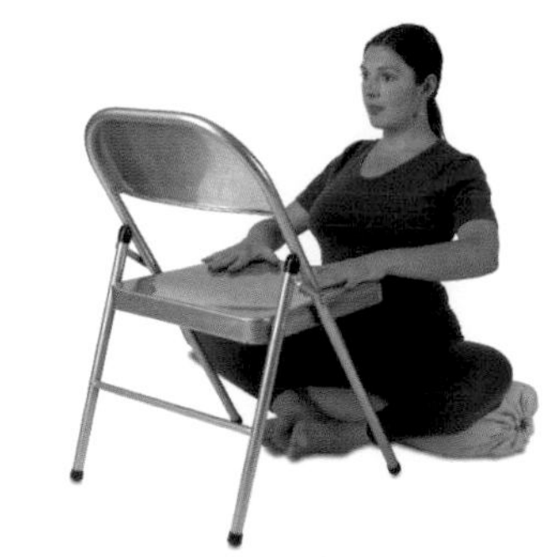
holding on to a chair, a trestle or something similar

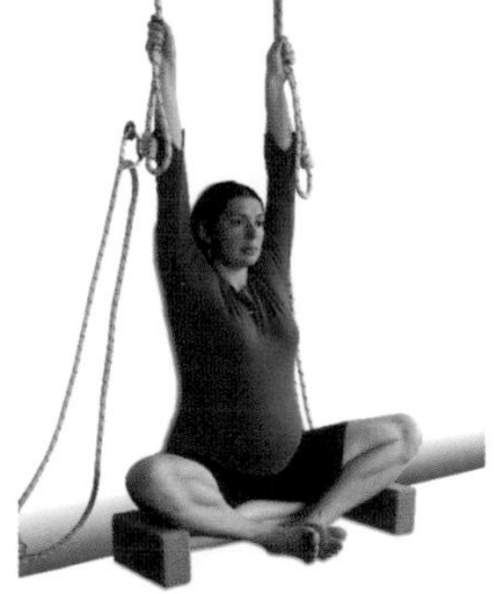
wall ropes and block

Upavishtha Konasana
Seated wide-angle pose

Upavishtha means "sitting." In this asana, you sit with your legs stretched at an obtuse angle, meaning between 90° and 180°.

When you're at the threshold of motherhood, you probably also have a few apprehensions, especially about delivery and the pain it involves. These increase as you enter the later stages of pregnancy and the day of your delivery draws near.

You need strength in your muscles to push the baby out, and your groin should be supple and prepared for the event. Your muscles should be trained to take some amount of pain.

Baddha Konasana and Upavishtha Konasana are the ideal asanas for this purpose. The lower part of the spine, the sacrum, gets tremendously pressurized in the actual process of delivery. These two asanas strengthen these parts, build up tolerance to pain, and maintain the required suppleness to bear the strain.

1 Sit in Dandasana (page 64) on a folded blanket 3 to 4 inches thick. Spread your legs apart and extend them sideways gradually, one by one, to avoid cramps. Increase the distance as much as you can.

2 Keep your soles firm and perpendicular to the floor, with the toes pointing upward. Be careful, because the normal tendency is to drop the feet inward.

3 Even though spreading your legs wide can cause pain in the hamstrings (back thigh muscles), continue the practice; the pain will soon disappear.

4 Keep your palms at the sides of your thighs.

5 Press your legs down and raise your waist and sides up. Because you're keeping your palms at the sides of your thighs, you have the added advantage of two points of support to raise your body upward.

6 Press your palms and legs down and raise your torso.

7 To come back, maintain the lift, bend your legs a little, and bring them back to the center without straining your groin.

CHECK YOURSELF

> *The back of your legs should be completely touching the floor.*

> *The back of the knees has a tendency to bend; stretch your hamstrings (back thigh muscles) and keep your knees down.*

> *Push your shoulder blades into your back ribs to open your chest and lift up its front, so that the gap between your diaphragm and lower abdomen increases. Keeping your palms at the sides of your thighs helps with this movement.*

> *If your spine feels heavy, use a rolled or folded blanket under your tailbone as shown.*

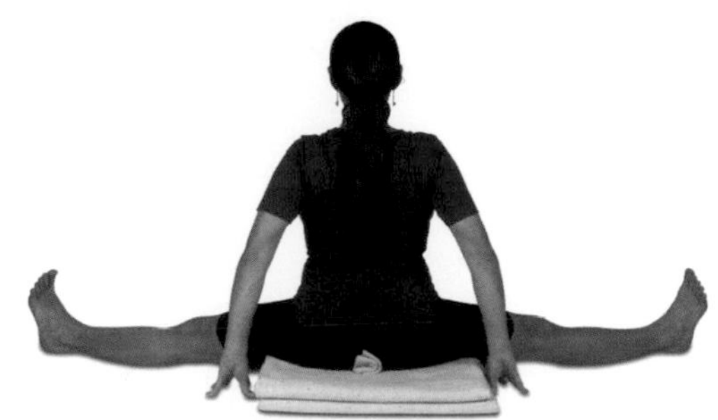

Extending the legs:

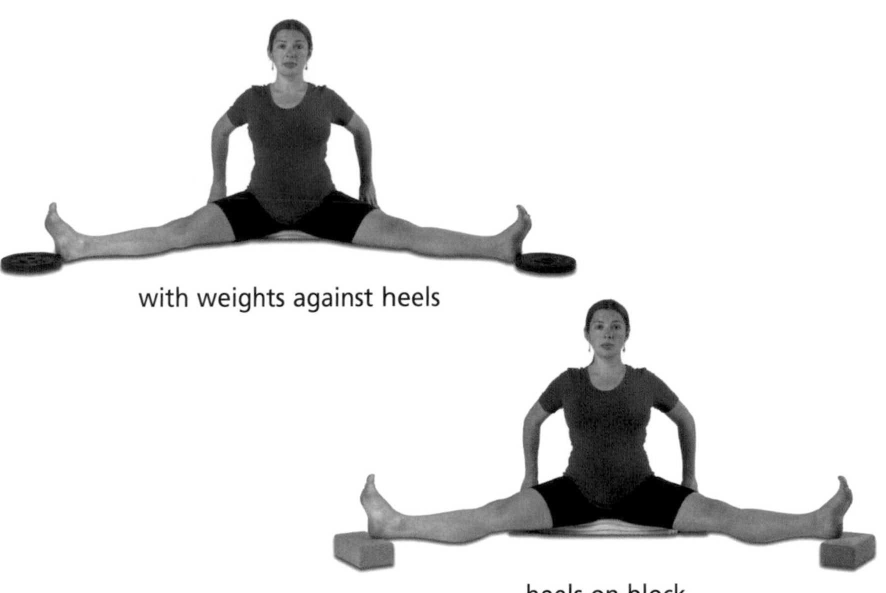

with weights against heels

heels on block

Opening the groin:

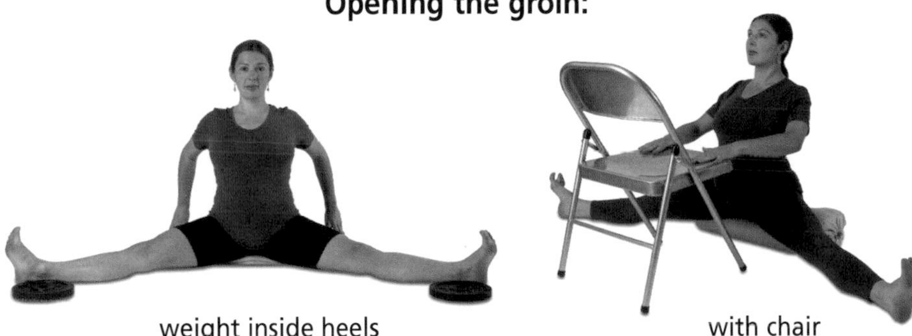

weight inside heels

with chair

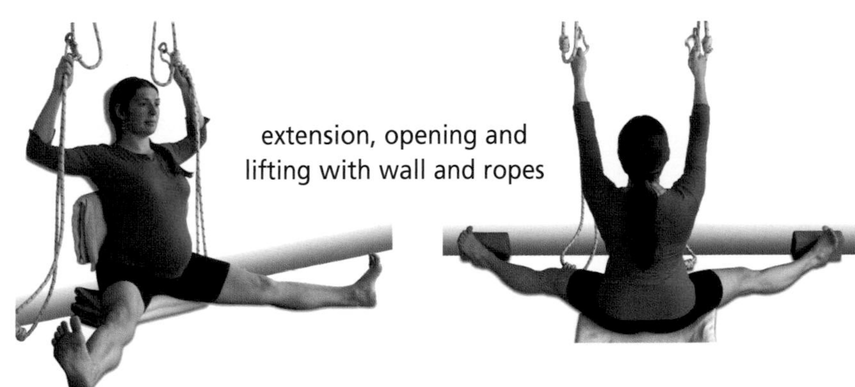

extension, opening and lifting with wall and ropes

Resting:

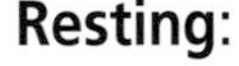

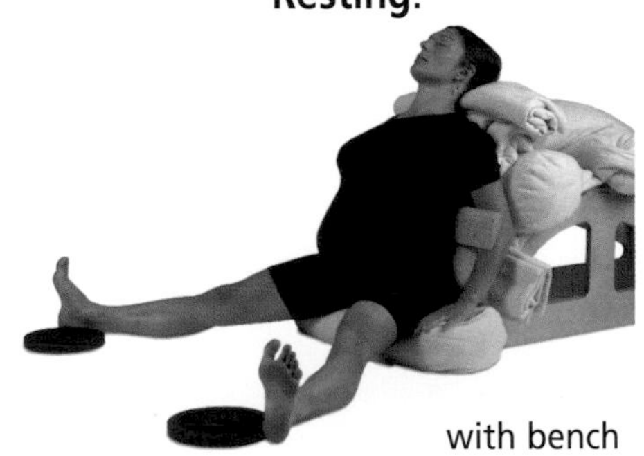

with bench

1st trimester: yes
2nd trimester: yes
3rd trimester: yes

Benefits

The benefits of Baddha Konasana and Upavishtha Konasana are more or less the same.

They both strengthen the muscles of the pelvic region and lower back, so practicing both is doubly beneficial.

If your groin is very stiff and you can't perform Baddha Konasana, with or without support of the knees, then Upavishtha Konasana is a great benefit for you. It's easier to perform and has similar effects, including:

- Improving the circulation of blood in the pelvis and abdomen
- Toning the kidneys, especially important for urinary problems in pregnancy
- Helping to reduce vaginal discharge

Contraindications

Avoid Upavishtha Konasana if the fetus has descended early.

Avoid if the cervix has dilated, or the cervix has been stitched up for these reasons.

Virasana
Hero pose

Vira means "brave" and "heroic." This pose resembles a warrior in a sitting position.

It is not uncommon for pregnant women to be reduced to tears because of severe pain and swelling in their legs. The swelling can restrict your movement, and the varicose veins on your calves and thighs can wreak havoc with your moods. It may seem that both your legs and back will buckle under the heavy weight they have to carry, perhaps for the first time.

Virasana is the asana for just this condition. It will bring back your courage, giving you relief from the pain and swelling. It will make you brave, as the name of the asana implies.

1st Trimester

During your first trimester, you should not find it difficult to sit on the floor. The inner sides of your calves will be adjacent to the outer sides of your thighs.

1 Kneel on the floor, keeping your knees together. If it's difficult to keep them together, keep them apart to avoid compression of the abdomen. Keep the edges of your outer thighs and hips in line.

2 Spread your feet 1 to 1½ feet apart, and turn them so that the soles face the ceiling. Keep your toes and feet in a straight line, extending backward.

3 Keeping your feet at the same distance apart, lower your buttocks until they rest on the floor, not on your feet. Take one or two breaths.

4 Keep your buttocks touching the floor.

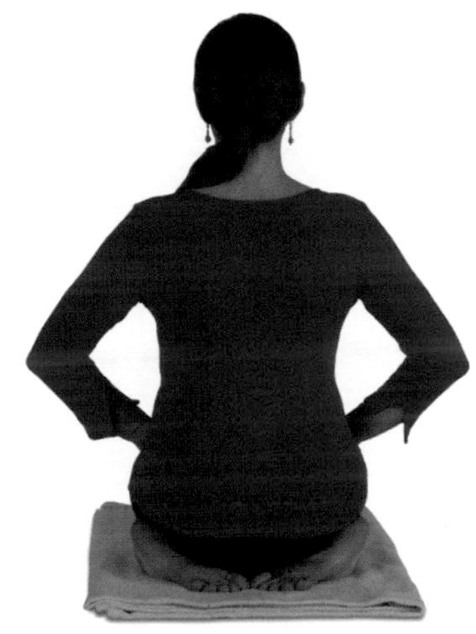

CHECK YOURSELF

> *Your body should not lean forward.*

> *Keep your groin and thighs down.*

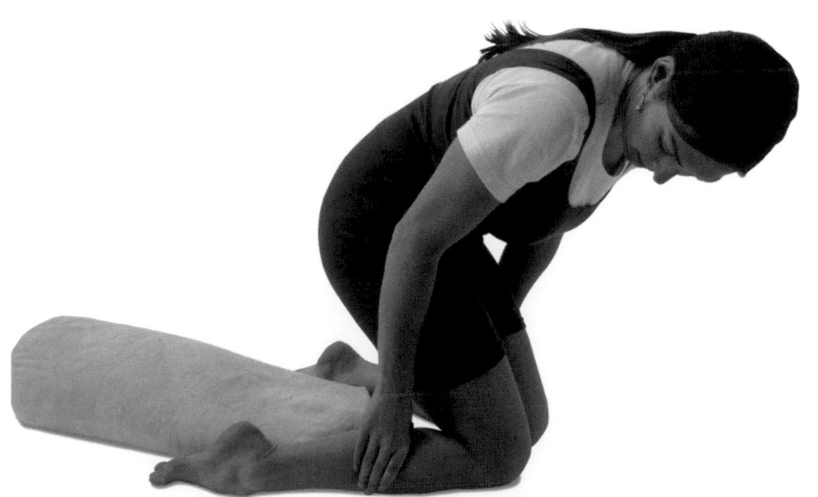

All Trimesters

1 If you feel pressure in your knees and ankles, sit on a folded blanket that is 3 to 4 inches high, a bolster, or a block, so that your buttocks are higher than your feet.

2 See below how to roll your calf muscle out to bring the shinbone down to the floor.

3 Your weight will now be evenly distributed on your knees, feet, and buttocks.

4 With your hands, press your inner heel lightly against the outer heel, lowering the outer edge of your foot.

5 Turn your palms downward and place your hands on your knees.

6 Keep the weight of your body on your thighs and raise your waist and the sides of your torso.

7 Keeping your chest expanded and your neck erect, look straight ahead.

8 Breathe normally and stay in this position for a minute, or as long as you can.

1st trimester: yes
2nd trimester: yes
3rd trimester: yes

Benefits
Reinstills courage
Prevents and removes pain and swelling in the legs
Counteracts fatigue
Helps correct overly concave lumbar (lower) spine
Improves kidney function
Reduces high blood pressure caused by kidney problems

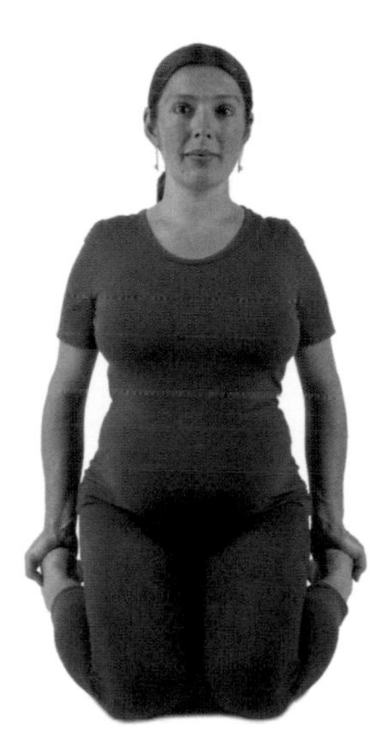

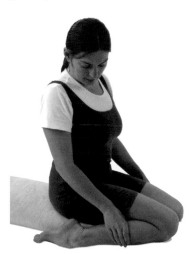

Virasana, kneeling

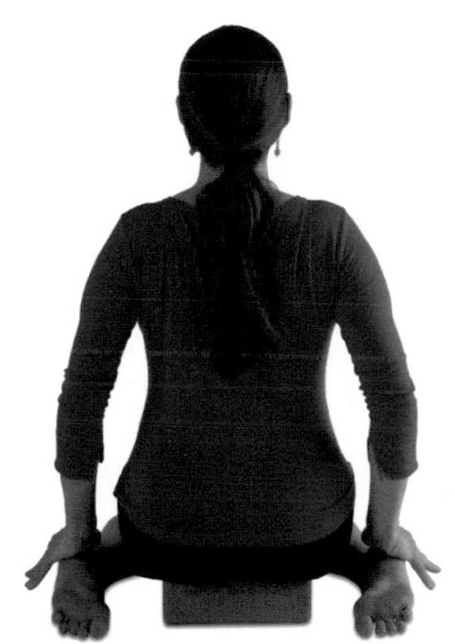

from the back on a block, taking the heels out

Coming out of the pose

Maintaining the extension of your torso, put your hands forward on the floor and slowly stretch one leg back at a time, extending only the heel. Repeat two to three times on both sides, until your legs are fully extended.

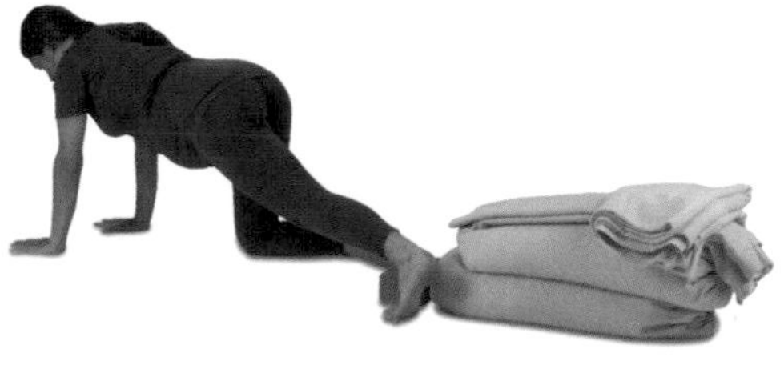

Help

If you can't extend your feet backward, keep them horizontal.

DETAILED DESCRIPTIONS OF ASANAS FOR ALL STUDENTS

Parvatasana from Svastikasana and Virasana

Mountain pose from cross-legged and hero pose

From Svastikasana

This asana relaxes the pelvis and back. Sit with your back against a wall if you feel tired.

1 Sit in Dandasana (page 64) at a height of 3 or 4 inches, bend your right knee, and put your right foot under your left thigh.

2 Bend your left knee and bring your left foot under your right thigh.

3 This is a simple cross-legged position, where your shinbones cross over in line with the center of your body and each foot is placed under the opposite thigh.

4 Sit upright on both buttock bones and lift your torso and chest, keeping your head straight.

5 To change your legs, stretch out in Dandasana and change the cross-leg position by bringing your left foot under your right thigh, and your right foot under your left thigh.

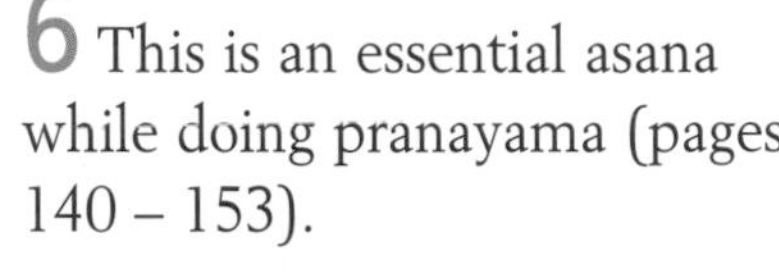

6 This is an essential asana while doing pranayama (pages 140 – 153).

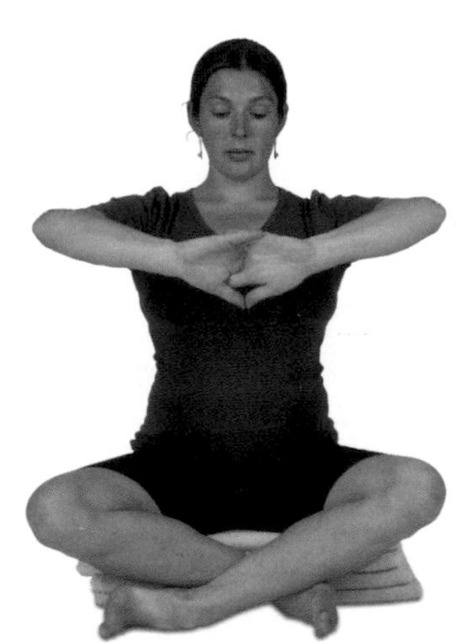

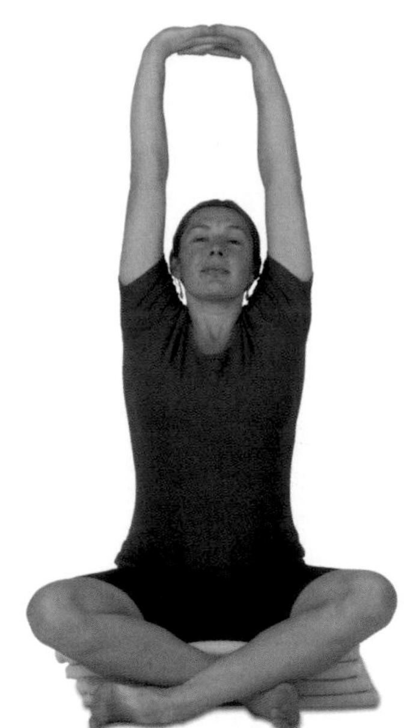

Svastikasana

From Virasana

1 In Virasana (page 72), make sure that you turn your feet backward and straighten them in line with your shins. Keep your knees together.

2 Interlock your fingers, turn your wrists and palms out, and extend your arms forward, in line with your shoulders.

3 Stretch your arms over your head, keeping your palms turned towards the ceiling.

4 Remain in this position for 20 to 30 seconds and breathe normally.

5 Use the belt as long as it is comforttable.

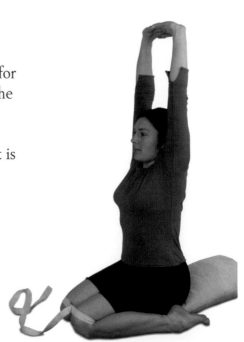

Virasana

CHECK YOURSELF

- *Straighten your arms from the armpits.*
- *Don't bend your elbows.*
- *Keep your shoulder blades in and your breastbone forward and up.*
- *Extend from the floating ribs (two lower ribs on either side) to the top of the chest, so that the chest cavity extends and expands.*
- *Keep your throat relaxed.*
- *Exhale, maintain the extension of the torso, and lower your arms.*
- *Change the interlocking of your fingers. By habit, you interlock your fingers keeping either your left or your right thumb uppermost. Notice their position when you raise your arms the first time, so that you can reverse it the second time. This gives a different stretch of the hands and arms and allows you to exercise unused muscles.*

1st trimester: yes
2nd trimester: yes
3rd trimester: yes

Benefits of Lifting the Arms in Parvatasana

Relieves backache

Relieves flatulence

Eases breathing

Lessens fatigue

Creates space in the abdomen for the safe growth of the fetus

Pashchima Namaskarasana and Gomukhasana (*below*) are especially good for: arthritis, stiffness in the neck, shoulders, elbows, and wrist

Reduces humpback

Gomukhasana from Virasana

1 Sit in Virasana (page 72) and entwine your hands like in Gomukhasana in Tadasana.

2 Proceed as indicated above in the technique for Parvatasana from Virasana and Svastikasana.

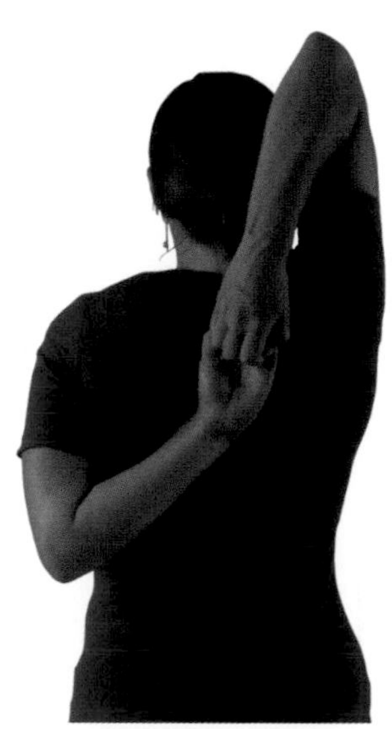

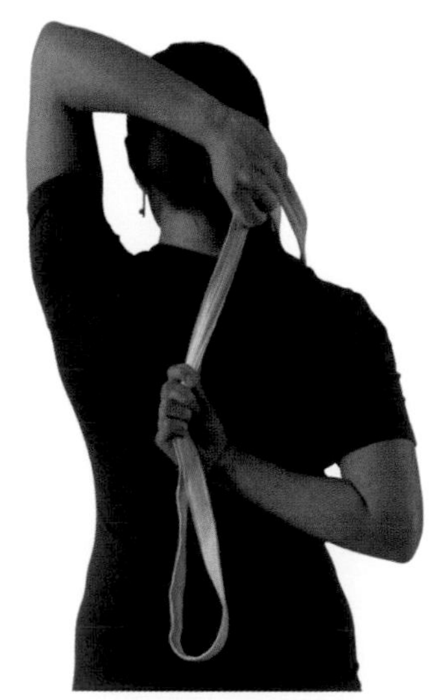

1st trimester: yes
2nd trimester: yes
3rd trimester: yes

Benefits

See Gomukhasana in Tadasana, page 37

HINT: Do the hand and arm work as in Gomukhasana in Tadasana, just as you did earlier in the standing poses.

Forward Bends
Pashchima Pratana Sthiti

Adho Mukha Virasana
Downward-facing hero pose

This asana is so comfortable that you can perform it from the first day of your pregnancy until the day you give birth to your baby.

1 Sit in Virasana (page 72).

2 Put your big toes together and place your feet horizontally.

3 Turn your calf muscles out and sit comfortably on your feet.

4 According to the stage of your pregnancy, use whatever support you need for your arms and forehead.

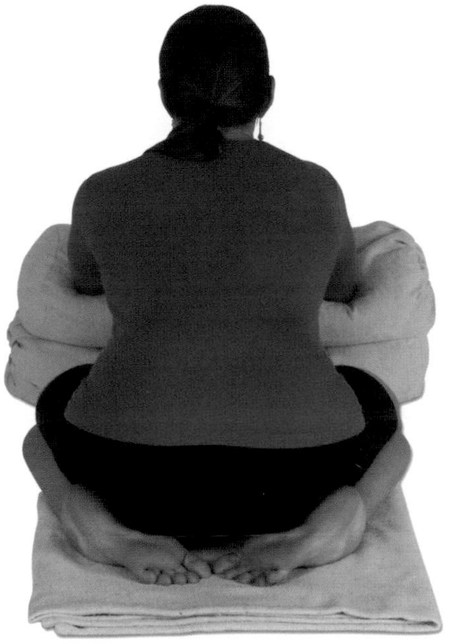

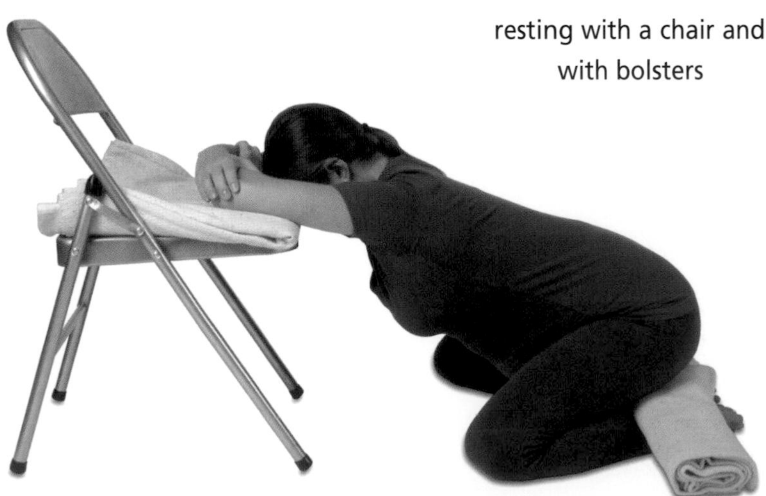

resting with a chair and with bolsters

1st trimester: yes
2nd trimester: yes
3rd trimester: yes

Benefits

- Rests the heart
- Eases breathing
- Allows your breathing to flow freely into your groin, lower back and spine, sides of the torso, and abdomen. You can even feel the breath in your inner thighs.
- Helps treat high blood pressure and diabetes
- Assists during labor: helps you breathe through contractions and relax between them

HINT: It is very relaxing if someone gently presses down the muscles to the left and right of the sacrum (bone plate between spine and tailbone). This allows your groin and hips to soften and your breath to flow into this area.

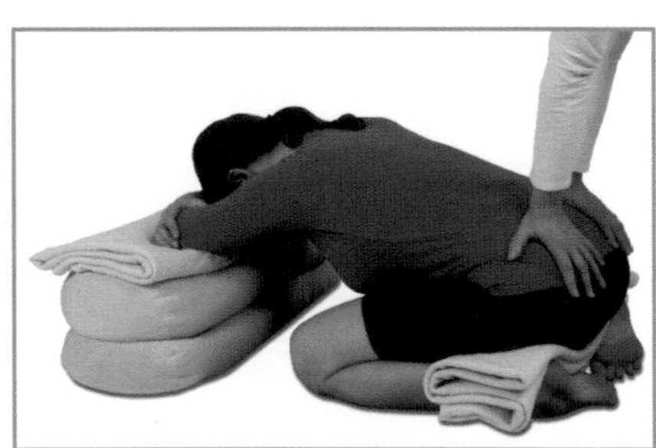

Malasana

Garland pose, with bolster and wall ropes

1st trimester: no
2nd trimester: yes
3rd trimester: yes

This upright pose keeps the birth canal upright for delivery.

1 Stand in Tadasana (page 32) with your feet 2 to 2½ feet apart, about two feet away from the wall.

2 Grip the lower ropes, bend your legs, and move your knees to the sides so the abdomen can find its place.

3 Keep your heels down and put your buttocks down on the bolster.

4 If your heels come up, take more support for your buttocks.

5 Don't lean backward; bring your body weight slightly forward.

6 Relax your head, shoulders, and back.

7 Concentrate on your breathing.

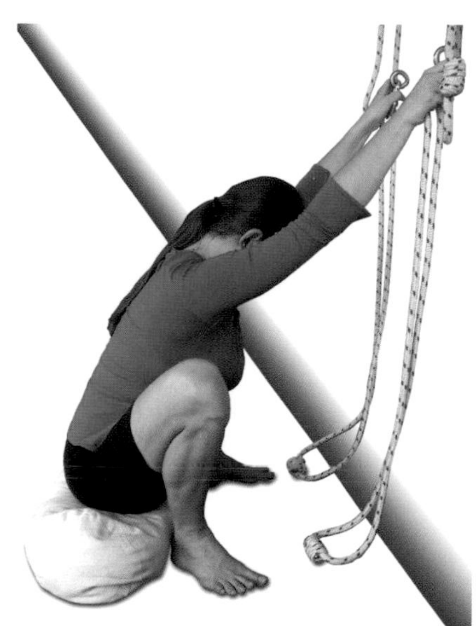

Benefits

Since your arms are lifted, breathing is much easier.

Your bent legs allow your pelvis and back to relax.

During delivery:
The birth canal is in an upright position, enabling the baby to find its way out more easily.

The pressure of the baby's head remains in a straight downward direction.

Malasana

Garland pose, sitting against the wall

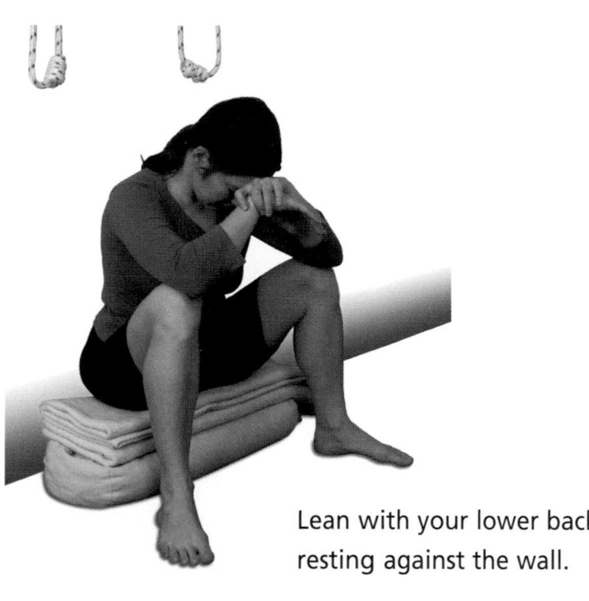

Lean with your lower back resting against the wall.

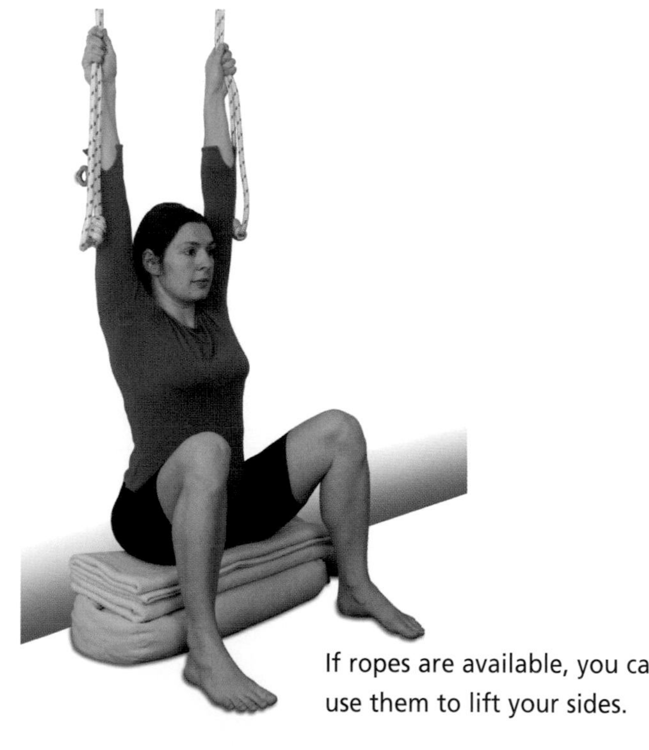

If ropes are available, you can use them to lift your sides.

Malasana
Garland pose, with trestle

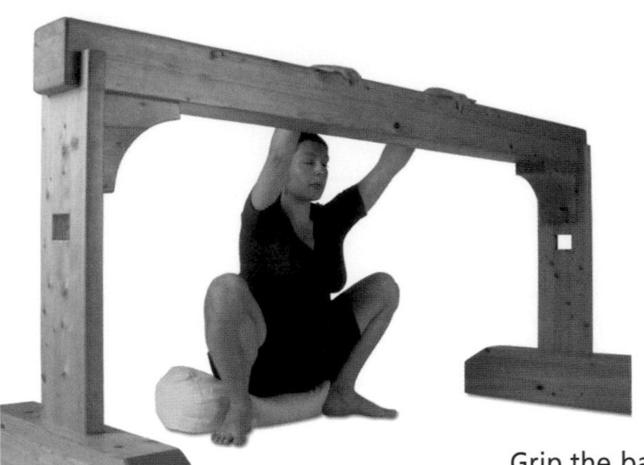

Grip the bar of the trestle.

Malasana
Garland pose, preparing for delivery

In the last weeks of your pregnancy, practice this pose with the person who will be with you during the delivery.

NOTE
Do not practice pushing before labor occurs!

1 Your helper sits behind you.

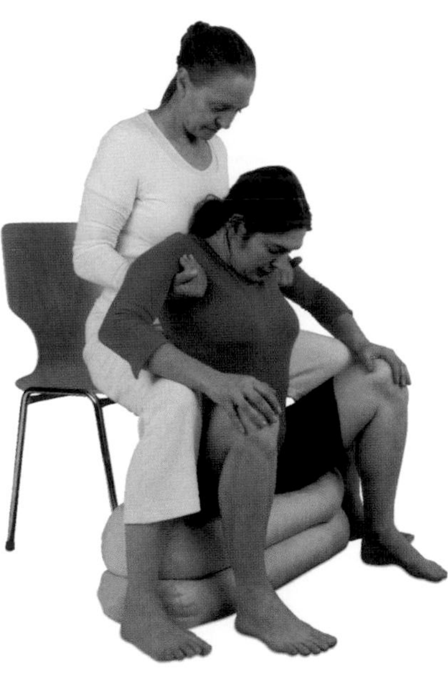

2 While closing your eyes tightly, put your chin down as in Jalandhara Bandha (page 80) and grip your knees. During push contractions, take a deep breath and softly push the baby down to the pelvic floor.

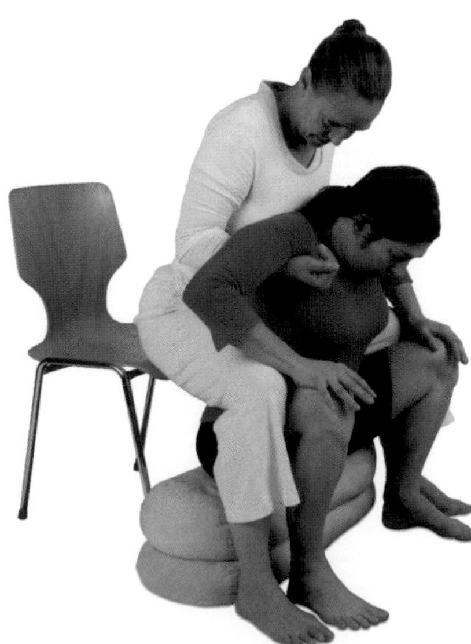

3 In between contractions, you can lean against your helper.

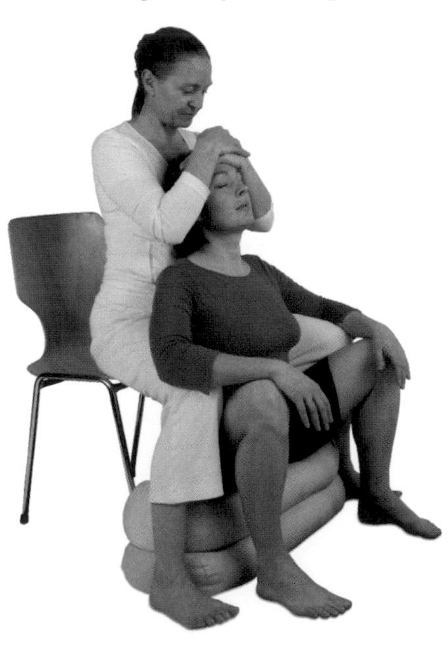

Maha Mudra

The great seal pose

1st trimester: no
2nd trimester: yes
3rd trimester: yes

Maha means "great" or "noble," and *mudra* means "lock," "seal," or "the act of sealing or closing." In this pose, the main openings of the body are sealed. One leg is bent near the lower abdomen, and the other is stretched out. The straightened foot is held with the palms or a belt, and the spine is raised by keeping the head down, thereby closing the throat, anus, and vagina—sealing the body at both the ends.

The spine is lifted by gripping and pulling the foot, which gives the spine firm support and helps it in its upward stretch.

Maha Mudra practices lifting the spine with support and controlling the contraction of the abdominal organs.

Maha Mudra is a mudra in Janu Shirshasana (page 82). This asana is the first in the chain to be performed before Shirshasana (and after it in reverse order). The asana chain is intended to strengthen the spine for Shirshasana.

Benefits

- Tones the liver, spleen, kidneys, and adrenal glands
- Helps return a slipped uterus to the correct position
- Expands the rib muscles, which expands the chest
- Lessens abdominal compression by lifting the bottom ribs
- Aids in treating nausea, vomiting, low spirits, and blackouts
- Tones the spinal muscles in preparation for Shirshasana
- Keeps the spine from collapsing and trains it to extend and stretch
- Improves digestion, also in preparation for Shirshasana; prevents the nausea that can occur during Shirshasana because of poor digestion

1 Sit on a support (folded blankets that are 3 to 4 inches high, or a bolster); this helps to avoid pressure and aids in lifting the spine and abdomen.

2 Sit in Dandasana (page 64).

3 Keep your left leg straight, bend your right knee, place the outer sides of your thigh and calf on the floor, and bring your heel close to the perineum. Your bent leg should be at a right angle to the extended one.

4 Hold your foot by hooking a belt around it.

5 Straighten both arms by locking your elbows.

6 Raise your torso by maintaining the grip and pressing your thighs to the floor.

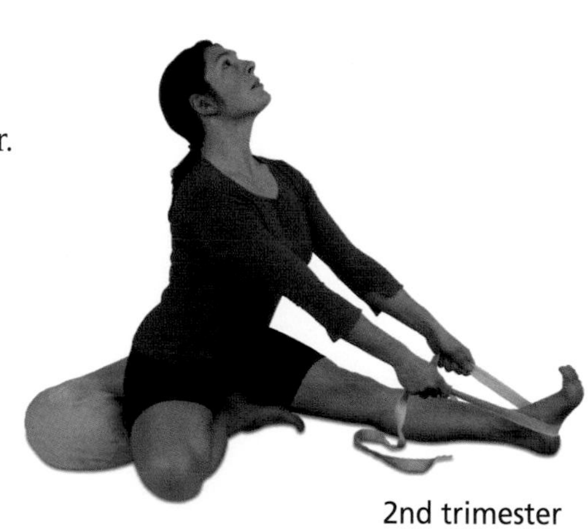

2nd trimester

7 Lower your head from the nape of your neck until your chin rests in the hollow of your collarbone.

8 Relax your head and forehead. Don't constrict your throat while you lower it, and close your eyes.

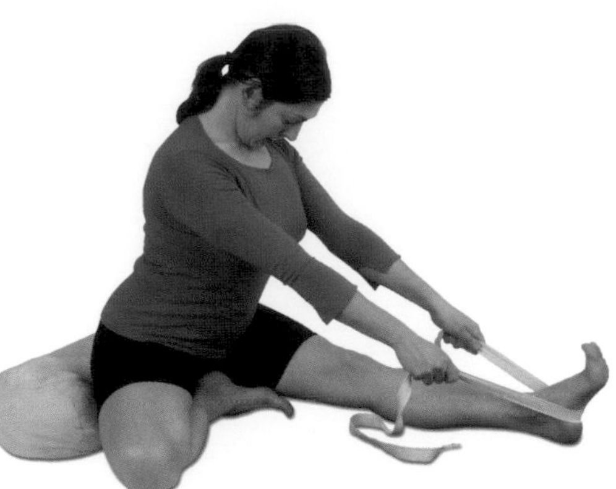

9 Exhale the air from your lungs and then inhale fully. Lift your abdomen from its base to the diaphragm and stretch your spine upward.

10 Remain in this final position for 3 to 5 seconds, holding your breath.

Here, what is known as Jalandhara Bandha occurs. *Jalan* means "net," and *bandha* means "bondage" or "binding." In Jalandhara Bandha, the neck and the throat are contracted and the chin rests in the notch between the collarbones.

During the practice of asanas, mudras, or pranayama, the brain is made to bow down, reducing its dominance over the practitioner. This provides for a silent mental state—a state of neutrality—and makes the breath quiet and subtle.

◇

Is your spine dropping as soon as you put your head down?

If you can't keep your spine lifted, your diaphragm drops, and you become short of breath, then avoid Jalandhara Bandha and perform the following technique instead:

1 Lift your head and bring it back.

2 Create space between your lower abdomen and the floating ribs (two lower ribs on either side).

3 Lift your breastbone.

4 Keep the sides of your chest up, not collapsing.

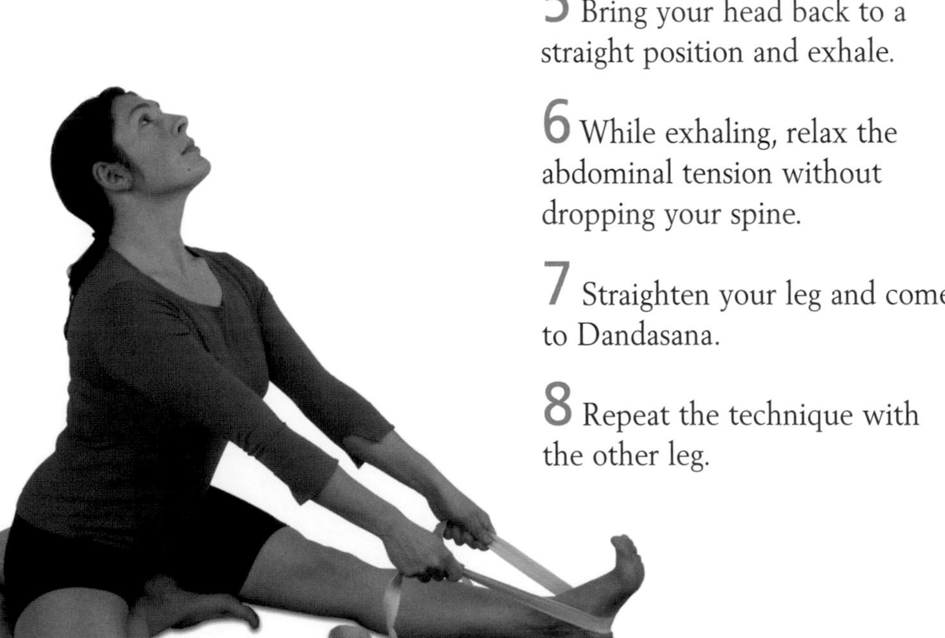

5 Bring your head back to a straight position and exhale.

6 While exhaling, relax the abdominal tension without dropping your spine.

7 Straighten your leg and come to Dandasana.

8 Repeat the technique with the other leg.

3rd Trimester

Sit on a support (a bolster or folded blankets that are 3 to 4 inches high) and put a chair or stool across your front leg, with your arms resting on it. Let your elbows rest towards your lower arms. Grip the ends of the belt that is around your foot.

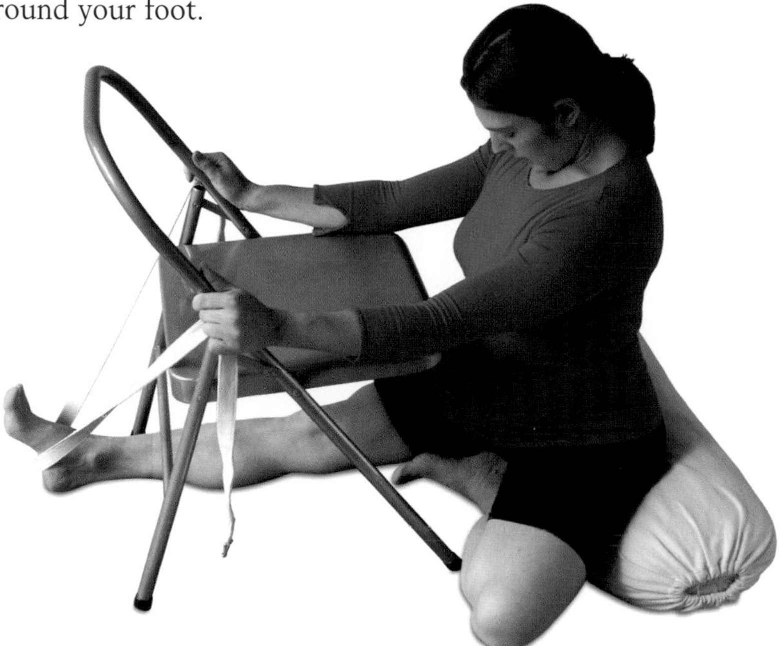

CHECK YOURSELF

- *Keep your chest expanded.*
- *Relax your eyes, forehead, tongue, and facial muscles.*
- *Don't tilt your body to one side.*
- *Increase the grip on your toe or foot to extend your spine.*
- *While exhaling, relax the abdominal tension without dropping your spine.*
- *Inhalation, retention, and exhalation complete one cycle; perform 5 to 8 cycles.*
- *After completing the cycles, raise your head, open your eyes, straighten your right leg, and come to Dandasana.*
- *Repeat the technique by keeping your right leg straight and bending your left knee.*
- *The retention of breath should be equal on both sides.*

Maha Mudra during Pregnancy

There are three bandhas in Maha Mudra: Jalandhara Bandha, Mula Bandha, and Uddiyana Bandha. When you're pregnant, you should perform Mula Bandha and Jalandhara Bandha, but not Uddiyana Bandha.

In Jalandhara Bandha, the neck is elongated and the throat is contracted, so that whatever breathing you do, the senses of perception and the mind are not tense and can be in a restful state.

Maha Mudra involves lifting the spine, maintaining its concave state, and lifting the sides of the chest. Though the base of the abdomen is raised in Mula Bandha, the abdominal muscles are not tightened inside nor drawn to the spine like in Uddiyana Bandha. The abdominal organs and the diaphragm are merely lifted.

Janu Shirshasana

Head on knee pose, concave back

Janu means "knee," and *shirsha* means "head." In the classical pose, your head is positioned alongside your knee.

The sitting poses help relieve many of the complaints of pregnancy: heaviness in the lower back and abdomen, gravitational pull on your spine, swelling in your legs, irritation in the genitalia, perspiration and body heat, and morning sickness.

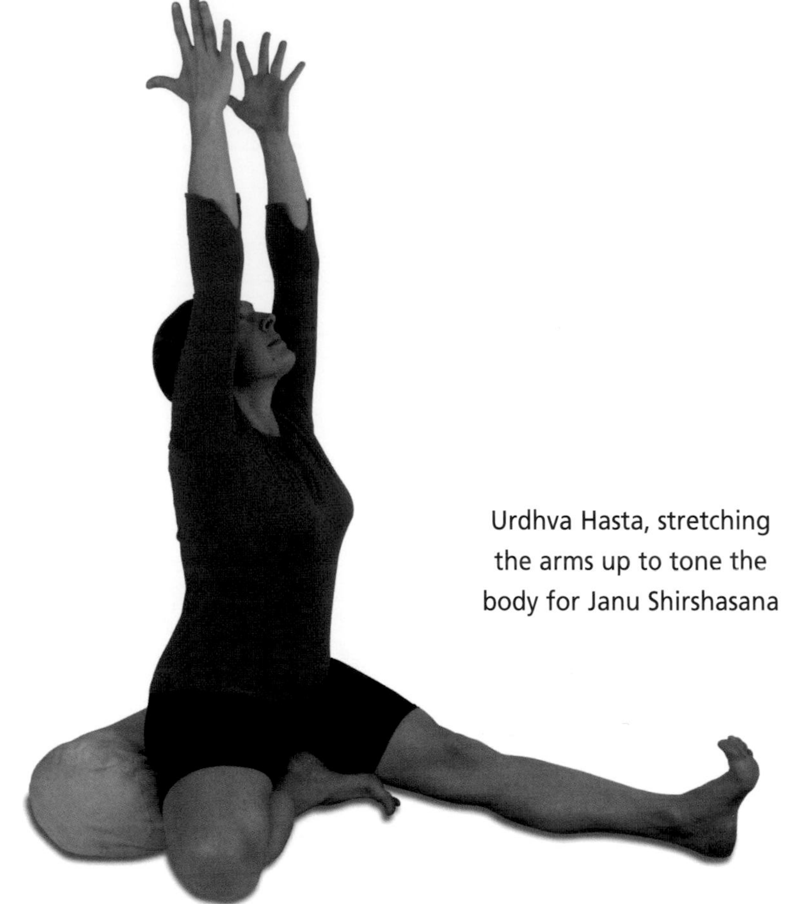

Urdhva Hasta, stretching the arms up to tone the body for Janu Shirshasana

1 Sit in Dandasana (page 64) on a support that is 3 to 4 inches high (folded blankets or a bolster), so that your buttocks are higher than your feet.

2 Bend your right knee and place your right heel near the right side of your groin; pull your right knee back.

3 Keep your left leg straight. The angle between your legs should be obtuse (between 90° and 180°).

4 Keep your weight on both buttocks and press your thigh and calf down.

5 Put a belt, scarf, or something similar around your left foot and hold both ends.

6 Inhale and stretch your arms up in Urdhva Hasta Dandasana (page 66).

7 Exhale, extend your arms forward, grip the belt, and lift your spine in Urdhva Mukha (page 90, step 6). Make your spine as concave as possible and lift your head.

8 Breathing normally, stay for 10 to 15 seconds, observing the points in "Check Yourself."

Coming out of the pose

Release your arms without dropping your extended spine, stretch the right leg out to Dandasana, and repeat on the other side.

1st trimester: yes
2nd trimester: yes
3rd trimester: yes

Benefits

Strengthens the spine and the muscles of the back and waist, so that the fetus remains well supported

Relieves heaviness in the abdomen, lower back, and tailbone and gravitational pull on the spine

Decreases swelling in the legs

Alleviates irritation in the genitalia

Reduces perspiration and body heat

Helps flush the bladder

Tones and activates the liver, spleen, and kidneys; lessens the feeling of sluggishness

This asana is a must if you suffer from a low, persistent fever.

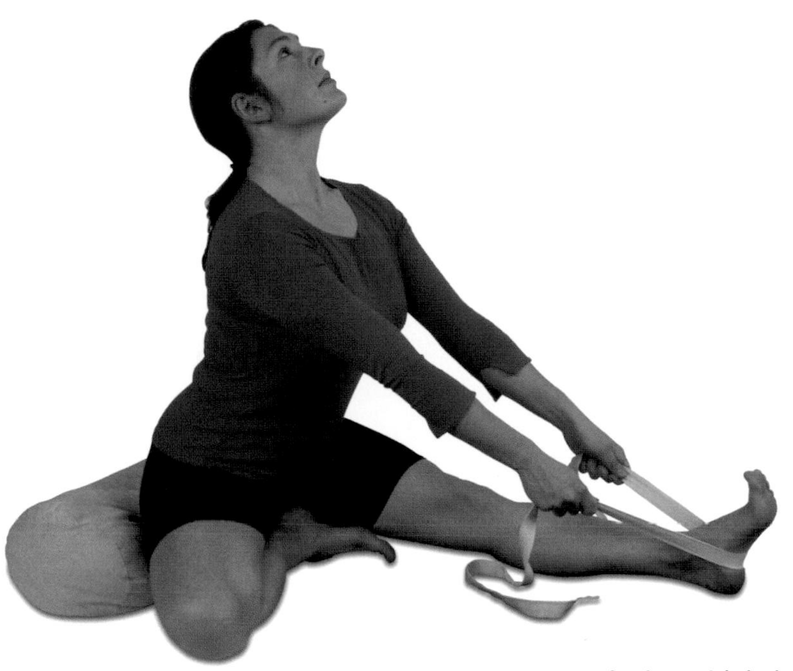

gripping with belt

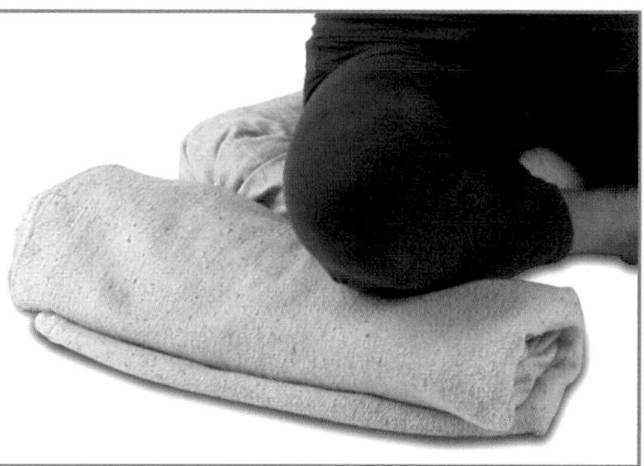

when the knee is not touching the floor: put a block or a blanket under the knee

CHECK YOURSELF

> *Keep your torso facing forward.*
> *Extend your spine from the base of your torso upward.*
> *Inhale and raise your head.*
> *Straighten both arms at the elbows.*
> *Create space between your lower abdomen and the floating ribs (two lower ribs on either side)*
> *Lift your breastbone.*
> *Keep the sides of your chest up; don't let them collapse.*

Upavishtha Konasana

Seated wide-angle pose, concave back

Upavishtha means "seated" or "sitting." In this asana, the legs are stretched in an obtuse angle while you sit.

For giving birth, you need muscle strength. Your groin should be supple and prepared for the event, and the muscles should be trained to take some amount of pain.

Baddha Konasana and Upavishtha Konasana are the ideal asanas for this purpose. The lower part of the spine and the sacrum get tremendously pressurized in the actual process of delivery. These two asanas strengthen these parts, build up tolerance to pain, and maintain the required suppleness to bear the strain of delivery.

◇

1 Sit in Dandasana (page 64) on a folded blanket 3 to 4 inches thick.

2 Spread your legs and extend them sideways. To avoid cramps, extend them gradually, first the right leg to the right side and then the left leg to the left side. Increase the distance as much as you can.

3 Keep your soles firm and perpendicular to the ground, with the toes pointing upward. Western women tend to drop the feet inward, and Eastern women tend to drop the feet outward, so be careful of this.

Even though spreading your legs wide can cause pain in the hamstring muscles, continue to practice—and with practice, the pain will disappear.

4 Hold the big toe of each foot with the thumb, index finger, and middle finger of the corresponding hand, keeping the thumbs on the outer side and the index and middle fingers on the inside of the big toe in Padangushthasana.

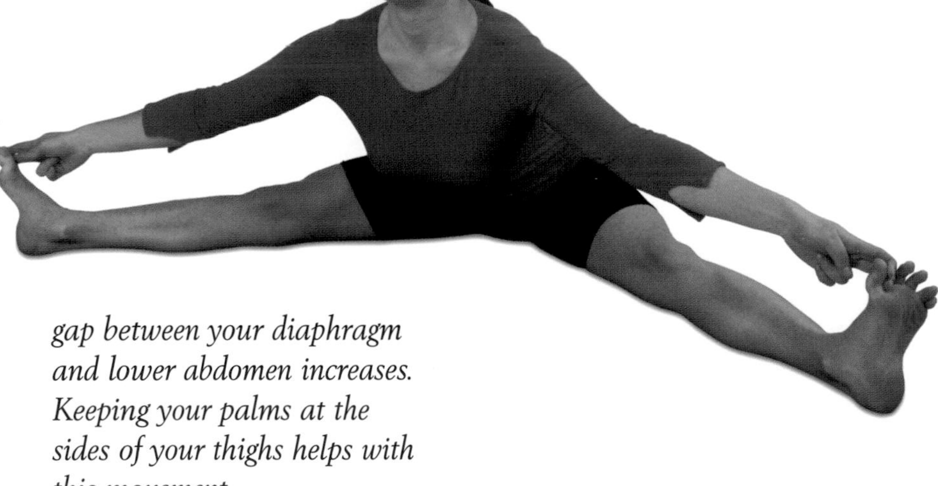

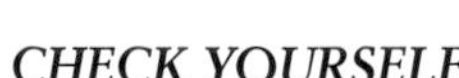

CHECK YOURSELF

> *The back of your legs should be completely touching the floor.*
> *The back of the knees has a tendency to bend; stretch your hamstrings (back thigh muscles) and keep your knees down.*
> *Push your shoulder blades into your back ribs to open your chest and lift up its front, so that the gap between your diaphragm and lower abdomen increases. Keeping your palms at the sides of your thighs helps with this movement.*
> *If your spine feels heavy, use a rolled or folded blanket under your tailbone as shown on page 85.*

5 When you can't reach the big toe, use a belt.

6 Although a nonpregnant woman could possibly now touch the floor with her forehead, nose, chin, or chest, this is not advisable for a pregnant woman. You should practice the pose in an upright and straight position in order to give maximum lift to the torso.

Help for the 2nd and 3rd Trimesters:

If you can no longer grip your toes or work with the belts:

- Keep your palms to the sides of your thighs.
- Press your legs down and raise your waist and sides up. With your palms to the sides of your thighs, you have the added advantage of two points of support, to raise your body upward.
- Press your palms and legs down and raise your torso.

1st trimester: yes
2nd trimester: yes
3rd trimester: yes

Benefits

The benefits of Baddha Konasana and Upavishtha Konasana are more or less the same. They both strengthen the muscles of the pelvic region and lower back, so practicing both is doubly beneficial.

If your groin is very stiff and can't perform Baddha Konasana, with or without support of the knees, then Upavishtha Konasana is a great benefit for you. It's easier to perform and has similar effects, which include:

- Improving blood circulation in the pelvis and abdomen
- Toning the kidneys, which is especially important for urinary problems in pregnancy
- Helping to reduce vaginal discharge

Contraindications

Avoid Upavishtha Konasana if the fetus has descended early, the cervix has dilated, or the cervix has been stitched up for these reasons.

Coming out of the pose

To come back, maintain the lift, bend your legs a little, and bring them back to the center without straining your groin.

Upavishtha Konasana, Resting in Adho Mukha

This variation is especially helpful for high blood pressure, kidney problems, and nausea.

1 You'll use a chair in two steps.

2 Sit on a support, spread your legs, and follow the technique for Upavishtha Konasana (page 84).

3 Put your hands on the chair in front of you.

4 Inhale, lift your spine, maintain the firmness of your buttocks and legs, keep your spine lifted, and bend forward.

5 Bring your lower arms onto the seat of the chair.

6 Rest your head on your lower arms or in front of them on the seat.

7 Keep your face and breathing relaxed.

8 You may rest here for up to five minutes.

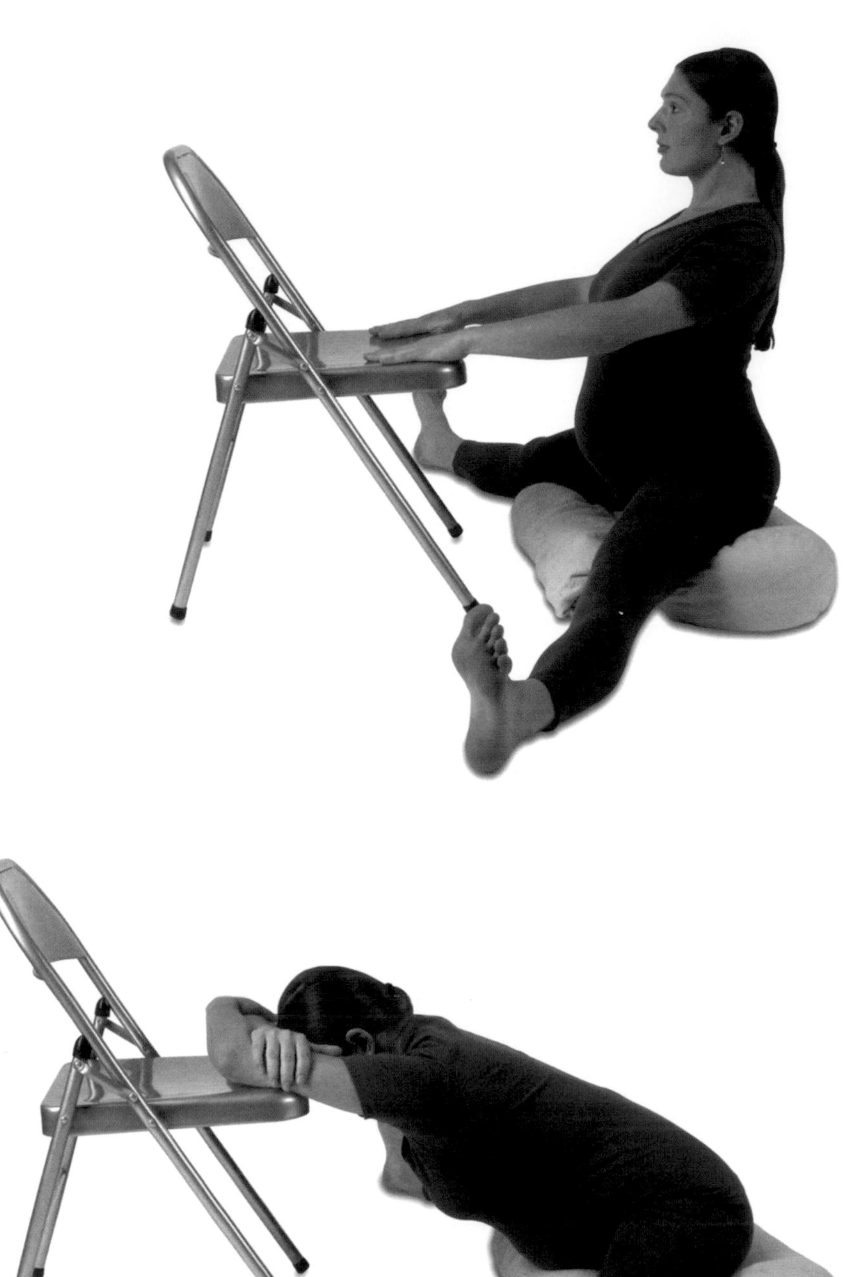

Pashchimottanasana

Intense west stretch pose, concave back

1st trimester: no
2nd trimester: yes
3rd trimester: yes

Benefits
Strengthens the spine
Massages and strengthens the abdominal organs
Stretches the pelvic region and stimulates blood circulation
Creates space for the fetus
Helps treat kidney disease and sluggish liver
Revitalizes the entire reproductive system
Relieves backache

This asana is also known as Ugrasana or Brahmacharyasana.

Pashchima means "west" which, when applied to the body, means "back." This asana involves a posterior extension.

In the Hatha Yoga Pradipika I:29, its effects are described as follows:
"Pashchimottanasana is the foremost of all asanas. Its effect is that the life force flows through the very intricate channels called *nadis*, gastric fire is kindled, and the stomach becomes free of all diseases." (5/1)

This asana stretches the pelvic region and stimulates blood circulation. The ovaries, uterus, and entire reproductive system are revitalized, and their efficiency enhanced. The pose also helps maintain a balanced attitude to sex. In humans, the spinal column is perpendicular to the ground, whereas in animals, it is parallel to the ground with the heart below it. Because of our upright position, the human heart is more prone to strain and disease.

In the full pose Pashchimottanasana, the spine is horizontal and parallel to the ground, so that the heart rests. Because you are pregnant, however, you will not do the full pose, but rather concentrate on the concavity in the first part of the pose.

1 Sit in Dandasana (page 64) and place your feet 1 to 1½ feet apart.

2 Inhale, lift your arms, and extend them upward in Urdhva Hasta Pashchimottanasana (see photo, page 88) so as to lift your torso away from your buttocks and legs.

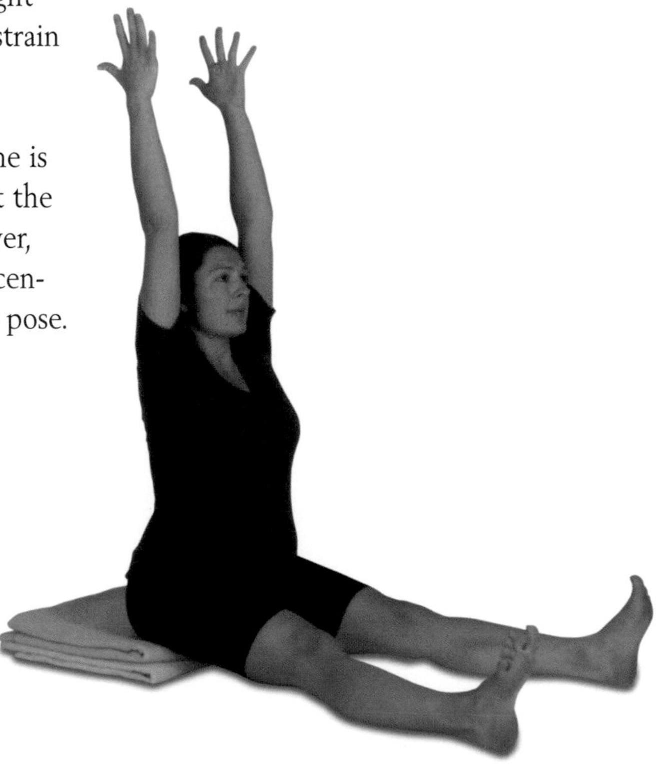

3 Maintaining the extension, exhale, and extend your hands forward to your feet. Have a belt around your feet and grip it in. Pull the outer edges of your feet towards you and extend your inner heels and the balls of your big toes.

4 Inhale and stretch your spine upward, making it concave. Raise your back, waist, and breastbone and lift your head.

5 Stretch your arms, lock your elbows, and tuck in your shoulder blades to open your chest and lift its front.

6 Breathing normally, stay in the pose for 20 to 30 seconds.

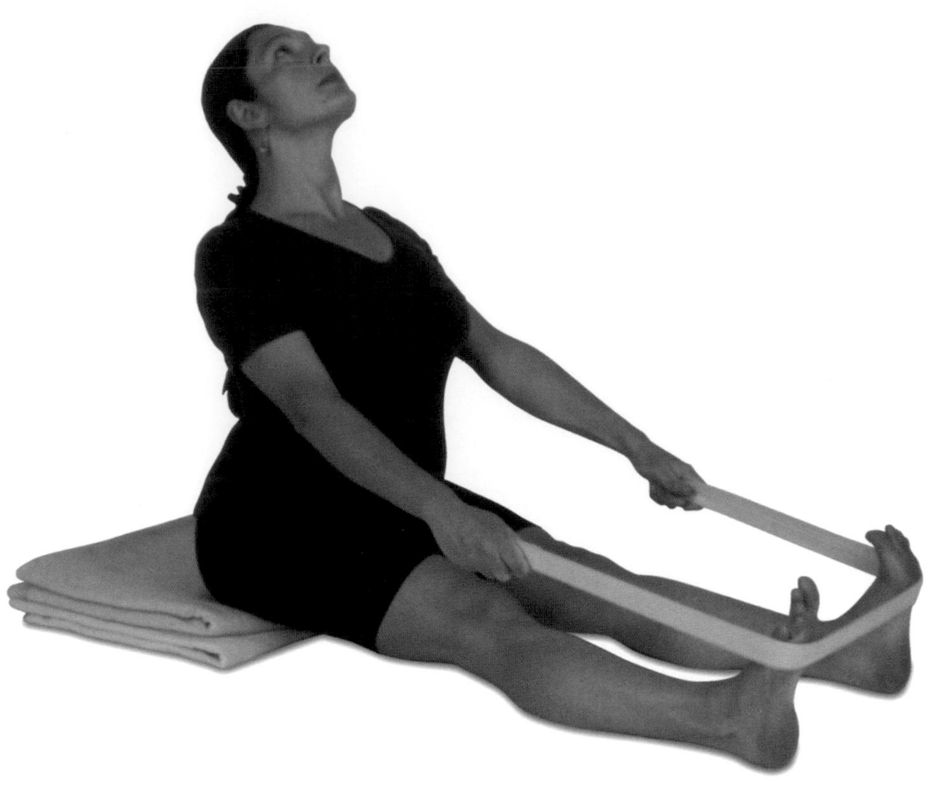

Coming out of the pose

Maintain the length and lift of your chest, inhale, and come back to Dandasana.

CHECK YOURSELF

- *Move your floating ribs forward and extend them towards your chest.*
- *Keep your stretched legs completely on the floor.*
- *Bring your inner legs and knees down.*

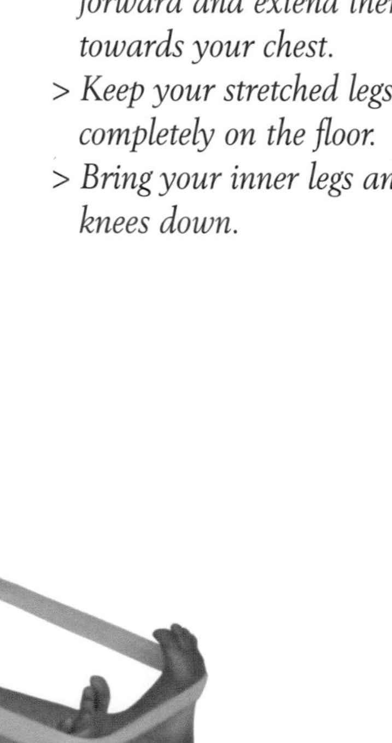

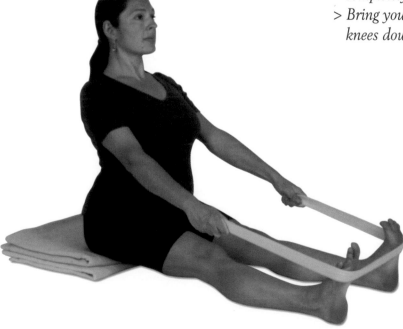

Trianga Mukhaikapada Pashchimottanasana

Three limbs intense west stretch pose, concave back

1st trimester: yes
2nd trimester: yes
3rd trimester: no

Triang means "three parts": foot, knees, and buttocks, and *mukhaikapada* means "the face and one leg." All these parts play different roles, along with the extension of the torso, to complete the pose.

1 Sit in Dandasana (page 64) on a 3-to-4-inch support.

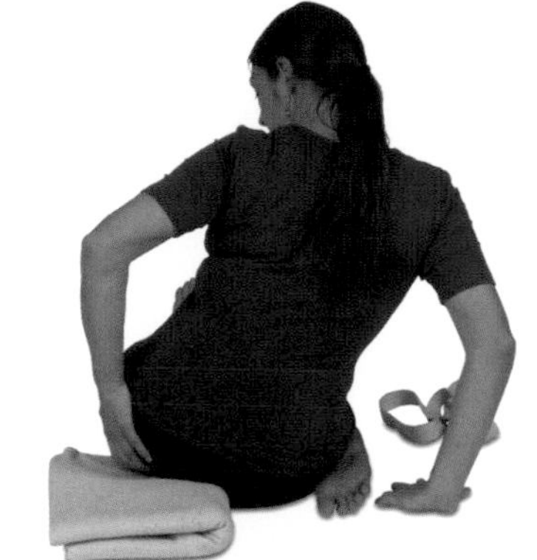

2 Shift your pelvis, so that the support is under your left buttock. Bend your right leg at the knee. Hold your ankle with your right palm and fold the leg back. Keep the toes of your right foot extending backward by the side of your right hip joint. Touch the inner side of your right calf to the outer side of your right thigh. The inner side of your right thigh should touch the inner side of your left thigh.

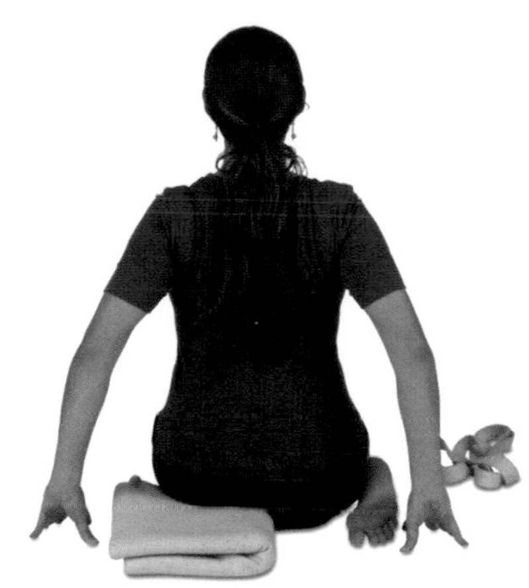

3 If you lean to the left, put more support under your left buttock.

4 Stretch your left leg forward.

5 Lift and extend your arms and hands upward in Urdhva Hasta Trianga Mukhaikapada Pashchimottanasana.

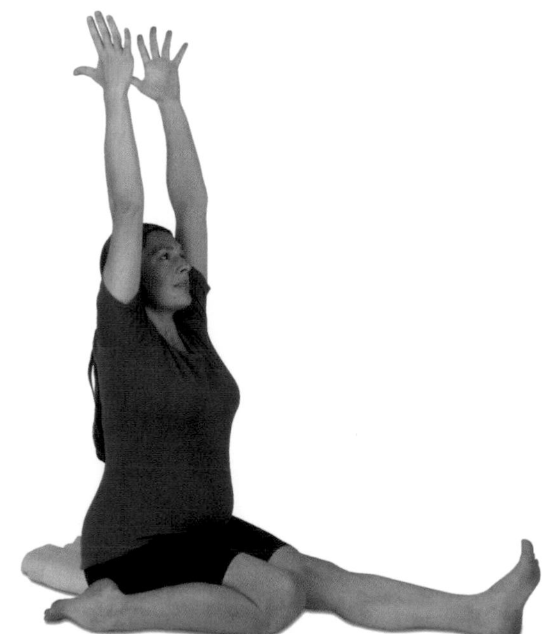

Benefits
Helps treat sprains in the ankles and knees
Improves flat feet and dropped arches, revitalizes the feet after a long day
Relaxes the groin and lower back
Lifts and tones the spine
Lifts the uterus, creates space for the fetus, and lessens heaviness in the pelvis; especially good for women who have had a miscarriage due to muscle weakness
Maintains the health of the reproductive organs

6 With an exhalation, extend your hands forward to your left foot, grip the foot with a belt, stretch your arms, lock your elbows, and tuck in your shoulder blades in Urdhva Mukha.

7 Lift your abdomen, chest, and breastbone. Raise your head and keep your spine concave.

8 Breathe normally and stay for 20 to 30 seconds.

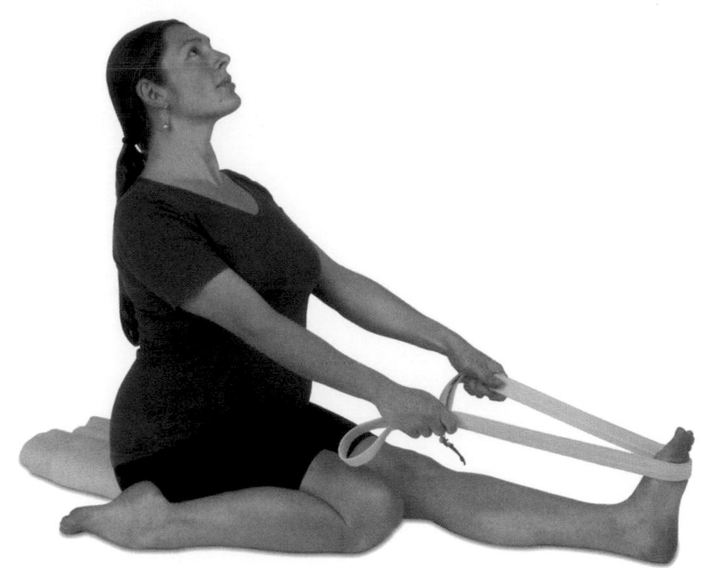

Coming out of the pose

Maintain the lift while coming back, stretch out your right leg to Dandasana, and repeat on the other side.

CHECK YOURSELF

- *Don't tilt your torso to the left; shift your weight to the right by bringing gravity to the middle of your right thigh.*
- *Extend the sides of your torso forward and up, lift your abdomen, chest and breastbone, raise your head, and keep your spine concave.*
- *Keep your left inner leg down and extended. Extend the inner arch of your left foot forward.*

1st and 2nd Trimesters: Beginners and Advanced Students

Practice in two parts: first, Urdhva Hasta (see step 5), and second, Urdhva Mukha (see step 6). If you still feel shaky, place your hands on either side of your hips.

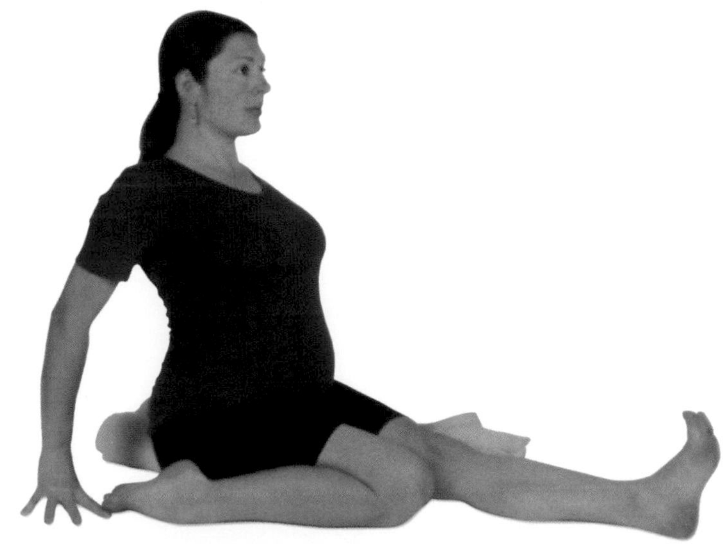

Twists
Parivritta Sthiti

Bharadvajasana 1
Torso twist 1 pose

1st trimester: yes
2nd trimester: yes
3rd trimester: yes

Twists without Compression

Even if you are fit and healthy during your pregnancy, back pain near your waist or tailbone is not uncommon. A spine that is not strong enough will become evident during advanced pregnancy, when your womb is heavier.

Some women experience back pain in the early stages of pregnancy, mostly in the waist region. In advanced pregnancy, it is the tailbone area that is most affected.

Bharadvajasana offers relief, but since it is a twisting asana, you may be somewhat anxious regarding its safety. It is important to understand that Bharadvajasana is not merely twisting, but twisting with a lift. You have to raise your spine straight up first, so that its concave state is retained, and then turn to the side. Most practitioners neglect this, unfortunately, which invites trouble in the form of body pain.

A compressed spine can never provide lateral movement. You have to raise your torso in such a way that you don't stoop, and only then turn to your side in Bharadvajasana, maintaining the axis of the spine without shifting. In other words, you don't merely rotate, but lift first and then rotate—a vertical lift and then a lateral twist.

As you twist, be careful that your chest does not narrow. Maintain the expansion of your chest and lift—don't compress—the floating ribs at the bottom corner of your torso. Never force the twisting movement, especially as it becomes more difficult as your pregnancy progresses.

Benefits

Bharadvajasana 1 (and on a chair) is a twist that we really recommend for pregnancy, because it does not compress the abdomen.

Strengthens the lower spine and firms the waist muscles

Works on the dorsal and lumbar (mid and lower) regions of the spine, removing stiffness and pain

Beneficial pose for slipped disks, since there is no compression of the spine, but rather a vertical extension

Relieves flatulence and constipation

In advanced pregnancy, helps treat digestion-related problems

Eases the pain of the baby kicking: if you feel the kick on the right side, rotate to that side, and vice versa.

Bharadvajasana 1

1 Sit in Dandasana (page 64), keeping a folded blanket, or bolster or block that is 2 to 3 inches high, under your buttocks.

2 Bend both legs and move your shins backward to the left, so that your feet are adjacent to your left hip.

3 Rest your buttocks on the blanket. Your feet should be lower than your buttocks. Lift your torso so that your spine is extended upward. Take one or two breaths.

4 Exhale and turn your torso to the right, so that your right shoulder moves to the right and your left shoulder comes forward. Turn your chest and abdomen to the right.

5 Place your right hand behind your right buttock and turn your spine more. Tuck your left shoulder blade in and revolve your right shoulder backward.

6 Take a breath or two. Turn your head and neck to the right and look straight ahead.

7 Breathing normally, remain in this position for 30 seconds.

Help

If you're heavy, or experience cramps in the buttocks (in the left buttock when you rotate to the right and vice versa), then use a higher support and a block for your hand.

This also ensures that your lower abdomen is not compressed and makes it easier to turn. During the last stage of pregnancy, your abdomen often becomes heavy on one side because of the shifting of the baby and its moving into position.

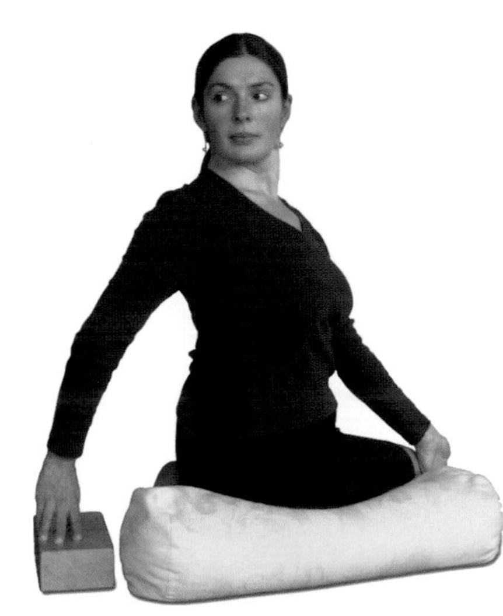

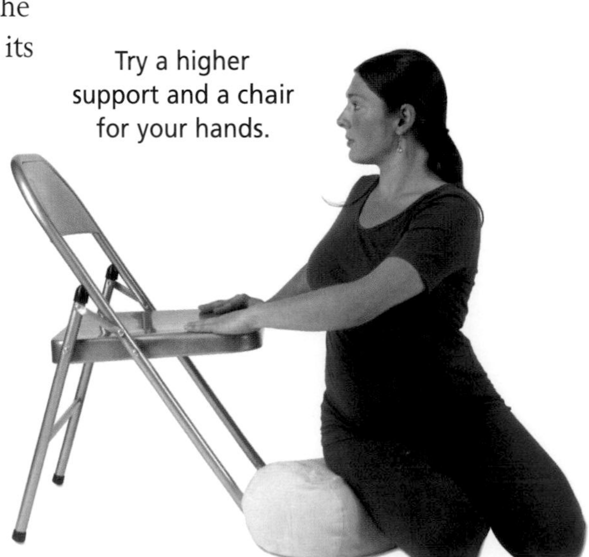

Try a higher support and a chair for your hands.

CHECK YOURSELF

- *Tuck your shoulder blades in and lift your breastbone.*
- *Keep your spine erect and turn on its axis.*
- *Keep your knee in the same position as you turn; it tends to move to the right.*
- *Don't lean backward; keep your right hip and right shoulder in line.*
- *Maintaining the lift and expansion of your chest, inhale, bring back your hands, bring your torso forward, and straighten your legs.*
- *Bend your legs and move your shins backward to the right side, adjacent to your right hip, and return to Dandasana.*

Practice next to a wall so that your hips can twist more easily:

1 Sit with your right hip touching the wall.

2 Place both feet near your left hip.

3 Place your right knee and thigh adjacent to the wall.

4 Place both hands on the wall in line with your shoulders.

5 Inhale, raise your torso, and turn it.

6 Change sides.

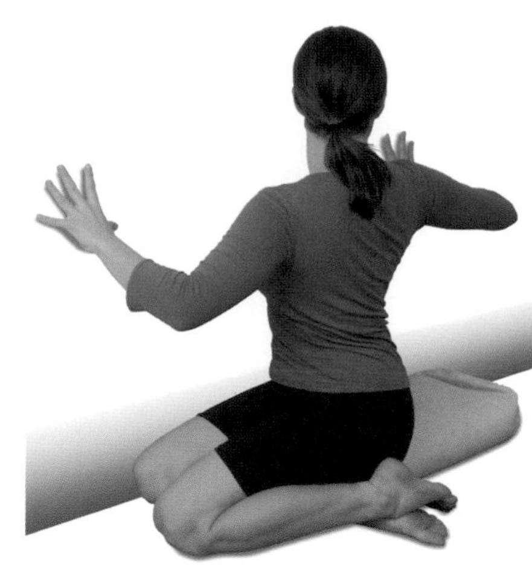

Bharadvajasana on a Chair

1 Sit on a chair sideways with your right shoulder against the back of the chair.

2 Place your thighs and feet parallel, slightly apart.

3 Sit erect and look straight ahead.

4 Inhale, and raising your torso, turn your chest to the right.

5 Hold on to the backrest of the chair.

6 Keep your torso lifted, your shoulder blades tucked into your back, and your shoulder bones rolled back.

7 Lift your breastbone, moving your spine in between your shoulder blades.

8 Exhale and turn your head to look over your right shoulder.

9 Repeat to the other side.

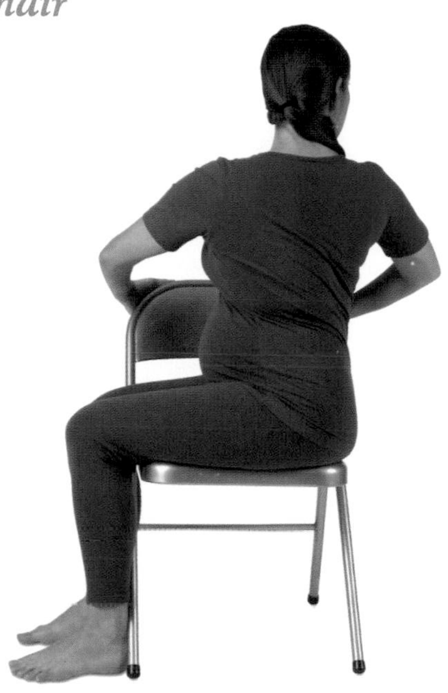

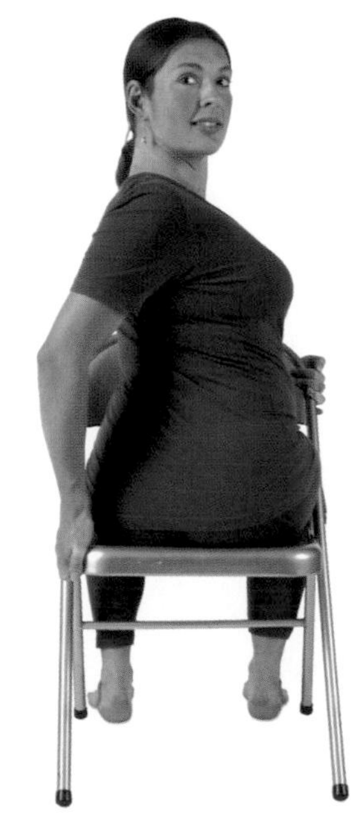

Coming out of the pose

Inhale, maintain the lift, release your hands, and come back.

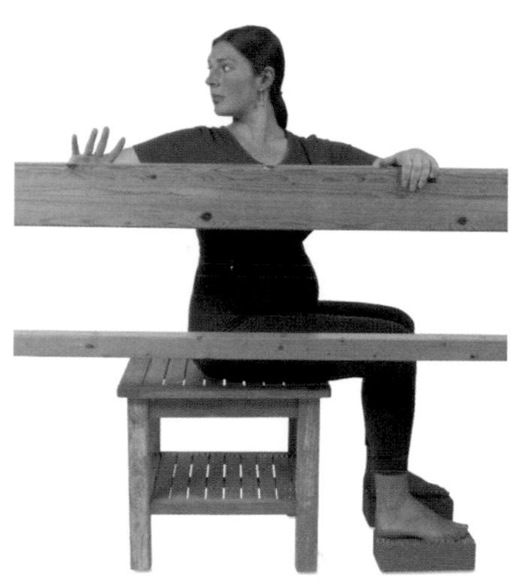

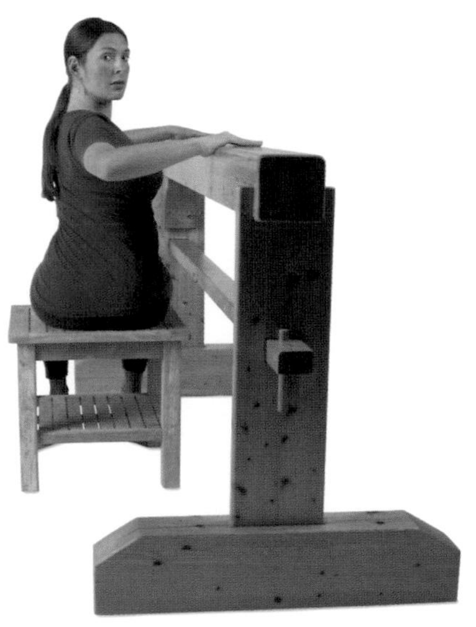

with trestle

Parshva Svastikasana, Parshva Ardha Padmasana (half Lotus seat), Parshva Virasana, Parshva Baddha Konasana, and Parshva Janu Shirshasana

Twisting poses

Here we reintroduce some of the basic asanas that you already know, but with an added twisting action. Some of the asanas not only twist and extend the sides, but are also a twisted forward bend with your head resting on a chair; they allow you to both twist and rest.

Follow the same technique as in Bharadvajasana, and remember:

- Inhale, raise your spine and torso, exhale, and turn your chest to the right.
- Remain seated while you twist.

NOTE

If you have a history of miscarriage, avoid all Parshvas in your 1st trimester.

Twisting in Svastikasana
on a raised surface with a chair, resting the head

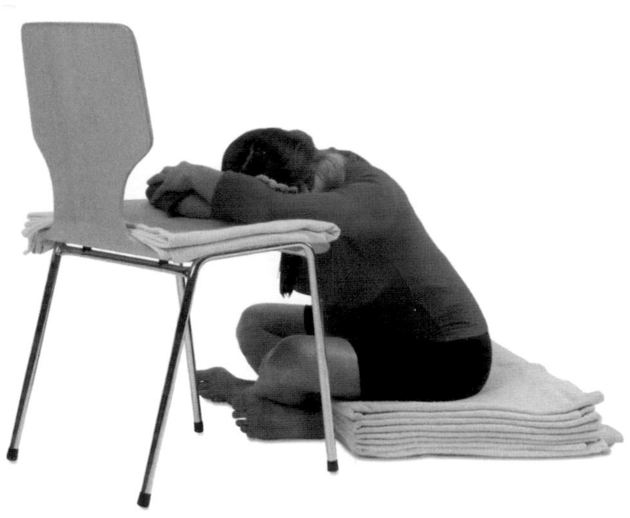

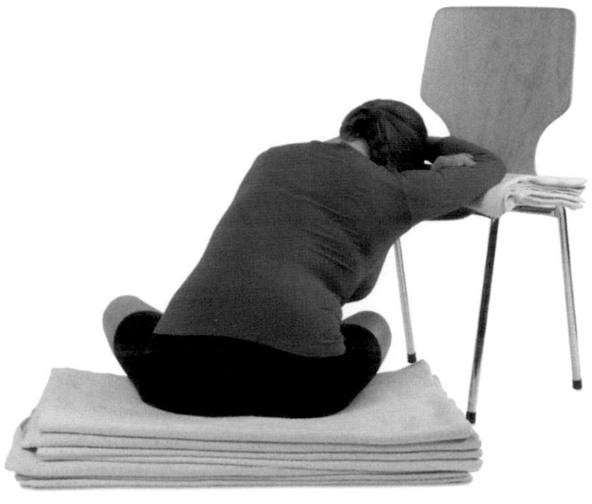

Twisting in Ardha Padmasana or Padmasana
on a raised surface with the wall

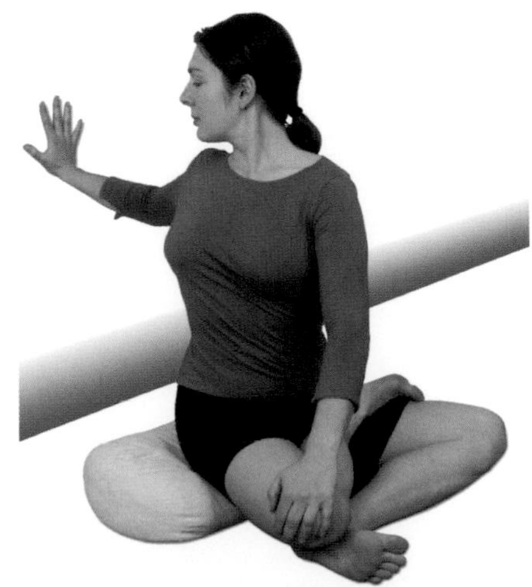

Twisting in Virasana
on a raised surface with the wall

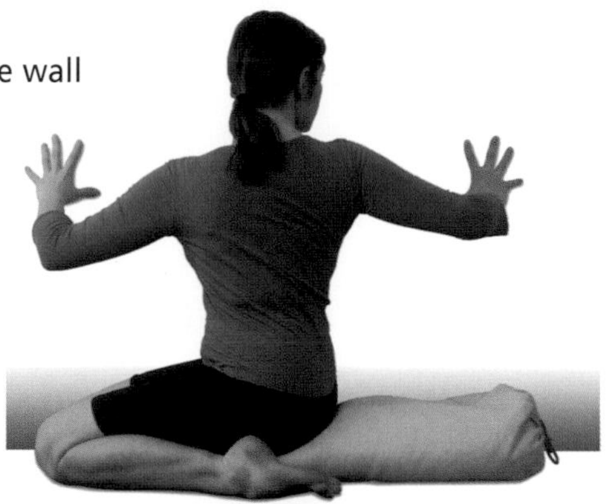

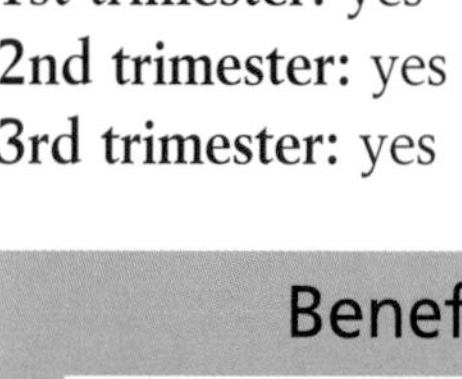

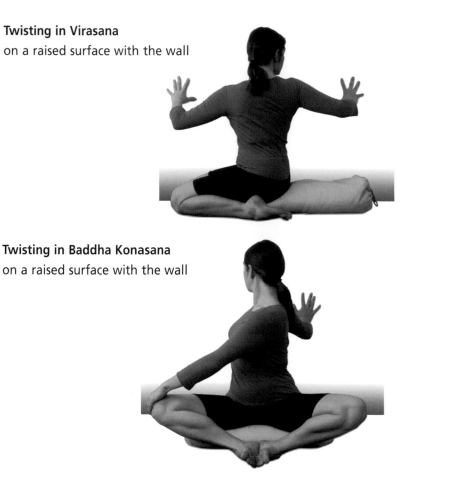

1st trimester: yes
2nd trimester: yes
3rd trimester: yes

Benefits

Provide relief from dizziness and fatigue

Help treat nausea, back pain, and toxemia

Assist in flushing the kidneys

Twisting in Baddha Konasana
on a raised surface with the wall

Twisting in Janu Shirshasana
on a raised surface with a chair, resting the head

1 Sit in Dandasana (page 64).

2 Spread your legs to Upavishtha Konasana (page 70).

3 Bend your left leg, move your heel towards the left side of your groin, and turn your sole up towards the ceiling.

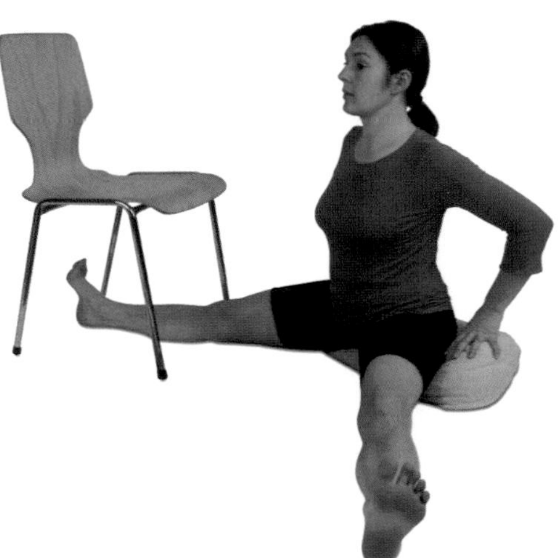

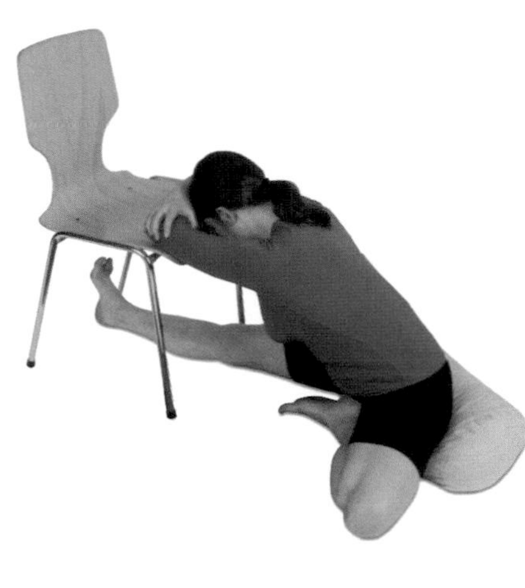

4 Extend your right leg, keeping the foot in the upright position of Upavishtha Konasana.

5 Pull the flesh away from your buttock bones, so that you can spread them.

6 Extend the sides of your torso, lift your breastbone, and turn to the right.

7 Put your lower arms on the chair and rest your head either on your lower arms or in front of them on the chair.

DETAILED DESCRIPTIONS OF ASANAS FOR ALL STUDENTS

Inversions
Viparita Sthiti

Introducing Inversions

Inverted poses are beneficial for your mental and physical health, especially during pregnancy. These asanas foster an attitude of detachment from habitual worries, and help you develop tolerance, moderation, and emotional stability. They nourish healthy thoughts and encourage harmonious growth for you and your baby. The asanas calm your mind, bringing freedom from mental tension and stress.

Although inverted asanas can be frightening at first for some, many pregnant women enjoy these poses the most and even perform them to the exclusion of others.

Weakness, fatigue, low spirits, and a feeling of heaviness are all common during pregnancy, caused by disturbances in the functioning of the different body systems. Inverted poses alleviate these complaints.

The poses bring about harmony among the circulatory, endocrinologic, and nervous systems and improve the health of the respiratory system. They help regulate blood pressure and improve blood supply, distribution, and circulation, which helps prevent varicose veins. Inverted asanas help maintain hormonal balance, enhance the functioning of the glandular system, and supply energy to the nerves.

The asanas play an important role in building up and rejuvenating brain cells. The brain needs one-sixth of the entire blood supply; inversions help keep the blood flowing to the brain without pressure on the arteries. This is why you'll feel both exhilarated and serene after practicing these poses.

The following inverted poses are suitable and beneficial to pregnant women:

- Shirshasana
- Viparita Dandasana
- Sarvangasana
- Halasana
- Setu Bandha Sarvangasana
- Viparita Karani

You'll be able to tell by your breathing whether you can continue practicing a particular asana. When the inversions cause your breathing to become heavy and labored, it's time to stop.

Up to the seventh month, you can probably perform all the inversions with no change in your breathing pattern. After that, although the exact timing depends on the size of your abdomen and your general constitution, you should drop the asanas in the following order:

Halasana: It's likely that you'll feel your first indication that it's time to stop while performing this asana. You'll feel choked, your face will redden, and the feeling of lightness disappears.

Sarvangasana

Shirshasana

Viparita Dandasana

Setu Bandha Sarvangasana

Viparita Karani

Two of the asanas, Setu Bandha Sarvangasana and Viparita Karani, can remain comfortable until the end of your pregnancy, right up to the day of your delivery.

Salamba Shirshasana
Headstand pose

1st trimester: yes
2nd trimester: yes, heels apart
3rd trimester: yes, feet apart

Sarvangasana and Halasana are prerequisites to learning Shirshasana, because it is essential to keep your spine straight. If you can't perform the previous two asanas properly, then it is quite impossible to do Shirshasana. If you have newly taken up the practice of Yoga during pregnancy, then you should practice Shirshasana only under the guidance of an expert teacher.

You should perform Shirshasana at or near the beginning of your Yoga practice, so that you're not tired. Always follow Shirshasana with Sarvangasana to avoid an irritated state of mind, and practice them both for an equal period of time. Alternatively, you can practice Sarvangasana for longer, but never Shirshasana for longer.

When you're pregnant, there are even more norms to follow; for example, you have to follow the following sequence, known as a chain:

- Before Shirshasana: Maha Mudra, Adho Mukha Shvanasana, and Uttanasana
- After Shirshasana, reverse order: Uttanasana, Adho Mukha Shvanasana, and Maha Mudra
- Continuation: Viparita Dandasana, Sarvangasana, Halasana, Setu Bandha Sarvangasana, and Viparita Karani

You should not perform Shirshasana with collapsed spinal muscles. It's important to strengthen and extend these muscles, so that there is no compression. Normally the problems encountered with Shirshasana are collapsed spinal muscles and sagging torso.

High blood pressure and heart palpitations are among the two most common problems during a woman's pregnancy. Prevention is always better than cure; to prevent a sudden rush of blood to the head, or a sudden rise in blood pressure, follow the chain of asanas for Shirshasana above.

Benefits

- Strengthens the thigh muscles
- Alleviates heaviness and fatigue
- Makes you feel fresh and energetic
- Helps treat toxemia
- Relieves severe vomiting, blurred vision, bleeding, vaginal discharge, swelling, varicose veins, and cramps
- Tones up the respiratory, circulatory, endocrinologic, and nervous systems. When these systems function well together, they improve the reproductive system and your ability to carry and nourish the fetus. As a result, the fetus will benefit from proper health and growth.

Many people believe the misconception that inverted poses endanger the brain and nervous system. Think about it: if that were true, then people who stand on their feet for hours at a time would develop thrombosis (blood clot). Just as this does not happen, standing on your head should not cause any harm, if done properly. You can learn to stand on your head as effortlessly as you stand on your feet.

1 When you first start to practice Shirshasana, we recommend that you work against the wall, or better still, at the corner of two walls. While performing Shirshasana against the wall will maintain your balance, using the support of a corner will also keep your torso and legs in line with your head.

2 On top of a sticky mat fold a blanket four times and place it in a corner, letting it touch both walls. Kneel on the floor as in Virasana (page 72), facing the corner.

3 Interlock your fingers to the base and keep your thumbs touching, forming a semicircular cup. Place your cupped hands 2 to 3 inches away from the corner. Your little fingers and thumbs should be parallel. Keeping your hands more than 3 inches away from the corner will cause the following errors to occur in the final position:

- Your spinal column will bend and lose its extension.
- Your stomach will protrude.
- The weight of your body will bear down painfully on your elbows.
- Your face will get red and your eyes swollen and puffy.

4 Rest your forearms on the blanket, with your elbows in line. Your wrists should be upright, with the inner bone of the forearms touching the blanket and the outer bone directly above.

5 The distance between your elbows should be the width of your shoulders, so that your arms remain straight. If the distance is too small, there will be painful pressure on your side ribs; if it's too large, your chest won't expand and there will be pressure on your cervical (upper) spine.

6 In this position, your palms, forearms, and the space between your elbows and chest form an equilateral triangle. Don't move your elbows and forearms once you've adjusted them.

7 Raise your buttocks so that your elbows and shoulders are in line and your head is in line with your palms, and breathe normally.

8 Exhale and place the crown of your head on the blanket, so that the back of your head remains parallel to the wall and ½ an inch away from your little finger. Keep the back of your head in the cup of your hands, and don't press your head between your wrists. Your ears should be parallel to each other. Remain in this position and take a few breaths.

9 Exhale and raise your knees, keeping your toes on the floor. Straighten your legs and bring your feet in. Your torso should be at a right angle to the floor.

10 Keep your legs firm and pull your kneecaps in. Stay in this position for a few seconds and breathe normally.

11 Bend your knees slightly, exhale, lift both legs with a jump, and support your back and buttocks against the wall. If your spine is leaning backward, extend it up. Your legs are still bent at the knees.

12 Lift your feet up and rest them against the wall and straighten your legs into Shirshasana. Your buttocks, the back of your legs, and your heels will be touching the wall. You should straighten your legs within a few seconds of jumping into head balance.

13 Try to take your buttocks off the wall and develop your ability to bear your weight on your arms, head, and torso. Constant use of the wall for support will lead to a bent spine, so you must eventually learn to leave it. Stay as long as you can—at least 1 minute—in this final position of Shirshasana, breathing normally and observing the points in "Check Yourself."

Before you start with Shirshasana, practice the following:

- Maha Mudra (page 79)
- Adho Mukha Shvanasana (page 62)
- Uttanasana (concave back), (page 60)

Afterwards, follow the technique for Shirshasana below.

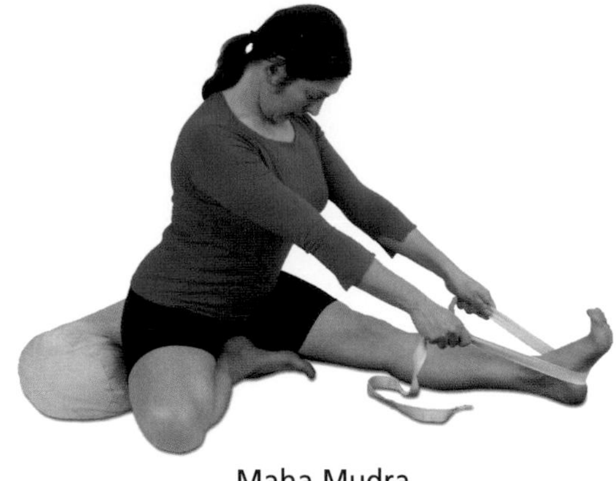

Maha Mudra

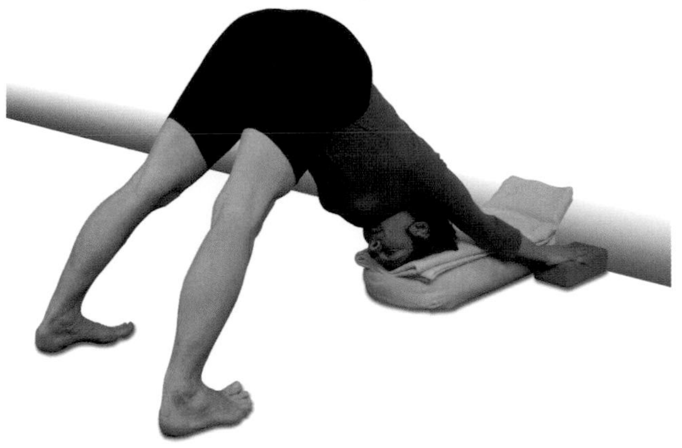

Adho Mukha Shvanasana

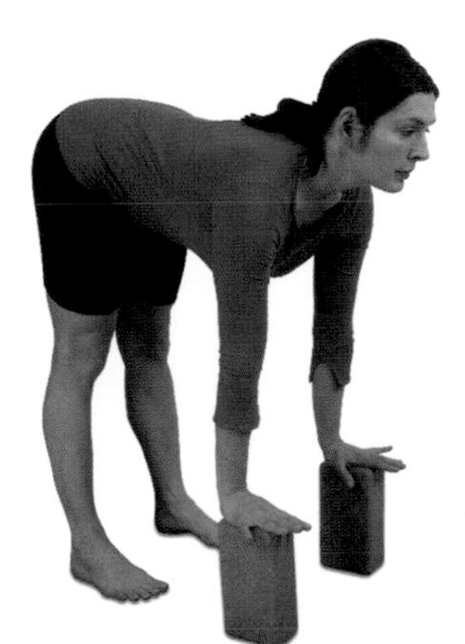

Uttanasana (concave back)

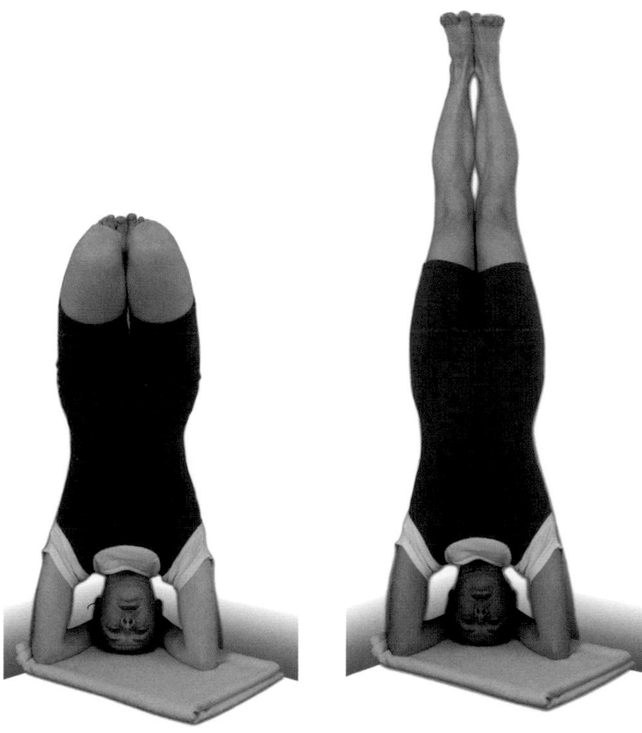

first months of pregnancy

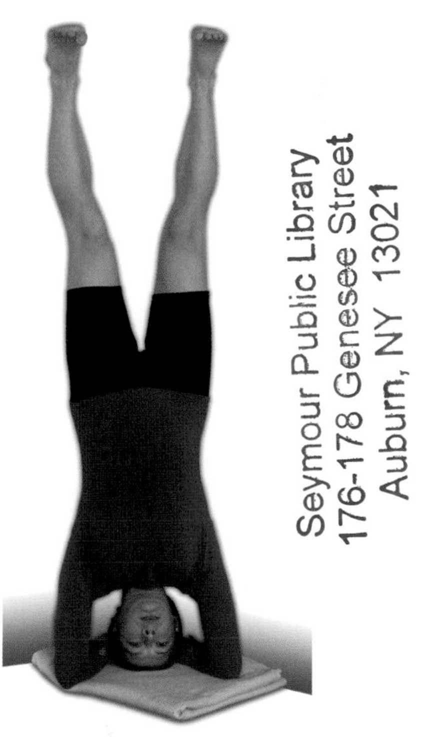

when the abdomen grows, feet apart

DETAILED DESCRIPTIONS OF ASANAS FOR ALL STUDENTS

CHECK YOURSELF

- *> Lift up your breastbone so that your cervical (upper) spine is not compressed and you don't feel the weight of your body on your head.*
- *> Lift your side ribs and broaden your chest so that the dorsal (mid) spine remains concave.*
- *> Keep your lumbar (lower) spine erect so that your abdominal muscles are stretched and your stomach does not protrude.*
- *> Keep your buttocks a little away from the wall so that your neck and the small of your back are balanced.*
- *> Support your heels against the wall so you don't lose your balance.*
- *> Take one foot 3 to 4 inches away from the wall and balance, keeping your legs straight. Tighten your buttocks and bring the other leg in line with the first.*
- *> Alternatively, you can keep your buttocks touching the wall.*

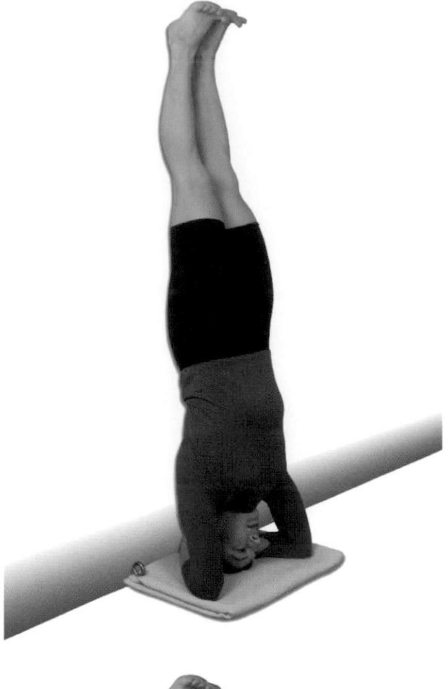

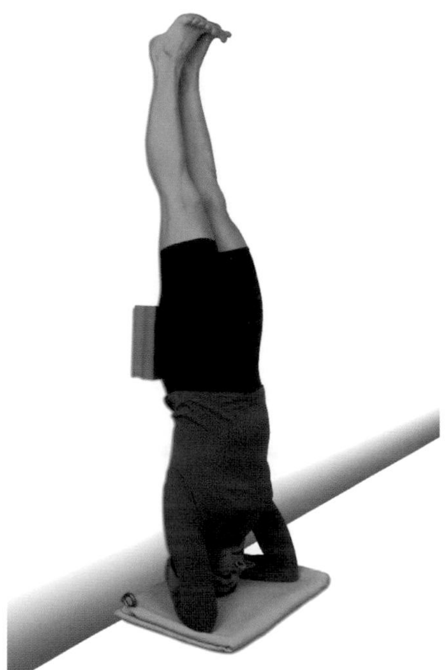

Help

If this is difficult, the teacher can place a pad in between the wall and your pelvis.

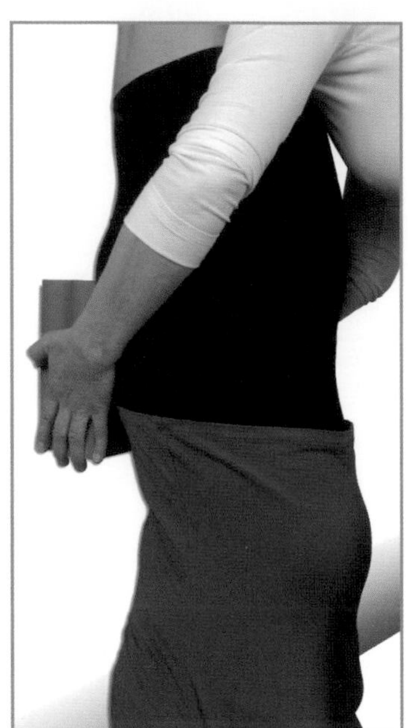

Coming out of the pose

Come down the way you began the pose by bending your legs and slowly taking your feet down.

Rest in Adho Mukha Virasana (page 76) and then start the sequence for after Shirshasana:
Uttanasana (concave back)
Adho Mukha Shvanasana
Maha Mudra

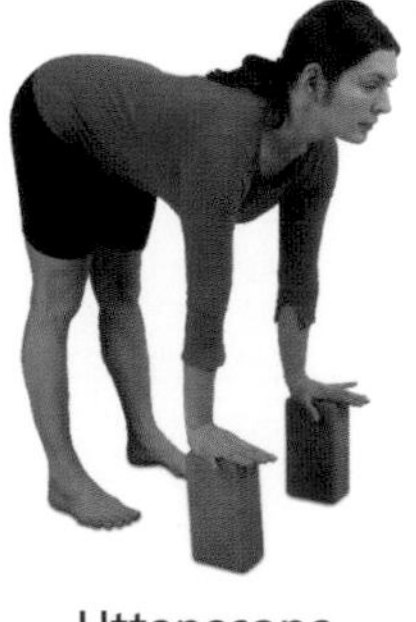

Uttanasana (concave back)

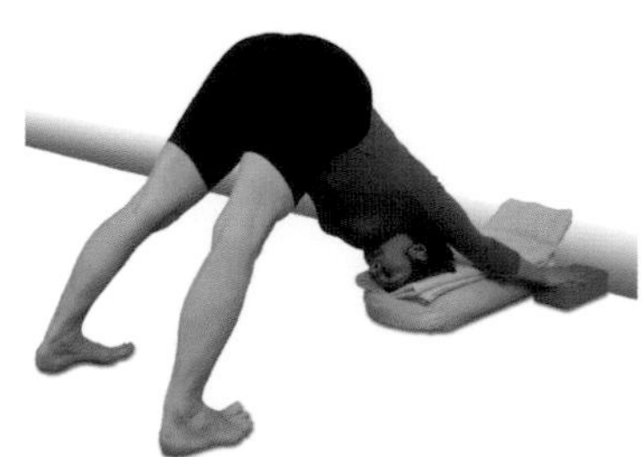

Adho Mukha Shvanasana

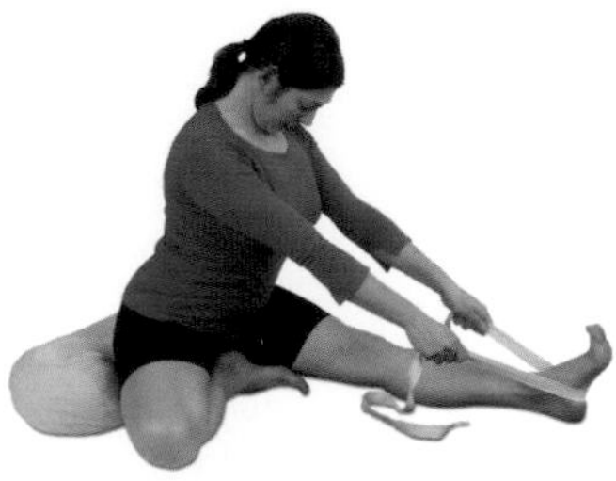

Maha Mudra

Special Instructions

When you're pregnant, you have to keep the lumbar (lower) spine in an ascended state, in other words continually lifting up, when you perform Shirshasana. Because your abdomen is heavy, your tendency will be to drop the lumbar region. It's important to lift your back, however, so that your abdominal muscles and those below the pelvic girdle do not get tightened.

You must also make sure that your spinal muscles don't collapse, which is an indication that your torso is not lifted up well enough.

1st Trimester

Your legs can be held up and together. In fact, this is beneficial at this stage of your pregnancy because it helps build up strength in the muscles.

2nd Trimester

As the fetus grows, you should vary the positioning of your legs: keep your toes together and your heels apart. This helps hold all your muscles together and helps support the waist muscles in ascending.

3rd Trimester

You may find that you need to keep your thighs apart, too. This lets the outer thigh muscles roll inward, keeping the groin supple. Be sure that you keep your thighs stretched up, to lessen the weight on your abdomen.

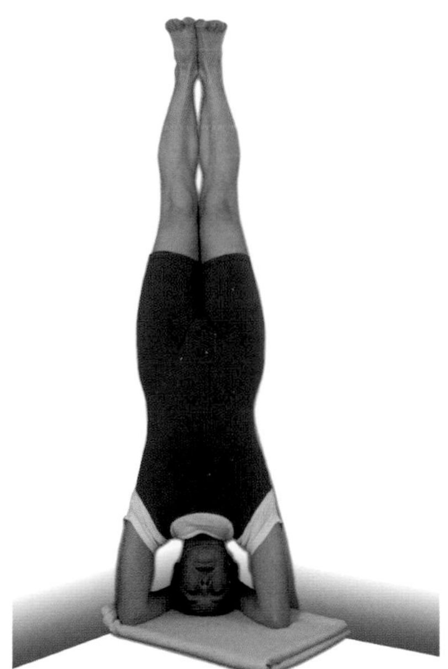

1st trimester

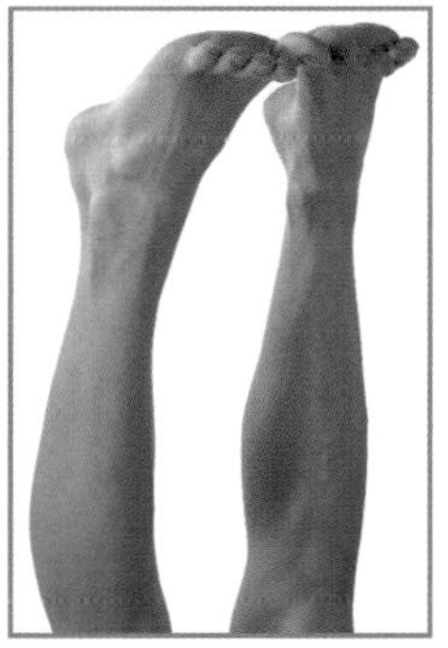

2nd trimester

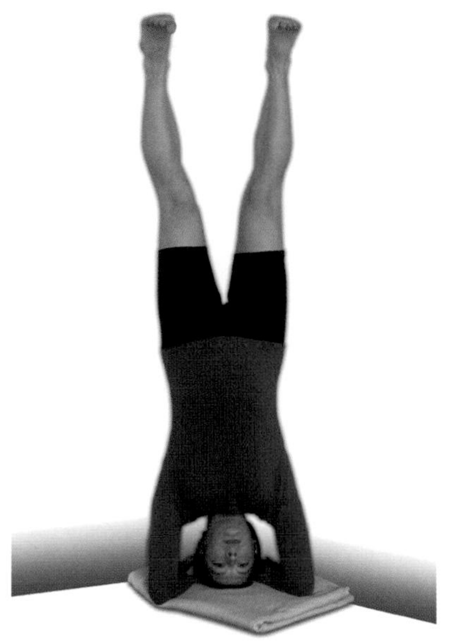

3rd trimester

Salamba Sarvangasana with chair
Shoulderstand pose with chair

Advanced Students
You can perform asanas without support in the first trimester only if you've gained proficiency in them before your pregnancy (at least five years of regular practice).

Beginners
If you're not already proficient in the asana in its unmodified form, then you should practice the modified version below with the help of a chair. You can continue it until your ninth month.

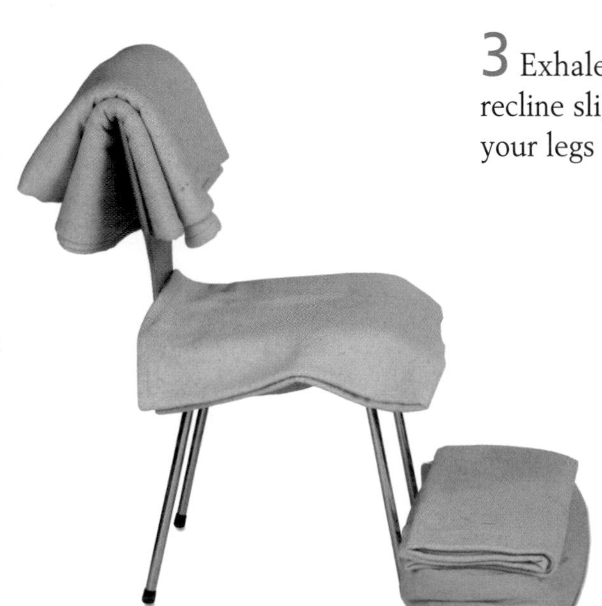

1 Put blankets over the seat and backrest of a chair and one or two bolsters in front of the chair.

2 Sit on the chair facing the back with your legs at the sides.

3 Exhale, and holding the chair, recline slightly backward and put your legs on the backrest.

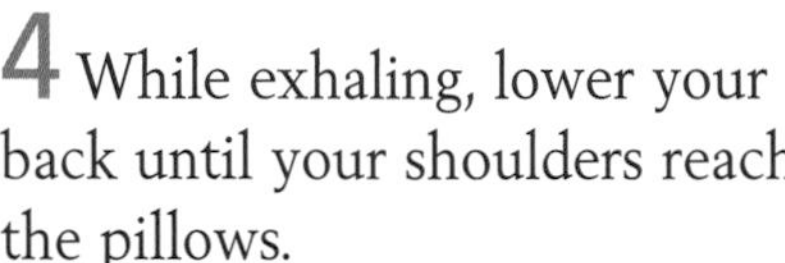

4 While exhaling, lower your back until your shoulders reach the pillows.

5 Pause and take a few normal breaths.

6 Put your arms underneath the chair, hold its back legs, and straighten your legs.

7 Stay in this final position for 5 minutes, breathing normally.

8 If you experience compression of the diaphragm, keep your legs apart.

9 You'll be safe in this form of Sarvangasana, because your lower back is supported and held up by the chair.

CHECK YOURSELF

> *Make sure that your back, from the waist to the buttocks, remains on the seat of the chair.*
> *Don't let your throat get compressed.*
> *Don't cave in your chest.*
> *Relax your face, eyes, mouth, and jaw.*

How to get into the pose

1st trimester: yes
2nd trimester: yes
3rd trimester: yes

Benefits

Calms the brain and nerves

Improves blood circulation in the chest area

Particularly beneficial to prevent toxemia during pregnancy

Relieves flatulence and constipation

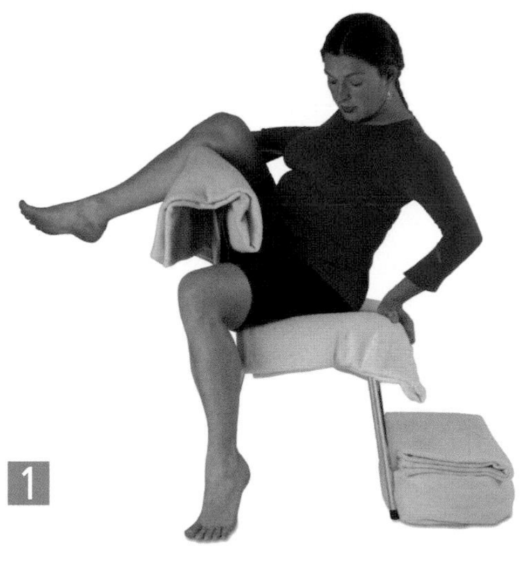

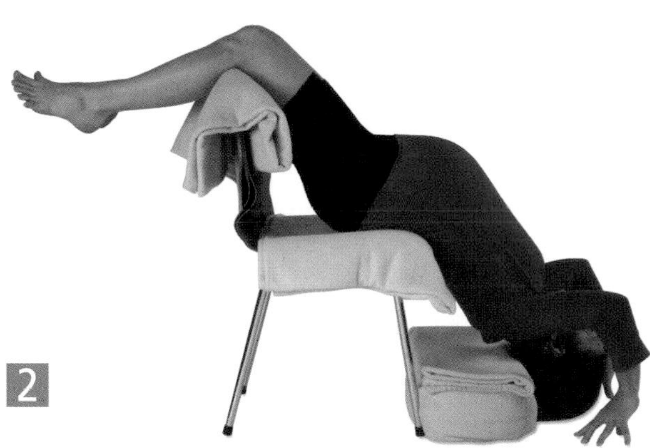

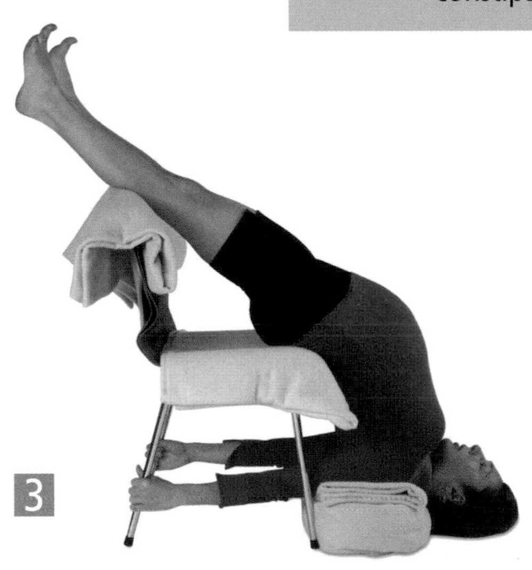

Coming out of the pose

1 Bend your knees.

2 Loosen your grip on the back legs of the chair and let go gradually, sliding down in the direction of your head smoothly.

3 Lie down on your back for a while.

4 To get up from the floor, first turn on your side and then get up.

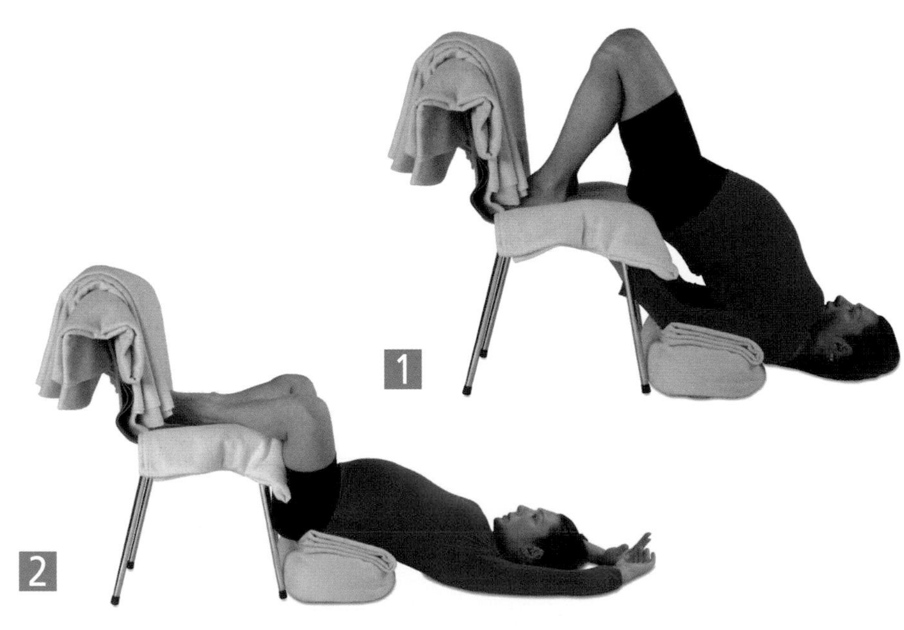

Ardha Halasana, Feet on Support
Half plough pose

1st trimester: yes
2nd trimester: yes
3rd trimester: yes

Beginners and Advanced Students

1 To make this asana safe and easy, have two chairs ready.

2 Sit on a chair, facing its backrest.

3 Slide down gradually onto your shoulder, using a bolster or a rolled blanket; hold on to the chair or have someone help you.

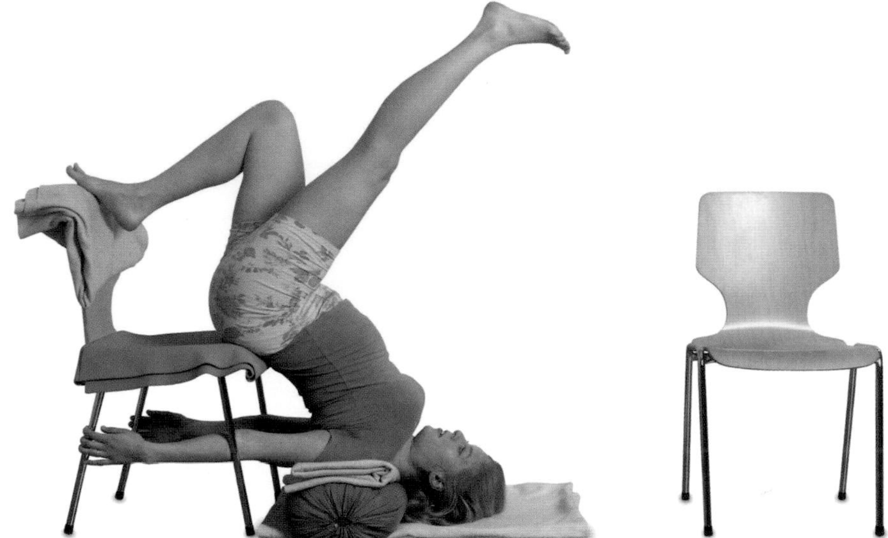

4 With bent knees, bring down your legs to the other side, onto a support such as a chair or box.

5 When your feet are firmly on the support, straighten your legs, bend your arms so that your elbows are inside the front legs of the chair, and support your back with your hands. Stay in the pose from 1 to 3 minutes. As you gain confidence, you can stay longer.

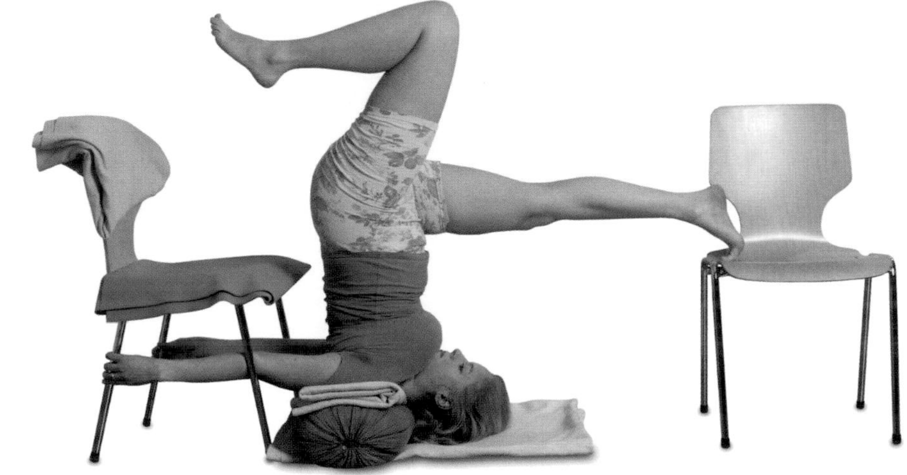

6 Keep your spine straight, make sure that your abdomen and chest are not compressed, and support your back with your hands; this should keep you from having a sensation of choking.

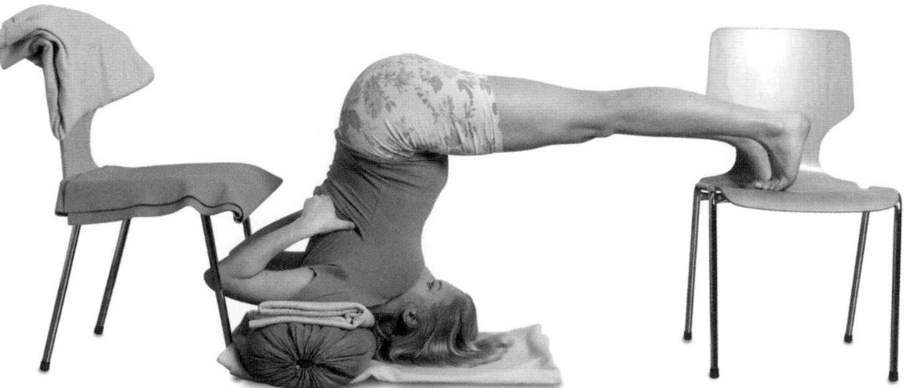

7 Keep your eyes open, looking at your navel. This frees you of tension, which is the way you should first learn to stay in this pose.

Coming out of the pose

Come back, grip the back legs of the chair, slowly lean your back against the seat, bend your legs, and slowly and gradually slide down. Rest your lower back on the pillow.

1st trimester: yes
2nd trimester: yes
3rd trimester: yes

Benefits

Strengthens and firms the spine, especially during the 1st trimester

Benefits those with a tendency to miscarry

Prevents sudden vaginal bleeding, especially during the early stages

Helps treat kidney problems, both as a regular precaution and during pregnancy

Corrects urinary problems

Calms down the brain and nerves, prevents sleeplessness

Ardha Halasana, Legs on Support
Half plough pose

Beginners and Advanced Students

1 Follow the technique on the previous page, with the variation that follows here.

2 Bring the chair or box closer, so that you rest your leg muscles. Your arms are held relaxed. Since the support keeps your spine raised, you don't have to make any effort to do so.

3 Keep your legs 6 to 8 inches apart if you feel that your uterus is being compressed.

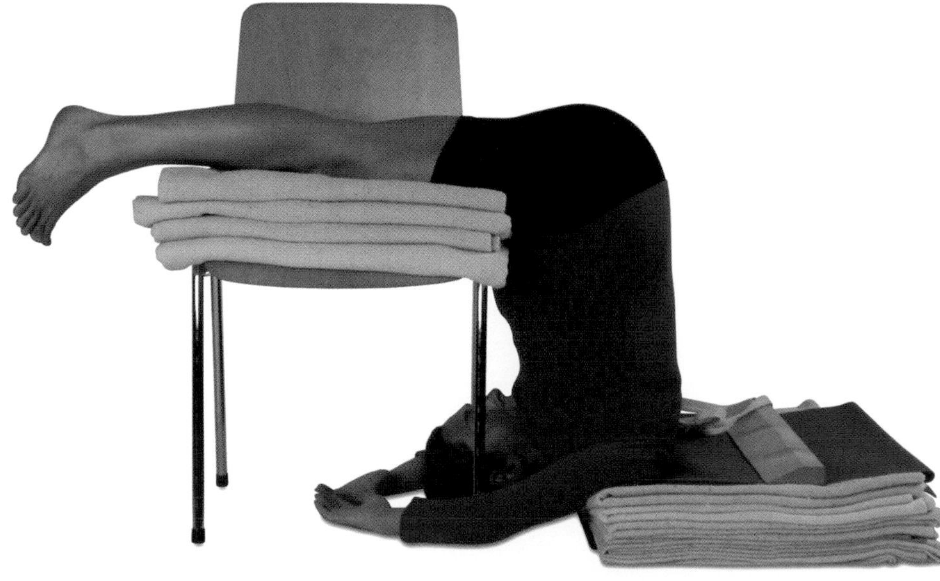

NOTE

In the advanced stages of pregnancy, you may find it difficult to rest your thighs on the chair. If that is so, rest your feet on the chair instead.

Ardha Supta Konasana, Legs Spread, Feet on Two Chairs
Half reclining angle pose

1st trimester: no
2nd trimester: yes
3rd trimester: yes

Benefits

Extremely beneficial for kidney problems and toxemia

Extremely beneficial for uterine complaints, such as pain and heaviness

Corrects the position of the uterus

Lessens vaginal discharge

Beginners and Advanced Students

As your pregnancy progresses, you can add this additional form of Ardha Halasana.

1 Sit on a chair in Sarvangasana (page 103). Have two chairs or a similar support behind you.

2 Put one leg after the other behind you onto the chairs.

3 Place the bottom of your toes on the support and straighten your legs.

4 Follow the technique for Ardha Halasana (page 104).

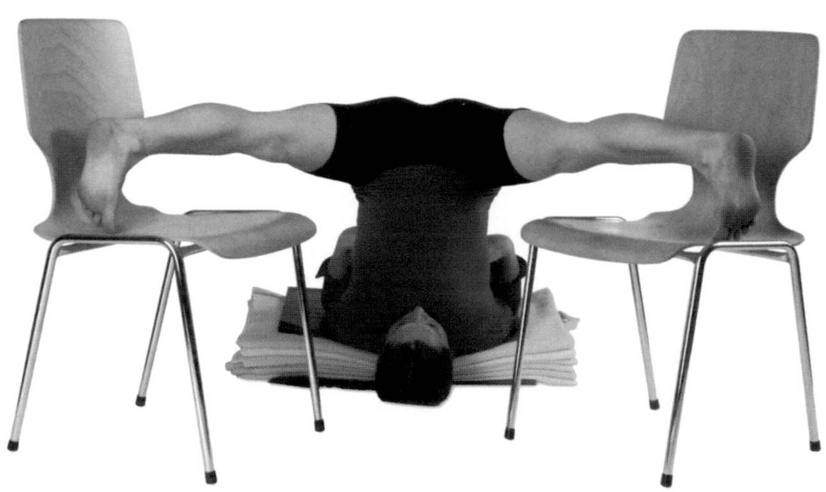

Ardha Supta Konasana, Legs Spread, Thighs on Two Chairs

1 Bring the support closer and rest your thighs and legs.

2 Follow the technique for Ardha Halasana.

NOTE
In the advanced stages of pregnancy, you may find it difficult to rest your thighs on the chair. If that is so, rest your feet on the chair instead.

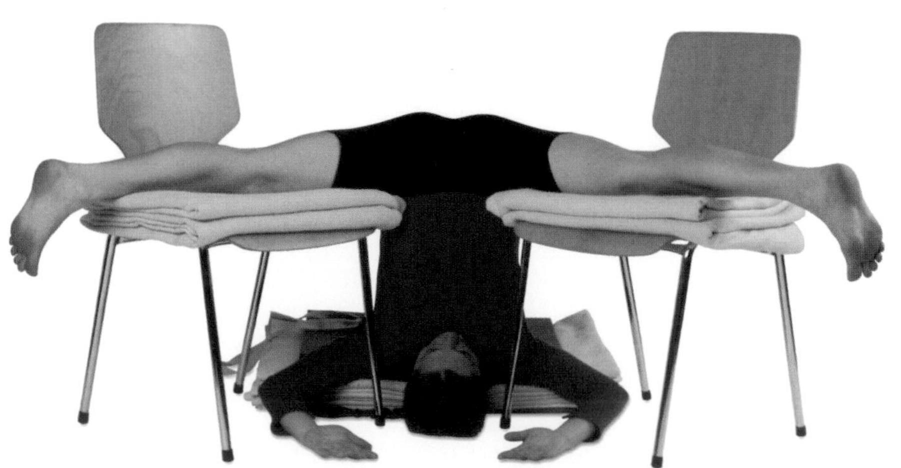

Setu Bandha Sarvangasana

Full bridge pose

Salamba Sarvangasana and Ardha Halasana, which have been demonstrated earlier in this chapter, are poses that scare many pregnant women, who therefore won't try them. If that includes you, then Setu Bandha Sarvangasana will not only build up your courage, but also compensate for the absence of Sarvangasana and Ardha Halasana. It is the one inverted asana that you should be sure to perform, even if you skip the others.

We recommend the practice of Setu Bandha Sarvangasana with props. Done this way, you can continue it throughout your pregnancy. In the later stages, if you feel a pull in the pelvic region, you can make a slight change in the method (*see Setu Bandha Sarvangasana Variations on page 109*).

◇

Technique 1: On a Bench

1st trimester: yes
2nd trimester: yes
3rd trimester: yes, as long as comfortable

This version is for the first and second trimesters. If, however, you feel the need to spread your feet, then you should follow Technique 2.

1 Place a folded blanket at the top end of a bench that is 10 inches high and a few pillows or folded blankets on the floor in front of it.

2 Lie lengthwise on the bench with your knees bent, keeping your head and torso on the bench. Breathe normally.

3 Exhale and slide down in the direction of your head until your head reaches the blankets on the floor.

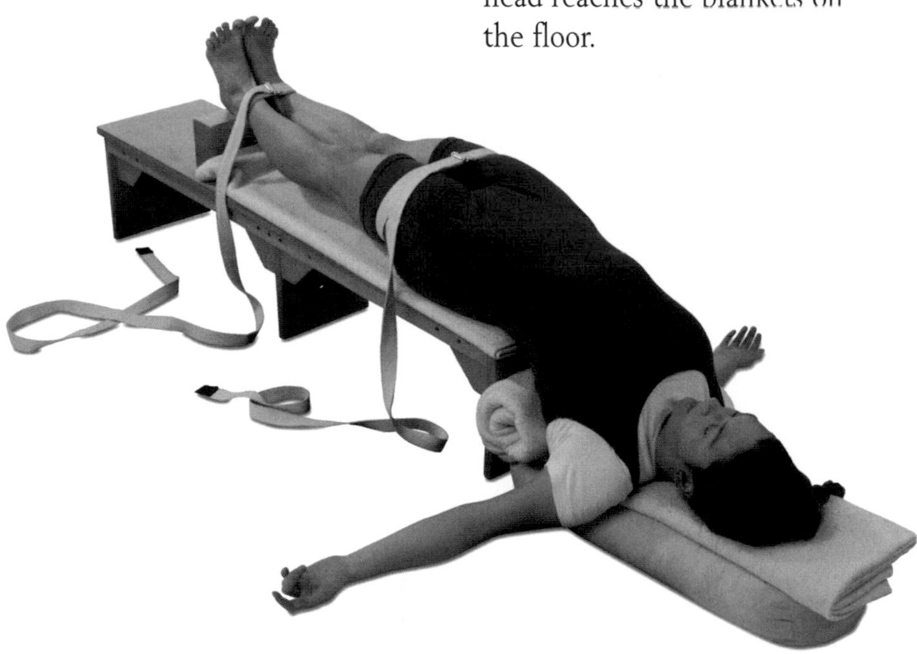

Benefits

- Creates a feeling of exhilaration
- Relaxes the diaphragm, which moves up and down freely in the increased space
- Removes heaviness
- Widens the pelvic girdle and eases abdominal tension
- Reduces vaginal discharge, headache, and lightheadedness
- Helps treat toxemia: if you have high blood pressure, perform this asana morning and evening.
- Promotes mental stability and balances mood
- Alleviates diabetes by regulating sugar level
- Aids the pituitary gland in maintaining hormonal balance (as do all the inversions), which benefits milk secretion

4 Slide down further until the back of your head and your shoulders also touch the blankets.

5 Straighten your legs so that your buttocks and legs remain on the bench.

6 Hold the sides of the bench. Keep your shoulders back and expand your chest.

7 Stretch your arms sideways and relax.

8 Breathing normally, remain in this final position for 3 to 5 minutes or as long as you are comfortable.

Coming out of the pose

Exhale, bend your knees, bring your feet in, and slide down in the direction of your head until your buttocks reach the floor.

CHECK YOURSELF

> Keep your face relaxed.
> Keep the back of your neck and your shoulders down.
> Keep your breastbone raised.

Technique 2: Supported

For the third trimester or when you don't feel comfortable with Technique 1.

1 Place bolsters and pillows as shown for Setu Bandha Sarvangasana, with legs bent on chair, for the 1st and 3rd trimesters.

2 Lie down with your back across the bolster and pillows (if the bolster is not enough) and a blanket under your head. Spread and extend your legs, as shown for the third trimester.

3 Keep your head rested and well supported.

4 Your spine is now effortlessly concave because of the support of the bolster and pillows, bringing freedom to the front of your torso.

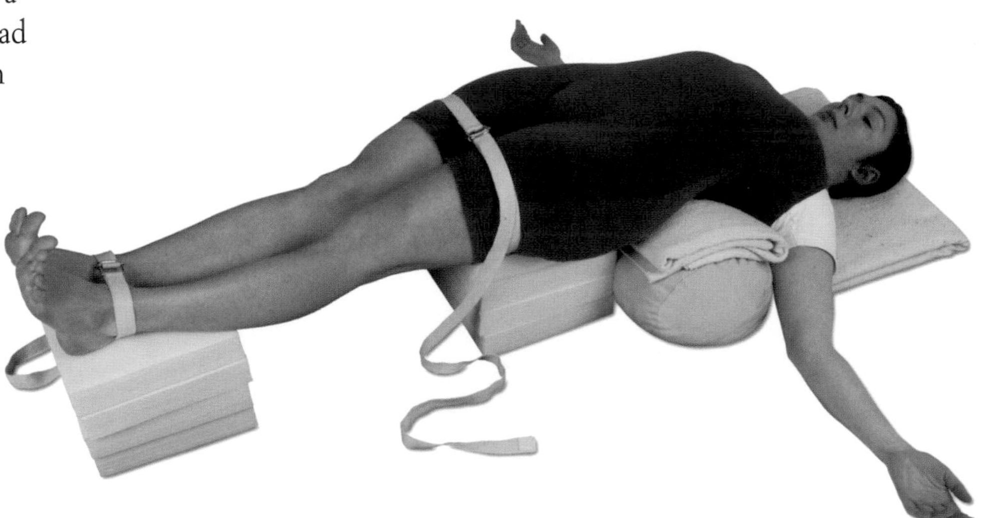

when no bench is available

SETU BANDHA SARVANGASANA: VARIATIONS

Setu Bandha Sarvangasana, on a Bench with Spread Legs

1st trimester: no
2nd trimester: yes
3rd trimester: yes

Towards the end of your pregnancy when your uterus is heavy, you may spread your legs farther apart. Place a belt around your upper thighs and around your feet in order to keep your spine and abdomen lifted.

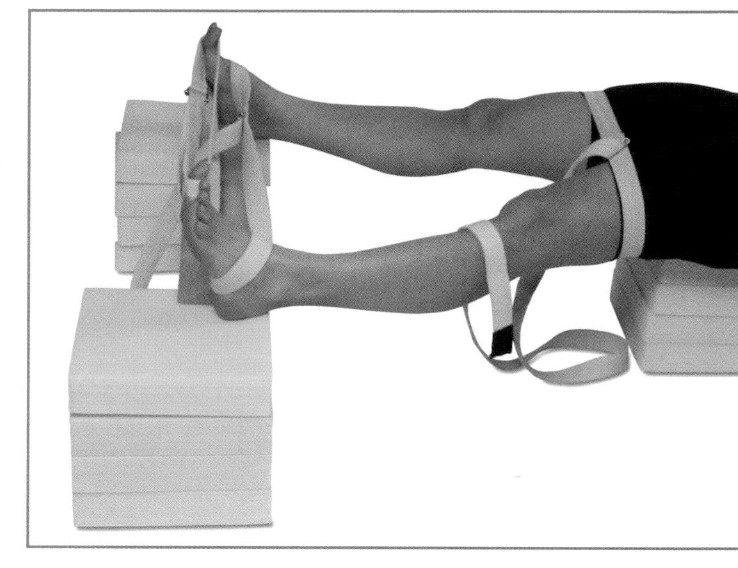

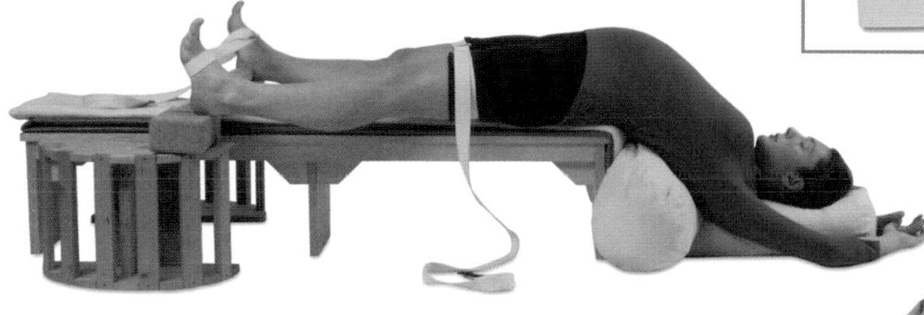

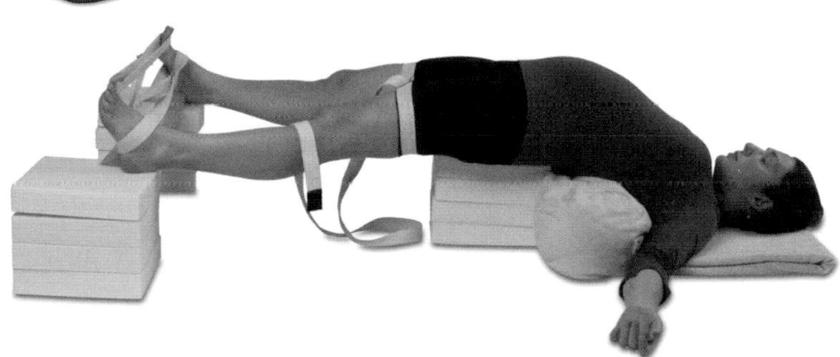

Viparita Karani Mudra, with Legs Bent on Chair

1st trimester: yes
2nd trimester: no
3rd trimester: yes

You can also bend your legs on a chair to increase the space in your chest and give more freedom to your heart.

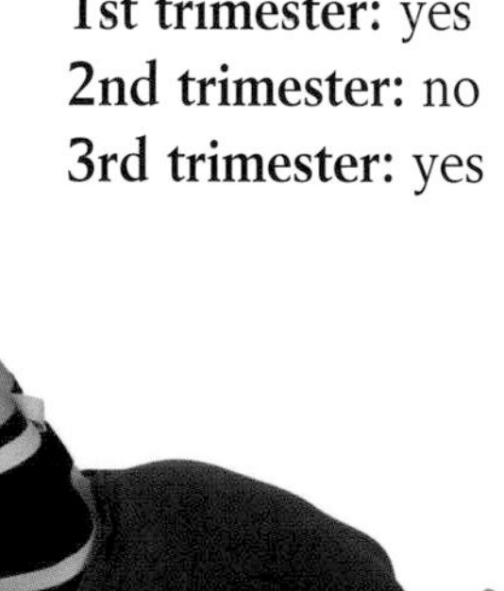

Baddha Konasana in Setu Bandha

Bound angle in bridge pose

1st trimester: no
2nd trimester: yes
3rd trimester: yes

This pose relaxes the groin, abdomen, diaphragm, and heart.

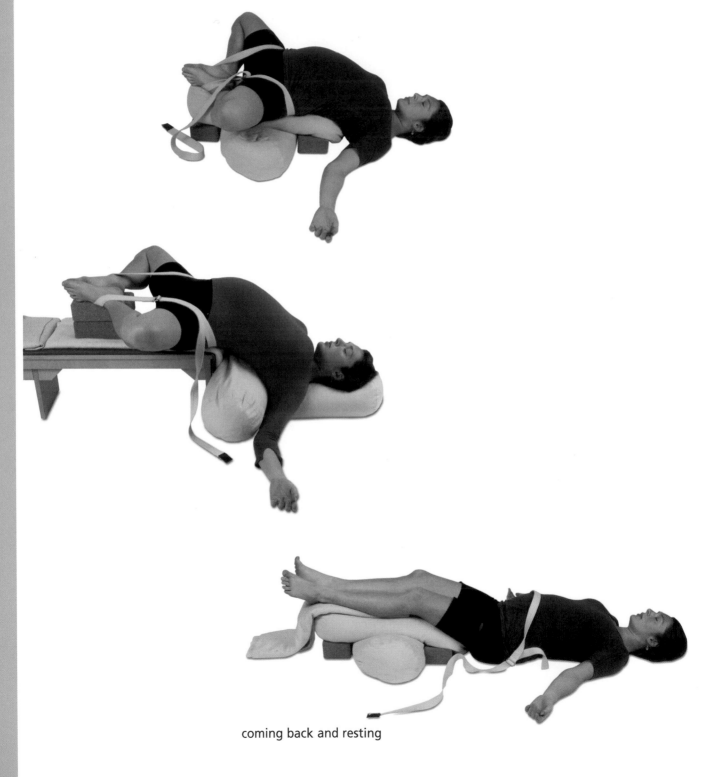

coming back and resting

Chatushpadasana
Four feet pose

1st trimester: no
2nd trimester: yes
3rd trimester: as long as comfortable

Chatushpadasana prepares you for the inverted poses because it works on lifting and expanding the chest. It affords direct contact with the shoulder blades, breastbone, spine, feet, and buttocks.

Benefits
Helps kidney function
Regulates menstrual periods and flow
Prevents bleeding during pregnancy
Strengthens the back muscles
Removes fatigue
Rejuvenates the nerves
Improves circulation in the chest
Develops self-confidence, willpower, and mental and emotional stability
Alleviates depression

Technique 1: With a Belt and Support

Practicing this asana enables you to do Setu Bandha Sarvangasana with ease.

1 Lie flat on the floor. Bend your knees, lift your pelvis, and rest your buttocks on a support.

2 Place your feet 1 to $1^1/_2$ feet apart. Loop a belt around your ankles and grip it.

3 Turn your heels slightly out so that the outer sides of your feet are pointing forward, press down your feet, and extend the bottom of your toes.

4 Raise your chest, thighs, and abdomen.

5 Keep the back of your head and your shoulders on the floor and your outer knees lifted.

6 Your extended arms allow your chest to expand easily.

7 Breathing normally, stay in the pose for 20 to 30 seconds.

Coming out of the pose

Maintaining the expansion of your chest, exhale and slowly bring your buttocks down to the support.

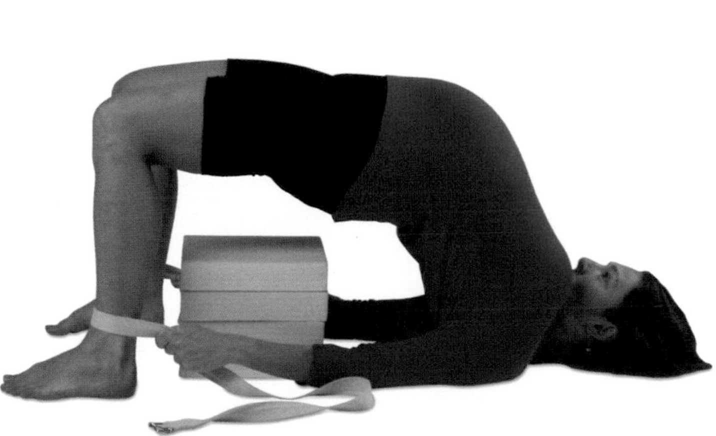

Help

If you are no longer able to grip the belt: Tuck your shoulder blades in, press your upper arms firmly into the floor adjacent to your chest, and extend your lower arms and your hands upward. Lift from here only.

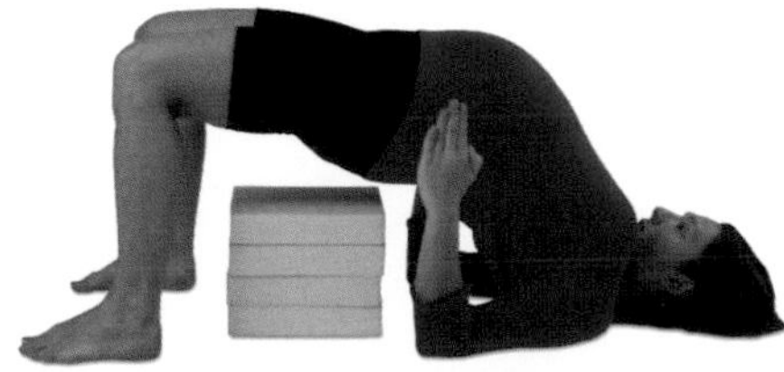

Technique 2: With a Chair

Practice this technique for as long as you feel comfortable.

1 Put three folded blankets on the floor in front of a chair. Lie down with your head on the floor and your shoulders supported.

2 Put your lower legs on the seat of the chair.

3 Grip the front legs of the chair and extending your arms, roll your shoulders away from your head and ears, press your upper arms down, and tuck your shoulder blades in to lift your breastbone.

4 Place your feet 1 to $1^1/_2$ feet apart on or against the seat of the chair, turn your heels slightly out so that the outer edges of your feet are pointing forward, press your heels down, and extend the bottoms of your toes.

5 Raise your chest, thighs, and abdomen. Tuck your shoulder blades in.

6 Keep the back of your head on the floor, your shoulders and upper arms down, and your outer knees lifted.

7 Breathing normally, stay for 20 to 30 seconds.

3rd trimester: with help of teacher

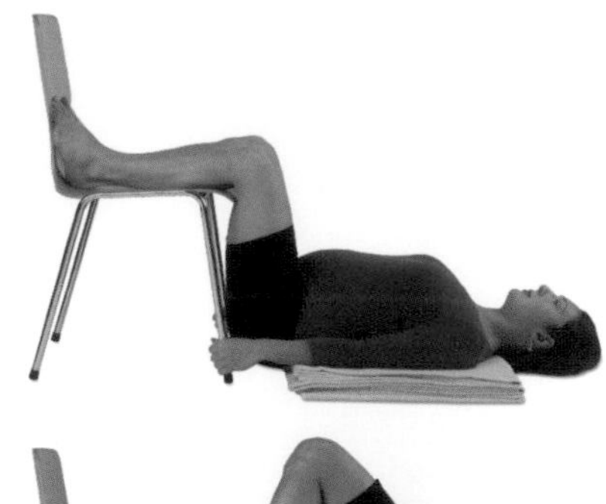

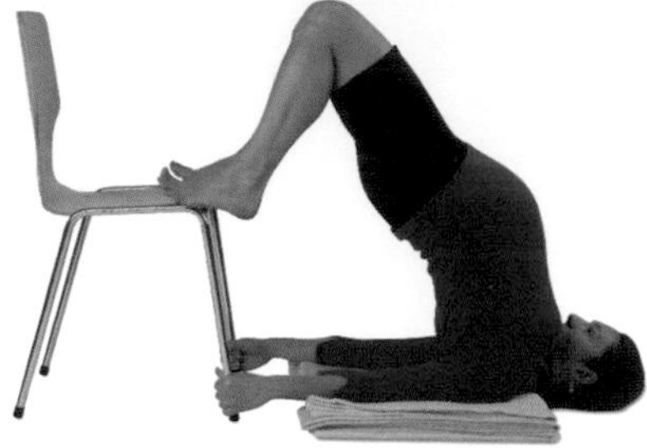

Coming out of the pose

Maintaining the expansion of your chest, exhale and slowly come down, resting your back on the floor.

Viparita Karani Mudra
Upward action seal pose

Viparit means "opposite" or "reverse." This pose is a mudra, or "seal" of a different kind than Maha Mudra (page 79).

The nine openings of the body can be sealed by several types of mudras, as explained in the Yogic texts. For example, the eyes, ears, and nose are sealed by Shanmukhi Mudra. In Maha Mudra, for instance, the anus is sealed in Mula Bandha, and the chin is locked in Jalandhara Bandha.

Now we come to Viparita Karani Mudra, where, according to the Yogic texts, the navel remains high and the palate remains low. Because the sun is considered to exist in the navel, and the moon in the palate, Viparita Karani Mudra is described as when the sun remains up and the moon down. This reverse position of the sun and the moon, that is, the navel and the palate, is found in inversions such as Shirshasana (page 97) and Sarvangasana (page 102). So it can be said that Viparita Karani is performed when any of these asanas is performed.

You can practice Viparita Karani Mudra while doing Sarvangasana when your buttocks are lowered onto your hands. By keeping your legs balanced and in line with the sockets of your buttocks, your chest is lifted and opened, and your navel is higher than your chest. Because your back is supported as it is in Sarvangasana, you don't lose your balance.

If you're pregnant, you'll find balancing on your hands to be strenuous. You can use a bolster, pillow, and blanket for support.

Beginners and Advanced Students: 1st trimester and advanced pregnancy

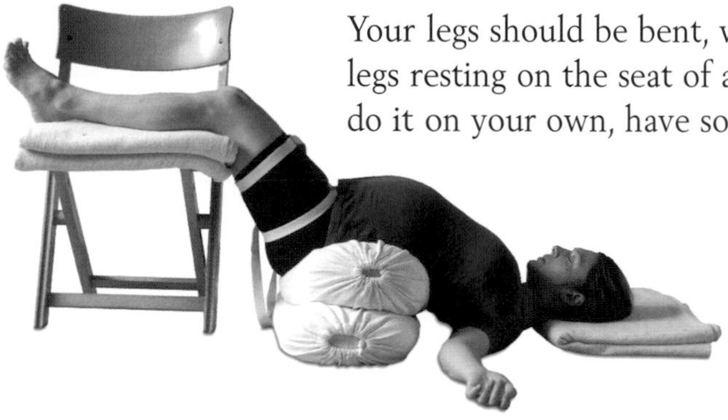

Your legs should be bent, with your lower legs resting on the seat of a chair. If you can't do it on your own, have someone help you.

Beginners and Advanced Students: 2nd and 3rd trimesters

1 Arrange the props as follows: Choose a flat bolster and put it against the wall under a flat pillow or blanket. This gives you a raised support of about 10 inches. Spread a blanket in front of it, so that the back of your head and your shoulders will stay on it.

2 Lie down on your back, keeping your buttocks near the edge of the bolster and your feet against the wall.

3 Exhale, raise your buttocks, and holding the ends of the bolster with your hands, place your buttocks on top. If you have practiced Sarvangasana before, you won't find it hard to raise your buttocks.

4 Shuffle and shift your buttocks up onto the support. Your body from your waist to your buttocks should remain on the support, and your dorsal (mid) spine should curve on its edge. This will bring your shoulders close to the edge of the support.

5 Straighten your legs against the wall so that your buttocks and the back of your legs remain in a complete state of rest, despite being inverted.

6 Exhale and roll your shoulders backward towards the wall to raise the sides of your chest. Spread your arms to the sides.

7 Stay in this final position for 5 minutes. Gradually increase the duration up to 10 minutes. Observe the points below:

- Don't allow your buttocks to slip off the edge. If that happens, readjust your position.
- Your body should bend and form curvatures at three places:
  1. Where your buttocks descend at the back edge of the bolster near the wall, sinking into the space between the bolster and the wall.

1st trimester: yes, with bent legs
2nd trimester: yes
3rd trimester: yes

Benefits

Brings significant change to the mind by calming it, allowing you to "see into your soul." The quieting of the brain and the chin-lock of the throat (Jalandhara Bandha) slow down and control your breathing. Diaphragm movement is slowed down, and your whole body quickly relaxes.

Cools down the nervous system, which in turn, because the nerves are in a state of non-stimulation, cools the body down.

Increases the gastric force (*agni*). This increases your appetite, which is a benefit if you have been unable to eat because of nausea and vomiting.

If practiced regularly, lessens swelling in the legs by eliminating water retention.

Brings speedy recovery and quick relaxation, which makes it a good mudra for beginning your Yoga practice when you're tired. The mudra not only prevents the thyroid and adrenal glands from over-activity, but it actually reduces their hormonal release, calming both body and mind.

Can be performed, along with Setu Bandha Sarvangasana, throughout your pregnancy.

2. Where your shoulders tuck into the front edge of the bolster
3. Lumbar region (lower back). Due to the fixation of your shoulders and buttocks, your lumbar region (lower back) curves on the end of the bolster and your entire torso spreads between the two "poles" formed by the shoulders and the buttocks.

- Keep your chest lifted.
- Your inhaling breath should move your chest from the back ribs to the frontal ribs, and your exhaling breath should move the sacrum (boneplate just above the tailbone) on the bolster, so that your abdomen does not become inflated.
- Keep your breastbone forward. Don't cave in your chest.
- Keep your legs together.

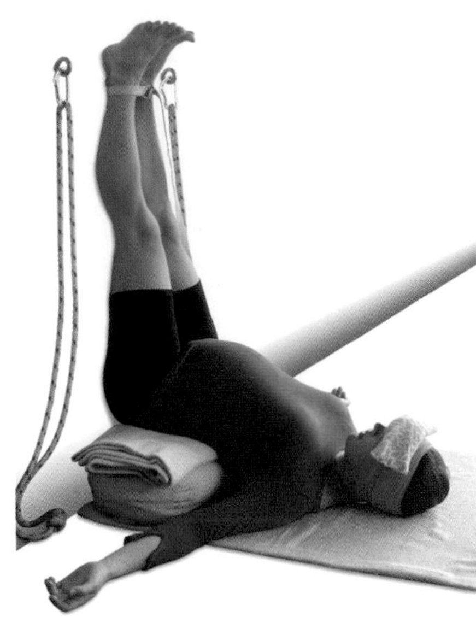

8 After getting into the right position, you can close your eyes and remain relaxed, breathing normally.

9 When you come back from the pose, open your eyes, bend your knees, keep your feet against the wall, and slide down until your buttocks reach the floor.

10 Roll to the right side first and then and sit up. Don't sit straight up.

Help

- If you have ropes affixed to a wall, then you can hold the rope and push yourself up on the bolster using the support.
- If you are heavy, you can have someone help lift you up on the bolster in position and tie a belt around your ankles.
- If you are thinner, try this technique:
  - Arrange the bolster as above.
  - Sit on one corner of it.
  - Lie down on your back, lift both legs up onto the wall simultaneously, and stay in position.
- In an advanced stage of pregnancy, you can keep your legs apart to lessen the pressure on your lower abdomen.
- If your head feels heavy, or you suffer from excessive vomiting or high blood pressure, then keep a folded blanket under your head. This will ensure that your head remains higher than your shoulders, or in other words, that your palate remains in a descending position. The raised position of your head calms the brain and eliminates anxiety.
- Relax your groin by folding your legs into Svastikasana, and then reversing your legs.

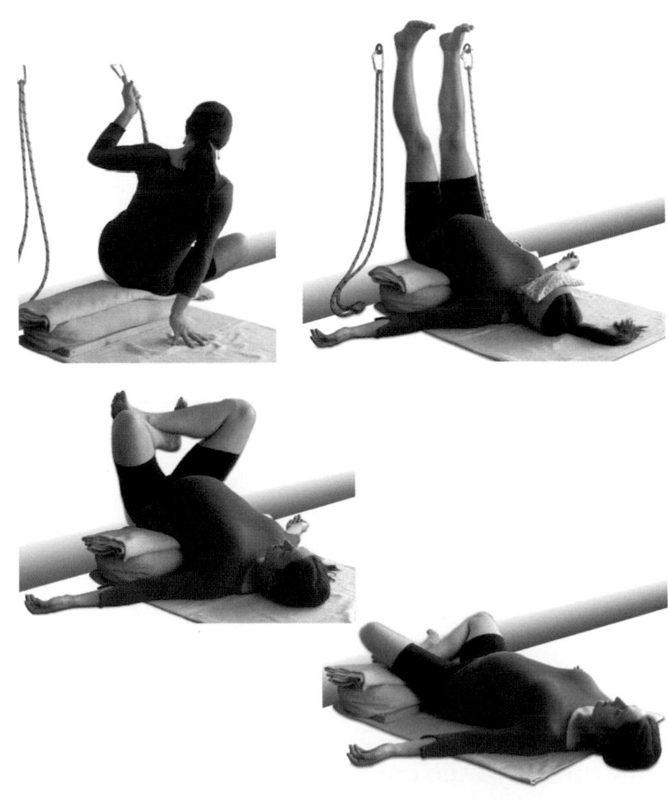

Asanas for Abdomen and Lumbar
Supta and Utthishtha Sthiti

Supta Padangushthasana 2
Reclining big toe 2 pose

1st trimester: yes
2nd trimester: yes
3rd trimester: yes

For this lying-down pose, have a belt, a rolled blanket/bolster, and a block ready.

1 Lie flat on the floor and put your heels on the block, which you have placed against the wall. Put the bolster next to your right hip on the floor and tie the belt so that it has a loop. Breathe normally.

2 Inhale, bend your right knee so that it points outward, and put the belt around your right foot. Extend your left leg, keeping your heel firmly on the block. Extend your right leg straight upward, stretching the hamstring (back thigh muscle).

3 Stretch your right leg so that it is perpendicular to the floor and move your left arm to the side in line with your left shoulder.

4 Take one or two breaths.

5 Exhale, keep your left leg outstretched, and pull your right leg sideways until it reaches the bolster.

6 Stay in this position for 10 to 20 seconds and breathe normally, observing the points in "Check Yourself."

Benefits

- Relieves sciatica and stiffness of the hip joints
- Soothes the nerves around the hips
- Opens the pelvic muscles, keeping the pelvic floor firm
- In advanced pregnancy, relieves pain in the region of the tailbone

CHECK YOURSELF
> *Don't lift the left side of your torso and your left buttock off the floor.*
> *Inhale, maintain the expansion of the chest, and lift your leg, bend it, and lower it to the floor. Put your right heel on the block, keeping your feet as far apart as the block allows.*

NOTE
In the 2nd trimester, you may rest your foot on the bolster. In the 3rd trimester, rest your outer thigh on the bolster. (See photos).

Utthita Hasta Padangushthasana 2

Standing big toe 2 pose

For this standing position, have a belt and a support for the lifted leg ready. If you're a beginner, have a stool or chair in front of the wall where you can put your foot temporarily.

We recommend that you rest your outstretched leg on a table or windowsill, as described below, which affords more curative value. Although similar to Supta Padangushthasana 2, this asana is done in a standing position, so that there is freedom of movement for the spine and more benefit for conditions such as weak hip muscles and backache.

1 Stand 2 or 3 feet away from the table or windowsill, with the right side of your torso facing it. Have the chair in front of the table or window as shown. Loop the belt around your right foot and stand in Tadasana.

2 Exhale, bend your right knee, and place your right foot (positioned as in Parighasana or Virabhadrasana 2) on the chair. Take one or two breaths.

3 Exhale and place your right foot on the table/support at right angles. Keep your left hand on your hip. Grip the belt firmly, extend your right arm, and lift your torso.

4 Stay in this position for 10 to 15 seconds, breathing normally, and observing the following points:

- Don't lift your right outer buttock upward. It has a tendency to lift, which can cause backache or cramp in the thighs.
- Keep your left outer hip and left outer ankle aligned.
- Straighten your torso by keeping your groin firm.
- Keep your torso and buttocks in one line.
- Lift your abdominal muscles and broaden your chest.
- Don't lift your shoulders or contract your neck.

5 Exhale and bend your right leg. If you want to feel safer, you can put your foot in the interim stage on the seat of the chair, and from there, bring your foot down to stand in Tadasana.

6 Feel the space this asana has created.

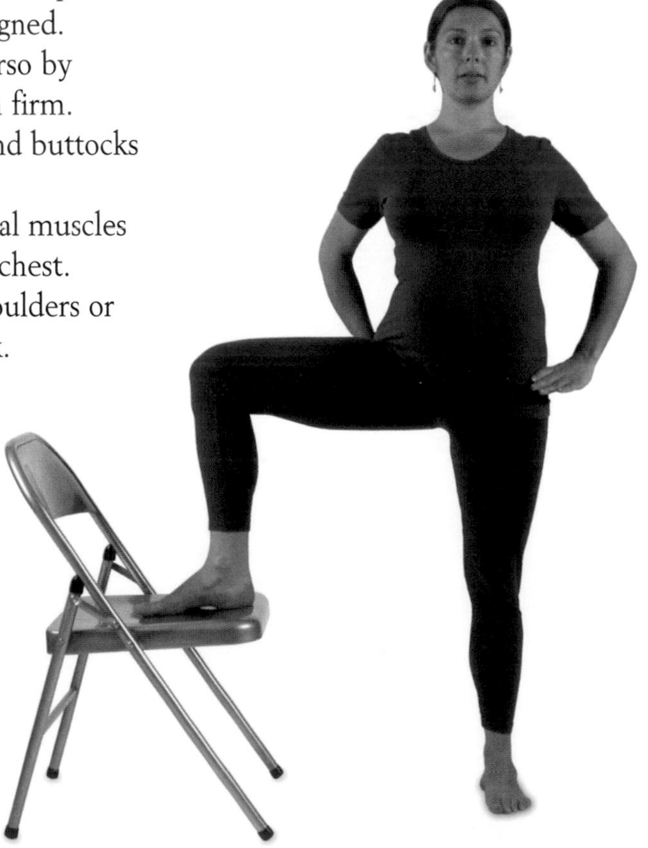

1st trimester: no
2nd trimester: yes
3rd trimester: yes

Benefits

Removes backache

Relieves rheumatism, lumbago, and sciatica

Opens the pelvic floor

Strengthens the spine

Help and Variations

- If you have a wall with wall ropes, you can also practice as shown here. Using wall ropes makes lifting the spine easier.

- Or, instead of pushing your foot against the wall, put your heel on the back of a chair.

- If your spinal muscles can't withstand the weight, then stand with your back against the wall. Put your foot on a stool or chair. In this variation, your back will have the support of the wall.

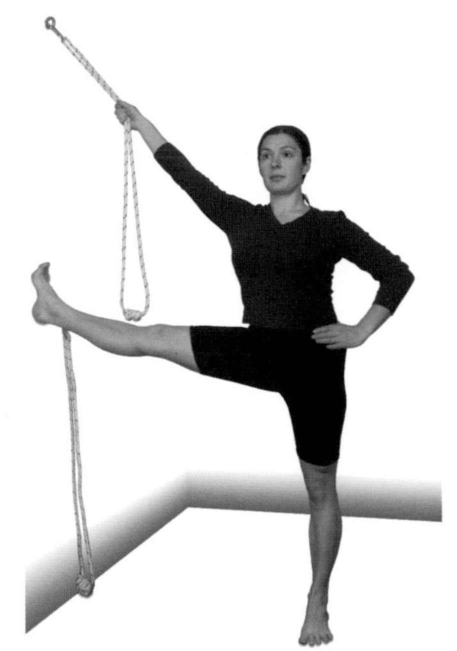

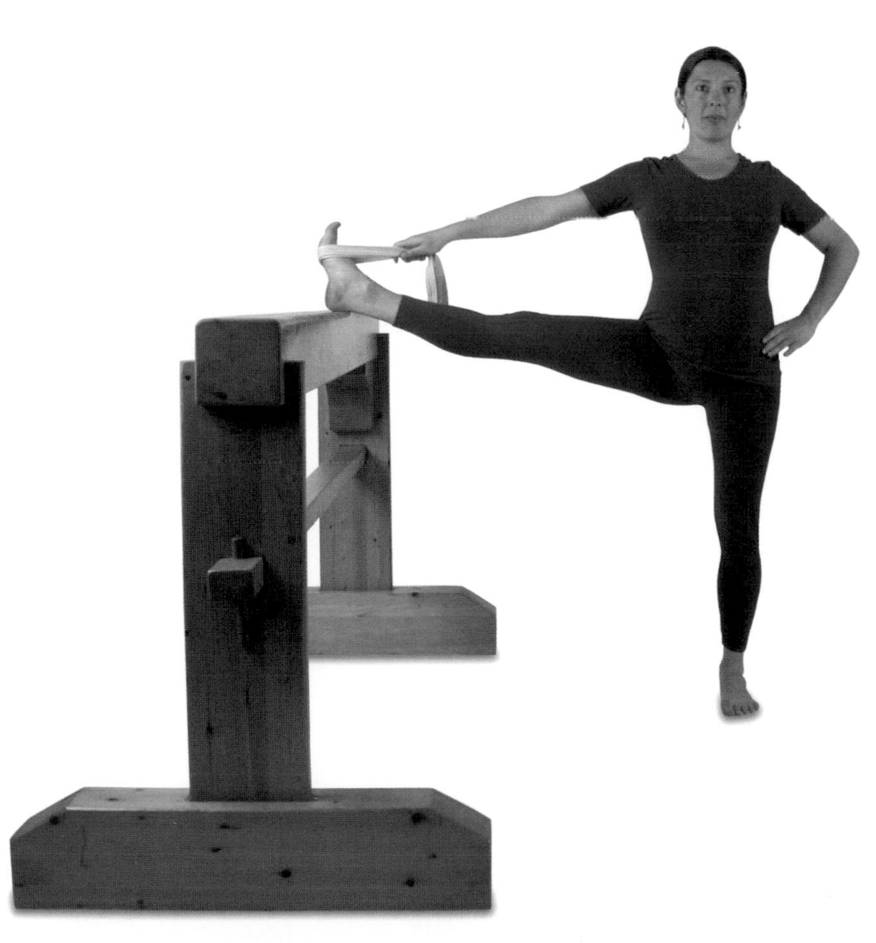

Back Bends

Purva Pratana Sthiti

Cross-bolsters, Resting in a Backward Extension

1st trimester: yes
2nd trimester: yes
3rd trimester: yes

You can follow this technique throughout your pregnancy, whenever you want to rest. You'll be able to breathe fully supported in this soft backward extension.

Usually in this pose, your heels are on the floor. As your pregnancy advances, however, and you may experience cramps or back pain, you can use blocks. In the photos, you can see the cross-bolsters with a block under the heels (and in the second photo, three blocks). Adjust your pose so that you don't feel any stress in your lower back.

1 Place a set of bolsters and pillows as shown.

2 Use a belt for your upper legs, and also your feet if you like, so that you don't have to stretch your legs intensively.

3 Lie down with your back across the bolsters (and pillows if the bolsters are not high enough) and a blanket under your shoulders and the neck, as shown.

4 If your head is hanging down and your neck shortens, then support your neck, taking care to keep your chin away from your sternum.

5 Your spine is now effortlessly concave thanks to the support of the bolsters and pillows.

Benefits

- Brings freedom to the frontal torso
- Spreads a feeling of exhilaration to the organs and nerves over the front of the spine
- Relaxes the diaphragm, which can move up and down freely in the increased space
- Can bring great calm and serenity to a pregnant woman who is feeling depressed
- Aids diabetes during pregnancy, by helping to keep sugar levels in check

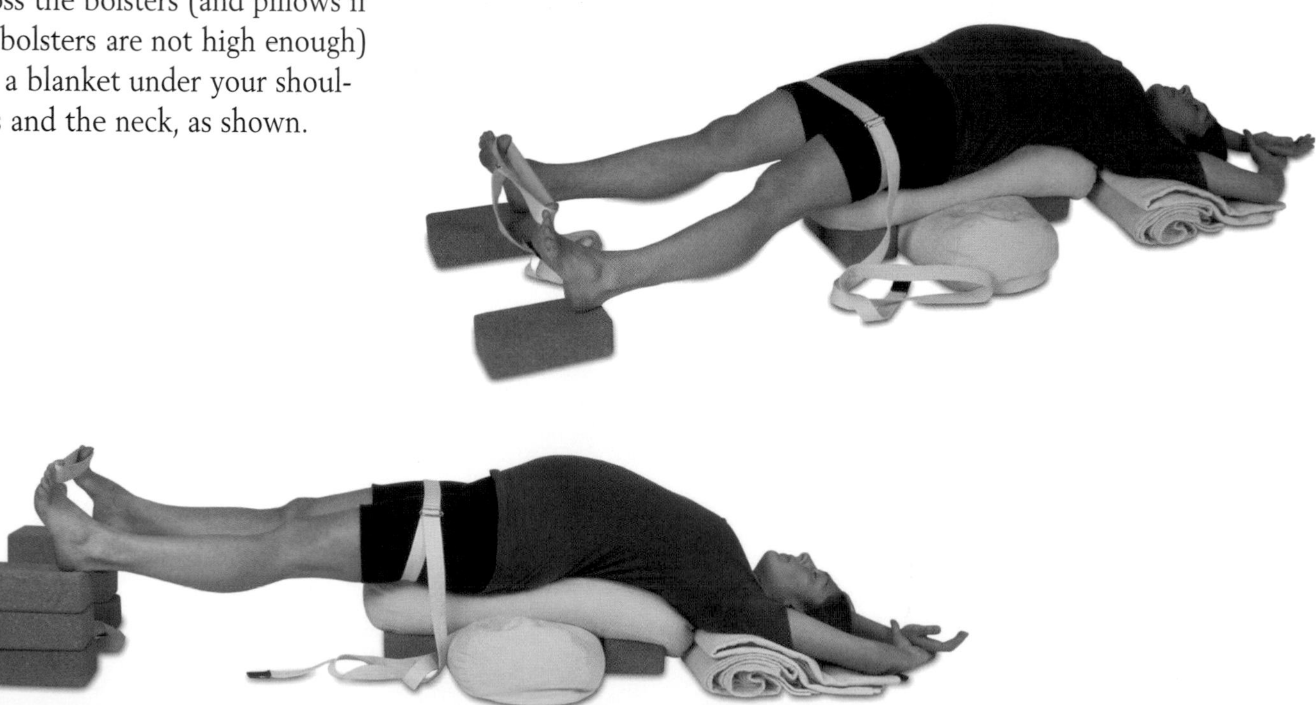

Bhujangasana, with Ropes
Cobra pose

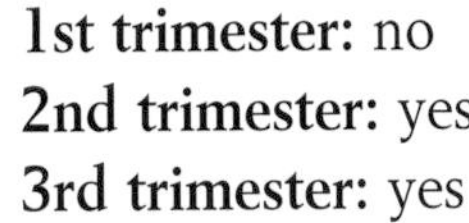

1st trimester: no
2nd trimester: yes
3rd trimester: yes

Benefits

See page 120

1 Stand in Tadasana (page 32) with your back to the wall, in between the two ends of the suspended rope. Make sure you are standing exactly in the center. Grip the rope firmly with your left and right hands, and walk your feet about 3 feet away from the wall until you stand in Tadasana. Keep your feet 1 to $1\frac{1}{2}$ feet apart, with your toes extending forward.

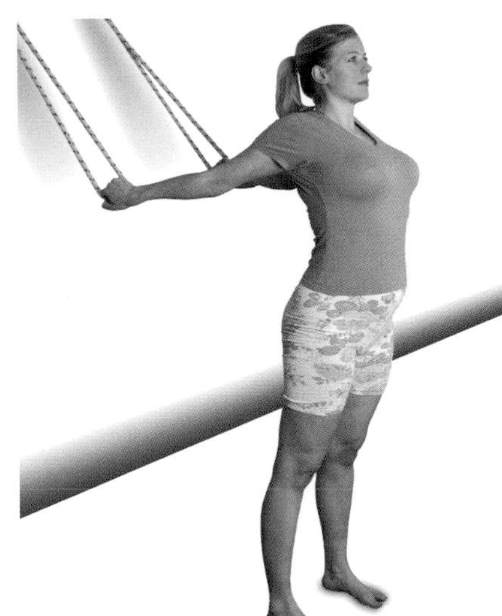

2 Grip the rope firmly, keeping your arms straight. Stand erect, and lift your abdomen, the sides of your torso, and your lower sternum. Take one or two breaths.

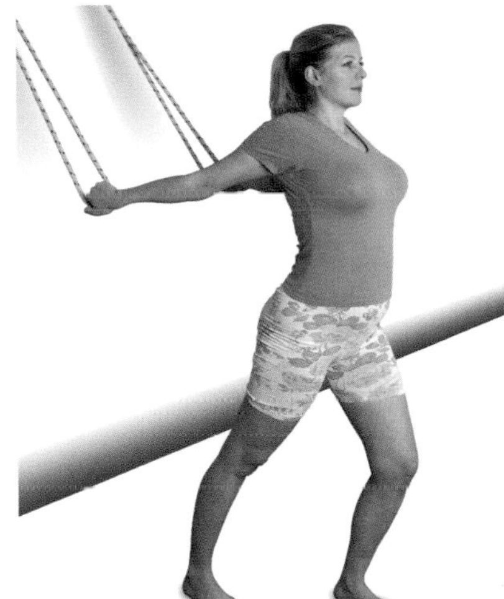

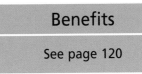

3 Inhale, raise your head, make your spine concave, and move your body forward as far as it will go. In order to be able to lean forward diagonally, move your feet a few inches back towards the wall.

4 Raise your head and come up onto the balls of your feet by straightening your arms. Keep your knees and elbows straight, let your palms face each other, and press the balls of your feet firmly onto the floor.

5 Exhale, tighten your buttocks and pull them towards the floor, take the buttocks into your body and lift your pelvic floor upward. Extend your torso further down to get a complete concave movement, and look up.

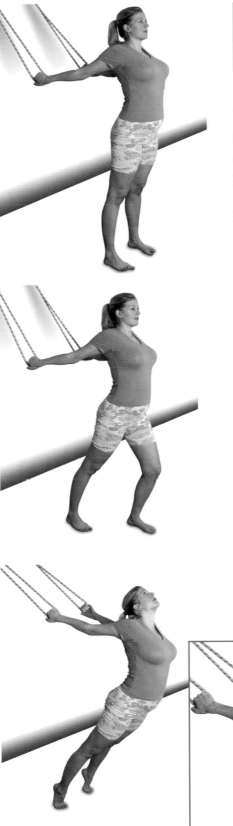

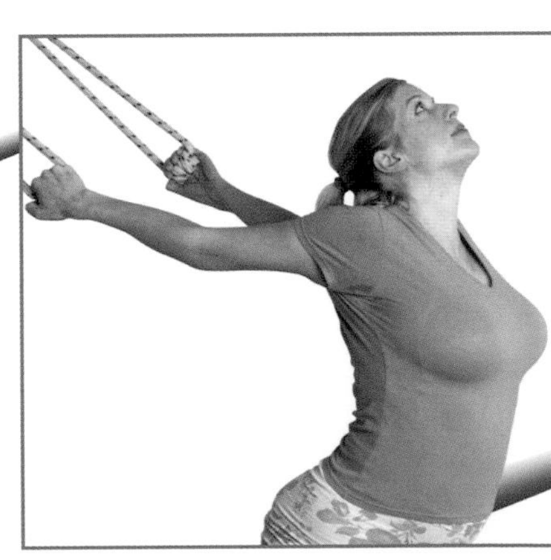

6 Tuck in the tailbone and the sacrum (bone plate between spine and tailbone), broaden your chest, and lift your abdomen towards your chest. Maintain a strong pull on your arms and keep your thighs firm.

7 Stay in this final position for 5 to 10 seconds and breathe normally.

8 Inhale, maintain the expansion of your chest, and walk your feet away from the wall until you are standing erect in Tadasana. Release your arms.

CHECK YOURSELF

> *Make sure that both arms are pulled evenly.*

> *Your movements should not be too fast or too slow.*

Bhujangasana, with Ropes, Chair, and Bolster
Cobra pose

This variation makes it easier to lift and to broaden your chest.

Benefits

- Gives confidence
- Relieves tailbone pain, especially in the last stages of pregnancy
- Relieves hip pain
- Lessens abdominal heaviness
- Rejuvenates the spine
- Creates space for the fetus to grow

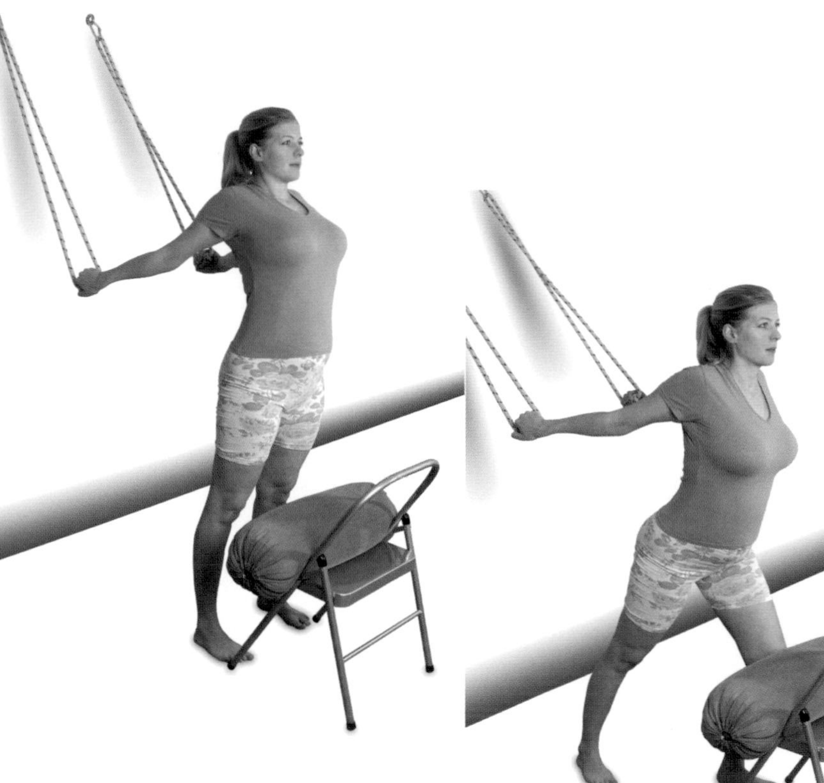

1 Measure the distance where you placed your feet in Bhujangasana with Ropes.

2 Prepare a chair with a sticky mat on top and a bolster crosswise.

3 Grip the ropes and stand in front of the chair.

4 Follow the instructions as given for Bhujangasana and bring your upper thighs onto the bolster.

5 Adjust the distance from your feet to the wall to ensure that you really are supported by the chair and bolster.

6 Keep your thighs firm.

Coming out of the pose

Inhale, maintain the expansion of your chest, and walk your feet forward until you stand erect in Tadasana. Release your arms.

Salamba Purvottanasana, with Trestle

Supported eastern intense stretch pose

1st trimester: no
2nd trimester: yes
3rd trimester: yes

Beginners and Advanced Students

This asana provides an immense lift and opening of the chest.

1 Grip the upper beam of the trestle by placing your forearms under and around it, as shown. Extend your hands and fingers forward.

2 Keep your feet parallel and your legs slightly bent.

3 Don't let your inner knees drop to the sides; keep your inner and the outer knees in line, facing the ceiling.

4 Breathe normally and stay for 30 to 60 seconds.

Benefits
Lifts the chest and its sides
Eliminates heavy and knotted feelings in the chest and upper back
Gives lightness
Creates physical and mental stability
Benefits the breast glands

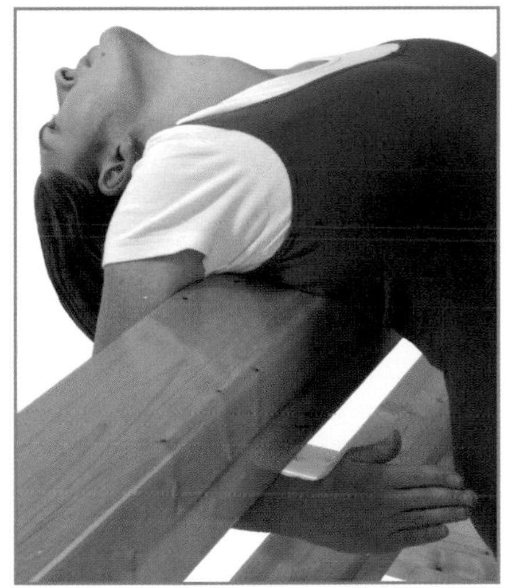

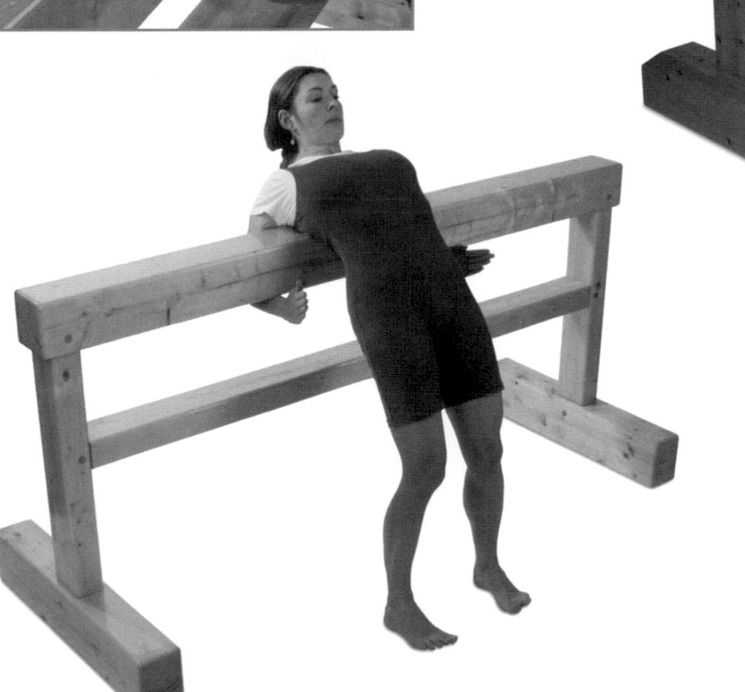

Coming out of the pose

1 To come back, put one lower arm after the other on top of the beam, and afterwards your hands, until you stand erect.

2 Maintain the lift of your breastbone and the opening of your chest while you rest in Tadasana (page 32).

Dvi Pada Viparita Dandasana, Fully Supported on a Bench and Chair

Two-legged inverted staff pose

1st trimester: yes
2nd trimester: yes
3rd trimester: yes

Benefits
Brings about a feeling of happiness
Builds self-confidence
Eliminates anxiety
Improves respiration and circulation

In this asana, the back is completely arched, supported by the crown of the head and the forearms on one end and by the feet on the other, so you have to hold yourself with almost no support.

Under normal conditions, you wouldn't use props either. Because you're pregnant, however, you should perform the asana with full support for your back. For that reason we recommend practicing with the appropriate props and modifications to the original technique.

Begin the fully supported variation of this asana together with a teacher as early in your pregnancy as possible, so that you'll be able to enjoy the freedom it gives in the last stages.

The backward spinal arch in this asana is a movement that rarely occurs in everyday movements; most household or other jobs involve bending your spine forward.

This pose counters the constant forward bending with a backward bend. The extension of the frontal spine caused by the backward bend creates space and thus freedom for the diaphragm to move.

Because the asana is performed with the lumbar (lower) spine and the buttocks well supported, your torso gets a full extension without strain on the spinal muscles. This lessens the load on the abdomen, bringing about improvement in crucial body functions such as respiration and circulation.

The chest expansion in this asana brings about a feeling of happiness. Practiced in this modified technique, it is particularly helpful if you are depressed, weak, or overly sensitive or emotional; it builds self-confidence and eliminates anxiety.

Before you start, keep in mind that:

- Going into the pose is difficult, so you need some amount of skill to perform it. Once you're in the pose, however, you can relax and enjoy its soothing and exhilarating effects.
- You can avoid any strain by understanding how to go into the pose.

1 Prepare a Viparita Dandasana bench or two chairs (page 237).

2 Place a folded blanket, or a bolster, or both, on the edge of the bench to protect your back.

3 Lie on the bench or on the chairs.

4 Hold the edge of the bench and expand your chest.

5 Keep the crown of your head resting on the bolster, or folded blankets.

6 Stay in this position for 3 to 5 minutes, breathing normally and observing the following points:

- Your chest should not cave in.
- Your head should not remain in a suspended state.
- Your face should remain relaxed.

Coming out of the pose

Exhale, bend your knees, slide your torso down to the floor, and lie flat on your back.

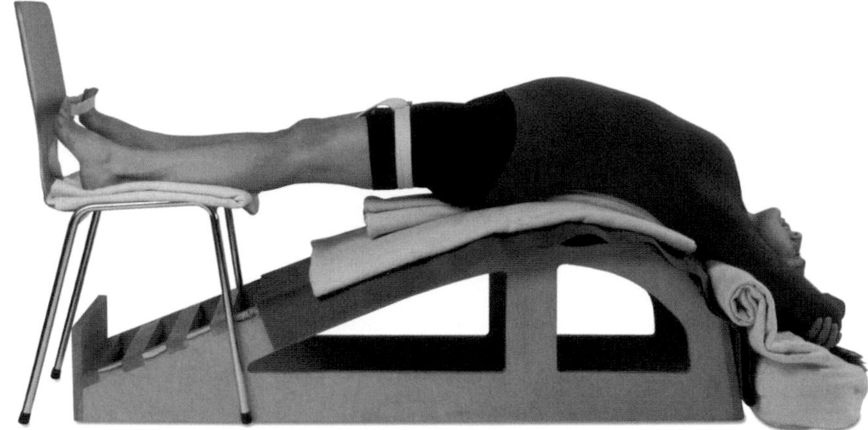

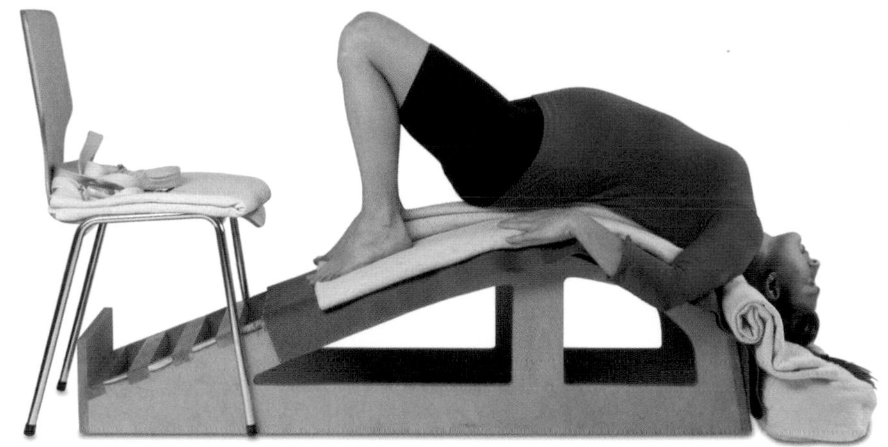

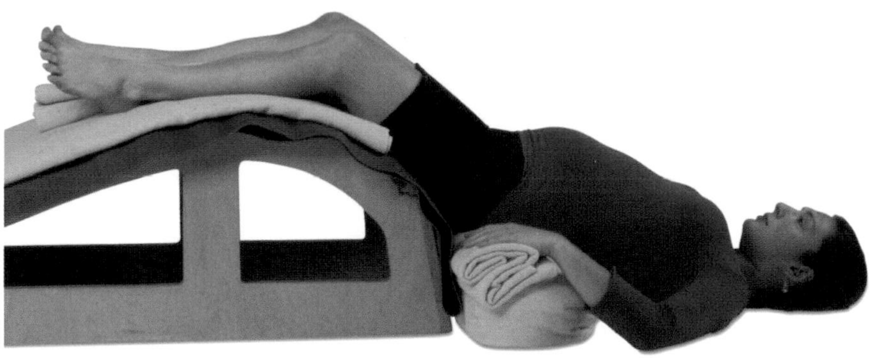

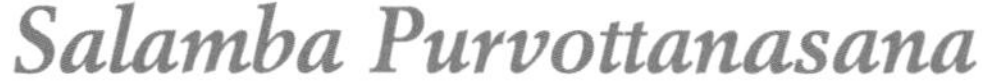

Salamba Purvottanasana

Supported eastern intense stretch

See Restorative Asanas, pages 126 – 139

Rope Asanas
Yoga Kurunta

Performing yogasanas with the aid of a rope has many advantages. It helps you do difficult asanas easily, safely, and smoothly without jerking. With regular practice, it develops a sense of direction in aligning the body.

Ardha Uttanasana, with Ropes and Chair
Half intense forward stretch pose

1st trimester: yes
2nd trimester: yes
3rd trimester: yes

In the chain of asanas to be performed before and after Salamba Shirshasana, this is the one that comes immediately before and after it.

Benefits

- Alleviates depression
- Calms the brain
- Lowers blood pressure
- Relieves stomach pain
- Strengthens the abdominal organs
- Helps the free flow of digestive juices
- Creates space for the fetus to grow and extend its limbs
- Lengthens and straightens the back of the cervix and the vagina, increasing blood circulation in that area

Technique
Please refer to this asana on pages 59 – 61.

Help
- For working in the concave position, practice with your hands on the chair.
- For more extension, stretch your hands over the back of the chair.

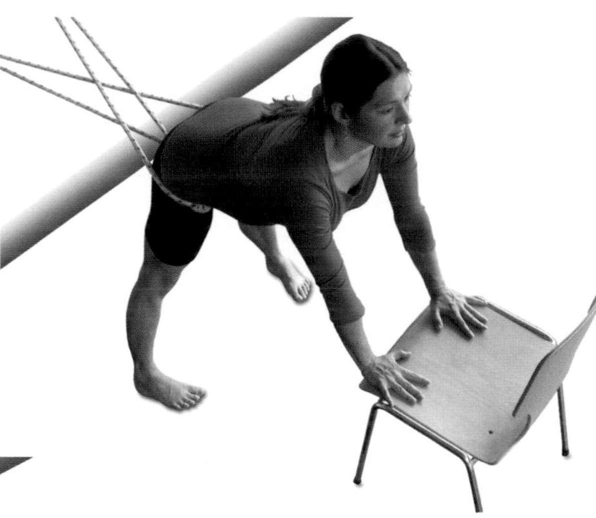

CHECK YOURSELF
> *Extend your dorsal and lumbar (mid and lower) spine.*
> *Open your chest.*
> *Turn your toes in and your heels out, in order to reduce abdominal pressure.*
> *Extend your bottom ribs.*
> *Don't bend your knees; pull your kneecaps and front thigh muscles up.*

Adho Mukha Shvanasana, with Ropes and a Support for the Head

Downward-facing dog pose

Adho Mukha Shvanasana (page 62) removes fatigue caused by the other standing poses. As in all inverted asanas, the heart is below the spine. In this prone asana, it rests away from the spine, which is a kind of resting position for it. When the heart is in an inverted position, you recover from mental and physical fatigue, and shortness of breath is alleviated. The body craves these asanas when it's tired.

You can rest even further by placing your forehead on a stool or chair (in advanced pregnancy) or on a bolster (first trimester and probably second trimester) and by using the support of ropes.

1st trimester: yes
2nd trimester: yes, as long as it is comfortable
3rd trimester: yes, with a chair or another support for your hands and head

Benefits

See page 63

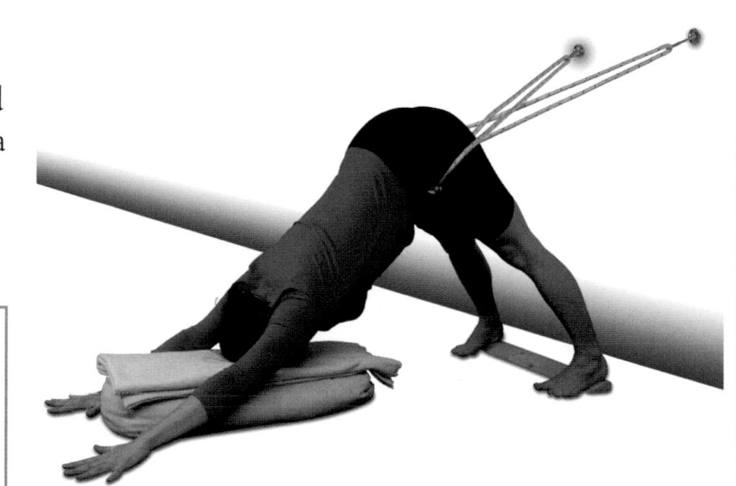

Special Instructions

- Place your feet 3 feet apart or on the edges of a sticky mat and put your heels on a slanted plank, with the outer edges of your feet in line with the outer edges of the mat.
- Lift your inner ankles.

Bhujangasana, with Ropes

Cobra pose

Page 119

Bhujangasana, with Ropes, Chair, and Bolster

Page 120

Malasana, with Bolster and Wall Ropes

Garland pose

Page 77

SEE ALSO

Adho Mukha Shvanasana, with Ropes, page 63
Sitting Asanas with ropes, pages 64, 66, 69, 71

Restorative Asanas
Vishranta Karaka Sthiti

Supta Baddha Konasana
Reclining bound angle pose

1st trimester: yes
2nd trimester: yes
3rd trimester: yes

Benefits

- Relieves pain, spasms, and burning sensation of the reproductive organs
- Tones the urinary system
- Protects against infection
- Helps ensure an easy delivery

When you're pregnant, it is common to experience a feeling of being knotted up inside, particularly in the abdominal region. This often comes with shortness of breath, anxiety, and tension. Practiced correctly, Supta Baddha Konasana is the right asana to overcome these feelings.

1st Trimester: Without Support

1 Lie flat on your back.

2 Bend your knees and bring your heels near your buttocks.

3 Spread your thighs and knees apart, bringing your heels and soles together.

4 Lower your knees as close to the floor as you can.

5 Place your arms over your head.

6 Stay in this position for 30 to 60 seconds, breathing normally. Gradually increase the duration to any length.

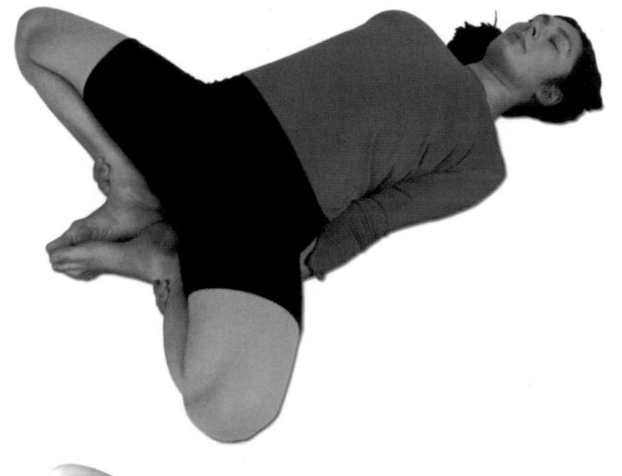

Coming out of the pose

1 Bring your arms down. Slowly come onto your elbows, lift your chest, and come back to Baddha Konasana (page 67).

2 Release your feet and stretch out your legs in Dandasana (page 64).

Entire Pregnancy

The variation below can take you through your entire pregnancy to the very last day. In advanced pregnancy, it may be difficult to keep your entire torso down. In that case, keep one or two bolsters under your chest and waist, and a pillow or blanket under your head. For more instruction on how to use the bolsters, see the variations below. For more relaxation, use a belt for your legs.

1 Sit in Baddha Konasana (page 67). Place a bolster lengthwise behind your back as mentioned above.

2 Put a belt around your lower back, through the groin, and around your feet. Pull your feet towards your pelvis.

3 Check that the bolster is straight.

4 Using the support of your elbows, lean back and recline your torso, shoulders, and head on the bolster. Support your head with a blanket. Make sure that your spine is placed evenly and lengthwise on the bolster.

5 Support your knees with rolled blankets or blocks. With your legs supported, extend your knees to the sides and lower them as close to the floor as possible.

6 Stretch your arms over your head in order to extend your abdomen and the abdominal muscles upward towards your chest. Turn your palms to face the ceiling.

7 Stay in this position for 30 to 60 seconds, breathing normally.

- Maintain the space you have created, and bring your arms to your sides.
- Gradually increase the duration to any length.

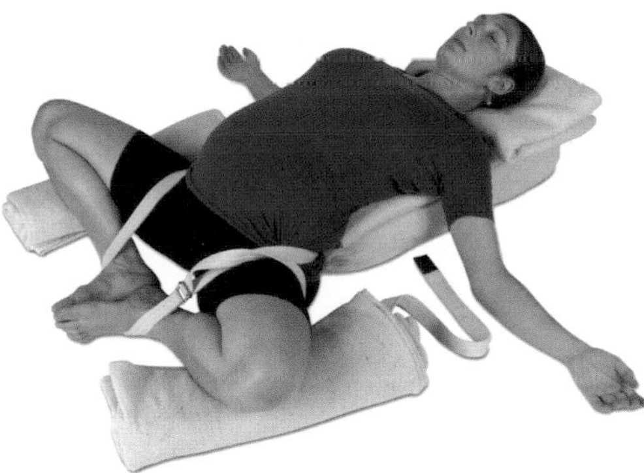

Coming out of the pose

While raising your knees off the ground, allow your groin muscles to relax, in order to avoid jerky movements and spasms.

Benefits

Supta Baddha Konasana is the finest of asanas, giving you a feeling of exhilaration. You can lie down safely in this pose for a prolonged period, especially with your back supported by blankets and pillows. The supine position, particularly with the pelvis in a broadened state, releases the crowded, heavy feelings of the abdomen. With your back supported, the pelvic region and thoracic diaphragm are released from inner knots. The supine position, however, offers much more—it relaxes the brain as well as the brawn.

Special Instructions

- Sometimes your ankles and the sides of your feet slip apart. In that case, rest your toes against a wall, place your palms underneath your thighs, and catch your ankles and pull them towards your thighs.
- If you are heavy, place a blanket that is 3 to 4 inches high or a bolster lengthwise under your back, so that your chest opens and your abdomen is at an angle.
- If you feel a strong pull in your lower back, use two separate belts, one tied around the ankle and thigh of each leg.

Bolster Variations

1 Place a slanted plank to support your back at the lower edge of your shoulder blades. This increases the opening of the chest, especially at the sides, and the area around the breastbone. In the photo you also see how to place and pull the belt.

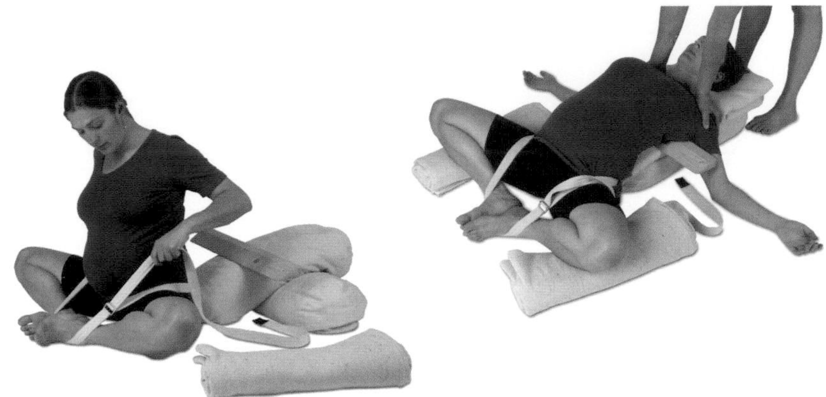

2 Place a bolster crosswise and a blanket for your head. This widens your diaphragm and spreads out your abdomen.

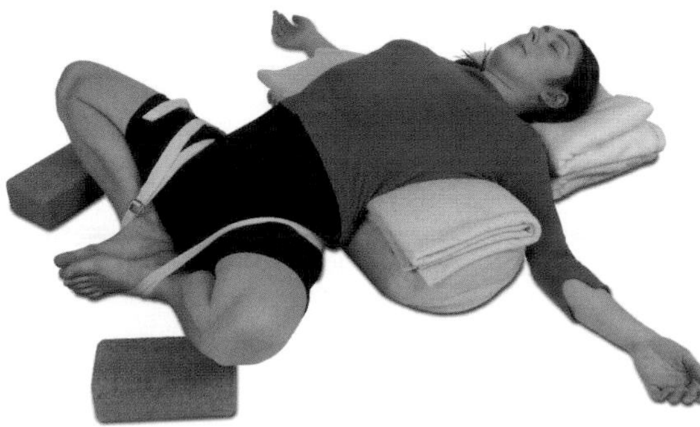

3 Use a block to support your feet. This gives a nice lift to the abdomen and more length in the lower back.

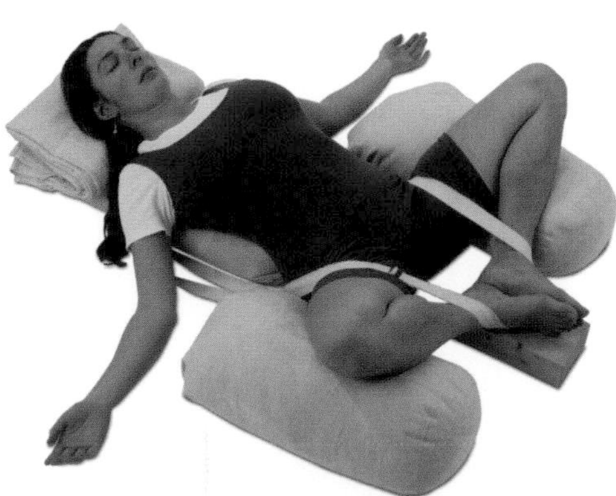

CHECK YOURSELF

When lying on your back:

> Don't raise your lumbar region (lower back).

> Keep the pelvic area broad.

> Keep your chest expanded.

> Allow your knees to go down towards the floor by moving them further sideways.

Free Breathing

When your muscles are spread out like a plateau, as they are in this asana, breathing becomes easier. The air moves in and out freely, without any obstacles.

People often ask how they should breathe during a particular asana. Usually, the answer is "normally." But normal breathing has its own varieties. The impetus can come from different centers of the body. You can use different parts of the body as foci to initiate breathing, for example, breathing in from the abdomen and breathing out from the head. This changes the effect of the breathing.

Supta Baddha Konasana is among the poses that make exhalation longer and deeper, because the body remains in a tension-free state. After a few long exhalations, the inhalations become effortless and deep as well. As the longer cycles continue, you find that the tension around your diaphragm decreases tremendously.

The free breathing and the specific pose combine to give you a feeling of a vast space within. You feel relaxed and remain in the tension-free state. You will reap the benefits of the asana by paying attention to all these changes, enjoying inner freedom and peace.

Supta Virasana
Reclining hero pose

1st trimester: yes
2nd trimester: yes
3rd trimester: yes

Supta Virasana, combined with Supta Baddha Konasana (page 126), helps you regain relaxation and bring back smooth, spontaneous breathing. Supta Virasana is the more difficult of the two, because you have to lean on your back in a bent-knee position.

Once you have mastered the pose, it soothes your system and lets the baby inside you rest quietly. The soothing effect also works on the abdominal region, diminishing flatulence and that itching sensation that often plagues pregnant women.

Benefits

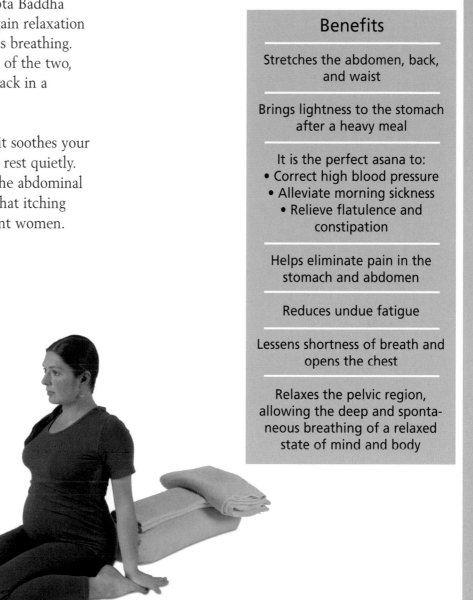

Stretches the abdomen, back, and waist

Brings lightness to the stomach after a heavy meal

It is the perfect asana to:
- Correct high blood pressure
- Alleviate morning sickness
- Relieve flatulence and constipation

Helps eliminate pain in the stomach and abdomen

Reduces undue fatigue

Lessens shortness of breath and opens the chest

Relaxes the pelvic region, allowing the deep and spontaneous breathing of a relaxed state of mind and body

1 Sit in Virasana (page 72). Put your palms on the soles of your feet. Take a few breaths.

2 If your weight has increased substantially or you have tension in your thighs and knees, it may be difficult for you to recline back far enough. Keep one or two pillows behind your buttocks to support your back and head, so that your thighs and buttocks rest on the floor and your chest is expanded.

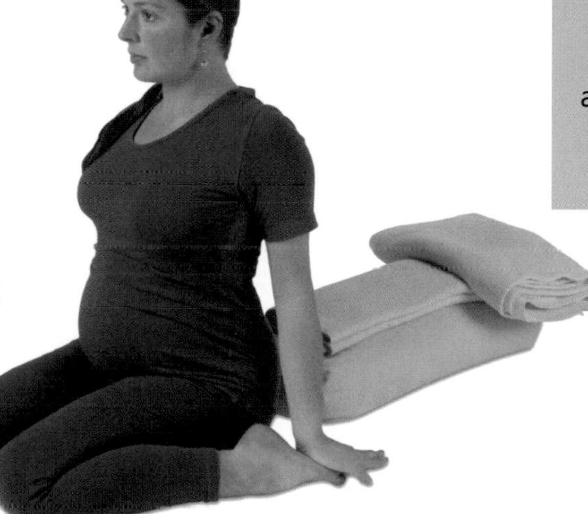

3 Exhale and lean your torso backward so that your back and waist lower towards the pillows or floor. Rest your elbows on the floor one by one and then your forearms as well.

Special Instructions for the Knees

At first, your knees tend to remain apart. With regular practice, however, it becomes easy to keep them together. If you still find it difficult, you can use a belt. It's important to keep your knees down; if necessary, use a folded blanket or a block underneath your buttocks to do so.

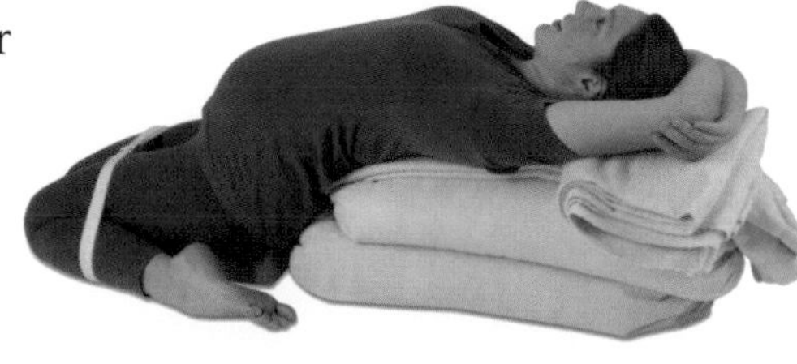

4 Lean back further until the back of your head is on the pillow.

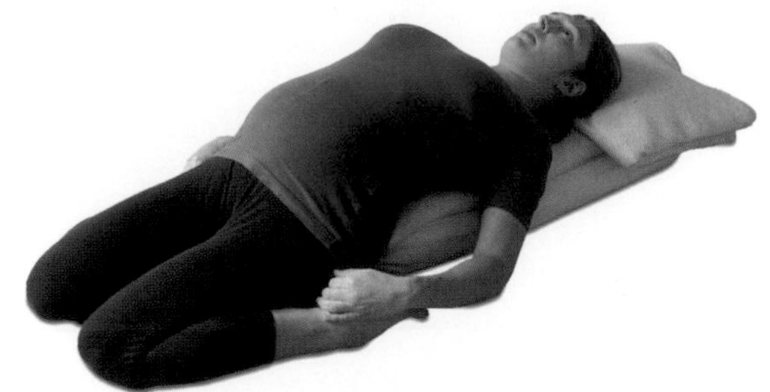

5 Release your back and place the back of your head on the blanket and your shoulders and torso on the pillow. Straighten your arms by the sides of your legs and stay for 15 seconds. Take a breath or two.

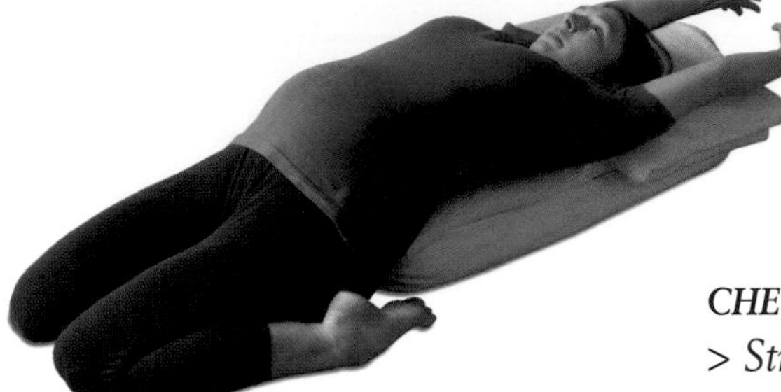

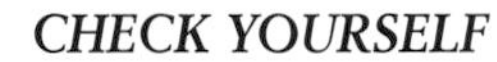

6 Grip your heels firmly, lift your sternum, and extend your arms over your head with the palms facing the ceiling.

7 Stay in this position for 30 to 60 seconds (and later as long as possible), breathing normally and observing the points in "Check Yourself."

8 After you have extended your arms, you can grip your elbows or place your arms at your sides.

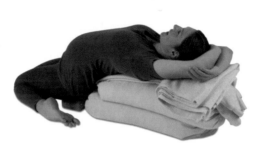

CHECK YOURSELF

> *Stretch the outsides of your arms so that your thighs and abdomen are massaged and pulled towards your chest.*
> *Don't lift your knees, buttocks, or shoulders from the floor.*
> *Tuck your shoulder blades in and open your chest.*
> *The front and back of your torso should be extended evenly.*

Coming out of the pose

Going into Supta Virasana is not at all difficult when you're pregnant; coming out is a different story, because it involves going against gravity. You want to get up in such a way that the baby inside is not jolted. It should be done gracefully, releasing your body and coming out with a minimum of sudden motions.
To come out of the pose, reverse the way you came into it. Exhaling lightens the body, so exhale and slowly raise yourself up. Keep your chest raised and don't let it cave in. If your knees are stiff, stretch your legs backward one by one, slowly extending your heels.

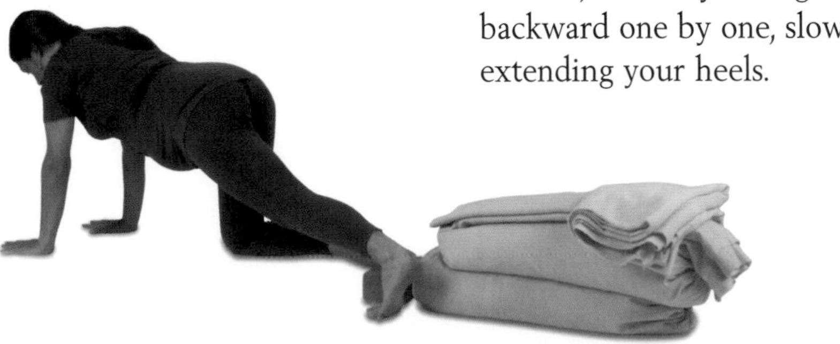

Help

If you can't sit on the floor, and your body is too stiff to lean back in Supta Virasana, you can start with an intermediate stage as shown here with bolsters and chair.

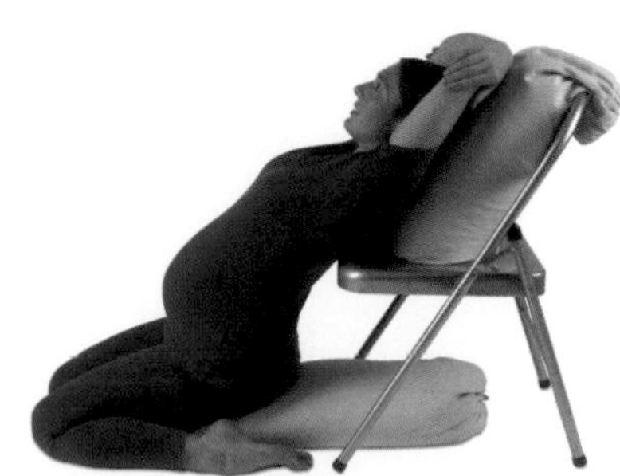

Supta Svastikasana, Matsyasana, or Ardha Matsyasana

Reclining cross-legged pose, fish pose, or half-fish pose

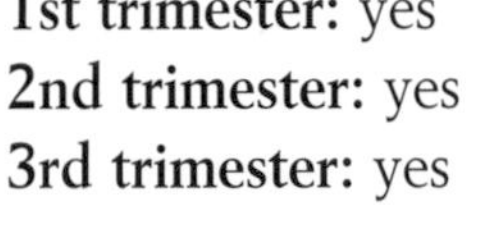

1st trimester: yes
2nd trimester: yes
3rd trimester: yes

1 Sit in Svastikasana (top photo) or Padmasana (middle photo), with a bolster lengthwise behind you.

2 Check that the bolster is straight.

3 Using the support of your elbows, recline back and lay your torso, shoulders, and head on the bolster. Support your head with a blanket. Make sure that your spine is placed evenly lengthwise on the bolster.

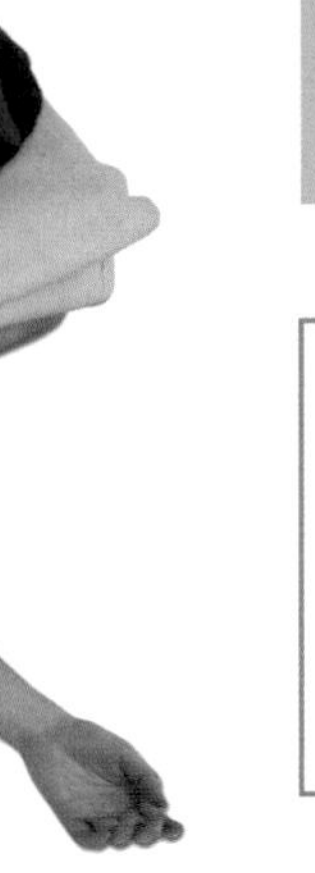

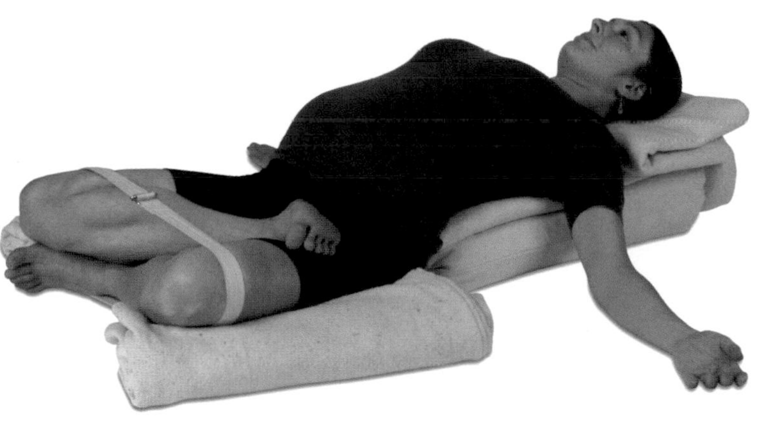

Benefits

- Relaxes the thyroid
- Relieves inflamed piles
- Widens and stretches the pelvis and abdomen, and extends the waist
- Helps treat stomachache, acidity, indigestion, ulcers, backache, and irritation of the liver, spleen, and gall bladder

Special Instructions

Follow the instructions given for Supta Baddha Konasana page 126.

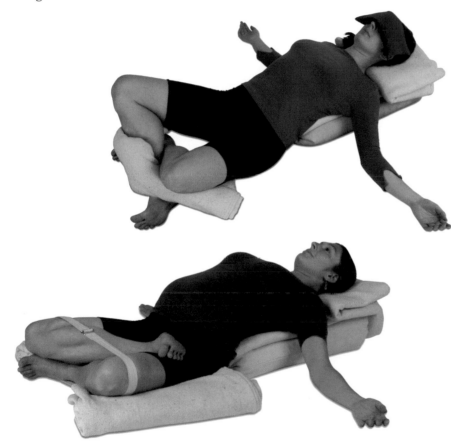

Coming out of the pose

After 30 to 60 seconds, come up as described in Supta Baddha Konasana, reverse your legs, and go back, breathing normally. Be sure to remain the same length of time on both sides. Later, you can extend the period of time.

Help

If you're having trouble keeping your legs and buttocks in position, you can tie a belt around your legs to support your knees. This also helps to soften and lift the abdomen.

If your abdomen still feels heavy, you can support your knees from the front with a rolled blanket, which lifts the abdomen even more.

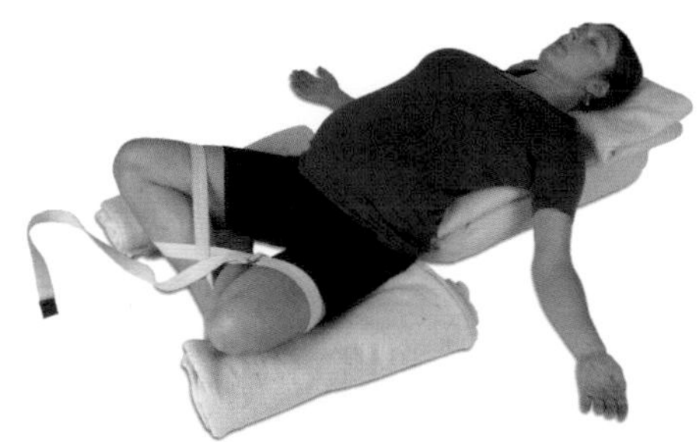

DETAILED DESCRIPTIONS OF ASANAS FOR ALL STUDENTS

See also the following inverted asanas:

Setu Bandha Sarvangasana, on a Bench with Spread Legs

Full bridge pose

Page 109

1st trimester: yes
2nd trimester: yes
3rd trimester: yes

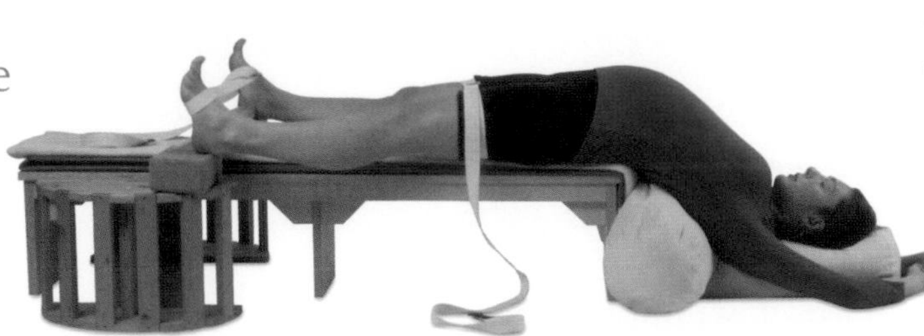

Viparita Karani, Legs Bent on a Chair

Inverted lake pose

Page 113

1st trimester: yes
2nd trimester: yes
3rd trimester: yes

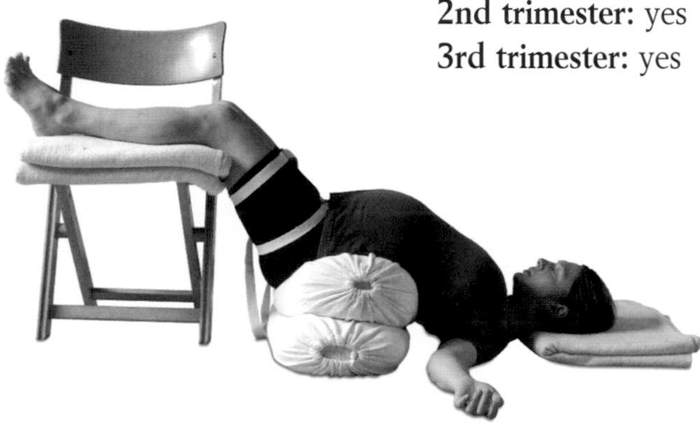

Viparita Karani Mudra

Upward action seal pose

Page 114

1st trimester: no
2nd trimester: yes
3rd trimester: yes

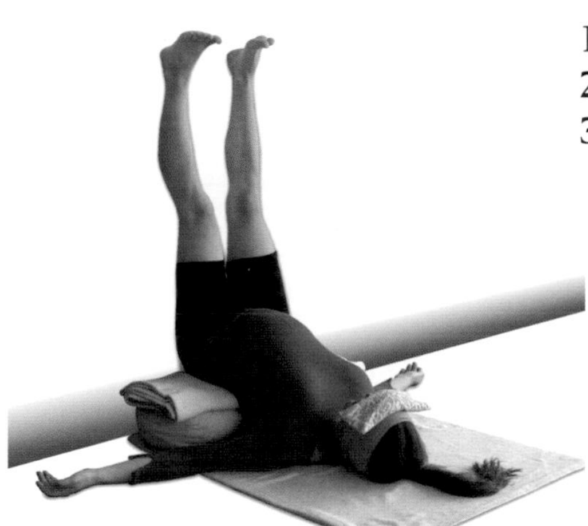

Salamba Sarvangasana, with a Chair

Shoulderstand pose

Pages 102 and 103

1st trimester: yes
2nd trimester: yes
3rd trimester: yes

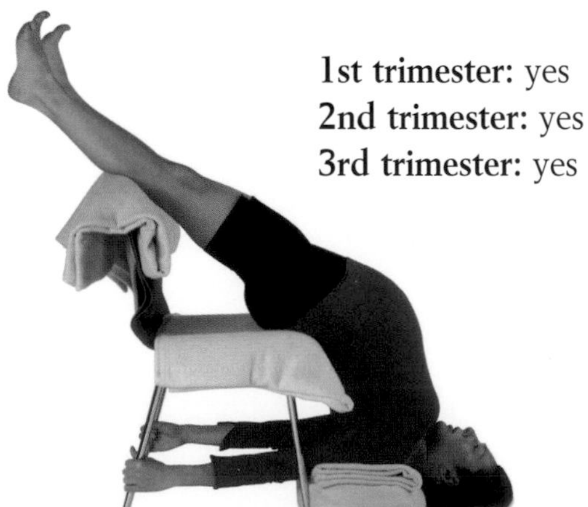

Salamba Purvottanasana

Supported eastern intense stretch pose

1st trimester: no
2nd trimester: yes
3rd trimester: yes

1 Place a table about 2 feet 6 inches away from the wall. Place two bolsters, one on top of the other, slightly recessed on the tabletop.

2 Sit on the very front edge of the bottom bolster, hold the edges of the table, and lie back over the second bolster.

3 Stretch your legs straight so that your toes are supported against the wall.

4 Let your arms extend out to the side with the palms facing up.

5 If your head falls back, place another blanket for support.

CHECK YOURSELF

> *Learn to spread your diaphragm.*

> *Broaden your chest by spreading your rib muscles.*

> *Keep your abdomen soft and below your chest level.*

> *Breathe smoothly, keeping the exhalation slightly longer than normal.*

> *Don't let your buttocks and feet slide down; you should feel your body securely held up on the bolster.*

> *If available, place a slanting plank horizontally on the top bolster to support your back at the lower edge of the shoulder blades (see photo). This gives an extra lift to the sides of the chest and the area around the heart.*

Benefits

- Lifts the spine and inner organs
- Lifts and widens the diaphragm and gives exceptional support to the heart
- Gives freedom in the chest and allows deep, smooth breathing
- Quiets the mind
- Relieves nervous tension

Contraindication

- Premature dilated cervix prolapse
- Bleeding and white discharge

Coming out of the pose

Bend your knees, exhale, and get up, lifting your torso.

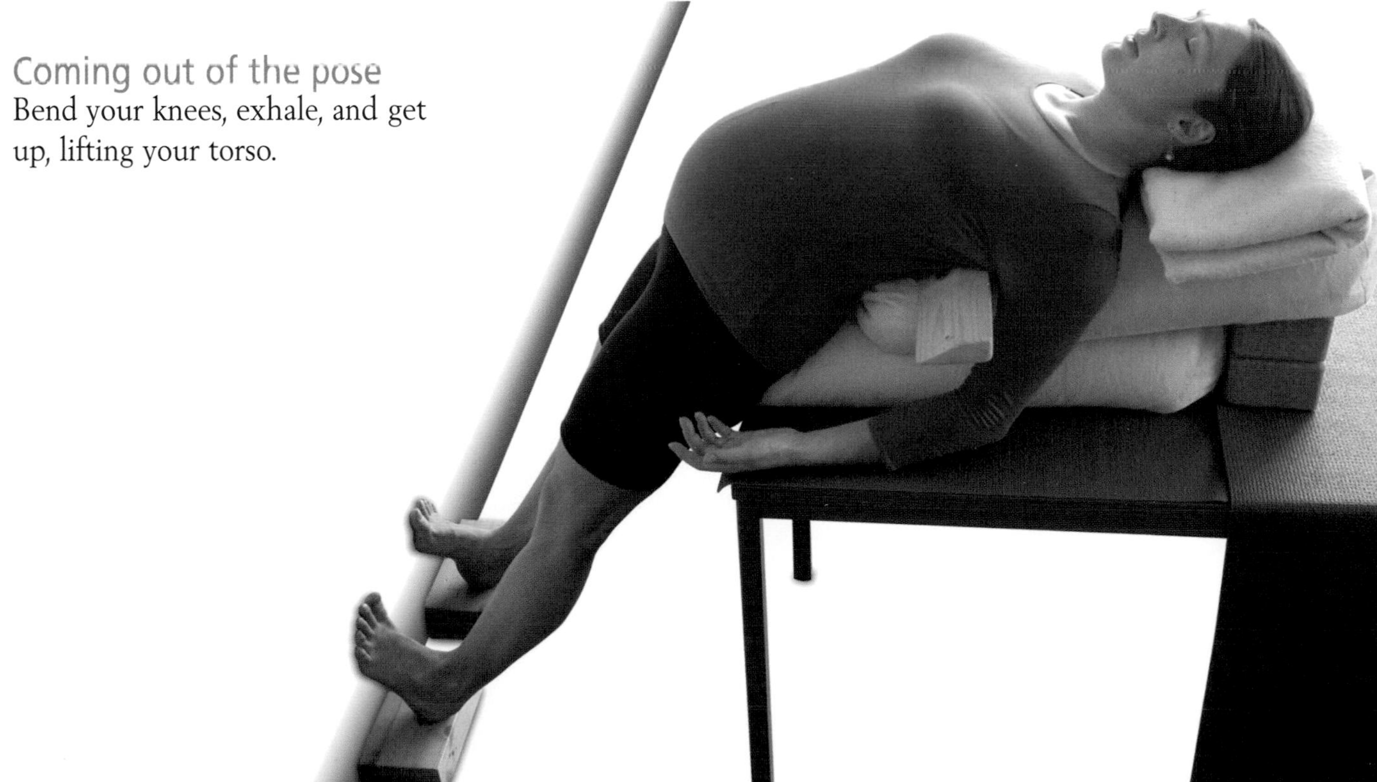

Cross-bolsters

Page 118

Shavasana

Corpse pose

In this asana, you lie motionless like a corpse, with your mind calm and still. This conscious relaxation of the body and mind invigorates both and removes all tension. The process is like recharging the battery of a car.

Although this asana appears simple, it is most difficult to master. The body and mind engage in a tug-of-war contest. By employing the art of introspection, Shavasana unites them and also connects asana and pranayama, leading you to the spiritual path.

Modified Technique with Bolster and Blanket

Adjusting Your Body

1 Spread a blanket on the floor. Place a bolster lengthwise for your back and a blanket for your head on top of the bolster.

2 Sit in Dandasana (page 64) with the bolster behind you.

3 Broaden and flatten your buttocks so that the flesh is not tight, especially in the small of your back (the region around the back of your waistline).

4 Lean your torso backward and start lowering your spine to the floor, making it convex so that the vertebrae come onto the bolster one after another. Don't move your buttocks or legs. Both sides of your torso should be spreading outward, from the center of your spine towards the sides of your body. The bolster supports your back from the waist to the head, so your chest remains at the same level as your abdomen, or a little higher.

5 Have a pillow or folded blanket under your head to keep it higher than your chest. Your body is in a descending plane from your head to your pelvis, avoiding tension in the head and heaviness in the chest, and facilitating breathing.

6 To keep the flesh of your buttocks from moving towards the sacrum, push the flesh to the sides and downwards. This relaxes the waist and lower back.

7 Release any hold on your legs and let your feet drop out to the sides.

8 Keep your chest relaxed, but don't cave it in.

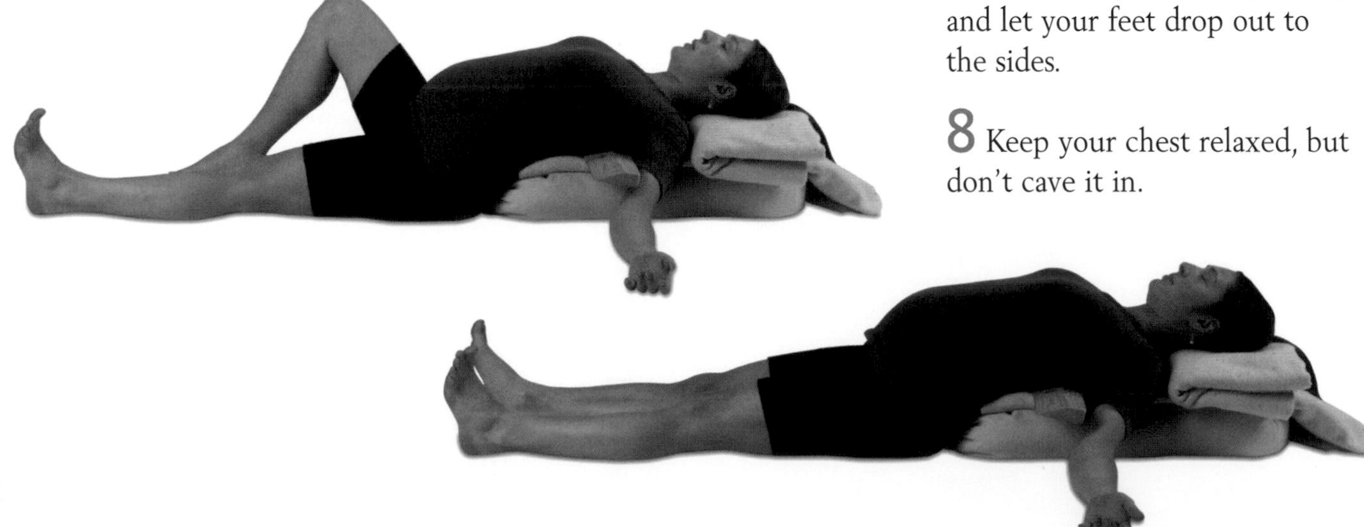

9 Relax your legs and drop your feet sideways to the ground, without disturbing the position of your legs.

10 Rest your extended arms at a 60° angle from your torso. Rotate your upper arms, elbows, and wrists so that your palms face the ceiling and your hands rest on the middle knuckle.

11 Make sure that the center of the back of your skull is resting on the folded blanket.

12 With your torso and limbs carefully and evenly placed, lower your upper eyelids down to the lower ones, release your eyeballs into their sockets, and relax any tension that might be around your eyes, temples, cheeks, and lips.

Head

1 With your hands, adjust the back of your head centrally on the floor. Keep the pebble-like projection at the base of the skull down.

2 Observe the following points:

- Don't tense your neck and throat.
- Don't press your chin against your throat.

Eyes and Ears

1 Close your eyes. Bring the upper eyelids downward gently without disturbing the pupils.

2 Keep your ears and eardrums relaxed; this can be adjusted by relaxing your lower jaw.

Nose

Keep your nose in a straight line, without tilting it to the side. The tip should face the middle of your chest.

1st trimester: yes
2nd trimester: yes
3rd trimester: yes

Benefits

Invigorates body and mind

Removes tension

Connects asana and pranayama and leads to the spiritual path

Arms and Shoulders

1 Broaden your spinal muscles keeping your shoulders away from your neck and your shoulder blades inwards.

2 Extend your upper arms from the sockets outward and place them on the floor without disturbing the position of your elbows. Bring the outer corners of your shoulders down.

3 Extend your forearms up to the wrists and place them on the floor so that your arms are at the same angle of 45° to 60° from the sides of your torso.

4 Keep your fingers relaxed and the skin of your palms passive.

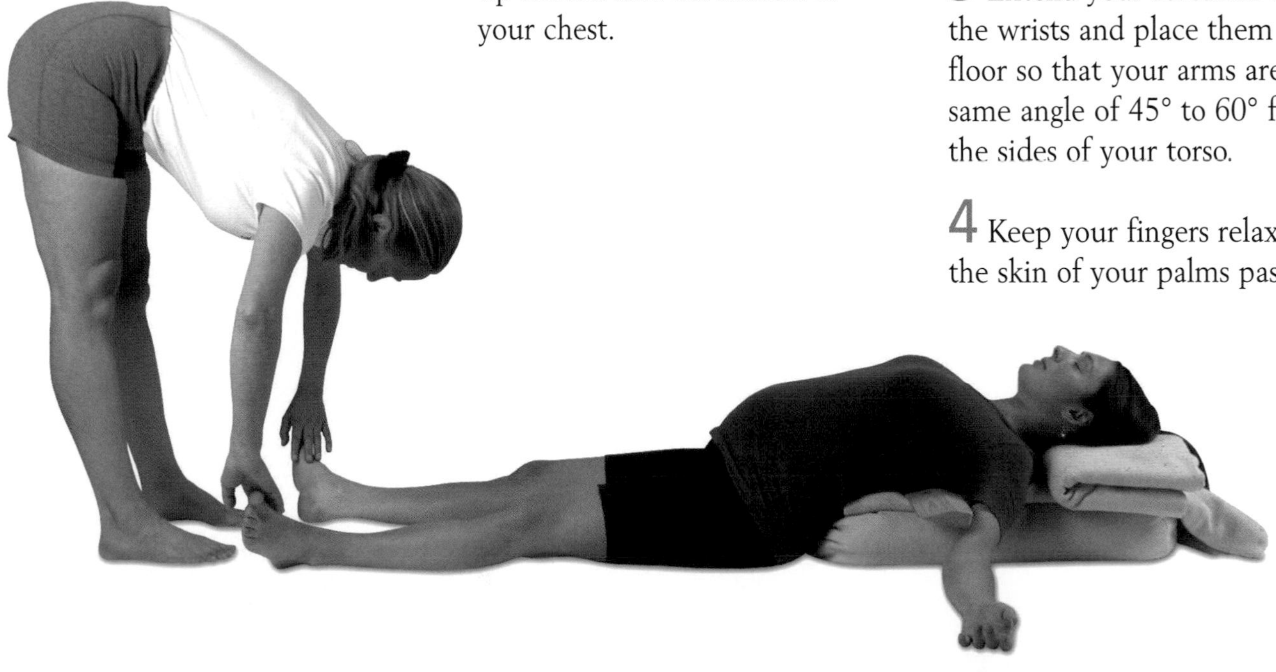

Final Position

1 The movement of breathing should not disturb your torso, limbs, and brain.

2 Remain in this final position of Shavasana.

Respiration

Don't do deep breathing. Breathing in Shavasana should be as subtle and smooth as the quiet flow of water in a river, so that the mind remains undisturbed.

During inhalation, don't:

- Jerk your head
- Tighten your throat
- Jerk your diaphragm
- Disturb the muscles at the back of your torso
- Cave in your breastbone
- Inflate your abdomen
- Tense your palms

During exhalation:

- Relax your brain
- Don't allow the air to touch the walls of the throat, causing irritation
- Don't release your diaphragm suddenly
- Keep your mind passive; let it watch and regulate the flow of exhalation
- Exhaling correctly results in a feeling of quiet surrender of the mind and body to Mother Earth, bringing a feeling of peace and oneness within oneself

◇

CHECK YOURSELF

> *Relax the skin of your forehead, your cheeks, lips, fingers, and hands, the sides of your torso, your buttocks, and your thighs.*

> *See that your palms are soft and relaxed.*

> *Keep your skin soft everywhere.*

> *Relax all your muscles.*

> *Drop the sides of the sacrum towards the floor to relax your buttocks.*

> *Don't lift your lumbar (lower) spine too far from the floor.*

> *Both sides of your torso near the spinal column should rest evenly on the pillows.*

> *Make sure that both sides of your body are evenly placed, and that half of it is not tilting to one side.*

> *Rest your upper shoulder blades on the blankets, but don't press them down, as pressure creates tension in the brain.*

> *Relax the skin of your facial muscles, which in turn relaxes the sensory organs.*

> *If there is any disturbance in your sensory organs, try to locate and relax it. Such disturbances are immediately reflected in the face and spread throughout the body via the nerves, tensing the entire system.*

> *Train yourself not to allow the thought process to arise:*
>
> - *If the brain is not at rest, the front of the head moves up from the chin as if the head and torso were separate.*
> - *If the brain is active, the eyeballs become hard.*

> *Drop your eyes downward. Direct your brain towards the center of your heart.*

> *The interrelation of the eyes, mind, and brain is very important: if the mind wanders, the brain moves upward and the eyes become unsteady.*

> *Draw in your eyes and ears and fuse them at the back of the brain. Let the energy flow towards the center of your chest, where external sounds cease to disturb.*

> *Surrender yourself, your body, and your mind to Mother Earth, so that you are calm and passive. This is total relaxation.*

Perfect Relaxation

In perfect relaxation, the mind remains unperturbed and an inward flow of energy is experienced. A new state of consciousness arises, with no movement and no resulting waste of energy. There is a feeling that the body has been elongated by several inches. This is freedom of the mind and freedom of the body.

Remain in this state of total relaxation as long as you can. From the state of silence, come back gradually to the active state. Don't disturb the silence of your mind or jerk your body suddenly and break its silence. Gradually bring your intellect, mind, and sensory organs, which have been submerged in a quiet, blissful state, back in contact with the world around you.

Coming out of the pose

1 Open your eyelids, but don't move your pupils up or down. Look straight ahead and continue experiencing the serene state while establishing contact with the external world.

2 Bend your knees and turn onto your right side by completely lowering your torso from the pillow. Don't turn your torso on the bolster, because the level will be awkward.

3 Press your left hand into the floor, look down, remain seated, and come up.

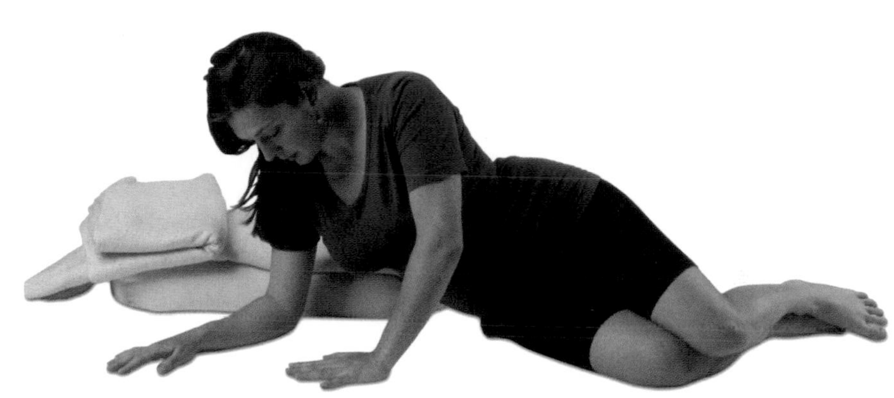

Notes

It may take some time for your mind to become steady and your body to become silent. With regular practice, you'll learn to release tension to experience the blissful state. In the beginning, you may fall asleep when you experience silence, but later you'll be able to be silent without falling asleep.

In the beginning, you may find it hard to adjust everything consciously. It will gradually become easier to observe and adjust everything simultaneously, so that your mind and body achieve rest quicker.

Later, as you master the asanas, you'll experience the nonexistent state of the body, the mind, the intellect, and the ego, and the self will be realized. The external world is there, but in this state, it seems nonexistent.

Special Instructions

- If it is difficult to relax your eyes in the beginning, wrap a soft bandage or cloth around your head, covering your eyes, ears, and the back of your head. The cloth should be folded four times, lengthwise.
- Although pregnant women are often advised to do Shavasana to help them relax, it is not all that easy for you to remove tension. Your bulky body makes it uncomfortable, and you may feel upset as a result. So bear in mind that these tensions have to be removed with other asanas before you can experience the relaxation of this asana.
- Especially in advanced pregnancy, you might prefer to perform inversions rather than Shavasana, since they bring the body and the mind to restfulness quickly.
- The best Shavasana, where you experience serenity, calmness, and a feeling of purity, can only come as a result of practicing other asanas accurately. The restorative asanas that we have dealt with in this section enable the body to be free of tension. Very often, you are unaware of the tension in your palms, fingers, soles, and toes, etc. Practicing these asanas removes these tensions and relaxes tight muscles.
- The feeling of nonexistence or emptiness created by Shavasana is not easy for you to face when you're pregnant. You may be nervous about confronting the state of solitude. Since your physical and mental condition is delicate, the best way to achieve positive quietness is to practice the other asanas in this section and then switch to Shavasana, so that the emptiness won't be negatively charged.
- If you do feel anxious, be sure to keep the blanket under your lumber region as shown in the second variation on the next page and breathe deeply and slowly, holding your breath for a second or two without any tension. This removes anxiety and relaxes your body faster. As anxiety decreases and you gain confidence, you don't need to focus attention on deep breathing. On the contrary, you can continue to breathe slowly, smoothly, and softly and you'll find that your breathing becomes subtle and easy.
- You should feel fresh, fearless, and positive after Shavasana. That is the parameter. You should not feel afraid, lonely, short of breath, or ready to burst into tears. If you do, you should concentrate more on the other asanas, before going on to Shavasana.

Variations

More relaxation for the back and abdomen

No. 1 In addition to the bolster that is lengthwise under your back, use a chair for your lower legs, which have to be fully supported. If the chair is too high, you can have one or two bolsters instead.

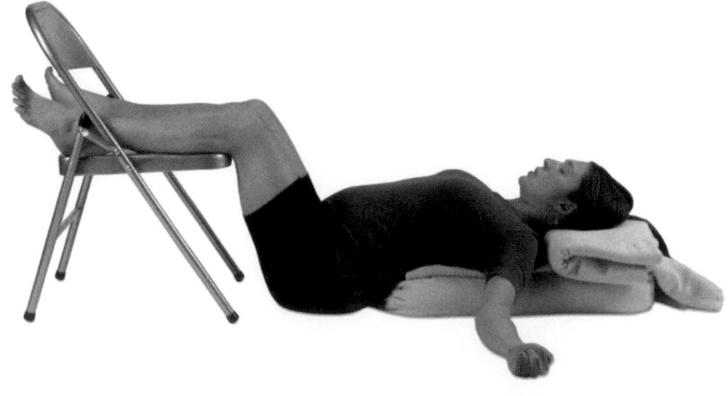

Make sure that your chest does not cave in and that your waist and buttock muscles relax down. This variation is also good for pranayama.

No. 2 Use two bolsters for your knees, a blanket folded three times for your chest and lumbar region (lower back), and a blanket for your head. Make sure that your chest does not cave in and that your waist and buttock muscles relax down, in the direction of the bolsters.

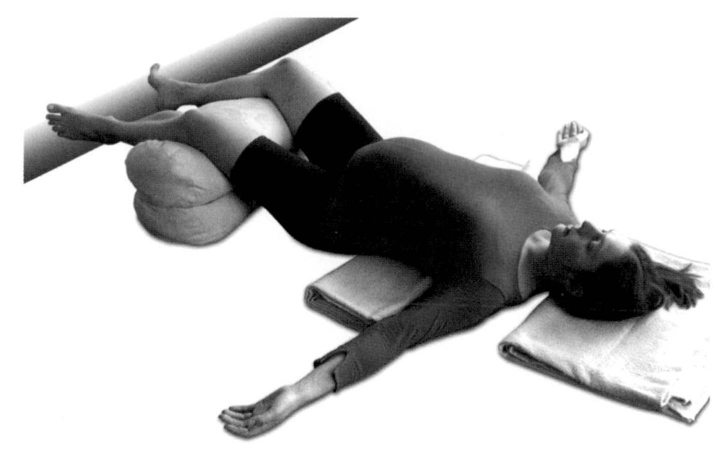

Advanced pregnancy: more height under the back

No. 3 To continue practicing Shavasana, you can put more height under your back (two to three bolsters as shown for Supta Virasana, page 129), to spread out the weight of your abdomen.

Last stage of pregnancy: pressure on the inferior vena cava, back discomfort

No. 4 In the last stage, when your uterus has become heavy, you may have problems lying on your back. This is because the baby is causing pressure on the inferior vena cava, the main vein that brings blood from the pelvis up to the heart. When this vessel is compressed, nausea, sweating, and dizziness are the result. If this happens, turn onto your left side and rest there to free the vein from pressure, as shown herc with a bolster for your bent leg.

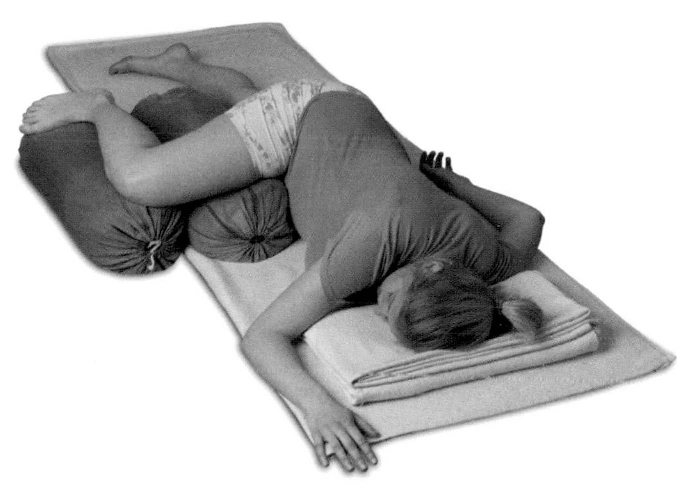

Breathing Techniques
Pranayama

Carrying a Spiritual Inheritance

For an expectant mother, practicing pranayama is as important as performing the asanas. Pranayama and the asanas together bestow physical and mental health on the mother and baby, and help the mother pass on a spiritual inheritance.

With the practice of Yoga, the mother unconsciously carries the pure, good, and auspicious imprints (*shubha samskaras*), which also affect the baby within. The foundation is laid in the womb itself for the child to develop on a morally, intellectually, and spiritually higher plane. This is the great importance of Yoga.

Vyasa Maharshi, Shakti (his grandfather), Ashtavakra, Vamadeva, Shuka, and others are examples of luminaries who reached intellectual maturity and spiritual accomplishment when they were still in their mothers' womb. The mothers of these great people were spiritually advanced in their own right. If a pregnant woman bears these examples in mind and practices Yoga seriously, she ensures that her offspring will benefit too.

The imprints of *yogabhyasa* (the practice of Yoga) remain deeply rooted in the hearts of the children. If the parents take to the practice of Yoga long before actual conception, the imprints of Yoga practice will be felt in the child. Therefore, it is also for the unborn child's sake that parents should take up the practice of Yoga.

Apart from this spiritual basis, Yoga undoubtedly helps you become physically stronger and healthier, and mentally calm , which ultimately helps the baby within to grow healthy as well.

Prana is energy; it is life itself, and breath. *Ayama* means "extension" and "expansion."

Pranayama means to make physical, intellectual, and spiritual energy become pervasive and comprehensive. Technically speaking, pranayama is a process of regulating, prolonging, and restraining inhalation, exhalation, and retention.

Its effect, however, is a process of *channeling* the energy, which renews awareness and sharpens intellectual powers. In the process of emptying your consciousness of unwanted, uncultured thoughts and emotions, pranayama kindles correct and polished thoughts, which lift you from the lower level of emotion and intellect to a higher one.

Chitta is the mind in its total sense and is composed of three categories: *manas*, the mind, *buddhi*, the intellect, and *ahamkar*, the ego or "I-ness".

The *chitta* and *prana*—consciousness and energy—are constantly in association. The prana is focused wherever the chitta is, and the chitta is focused wherever the prana is. The vehicle of chitta moves on two powerful forces: breath and desires. Therefore it is directed either in the direction of the breath or in the direction of desires. If breath prevails, then desires are controlled and consequently, the senses and the mind. If desire prevails, then breathing becomes uneven and the mind gets agitated. Pranayama is a technique through which breathing is controlled, disciplined, and directed in order to master desires.

A variety of pranayama exist to control the desires that disturb us at different stages of life, in different states of mind, and at different levels of physical, mental, intellectual, and spiritual ability.

If you would like to take up the practice of pranayama during your pregnancy, please note the guidelines below:

- Don't practice pranayama to the exclusion of asanas, because it is only through the practice of asanas that you gain control over your body, including:
  - The freedom and control that you need when moving your chest for proper breathing
  - The firmness you need for the lift of the spine
  - The movement and freedom that you need for the chest, neck, throat, spine, sternum, and collarbone to perform Jalandhara Bandha
  - The ability to perform Shavasana correctly
- Practice pranayama after your morning hygiene routine including brushing your teeth, washing, and using the toilet.
- Try to practice on an empty stomach; if you can't, then have a cup of tea, coffee, or milk.
- Wait at least four hours after a full meal before practicing.
- You can have a meal one hour after practicing.
- The best time to practice is in the morning before sunrise, or the evening after sunset. If you can't, then practice after doing the asanas or whenever convenient.
- If you practice pranayama first, then wait at least half an hour before practicing the asanas.
- If you practice asanas first, then you can do pranayama after a shorter period. Wait for fifteen minutes in between; you can use this interval to practice Shavasana.

Introducing Pranayama

Although there are many varieties of pranayama, we will deal with two types that can best guide you, when you're pregnant, to ease tension, anxiety, and pain, and to learn to take whatever comes with calm.

Pranayama is based on inhalation (*puraka*), exhalation (*rechaka*), and retention (*kumbhaka*).

Ujjayi Pranayama and Viloma Pranayama

Both of these pranayama can be done either in a lying-down or sitting pose, so you can either lie down in Shavasana, or sit in Padmasana, Svastikasana (cross-legged pose), Virasana, or even Baddha Konasana.

Ujjayi Pranayama

Ujjayi means "an ascending conquest without failure." It is the kind of pranayama that develops and improves your respiratory capacity progressively and gradually, eventually improving the nerves and increasing both willpower and intellect.

Ud means "upward," "superior in rank," or "expanding." It indicates the sense of power and preeminence. The second part of the word, *jayi*, means "victory" or "conquest." In the Yogic world view, this refers to the conquest and restraint of the chitta. In Ujjayi Pranayama, the lungs expand and the chest thrusts out like a mighty conqueror. The intellect is enhanced, so that buddhi, like a commanding chief, rules, controls, reasons, and applies its energy to determine what is right and wrong, true and untrue, real and unreal, permanent and temporary.

Ujjayi Pranayama involves deep breathing that controls every movement of the muscles as they expand and contract. It is a process in which you search for, tone, and regulate the movements of the chest and abdomen, and achieve clarity in these movements.

Viloma Pranayama

Viloma means "going against the natural order of things," "reverse," or "contrary." In the natural cycle of breathing, you inhale and exhale evenly, maintaining the continuous of flow of breath. In Viloma Pranayama, this continuous process is interrupted. *Vi* denotes "disjunction" or "negation," and *loma* means "hair." Viloma means "against the hair." It indicates a kind of opposition, stopping the natural flow or wandering of the mind.

A person who does not want to control the movements, temptations, emotions, and disturbances of the mind allows his or her mind to sway uncontrolled like a boat caught in the wind at sea. Such a mind remains uncontrolled, unconditioned, and untrained. The mind of the common man is of this type—like the hair on the skin, which falls in a certain direction. Moving the hair against its direction is painful, and so is trying to change the wandering nature of the pleasure-seeking mind.

In Viloma Pranayama, inhalation and exhalation are not a continuous process. The flow is checked and interrupted by several pauses. This pranayama is comparable to climbing up or down a tall ladder, with a pause at each step. During the pauses, the breath is neither let in nor out.

This pranayama has two variations. The first is done with interrupted inhalation, and the second with interrupted exhalation. The several pauses during either inhalation or exhalation make the motion and action of respiration more sensitive and clear. The action of respiration is sharpened and becomes more intensive.

The interruptions increase the duration of each inhalation and exhalation; this improves the intake of oxygen and the disposal of carbon dioxide, energizes the physiological body, and invigorates the circulatory system.

Positions for Pranayama

Sthirasukhamasanam

"Choose the position that will give you physical steadiness and mental tranquility."
(Patanjali, II:46)

1 Lying down in Shavasana (page 134) for a restful state

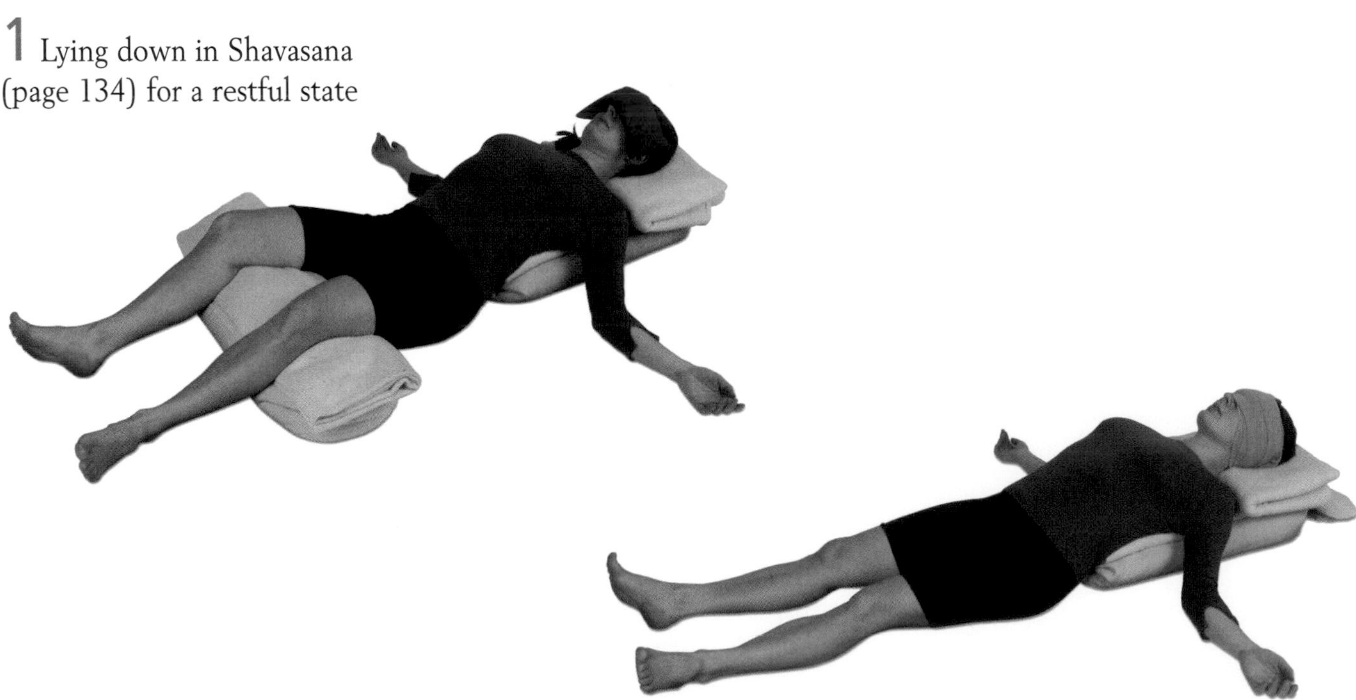

2 Sitting against the wall with legs in Svastikasana to keep the spine erect and the mind alert, steady, and thoughtful. Use blanket support for your knees. For a better lift, you can keep your hands close to your hips on the support.

3 Sitting against the wall with legs in Baddha Konasana, aerating the pelvis and widening the diaphragm. Use a blanket or block to support your knees. Hands either on the thighs or cupped close to your hips on the support.

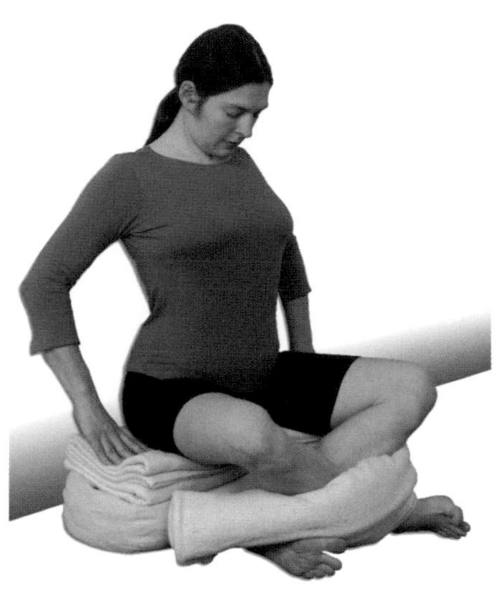

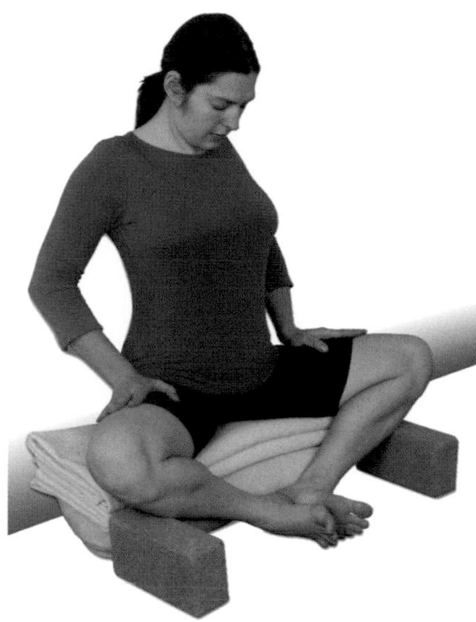

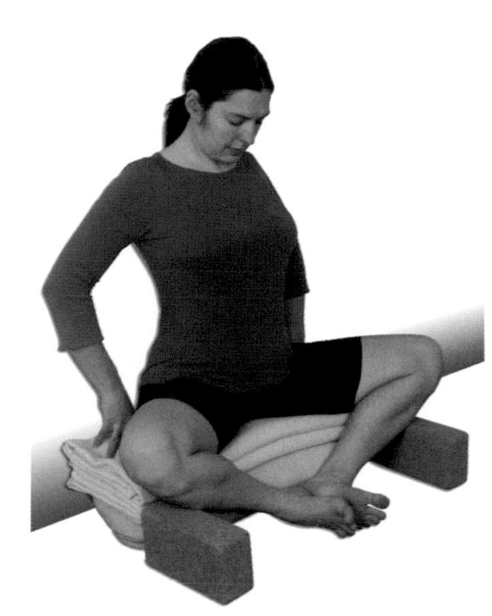

4 Sitting on a chair with a bolster in the back, to open the chest and diaphragm

5 Sitting on a chair holding the backrest for an easier lift

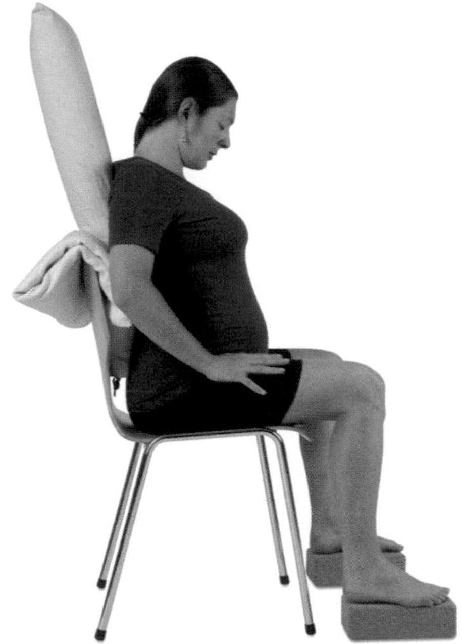

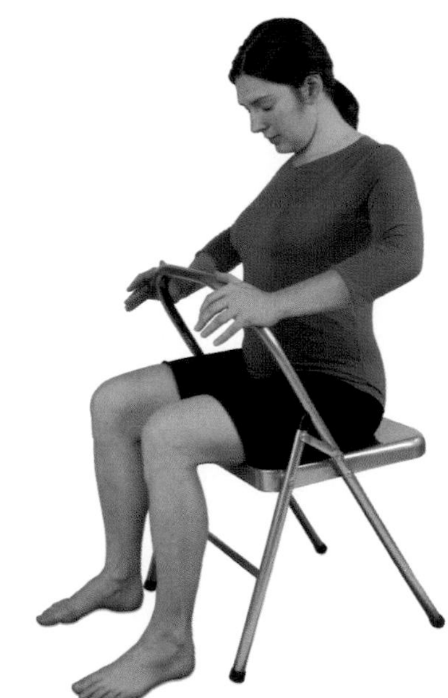

6 Sitting on a chair with the trestle along your back to widen the diaphragm and lift the spine and the internal organs. A very good choice in the last stages of pregnancy or when anxiety is inhibiting exhalation.

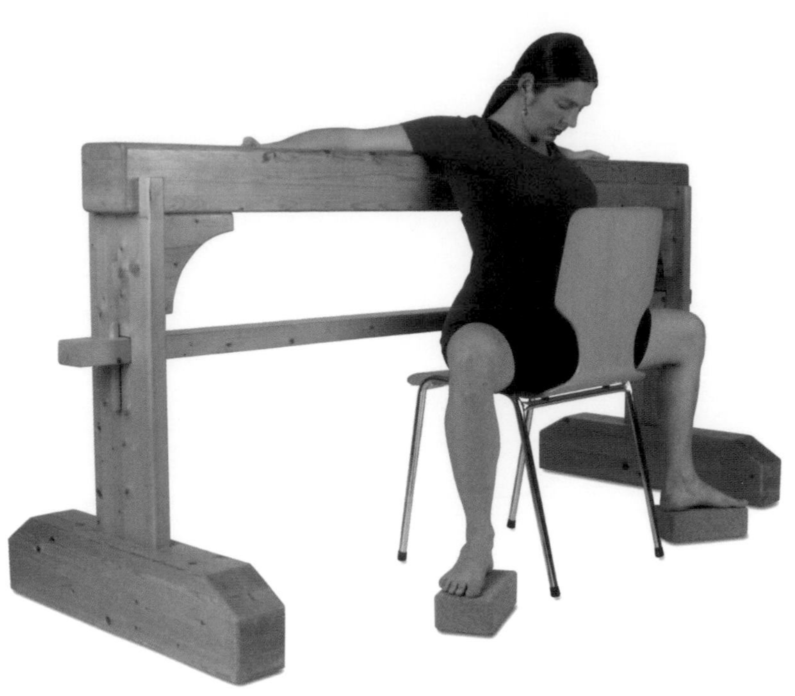

◇

In all positions for pranayama and relaxation, you can wrap a bandage around your head. The bandage should cover your ears, eyes, forehead, and part of the neck. The skin on your forehead should not be lifted towards the crown of your head, but should descend downward towards your eyes. This is necessary to allow the frontal brain and the senses of perception to rest in a quiet state. Tie the bandage only as indicated and tuck in the end on the side. The technique is shown in the photos below.

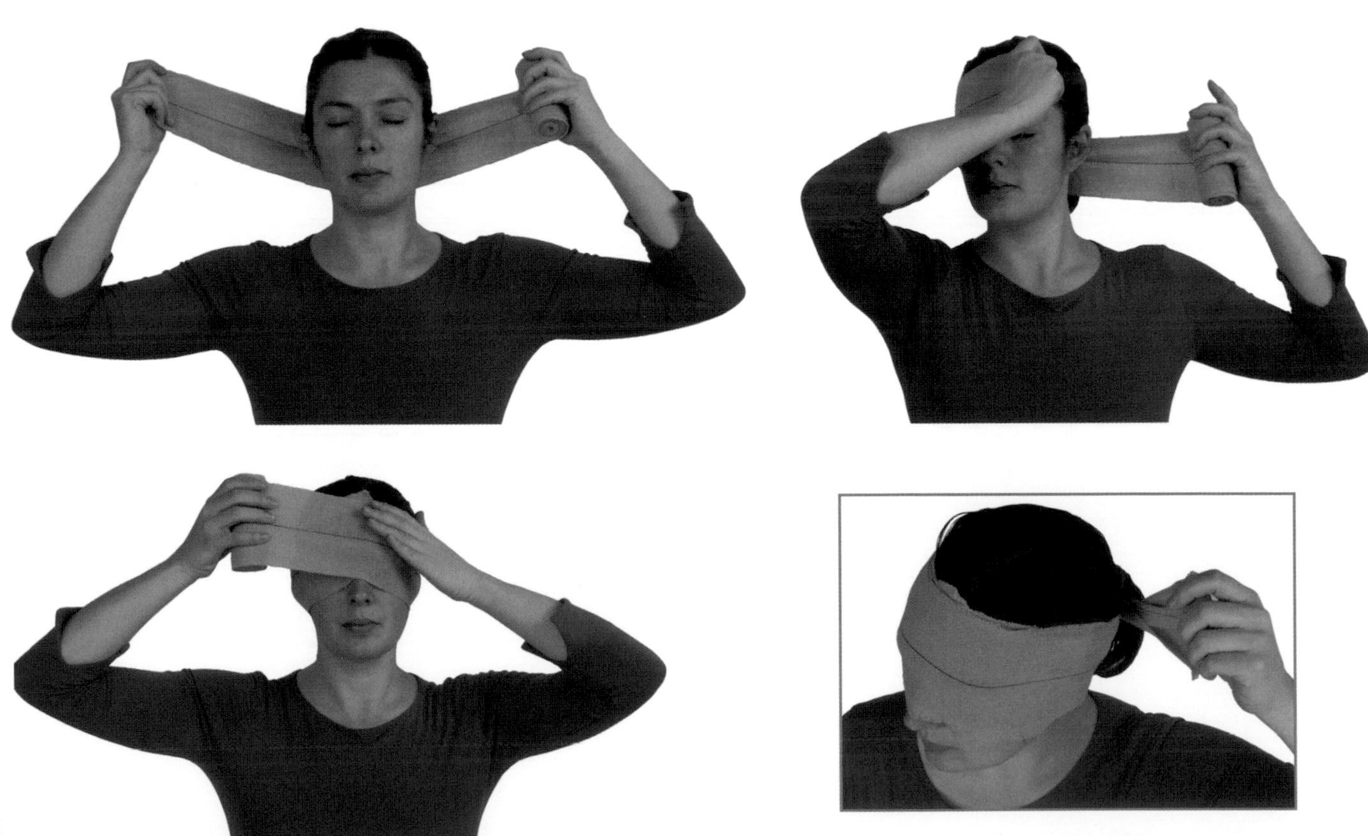

A Word to Beginners

Begin with the pranayama in the lying-down positions like Shavasana (page 134) and Supta Baddha Konasana (page 126). The sitting poses are not recommended in the first and second trimesters, because the combination of sitting and doing the pranayama might cause too much tension. In your third trimester, after having toned your body, you can start with the sitting poses to prepare for the delivery.

◇

Instructions for the Sitting Poses

Svastikasana is the best pose for you because your legs are crossed, which gives the body firmness and stability. In this pose, it's easy to keep your spine erect and your mind alert. The base of the spine and the perineum remain off the ground, giving a feeling of weightlessness and a steady, thoughtful state of the mind. The base of your torso becomes light, giving the chest area freedom to expand in pranayama.

- When you practice pranayama, your facial muscles, ears, eyes, neck, shoulders, arms, and thighs can get tight or strained. It is essential to keep them completely relaxed.
- Whatever sitting pose you choose, make sure that your spine is well stretched and concave, and that your body is erect.
- Your legs should stay as immovable as a root, so that the trunk above remains firm and strong.
- Balance the cervical (upper) vertebrae on the tailbone and maintain both at right angles to the floor, so that your torso does not lean forward or backward.
- Rest your seat in a balanced position between the anus and the perineum.
- Stretch your spine vertebra by vertebra and extend upward, in the direction of your head. You should feel the extension from the base to the top as though you're climbing a ladder step by step. First correct the position of your spine, and then adjust the other parts of the body.
- Normally, the sacrum sags and sticks out, which affects the flow of energy at the base of the spine. So you have to pull it in and lift it up, thus reversing the process of sagging energy.
- The lumbar (lower) spine often caves in, resulting in a convex dorsal (mid) spine and collapsed chest; it must be re-educated by creating space between your waist and chest to enable your torso to extend vertically up.
- The dorsal spine is usually convex, which keeps the lungs dropping within the thoracic cavity. It must be made concave, so that your inner organs function well.
- The cervical spine must be pulled slightly back and then extended up for proper alignment of the body and integration of the mind. Otherwise dullness sets in.
- The spine, with all its natural curvatures, has to remain erect without undue concavities or convexities, so that energy and life force may flow freely throughout the body.

Wall Support

We recommend using the support of the wall as you learn to sit in these poses. It will help you raise your lower spine without having to move it abruptly, and help you feel more comfortable and breathe freely.

Shoulders

- The lower part of your shoulder blades should be pulled into your chest and away from your spine in order to broaden the chest cavity.
- Your shoulders should be extended sideways away from your neck, not be tensed up or raised towards your ears.

Chest

- Tuck in and roll up your back ribs so that the frontal ribs lift and broaden, creating space for the rib muscles to extend. Expand your chest.
- Lift your breastbone.
- Your floating ribs (two lower ribs on either side) should expand towards the sides, so that your diaphragm can move with ease.
- Develop your ability to extend your rib muscles upward and expand them sideways during inhalation, and relax them towards the center in exhalation. Try to do this without jerky movements, aggressiveness, or sudden contraction.

Jalandhara Bandha

When you practice pranayama in a sitting pose, Jalandhara Bandha is essential. *Jala* means "net," and *bandha* means "bondage" or "binding." This bandha regulates the flow of blood and prana to the heart and to the glands in the neck and brain.

In Jalandhara Bandha, your neck and throat are contracted, and your chin rests in the notch between your collarbones. Once your have mastered Salamba Sarvangasana, this is easy.

Until then, don't force your neck muscles down; just lower your head from the nape of your neck as far as you can comfortably. At the same time, lift your breastbone and don't cave in your chest. During inhalation, your head has a tendency to lift up; be careful with every inhalation that this does not happen.

From the physical point of view, Jalandhara Bandha prevents strain on the heart during pranayama. From the psychological view, however, it has a deeper significance. The brain is considered to be the seat of the ego. In Jalandhara Bandha, the brain is lowered, thereby reducing its dominance during pranayama. The brain is made to bow down in salutation to one's own soul, which is part of the universal soul. Your breath becomes quiet and subtle, and you experience a state of neutrality.

Eyes

- Your eyes should be closed completely, but not tightly. Your eyelids should exert only very light pressure on your eyeballs. Keeping your eyes open in Pranayama will disturb your practice and cause a burning sensation in the eyes.
- Your eyes should look inward and watch the subtle movements of your body and breathing. Don't let your pupils roll up towards your forehead, because that starts the thought process. Focus your pupils on the seat of the self.

Ears

- Keep your ears relaxed. If they contract or are subjected to tension, your lower jaw will also contract and your temples will be tensed. This will cause headache and heaviness of the head.
- Listen to the sound of inhalation and exhalation. The sound should be smooth, clear, steady, long, and pleasant. The inhalation and the exhalation should be of equal tempo and rhythm. Your ears should remain alert throughout your practice so that the moment the sound becomes ruffled or harsh, you can immediately correct it.

Nose

- Breathe through your nose, not through your mouth.

- The septum, which divides the nose, should always be kept straight.
- The mucous membrane should be soft and not tensed, so you can register the sensations of inhalation and exhalation. If the membrane is tough and hard, sufficient air does not pass through. This makes the lungs inactive.

Tongue

- Your tongue should be relaxed and rested on your lower jaw. It tends to touch the upper jaw, but you should try to break this habit. If your tongue is not relaxed, then saliva accumulates and hinders the flow of breath.
- Saliva is produced in the beginning, but you should swallow it only after exhalation (not after inhalation and not during the process of breathing).

Mouth

- Don't clench your teeth.
- Loosen your lower jaw from the upper jaw.
- Keep your lips relaxed.

Throat

- Relax your throat.
- Avoid jerky and forceful inhalation, which can cause irritation.

Arms

Relax your arms in their sockets so that they remain loose.

Jnana Mudra

Rest the back of your wrists on your thighs. Join the tips of your thumbs and index fingers, forming them into a circle. Relax the other three fingers. (Normally when Jnana Mudra is shown, these three fingers are extended; in pranayama, however, they should be kept loose). Your palms should remain soft and the back of your wrists should rest on your thighs.

Jnana Mudra indicates the experience of supreme knowledge. It symbolizes the union of the individual soul (represented by the index finger) with the Supreme Being (represented by the thumb).

Brain

Keep your brain calm and passive, yet alert. Don't tighten the skin of your head. The function of the brain is to watch closely the subtle movements of breath and the actions of the body, and to send messages to the parts of the body where adjustments are needed (acting here as the controller). It also receives messages from all over the body informing that the adjustments have been made (acting here as the receiver).

It may seem impossible to keep the brain both passive *and* alert enough to perform the necessary actions. During pranayama, however, with regular and persistent effort, it is possible to perform these apparently contradictory actions with case. Once you have learned how to do so, the actions become automatic and the brain, torso, chest, and mind all function spontaneously.

Ujjayi Pranayama 1, in Shavasana

Expanded conquest of life-force energy 1, in corpse pose

1st trimester: yes
2nd trimester: yes
3rd trimester: yes

1 Lie down on a blanket with a bolster underneath your back.

2 Relax your body and quiet your mind as explained in Shavasana.

3 Begin the pranayama. Exhale completely, emptying whatever air is in your lungs.

4 Relax your diaphragm so that it is soft. Deflate your abdominal organs, but don't forcibly press them in. Keep them in contact with your spine.

5 Inhale slowly, quietly, deeply, and steadily. As you begin inhalation, keep your mind quiet; a disturbed and anxious mind, polluted with thoughts, will increase the speed of your breathing and create jolts in the body.

6 Fill your lungs completely with air, from the floating ribs to the top brim of the chest. This is called *puraka*. Observe the following points:

- Keep all other parts of your body relaxed.
- Keep your chest cavity separated from your abdomen so that the abdomen remains relaxed.
- When your lungs are full and you can't take in any more air, you'll experience a natural pause for a second or two. Your brain is likely to become tense and hard, so maintain your position in such a manner that your chest does not get overinflated and your brain cells remain in a deflated state. The natural pause will allow this change to occur in the brain.
- Don't allow your ribs to collapse, and keep your grip on your diaphragm.
- Keep your chest held up without tightening your throat.

7 Exhale slowly, quietly, and steadily, until your lungs are empty. This is called *rechaka*. Sudden exhalation will cause body tremors. To avoid these tremors and check the sudden outrush of breath, consciously hold your chest high and lead the outgoing breath steadily and smoothly. Make sure your rib muscles don't get compressed.

8 This completes one cycle; do 8 to 10 cycles.

9 After completing the last cycle, lie in Shavasana and breathe normally.

Benefits

The basis of all pranayama is reflected in this one, as are the corresponding benefits:

Generates vital energy

Aerates the lungs

Tones and soothes the nervous system

Steadies the wandering mind

Alleviates exhaustion

Heals respiration problems such as burning in the chest and shortness of breath

Special Instructions

- Although you should perform 8 to 10 cycles of Ujjayi Pranayama, it can be difficult to perform the cycles continuously. Your diaphragm and abdomen may become tightened, which causes the cycles to occur too fast.

- To counteract this, alternate cycles of Ujjayi and normal breathing. After each Ujjayi cycle, do some normal inhalation and exhalation, which allows the diaphragm muscles to recover and the next Ujjayi cycle to go smoothly.

Respiration in Ujjayi Pranayama 1

***Puraka* (Inhalation)**

- Breathe through your nose. Feel the touch of your breath on your palate. If it's soothing, the sound is like the syllable "sssa." If it's irritating to the throat, it causes you to cough and does not allow your lungs to fill properly.
- When you inhale, fill the lower part of your lungs first, then the middle, and lastly the upper part.
- Expand and extend your rib muscles sideways from the breastbone to the sides of your torso, and upward from your floating ribs (two lower ribs on each side) to the top of your chest simultaneously, so that your chest is broadened all the way around.
- Raise your back ribs slightly towards your front ribs.
- Open your chest gently from the center outward, as if it were a flower opening, with the pressure of the incoming breath being the centrifugal force.
- Inhalation, and the extension and expansion of your chest, should be simultaneous.
- After inhalation your head and chin tend to rise; make sure this does not happen.

Rechaka (Exhalation)

- Keep your brain, throat, and sensory organs relaxed, exhale fully, and then inhale quietly and deeply.
- Exhale gently through your nose, without straining your throat and without suddenly dropping your rib muscles and breastbone. The expelled air will make a "huuum" sound at the base of your throat.
- At the beginning of the exhalation, your top ribs remain firm. Relax them only when you reach the middle of the exhalation.
- Exhalation causes a certain amount of tension in the diaphragm. Stretch it sideways to soften it; tension in the diaphragm strains the heart.
- Keep your abdominal organs parallel to your spine.
- As you exhale, the sides of your torso should not collapse. Your chest should deflate slowly and gradually from the sides to the center with centripetal force, like a lotus closing its petals after sunset.
- Don't allow your chest to contract inward during exhalation.
- Both puraka and rechaka should be done consciously, with alertness.

Ujjayi Pranayama 2

1 Sit or lie down, in the pose you have chosen.

2 Keep your spine erect, raise your breastbone, lower your head, and perform Jalandhara Bandha.

3 Place the back of your wrists on your thighs and your palms in Jnana Mudra. Keep your fingers loose.

4 Close your eyes and draw them inward.

5 Exhale slowly and completely.

6 Take a slow, deep, and steady breath through your nose. You should feel the incoming air on your palate and hear a "sssa" sound. The sound should be soft, and you shouldn't try to elicit it forcefully. Keep your tongue loose, resting on your lower jaw.

7 Fill your lungs completely with an inward breath, extending and expanding your chest. Deep inhalation is a conscious effort to breathe in fully by expanding your chest deliberately and gradually from the bottom to the top, and outward, like a fountain, spreading up and sideways. Don't inflate your abdominal area, but keep it in contact with your spine. Your chest moves up like a hill, and your abdomen remains like a valley.

8 Observe the following points:
- Don't tense your brain, eyes, or temples.
- Your diaphragm should be firm, so that your chest does not feel tension.

9 Release the pressure on your abdominal organs. Exhale slowly, deeply, and completely, observing the following points:
- Release the tension on your rib muscles, breastbone, and diaphragm gradually.
- Do so only after 1 or 2 seconds of exhalation, to avoid injury to your heart or lungs.

10 Before inhaling again, wait for a second in normal retention. Retention is the gap between inhalation and exhalation, and between exhalation and inhalation. It takes place unconsciously. In retention, don't pull your abdomen in. (It is pulled in for Uddiyana Bandha, which pregnant women don't perform.)

11 The following is the complete cycle of Ujjayi Pranayama 2:
- *Puraka* (inhalation): full and complete
- *Kumbhaka* (retention): 3 to 5 seconds
- *Rechaka* (exhalation): full and complete
- *Kumbhaka* (normal retention): 1 second

12 Before going into the next cycle, take two or three normal breaths with normal inhalation and exhalation.
In normal inhalation:
- Expand your middle ribs more than the top and bottom ribs.
- Extend and expand your chest as fully and naturally as possible, without tension or pressure on the brain, rib muscles, or diaphragm.
- Hold up your breastbone.
- Keep your diaphragm soft and lifted, so that there is no stress on the lungs or the chest muscles.

13 Inhale and exhale in the Ujjayi manner.

14 Do 8 to 10 cycles this way, without increasing the length of the retention.

15 After completing the last cycle, breathe normally and remain still in this position for some time. Then slowly raise your head and open your eyes quietly.

Benefits

Ujjayi breathing:

- Strengthens your body physiologically and gives a sense of steadiness
- Supplies plentiful oxygen
- Increases lung capacity and opens and activates the air sacs
- Creates a filtering action
- Increases endurance
- Reduces anxiety
- 1st trimester: eliminates tiredness, low energy, and nausea
- 3rd trimester: gives vitality and energy
- Delivery: can be a great help, if you have practiced during pregnancy

16 You can now either lie down in Shavasana or switch to Viloma Pranayama.

Notes

Don't release the Jalandhara Bandha after each cycle. Continue it even during normal breathing and release it only when you have finished pranayama. When keeping your head in a straight position, don't open your eyes or allow your body to collapse.

Viloma Pranayama Stage 1, Interrupted Inhalation
Interrupted inhalation pose

1st trimester: yes
2nd trimester: yes
3rd trimester: yes

1 Lie down correctly in Shavasana.

2 Exhale, emptying your lungs.

3 Inhale through both nostrils, feeling the touch of the air on the membrane of the nostrils. Follow the instructions for Ujjayi Pranayama 1. Remember, though, that here the inhalations are with interruptions.

4 Inhale for 2 seconds, and hold your breath for 2 seconds. Again: Inhale for 2 seconds, and hold your breath for 2 seconds. Continue this process until your lungs are full.

Feel the movement of your chest from the bottom of the floating ribs upward, up the ladder of the chest, to the top. After inhalation, retain and stabilize the lift of your chest.

5 Exhale slowly, deeply, and continuously until your lungs are empty, following the instructions given in Ujjayi Pranayama 2. When you exhale, hold your chest up and release the air slowly through your nostrils, gradually releasing the tension from the bottom of your chest.

6 This completes one cycle. In the beginning, practice 6 – 8 cycles.

7 The complete cycle of Viloma Pranayama Stage 1 is as follows:
- Inhalation – retention, inhalation – retention, repeated until your lungs are full. The last retention is a little longer than the previous ones.
- Complete exhalation without a break.

8 After the first 2 seconds of inhalation, your chest expands and extends, and your diaphragm remains firm. Thereafter, during retention, don't release your chest, diaphragm, or breastbone. Retention should not cause any pressure or tension in the brain, and it should not inflate your abdomen.

9 On average, you'll be able to do 4 – 5 retentions. Later, when your inhalation time increases, the retention time will also increase. The inhalations and retentions should be of equal duration.

10 Because it is difficult to do retention with each cycle, you can alternate one cycle of Viloma Pranayama Stage 1 with one cycle of Ujjayi Pranayama 1 (deep breathing), and continue this method for the entire duration of your pregnancy.

Sitting Poses

1 After mastering this pranayama in Shavasana, you can also do it in a sitting postion. Towards the end of pregnancy, sitting pranayamas become easier to do. During early pregnancy, however, when you may have morning sickness, it's better to do them semi reclining, with the support of bolsters or other props.

2 In sitting poses, keep your spine erect. Lower your head and do Jalandhara Bandha.

3 Follow the same techniques as above.

Viloma Pranayama Stage 2

Interrupted exhalation pose

1 Lie down in Shavasana (page 134).

2 Exhale, emptying your lungs. Don't raise your head.

3 Inhale slowly, steadily, deeply, and rhythmically. After a complete inhalation, pause for a while, observing the following points:
- Don't raise your head.
- Keep your breastbone up.
- Keep your diaphragm firm, so that you don't exhale suddenly.

4 Exhale for 2 seconds, and pause for 2 seconds. Again, exhale for 2 seconds, and pause for 2 seconds. Continue in this manner until your lungs are completely empty. Release your chest from the top to the bottom.

5 After the last exhalation, don't retain the breath, but do a cycle of Ujjayi Pranayama 1 (page 148). Alternate cycles of Viloma Pranayama Stage 2 and Ujjayi Pranayama 1.

6 Practice 6 – 8 cycles.

7 The complete cycle of Viloma Pranayama Stage 2 is as follows:
- Complete inhalation
- Exhalation – retention, exhalation – retention, repeated until your lungs are empty.
- Last exhalation – no retention

8 During retention, your chest is firm, but it does not expand or constrict.

9 After complete exhalation, always relax your head.

Sitting Poses

- As in stage 1, you can do stage 2 in a sitting position, after you have mastered it in Shavasana.
- In sitting positions, you must perform Jalandhara Bandha to avoid straining your heart.
- Follow the same technique as above.

Special Instructions

- The number of pauses in inhalation (stage 1) and exhalation (stage 2) should be equal. The interrupted exhalations and retentions in stage 2 should be equal in length.

- Here also, if it is difficult to perform several cycles of stage 2 at one stretch, you can alternate cycles of stage 2 and Ujjayi Pranayama 1.

Beginners

1st trimester: no
2nd trimester: no
3rd trimester: yes

Advanced students

1st trimester: yes
2nd trimester: yes
3rd trimester: yes

Benefits

Breath finds the most remote places.

Ujjayi Pranayama strengthens physiologically and creates a sense of steadiness.
Viloma Pranayama strengthens mentally and creates a sense of exhilaration.
Both give a feeling of ease and lightness, especially in the third trimester.

Viloma Pranayama Stage 1

Energizing

Relieves:
Fatigue
Strain
Weakness
Low blood pressure

Increases courage and endurance

Viloma Pranayama Stage 2

Cooling

Relieves:
Nausea
High blood pressure
Heaviness in the abdomen

Soothes and quiets the mind and brain

Reduces overactivity

Recommended Combinations of Pranayama Techniques

Practice the first sequence below followed by the second sequence, and then return to the first one again, and so on.

If you prefer, you can always practice the sitting pranayama while lying down, until you feel ready to begin practicing sitting up.

◇

1st Sequence

1st day: Ujjayi Pranayama 1 in Shavasana with Viloma Stage 1, sitting
2nd day: Viloma Stage 1 in Shavasana with Viloma Stage 2, sitting
3rd day: Viloma Stage 1 in Shavasana with Ujjayi Pranayama 2, sitting

2nd Sequence

1st day: Ujjayi Pranayama 1 in Shavasana with Ujjayi Pranayama 2, sitting
2nd day: Viloma Stage 2 in Shavasana with Viloma Stage 1, sitting
3rd day: Viloma Stage 2, in Shavasana and sitting

Note Regarding the 3rd Trimester

Towards the end of your pregnancy, you should concentrate more on pranayama. In fact, by the very nature of your needs at this time, you might find the pranayamas easier than the asanas. You can reduce the duration of each inhalation and exhalation, as well as the duration of each cycle of pranayama. Therefore, you could practice in two shorter sessions, one in the morning and one in the evening.

CHAPTER 3

The Beginning of Your Pregnancy

Before You Conceive and the First Trimester

When you have decided to get pregnant, it's very important that you maintain or reach health conditions that will ensure a healthy pregnancy (*see section below*). During the first three months (up to the 14th or 16th week after conception), your health is equally—if not more—important, to protect the pregnancy.

The health of the thyroid gland is especially important. Deficiency in its secretions and enlargement of the gland (goiter) can result in miscarriage.

The following asanas are among the most beneficial for this stage. Practice them, if you can, under the guidance of an experienced Iyengar Yoga teacher.

- Salamba Shirshasana (page 97, with precise alignment)
- Salamba Sarvangasana (page 102, with precise alignment)
- Setu Bandha Sarvangasana (page 108, supported)
- Janu Shirshasana (page 82, concave back and bottom chest lifted, after you have conceived)

◇

Health Conditions for a Healthy Pregnancy

- Blood that is rich in hemoglobin
- Normal blood pressure
- Moderate weight gain (up to 22 pounds considered normal)
- No albumins in the urine
- Healthy thyroid gland
- Daily practice of relaxing and restorative Yoga asanas and pranayama. These soothe the nerves and the endocrinologic system, and gently strengthen blood circulation in the pelvis, reproductive organs, and spine.

Once You're Pregnant: Asanas to Stop

The following asanas, which have a lifting and wringing action, could endanger the embryo by thinning the inner lining of the uterus.

• Parivritta Trikonasana and Parivritta Parshvakonasana

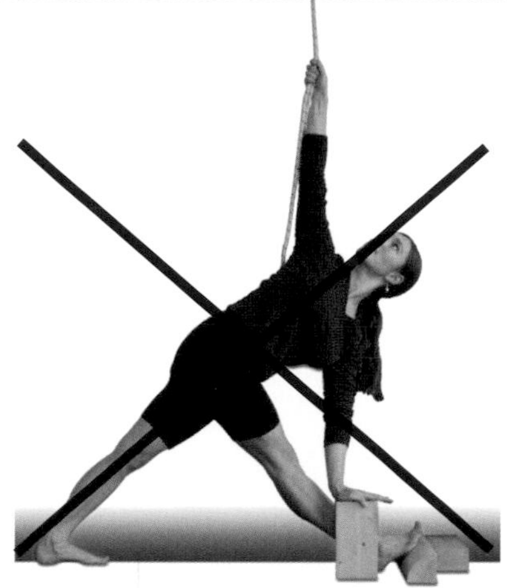

• Marichyasana

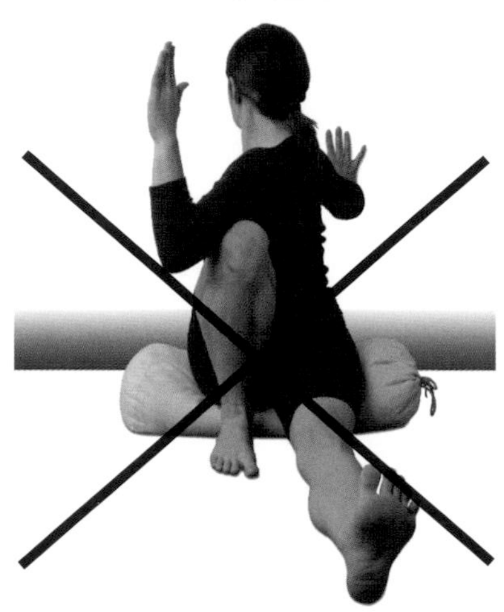

• Ardha Matsyendrasana

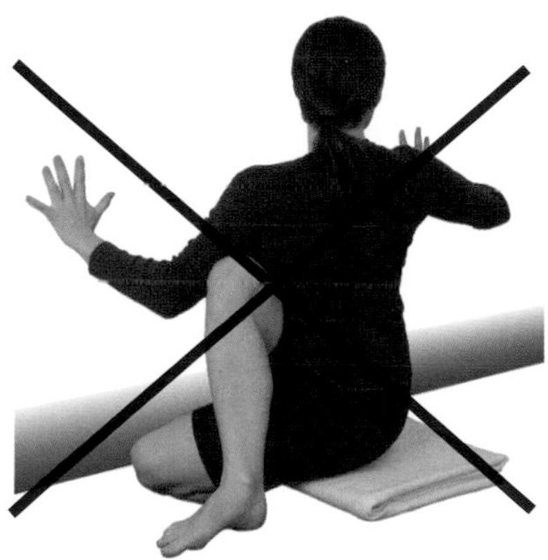

• Dhanurasana and Urdhva Dhanurasana

These also endanger the embryo by lengthening and thinning the inner lining of the uterus.

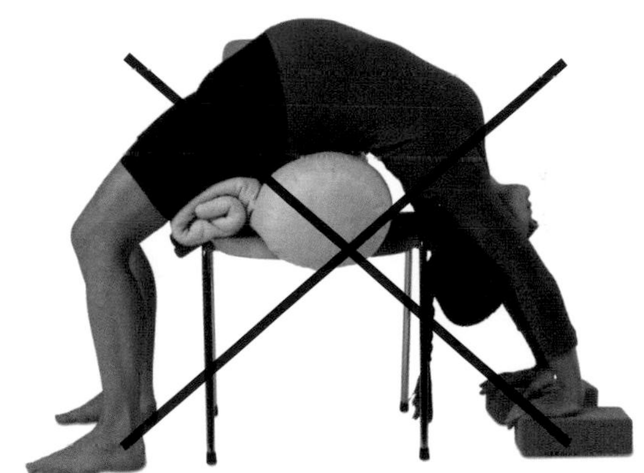

• Urdhva Prasarita Padasana

Puts too much pressure on the pelvic floor and might cause miscarriage.

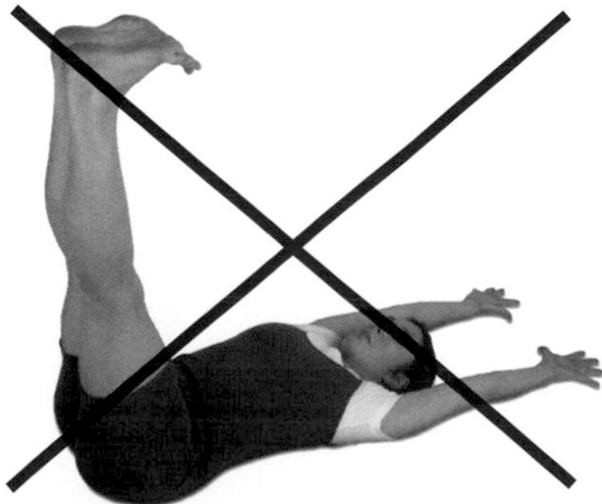

• Pashchimottanasana

Compresses the fetus.

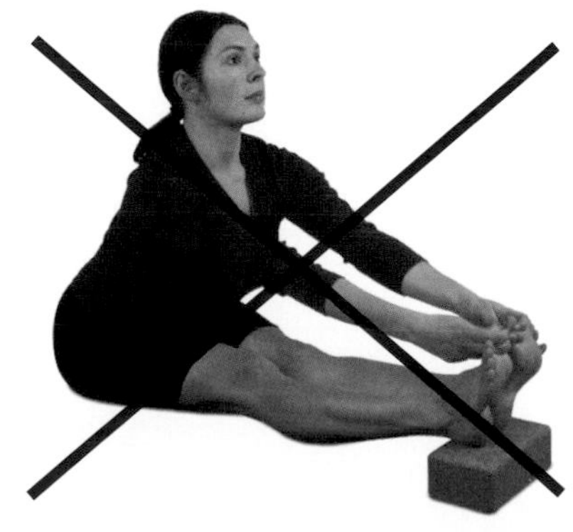

Possible Problems in Early Pregnancy

Yoga offers you help for all the problems listed below. The asanas we recommend in this book are easy and safe.

- Morning sickness
- Heaviness
- Weakness and fatigue
- Shortness of breath
- Thyroid problems
- Heartburn
- Diabetes or gestation diabetes
- Poor discharge of bile or poor liver function
- Constipation
- Swollen feet or legs
- Varicose veins
- Back pain
- High blood pressure
- Toxemia
- Headache
- Dizziness
- Numbness
- Vision problems
- Urinary problems

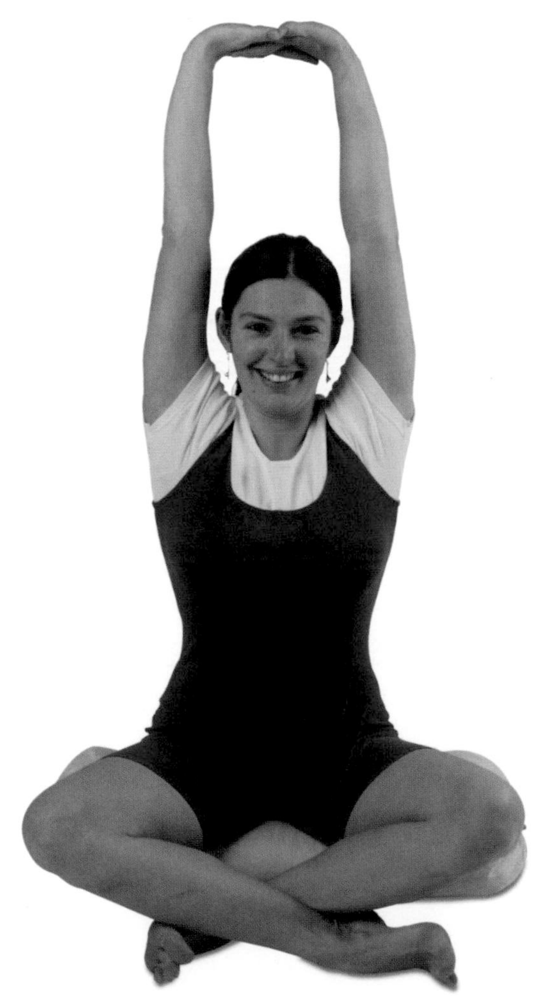

Sequences for Common Problems in Pregnancy

Problems and constitutions vary from woman to woman, so we recommend the various sequences that appear below.

Sequence 1: Prematurely Dilated Cervix

For the condition of prematurely dilated cervix, we recommend the following asanas, which help lift the pelvic floor and pelvic organs. You can enjoy these benefits safely, even if your cervix has been stitched, by following the guidelines below:

- Always practice under the guidance of an experienced Iyengar Yoga teacher.
- Follow the sequence as given without adding further poses, especially standing poses and poses that encourage the opening of the pelvic muscles, such as Baddha Konasana and Upavishtha Konasana.
- In this sequence, asanas that you would normally practice with the feet apart are performed with the legs and feet together, and if possible, using belts and/or blocks.

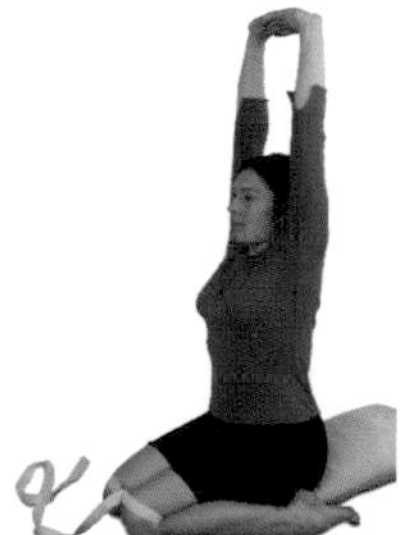

1 Parvatasana from Virasana (and Svastikasana), *page 74*. Perform from Virasana **only**, sitting on a block or firm support.

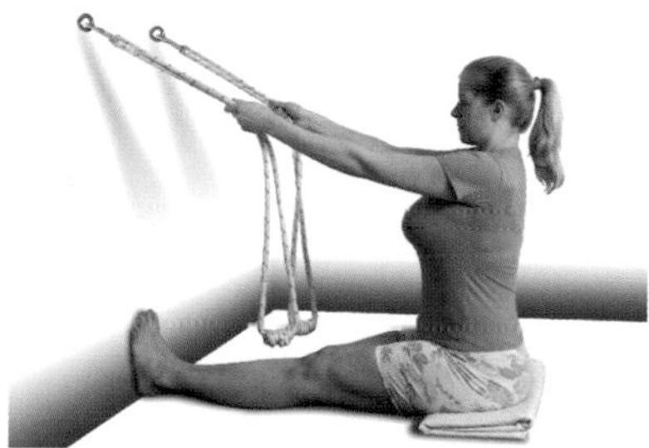

2 Dandasana, *page 64*. Practice with legs together, feet against wall.

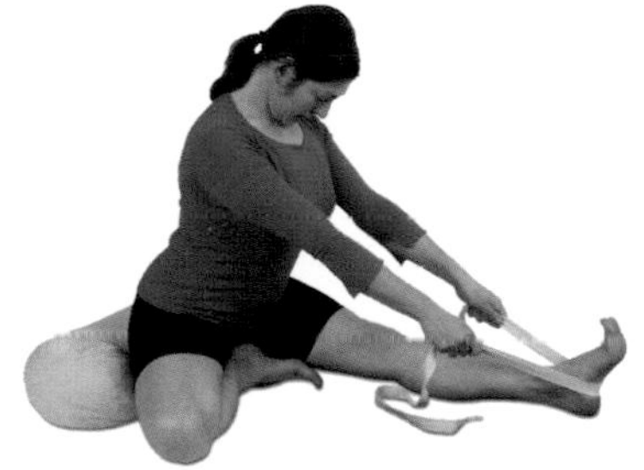

3 Maha Mudra, *page 80*

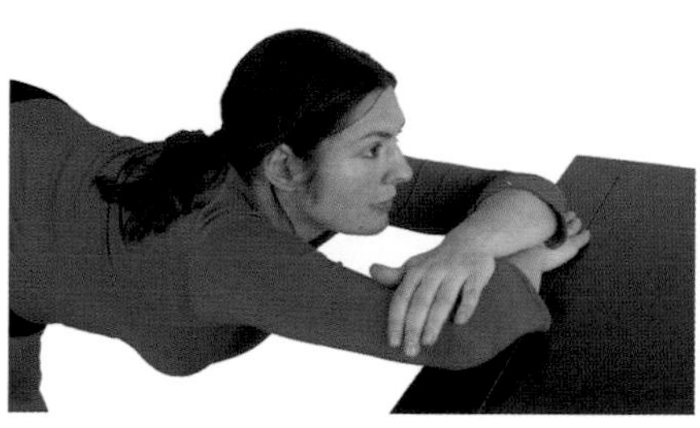

4 Ardha Uttanasana, *page 60*. Practice **only** with feet together, concave back, and head lifted.

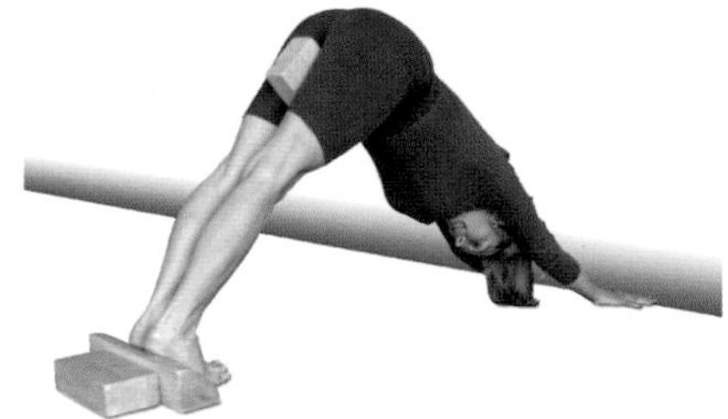

5 Adho Mukha Shvanasana, *page 299*. Practice with feet together and heels on firm support.

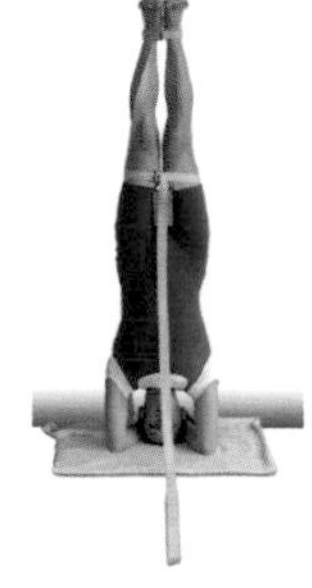

6 Salamba Shirshasana (in corner or against wall), *page 339*. Practice with feet together, and with belt(s) and/or block.

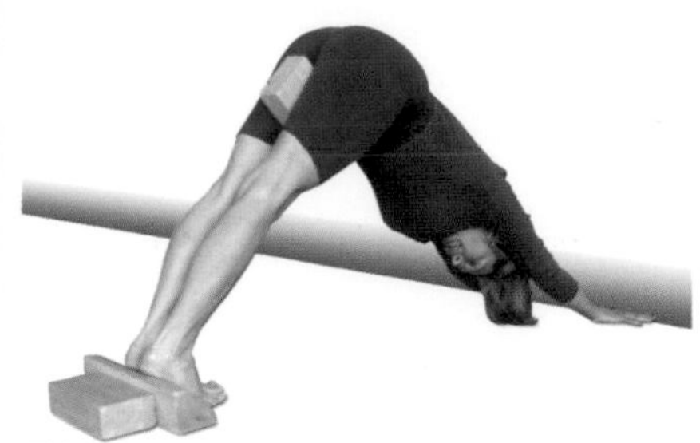

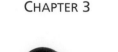

7 Adho Mukha Shvanasana, *page 299*. Practice with feet together and heels on firm support.

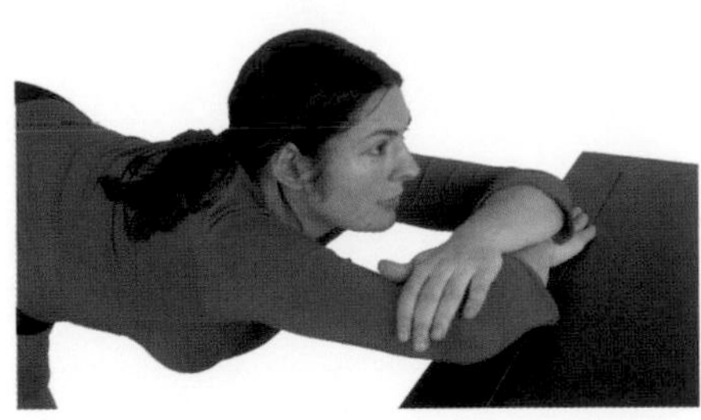

8 Ardha Uttanasana, *page 60*. Practice **only** with feet together, concave back, and head lifted.

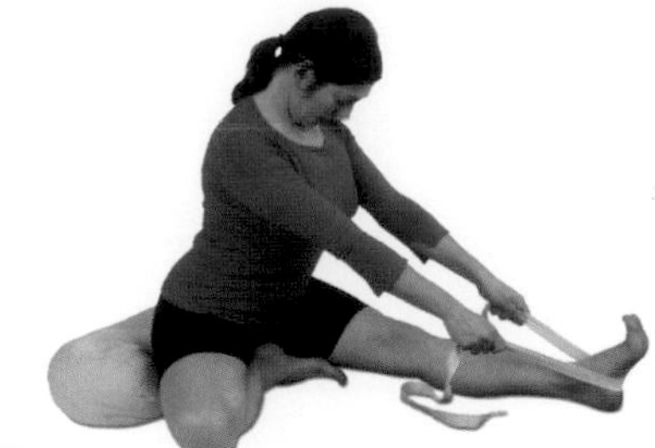

9 Maha Mudra, *page 80*

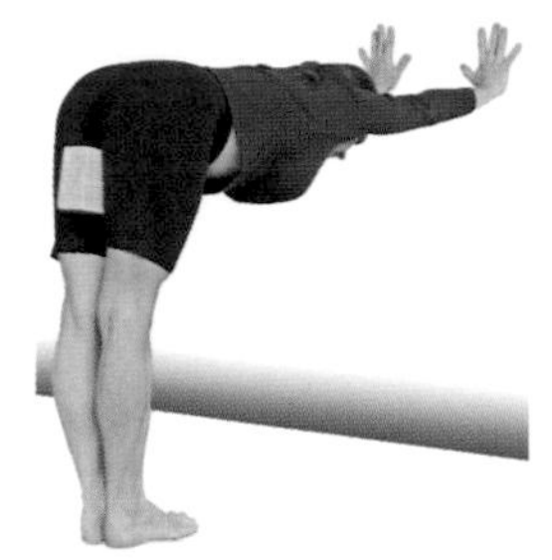

10 Ardha Uttanasana, *page 292*. Practice **only** with feet together, concave back, block between thighs, and hands against wall.

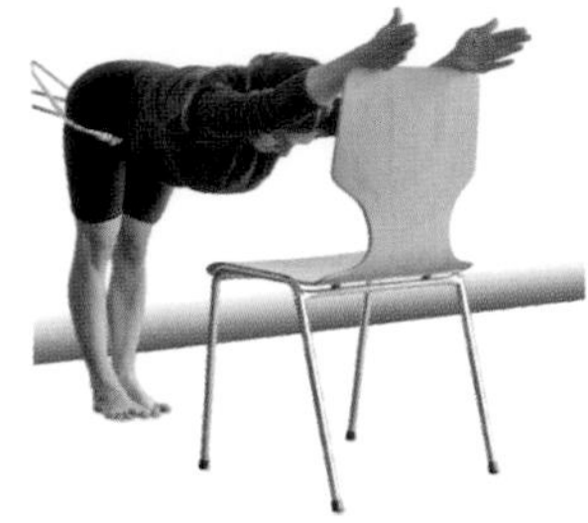

11 Ardha Uttanasana, *page 124*. Practice **only** with feet together in ropes, and hands on backrest of chair.

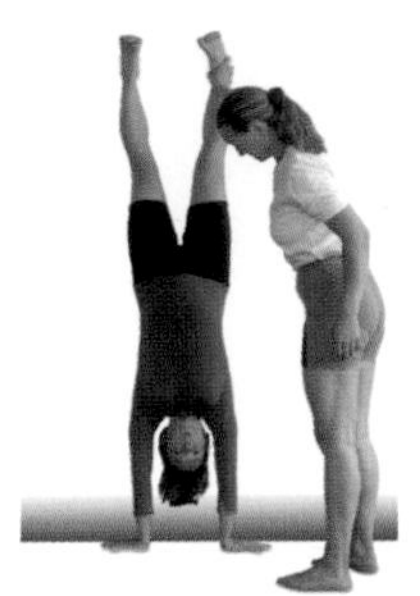

12 Adho Mukha Vrikshasana (with teacher/helper), *page 226*. Practice with feet together and do not jump!

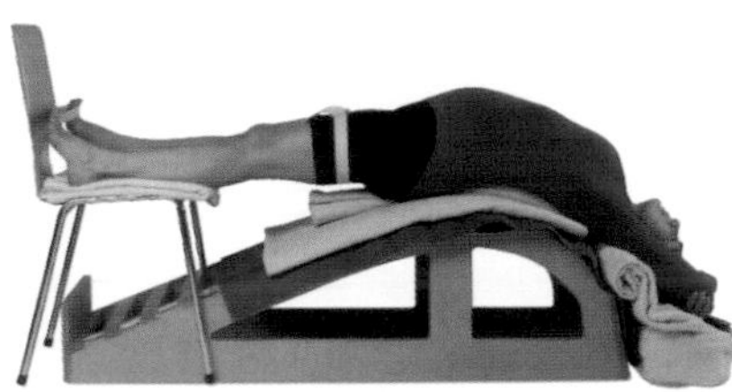

13 Dvi Pada Viparita Dandasana (fully supported, Viparita Dandasana bench, L-shape), *page 123*. Practice with feet together and belts.

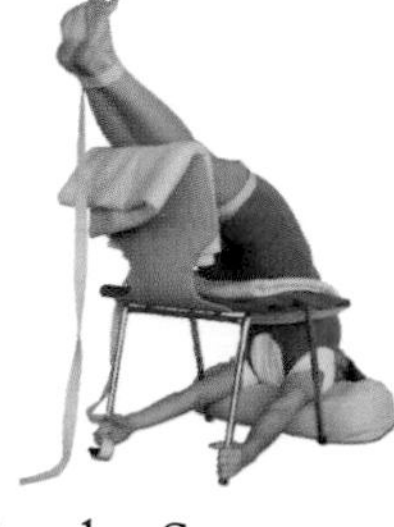

14 Salamba Sarvangasana (chair), *pages 103 and 330*. Practice with feet together, and belts and/or block.

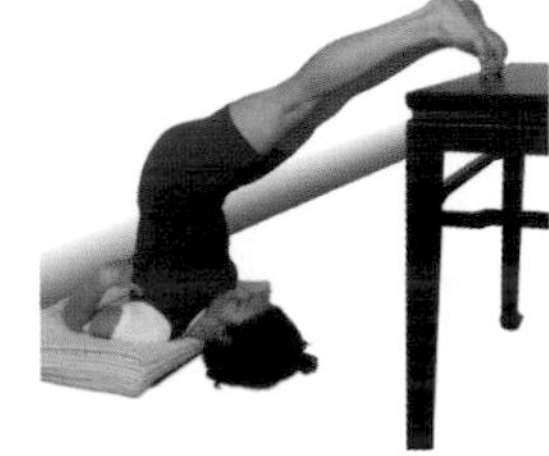

15 Ardha Halasana (toes on table), *page 332*. Practice with feet together.

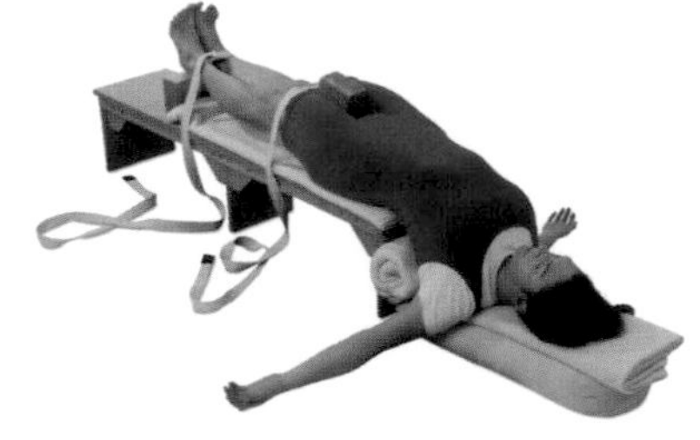

16 Setu Bandha Sarvangasana (bench or similar height), *pages 108 and 334*. Practice with feet together, and belts and/or blocks.

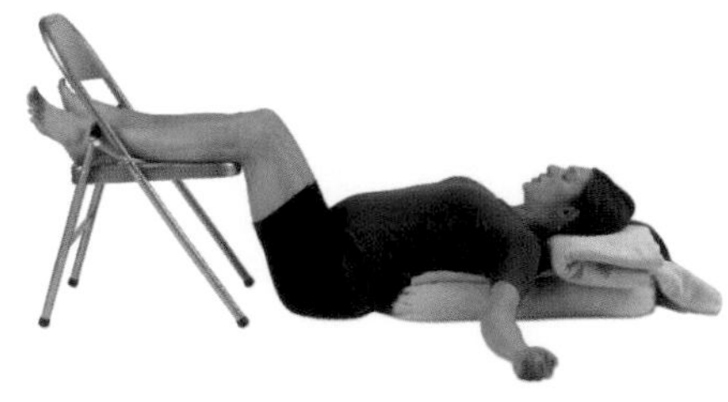

17 Shavasana, Variation 1, *page 138*. Practice with lower legs on chair.

NOTE

How to use belts and block, see also pages 330 and 334

Sequence 2: Dizziness, Fatigue, and Headache

This sequence helps treat a wide array of conditions that are common in pregnancy, including problems with constipation, bile problems or poor liver function, urinary function, and vision.

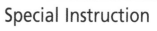

Special Instruction

- If you suffer from dizziness or vision problems, don't look down.
- If you have a history of miscarriage, avoid all Parshvas in your 1st trimster.

Beginners and Advanced Students

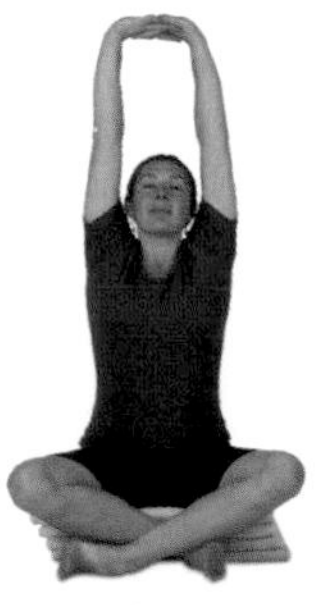

1 Parvatasana from Svastikasana (change legs), *page 74*

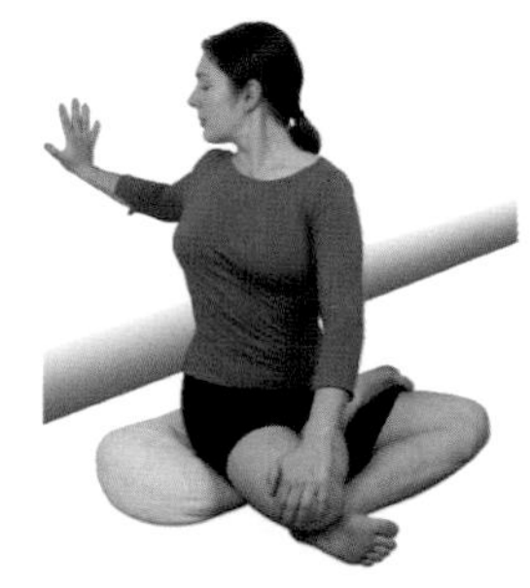

2 Parshva Padmasana, *page 94*, or Parshva Svastikasana (chair or wall, change legs)

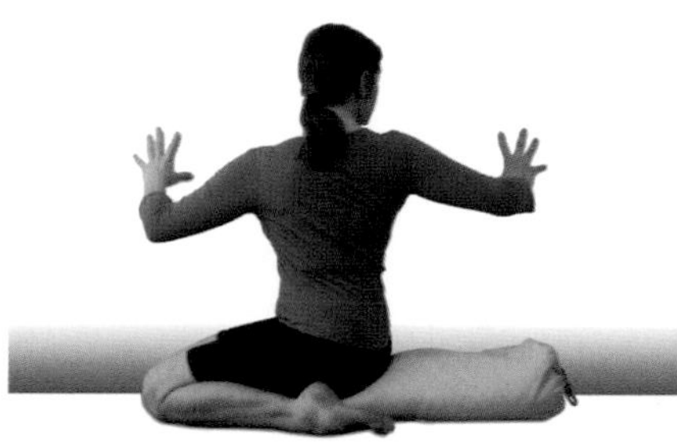

3 Parshva Virasana (chair or wall), *page 95*

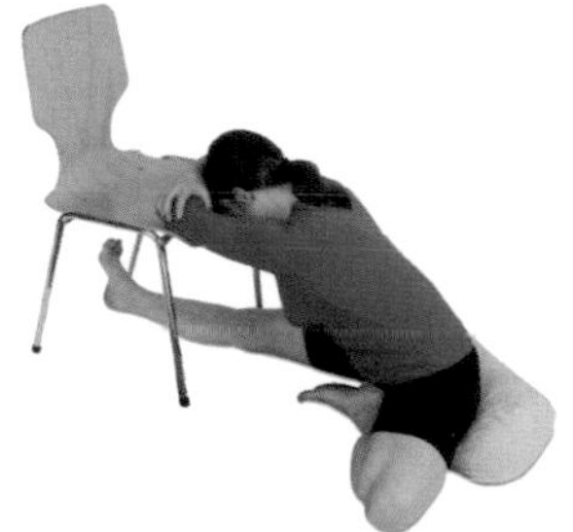

4 Parshva Janu Shirshasana, (chair), *page 95*. Instead of practicing with a slight forward bend, you can do it upright.

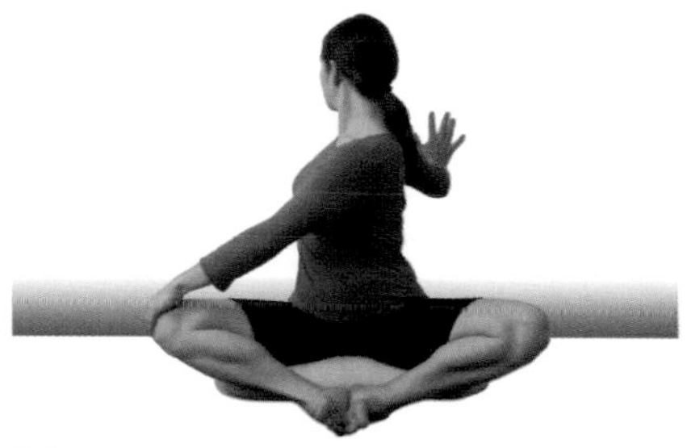

5 Parshva Baddha Konasana (chair or wall), *page 95*

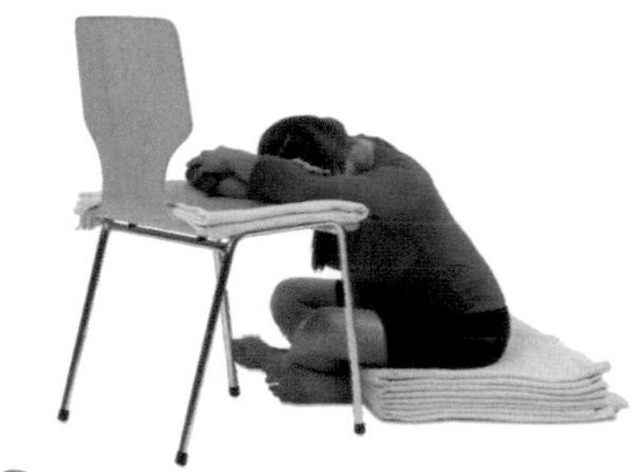

6 Parshva Svastikasana (chair), *page 94*

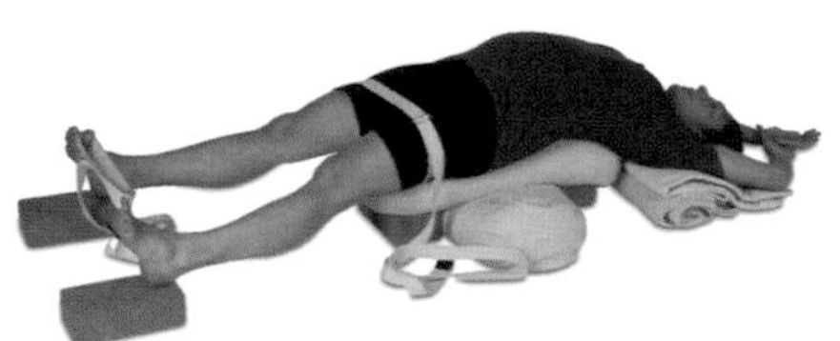

7 Cross-bolsters, *page 118*

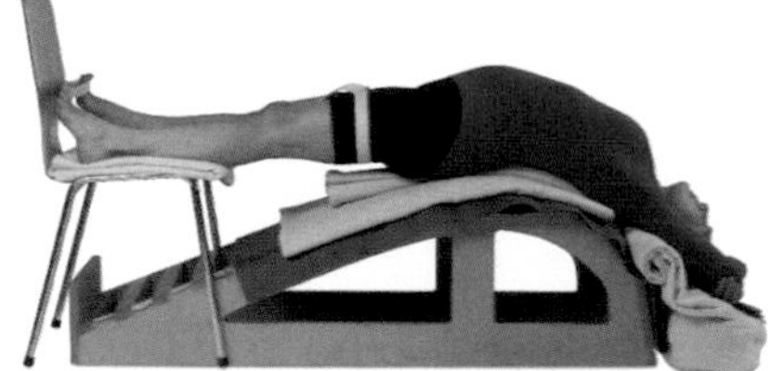

8 Dvi Pada Viparita Dandasana (L-shape, on Viparita Dandasana bench), *page 123*

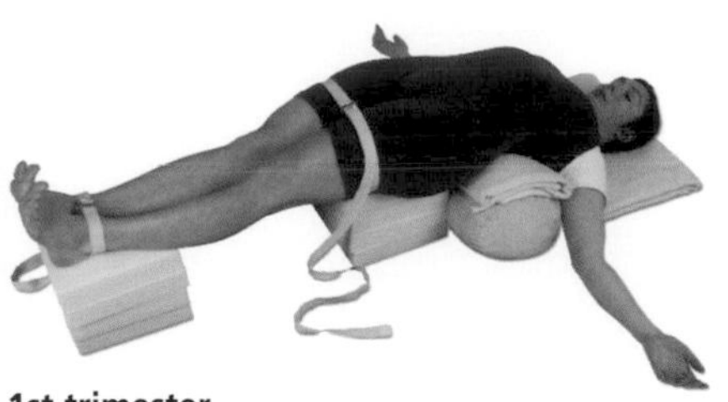
1st trimester

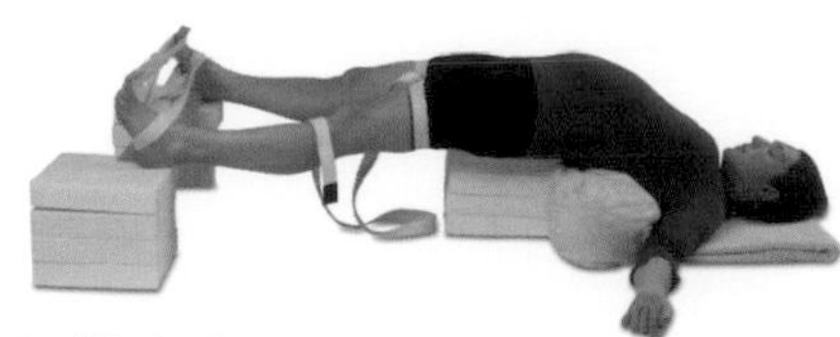
2nd/3rd trimester

9 Setu Bandha Sarvangasana (bench or similar heights), *pages 108 and 109*

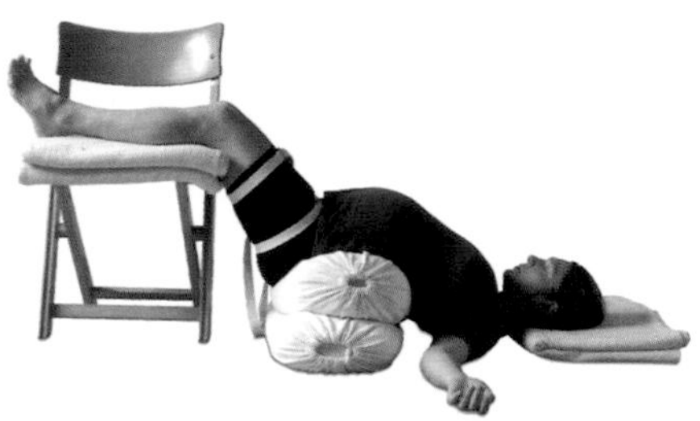

10 Viparita Karani, *page 113.*
1st trimester: legs bent on chair

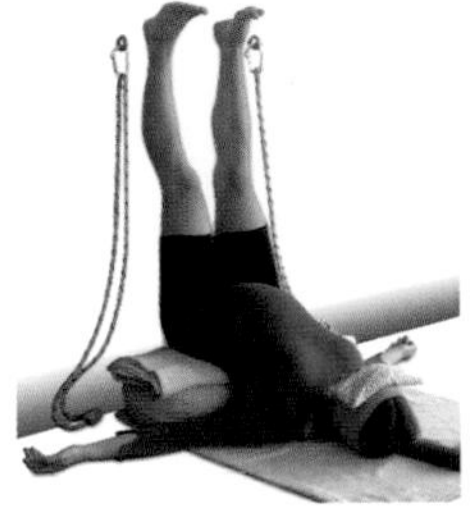

2nd and 3rd trimesters: legs straight

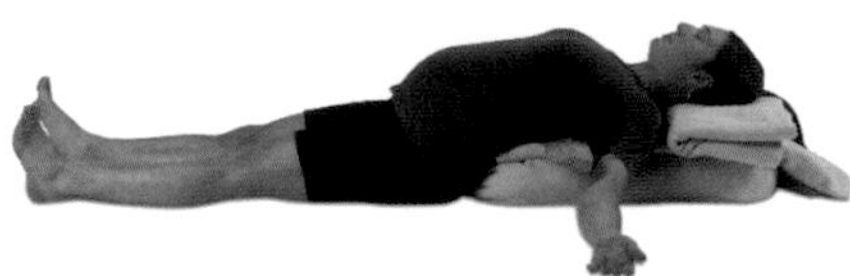

11 Shavasana (bolster/s), *page 134*

Sequence 3: High Blood Pressure

Beginners: 2nd and 3rd trimesters (1st trimester, follow the Sequence for First Trimester and throughout Pregnancy in Chapter 4)
Advanced students: throughout pregnancy

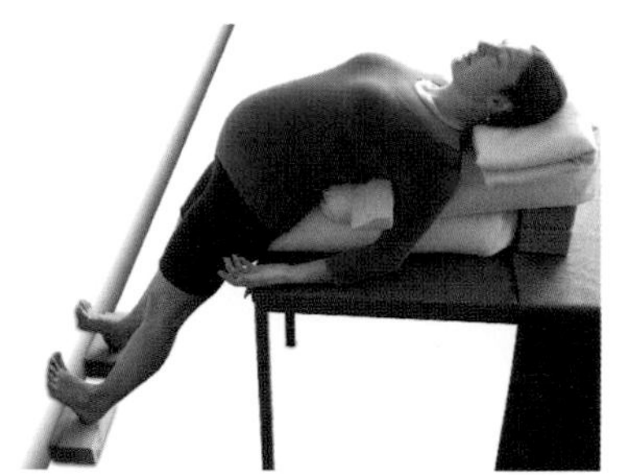

1 Salamba Purvottanasana, *page 133* (support, 2nd and 3rd trimesters only)

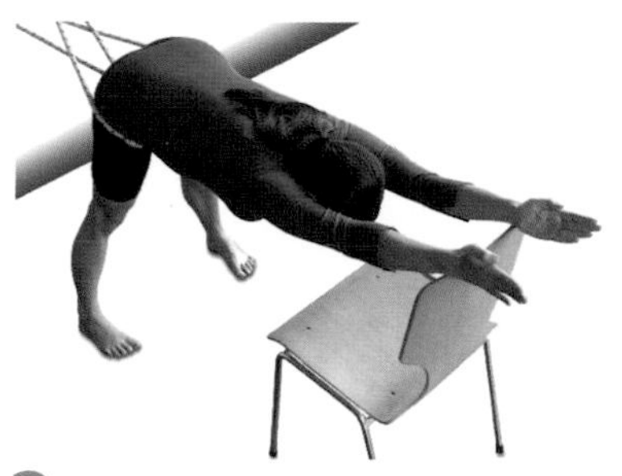

2 Ardha Uttanasana, *page 124* (ropes and support for head)

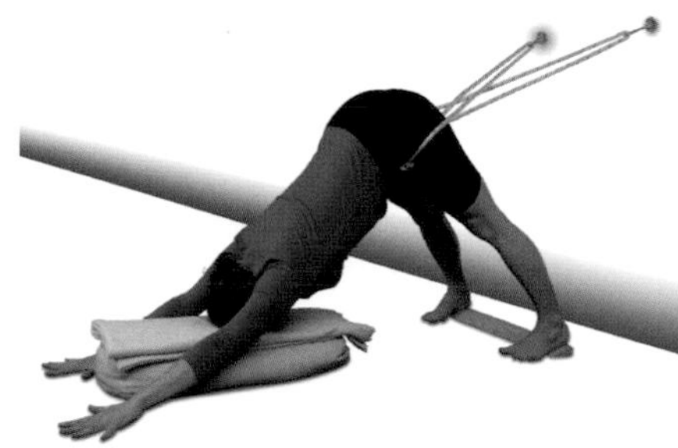

3 Adho Mukha Shvanasana (wall ropes and support for heels and head), *page 125*

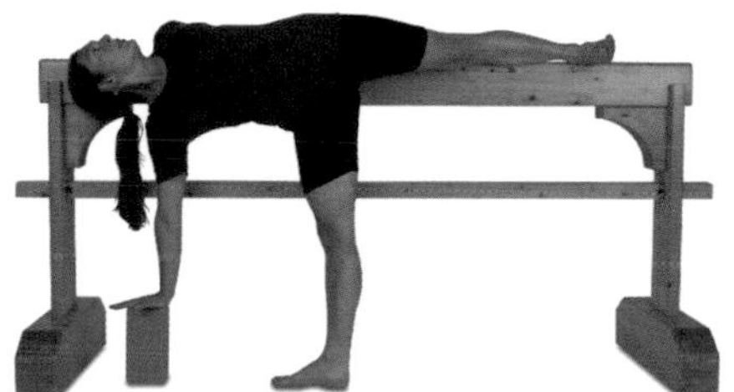

4 Ardha Chandrasana (trestle or similar support), *page 48*

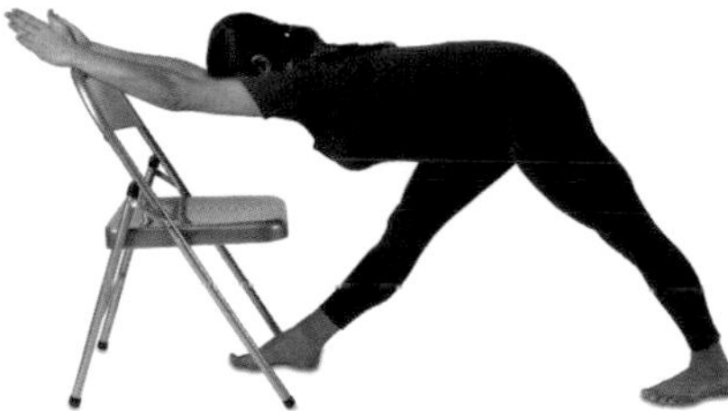

5 Parshvottanasana, *page 51* (hands on support, or head resting like in Prasarita Padottanasana, *page 58*)

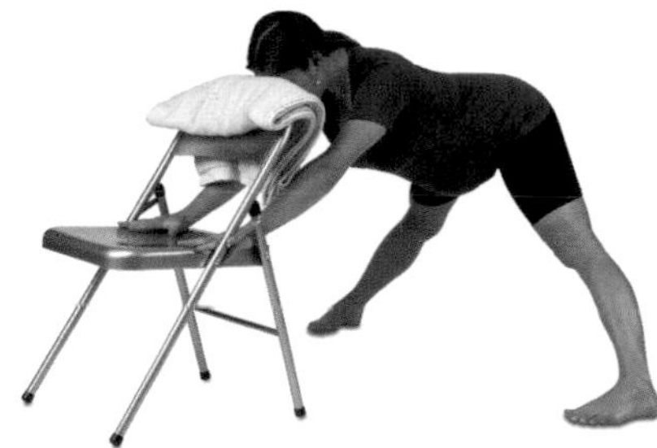

6 Prasarita Padottanasana (head resting), *page 58*

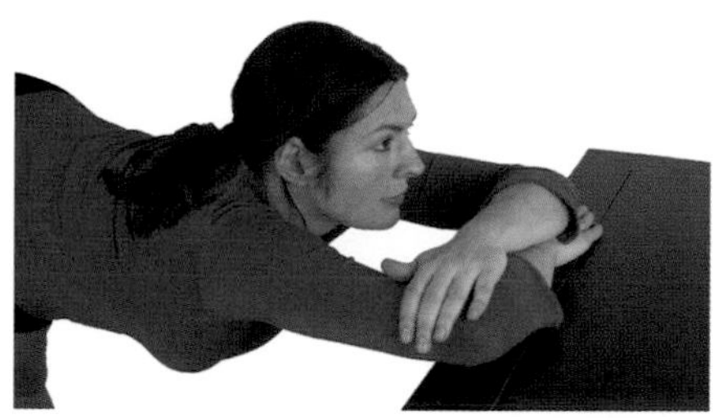

7 Ardha Uttanasana (hands on support), *page 60*

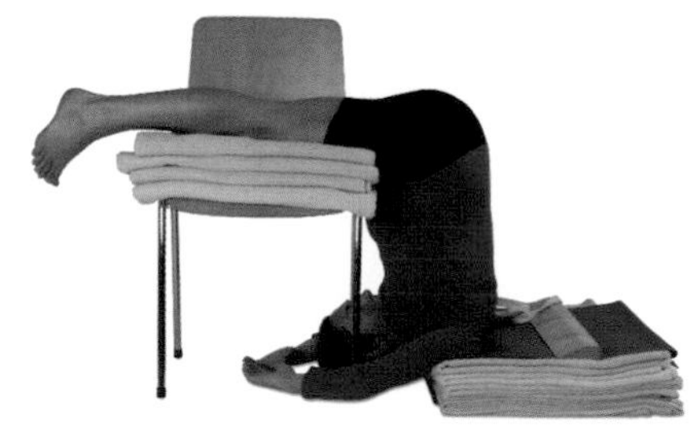

8 Ardha Halasana (chair or stool), *page 105*

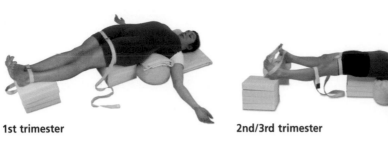

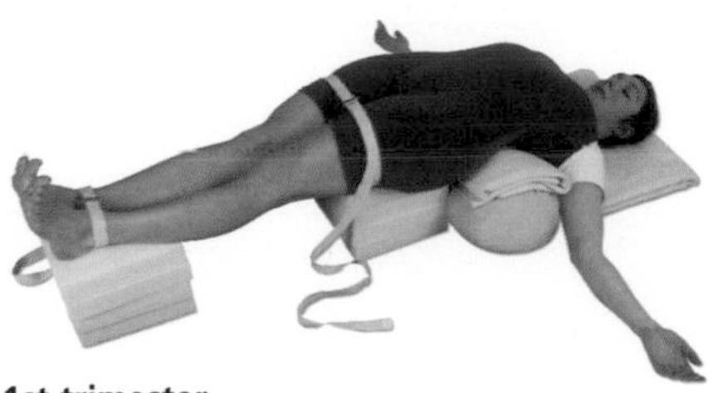

1st trimester

2nd/3rd trimester

9 Setu Bandha Sarvangasana (bench or similar height), *pages 108 – 109*

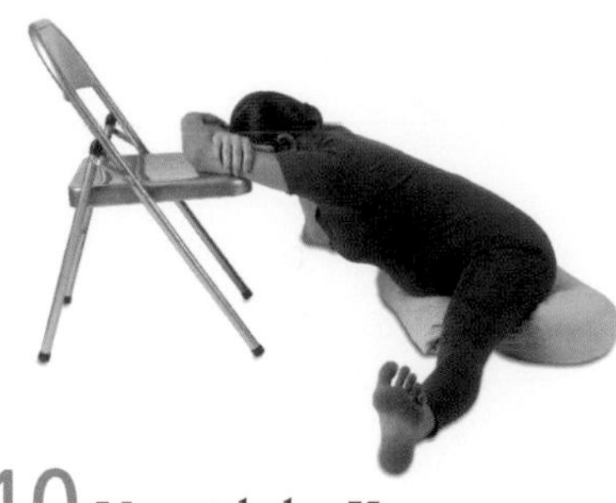

10 Upavishtha Konasana (sitting on bolster, head and arms resting on chair), *page 86*

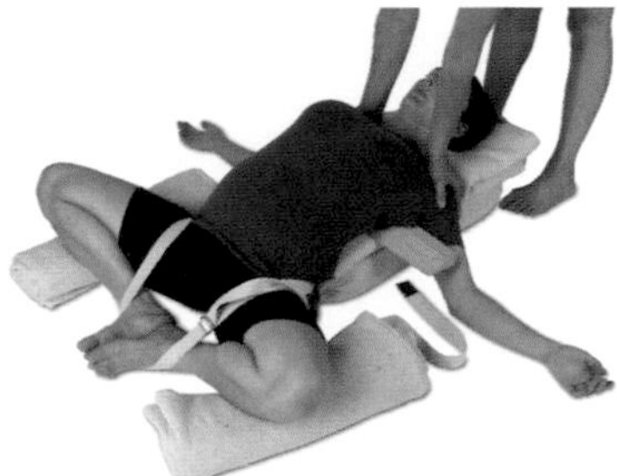

11 Supta Baddha Konasana (bolster lengthwise, slanted plank), *page 128*

and/or

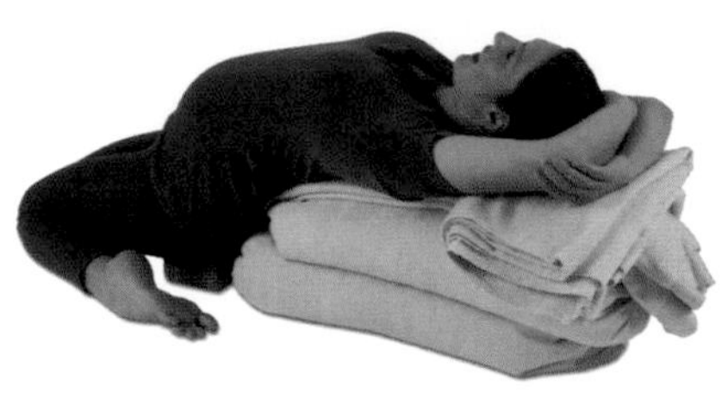

12 Supta Virasana (bolster/s), *page 130*

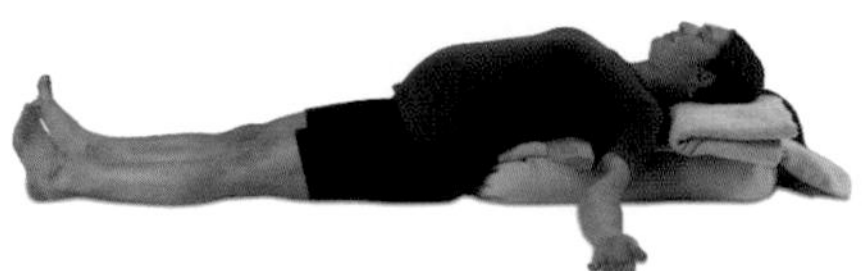

13 Shavasana (bolster/s), *page 134*

Sequence 4: Diabetes

If you have diabetes, you shouldn't exercise intensely. Your sequence should be reduced to one that gives relief and has positive effects on the pancreas, such as the following:

Beginners: 2nd and 3rd trimesters (1st trimester, follow Sequence for 1st Trimester and throughout Pregnancy, Chapter 4)
Advanced students: throughout pregnancy

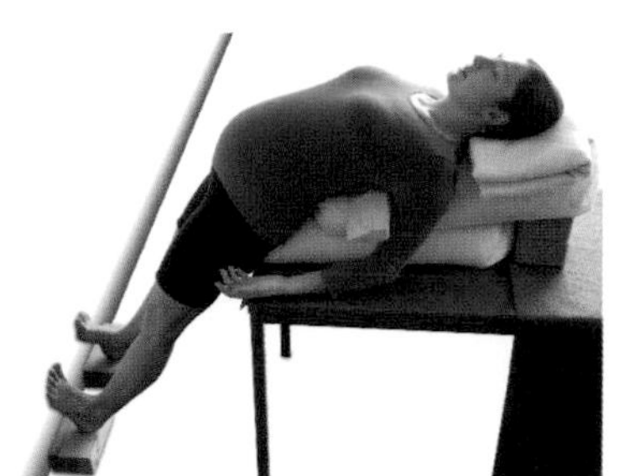

1 Salamba Purvottanasana (2nd and 3rd trimesters only), *page 133*

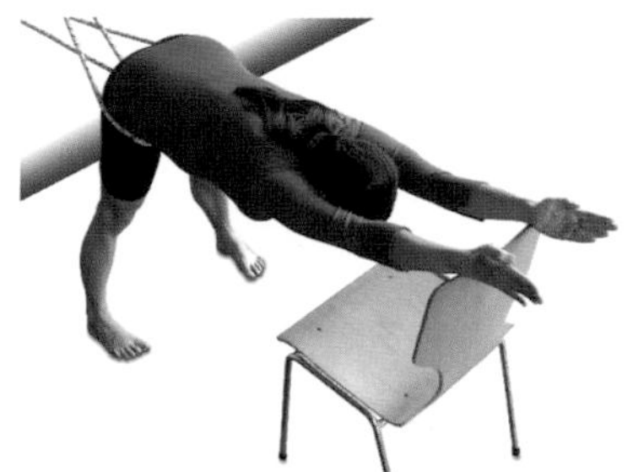

2 Ardha Uttanasana (with ropes and chair), *page 124*

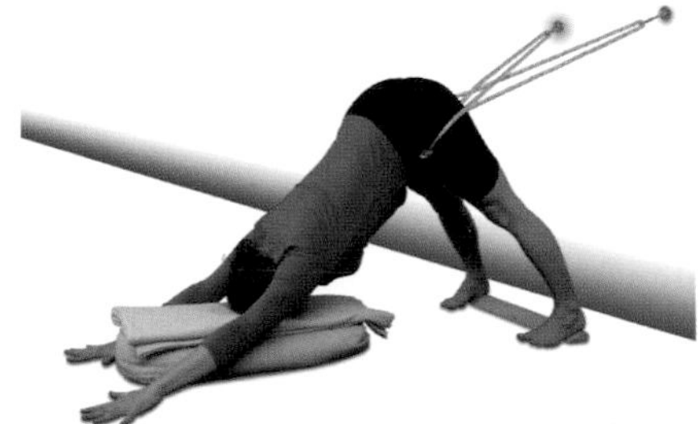

3 Adho Mukha Shvanasana (wall, ropes, and support for heels and head), *page 63*

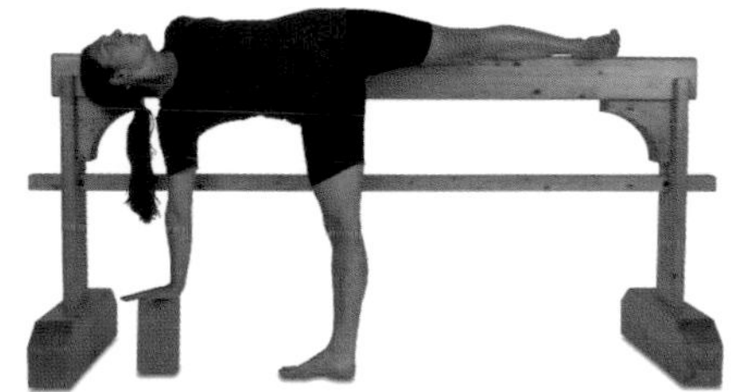

4 Ardha Chandrasana (trestle or similar support), *page 45*

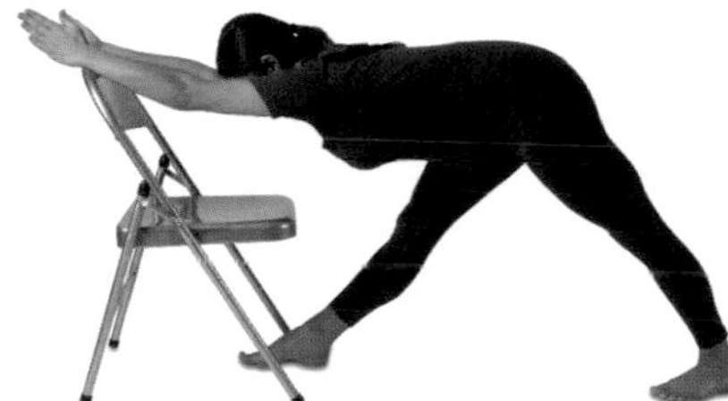

5 Parshvottanasana (hands on support), *page 51*

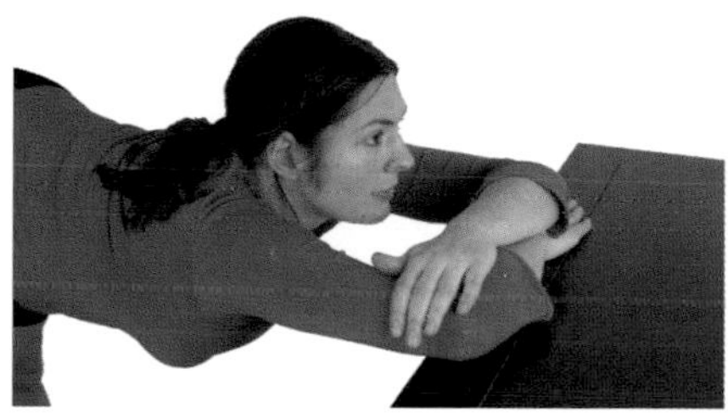

6 Ardha Uttanasana (hands on support), *page 60*

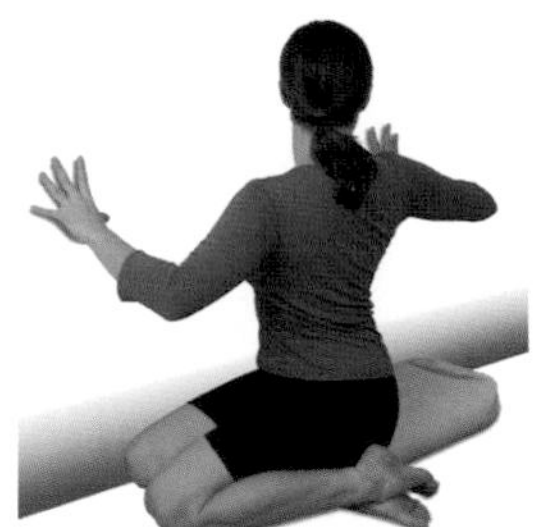

7 Bharadvajasana 1 (sitting on bolster or chair), *page 93*

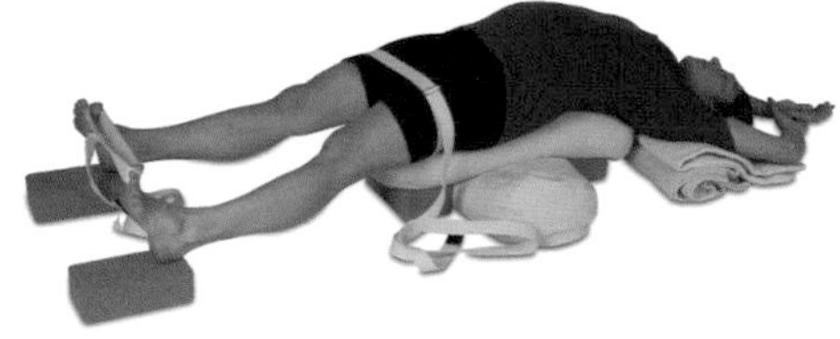

8 Cross-bolsters, *page 118*

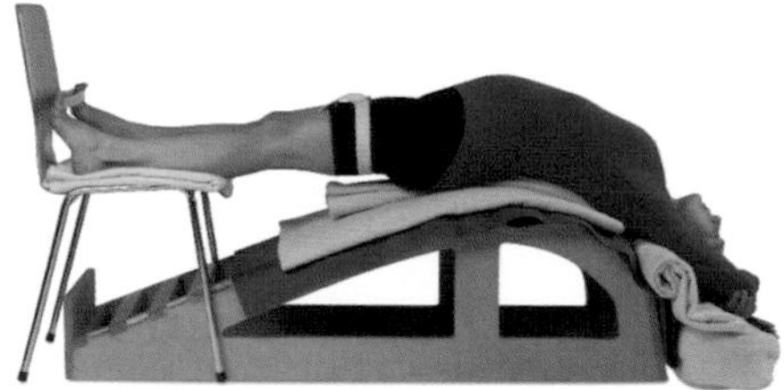

9 Dvi Pada Viparita Dandasana (L-shape, on Viparita Dandasana bench), *page 123*

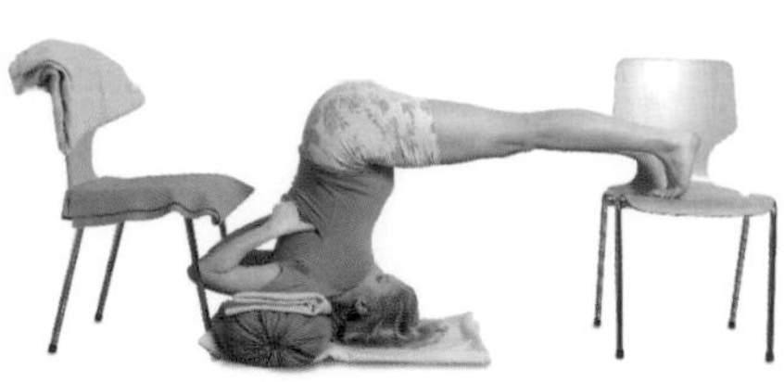

10 Ardha Halasana (chair or stool), *page 104*

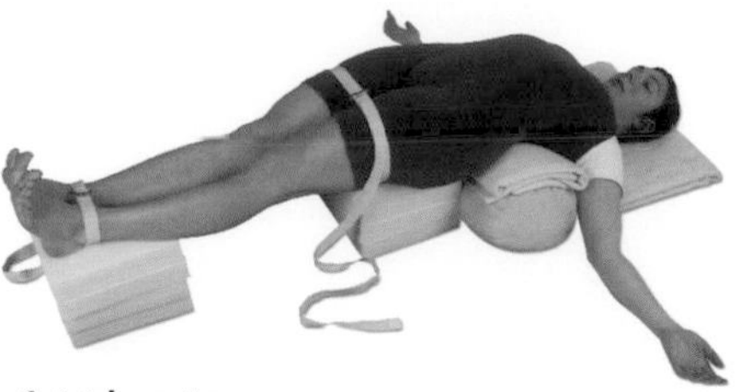

1st trimester

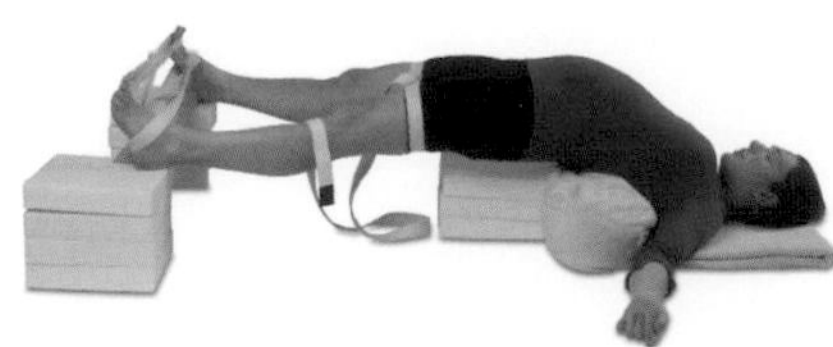

2nd/3rd trimester

11 Setu Bandha Sarvangasana (bench or similar height), *pages 108 – 109*

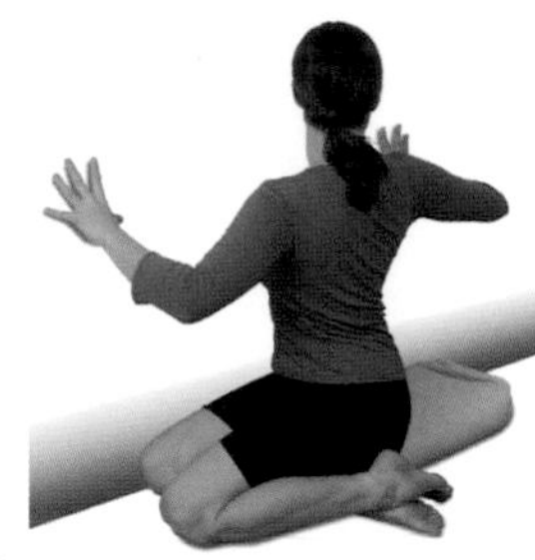

12 Bharadvajasana 1 (sitting on bolster or chair), *page 93*

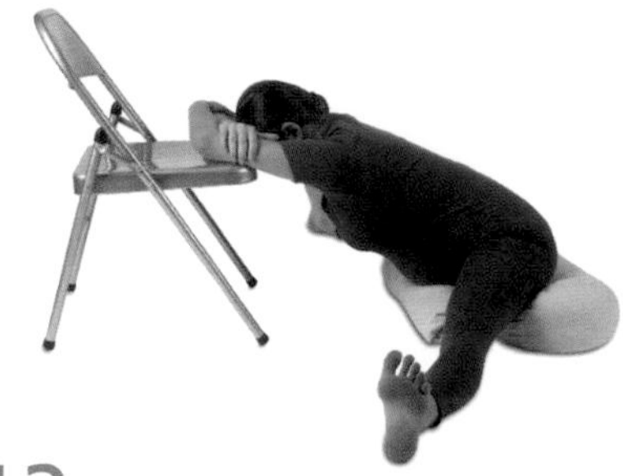

13 Upavishtha Konasana (sitting on bolster, head and arms resting on chair), *page 86*

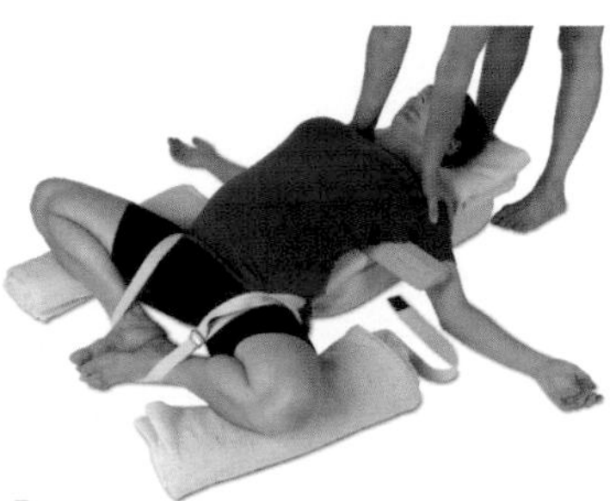

14 Supta Baddha Konasana (bolster lengthwise, slanted plank), *page 128*

and/or

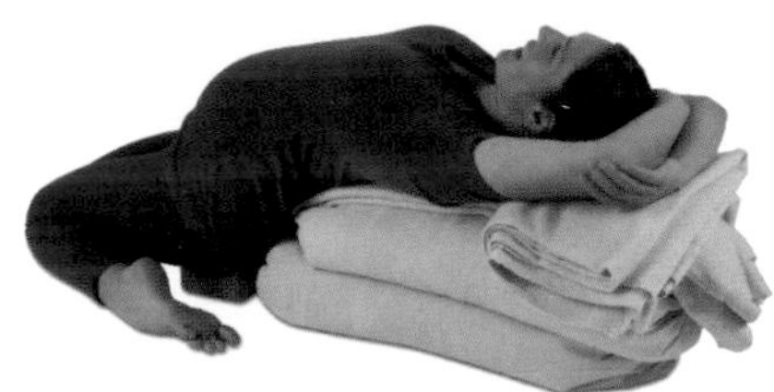

15 Supta Virasana (bolster/s), *page 130*

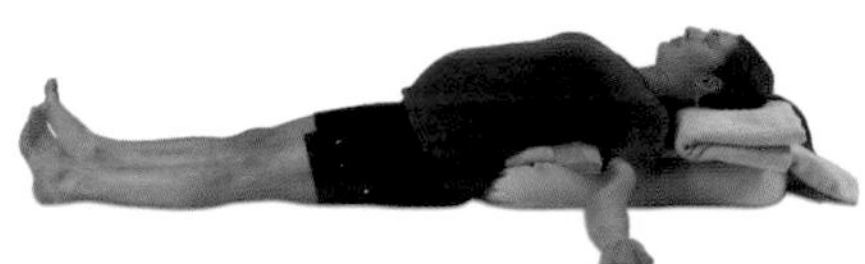

16 Shavasana (bolster/s), *page 134*

Sequence 5: Tension, Heartburn, and Shortness of Breath

This sequence is a restorative one for after a long day; it relaxes the pelvis, legs, and lymphatic system.

Beginners and advanced students: throughout pregnancy

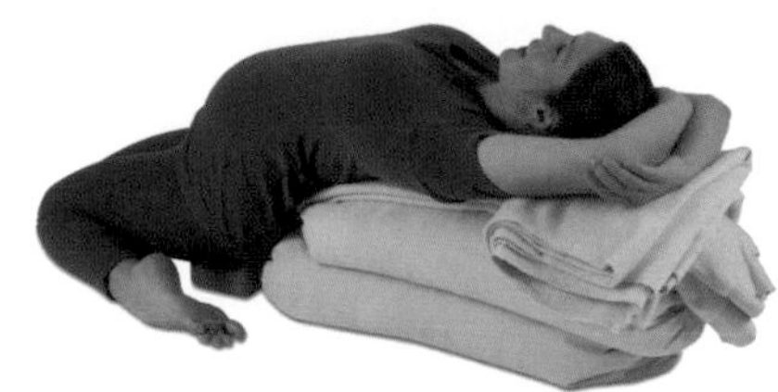

1 Supta Virasana (bolster/s), *page 130*

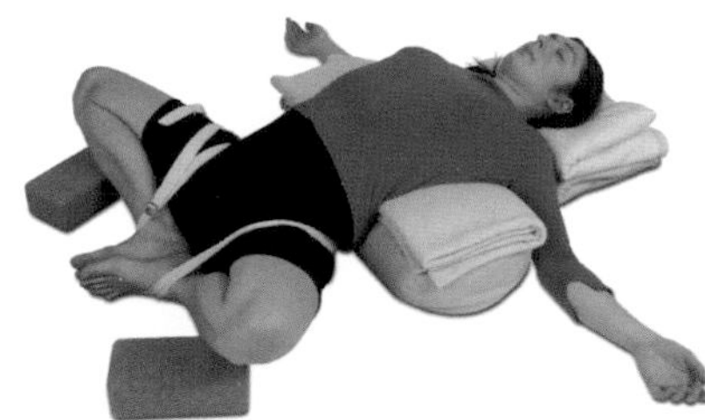

2 Supta Baddha Konasana (bolster crosswise), *page 128*

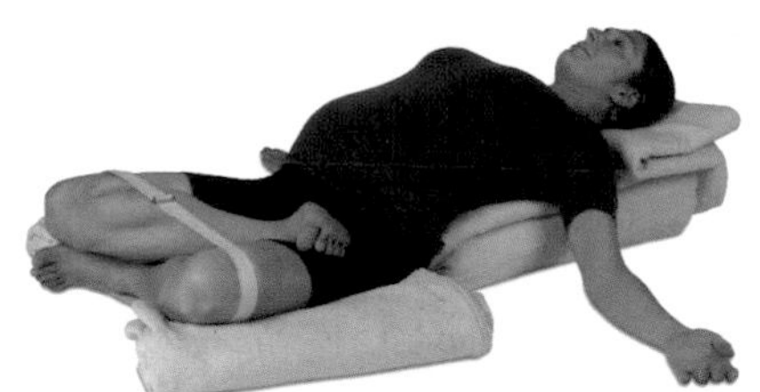

3 Matsyasana (bolster/s), *page 131*

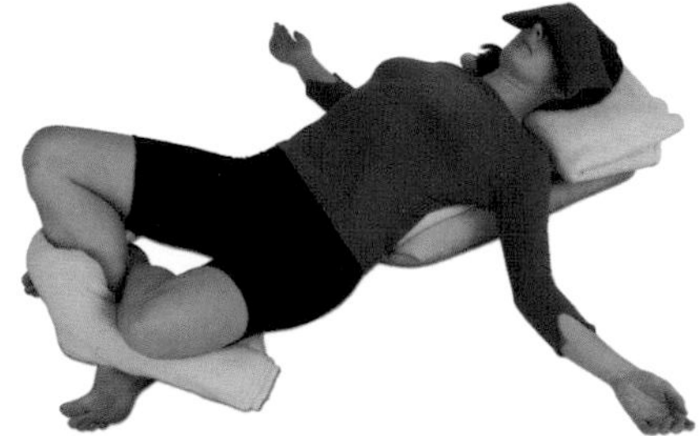

4 Supta Svastikasana (bolster/s), *page 131*

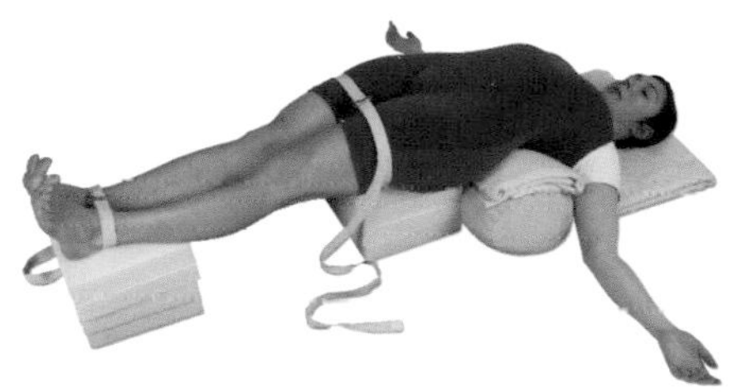

1st trimester

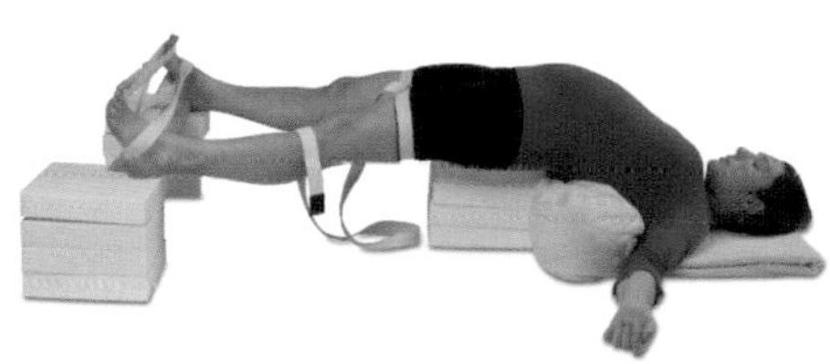

2nd/3rd trimester

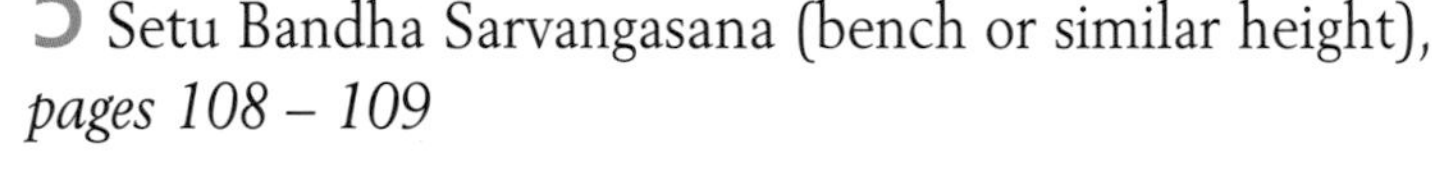

5 Setu Bandha Sarvangasana (bench or similar height), *pages 108 – 109*

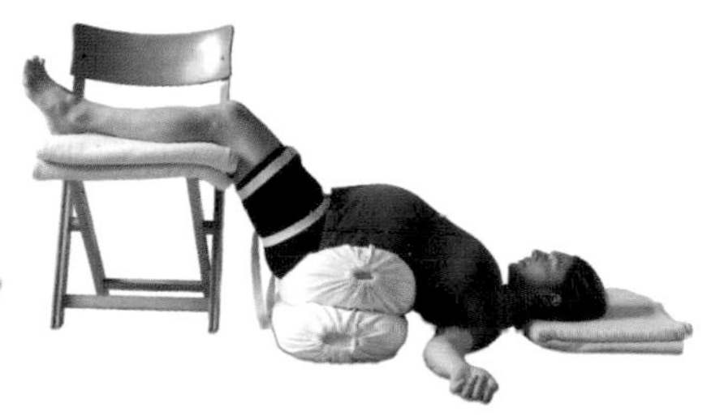

6 Viparita Karani (legs bent on chair, 1st trimester), *page 113*

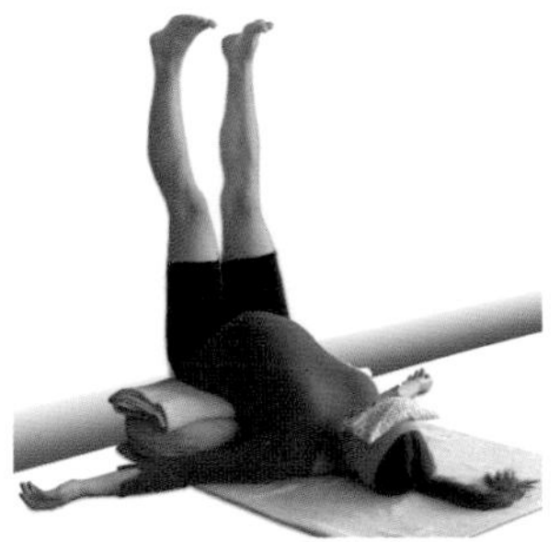

7 Viparita Karani (2nd and 3rd trimesters), *page 114*

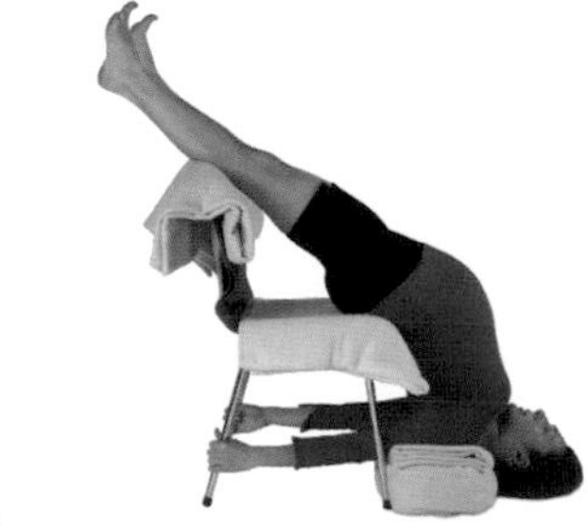

8 Salamba Sarvangasana (chair), *page 103*

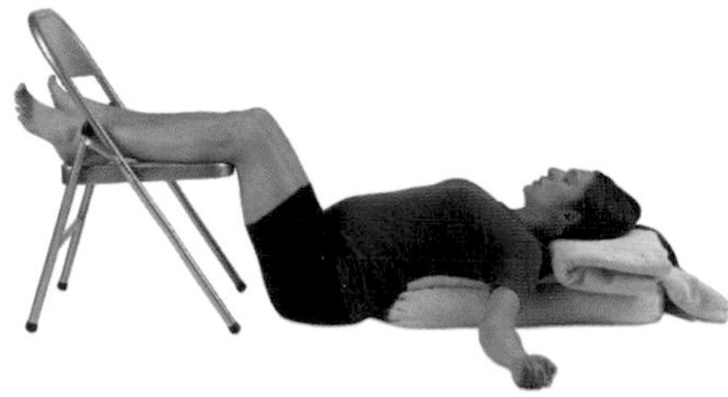

9 Shavasana (bolster and knees on bolster), *page 138*

Sequence 6: Back Pain

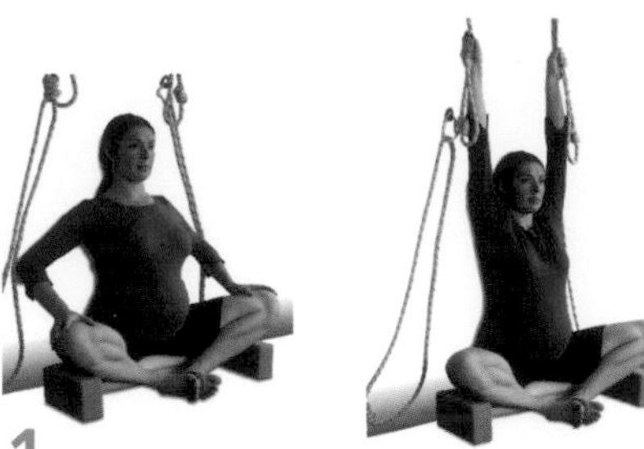

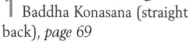

1 Baddha Konasana (straight back), *page 69*

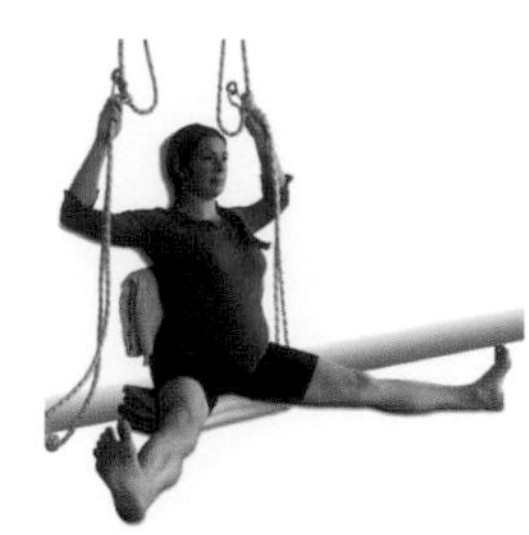

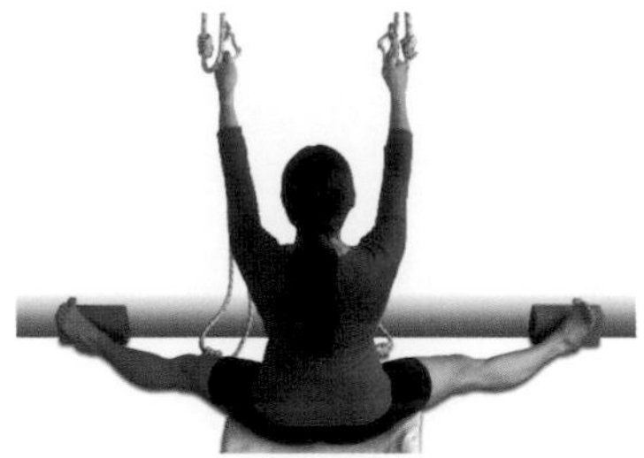

2 Upavishtha Konasana, *page 71*

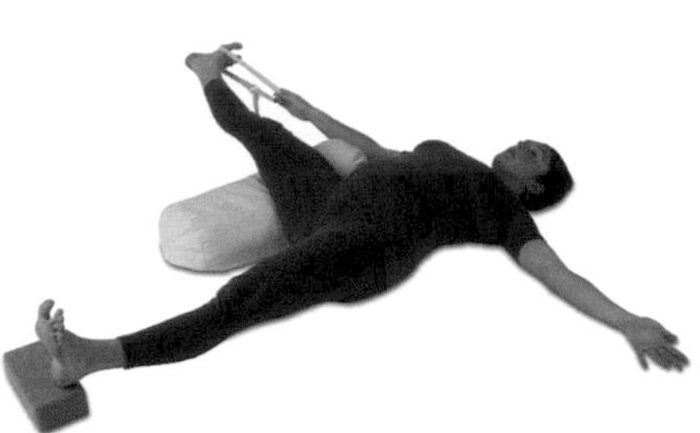

3 Supta Padangushthasana 2, *page 115*

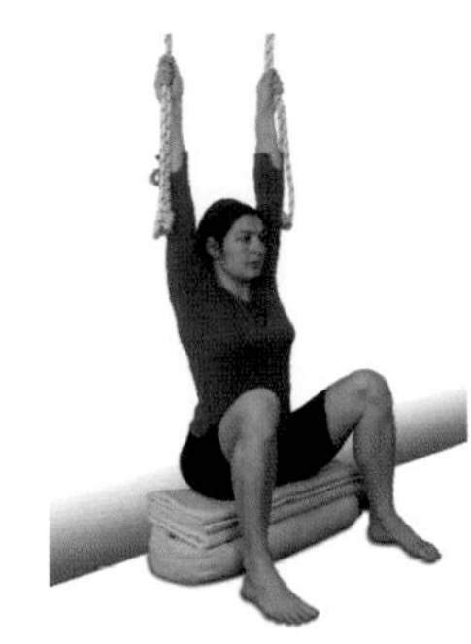

4 Malasana (gripping the ropes), *page 77*

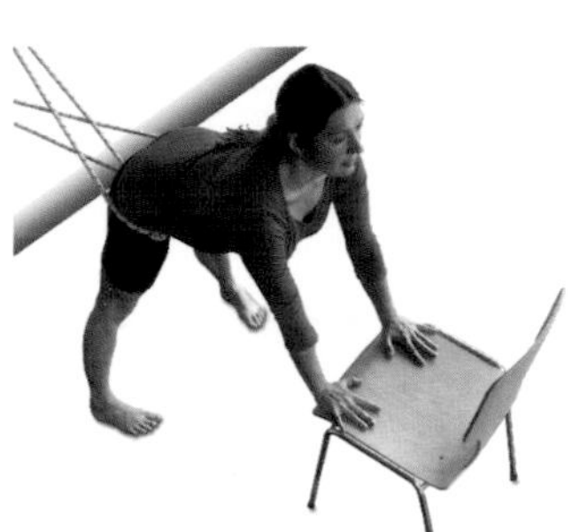

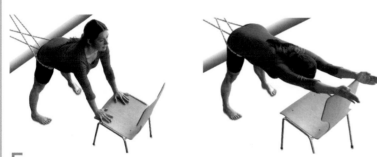

5 Ardha Uttanasana (with ropes and chair), *page 124*

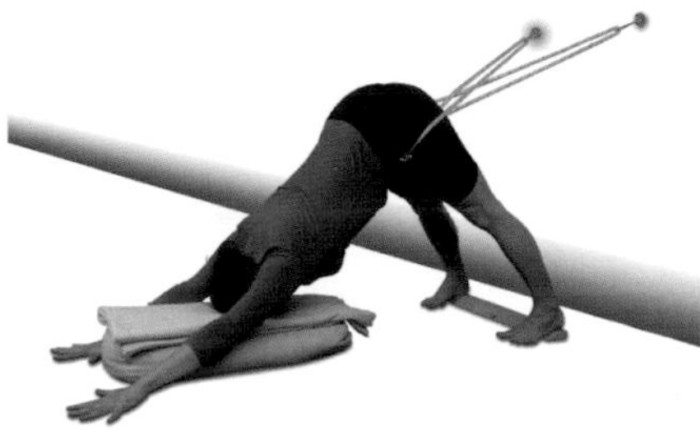

6 Adho Mukha Shvanasana (wall ropes and support for heels and head), *page 125*

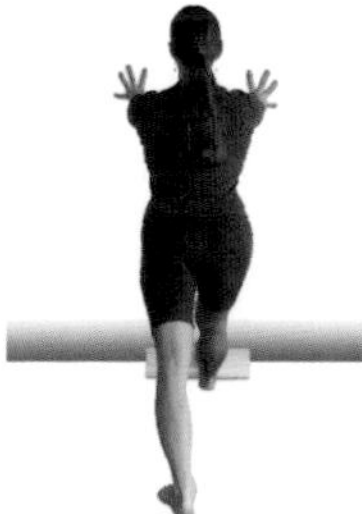

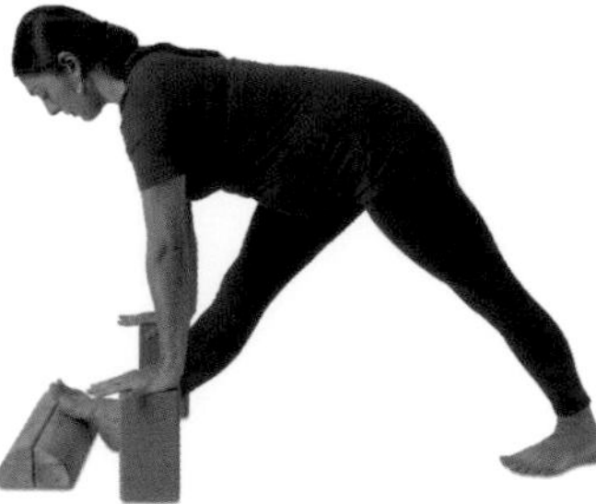

7 Parshvottanasana (hands against wall), *page 285*, (front foot on support), *page 51*

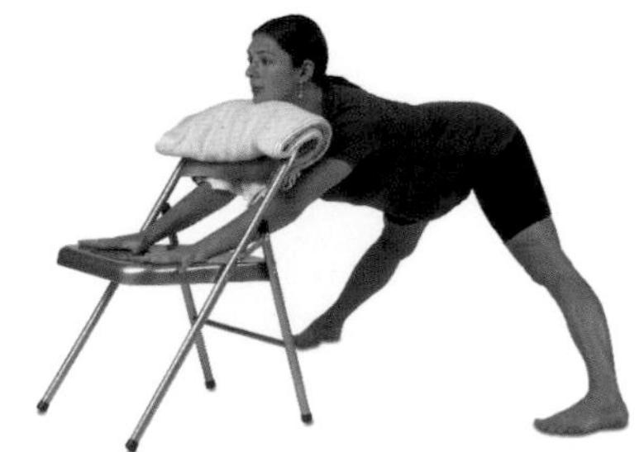

8 Prasarita Padottanasana (concave back), *page 58*

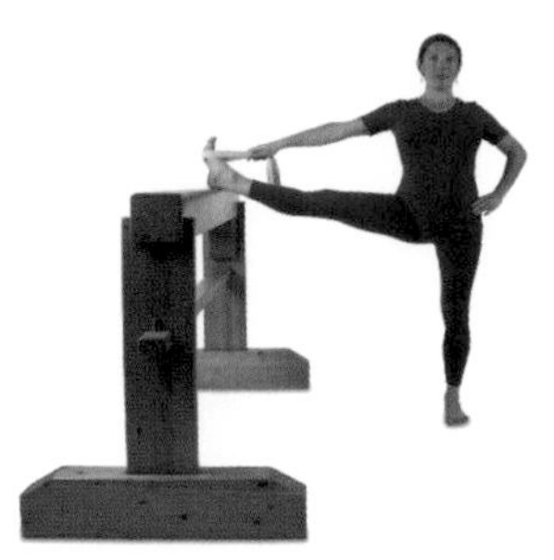

9 Utthita Hasta Padangushthasana 2 (2nd trimester only), *page 117*

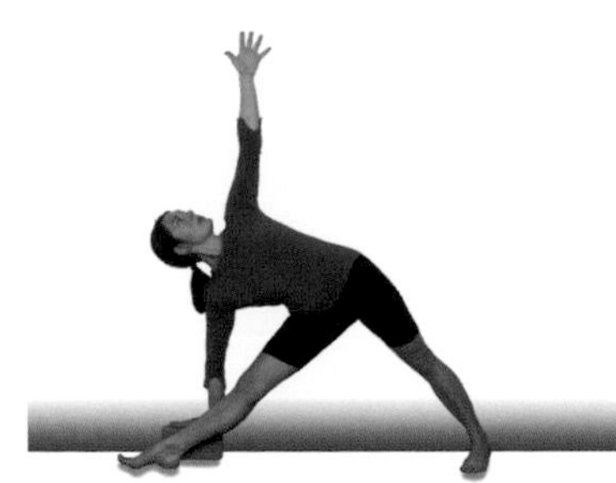

10 Utthita Trikonasana (wall/trestle), *page 39*

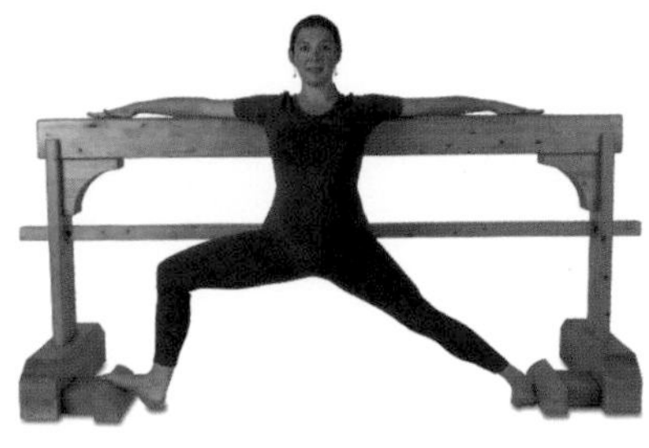

11 Utthita Parshvakonasana (wall/trestle), *page 43*

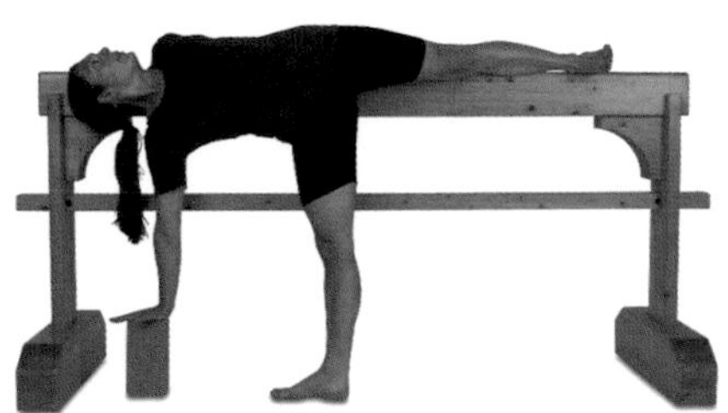

12 Ardha Chandrasana (wall or trestle), *page 48*

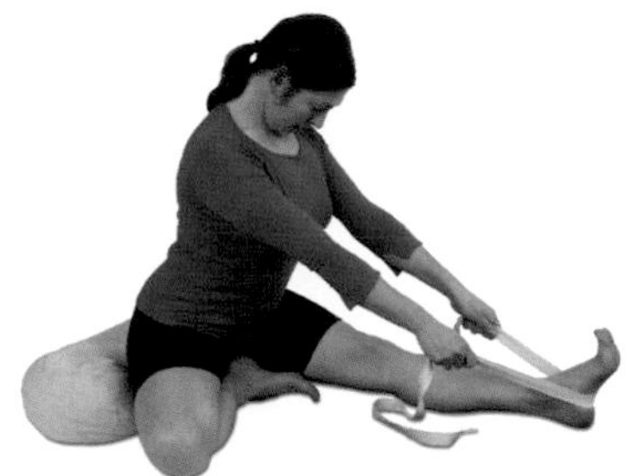

13 Maha Mudra, *page 80*

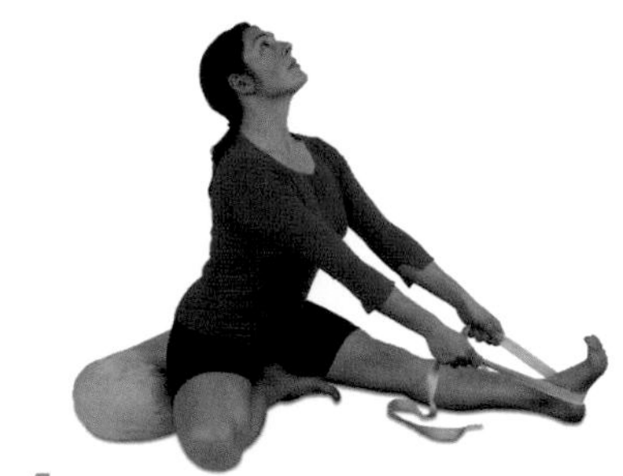

14 Janu Shirshasana (concave back), *page 83*

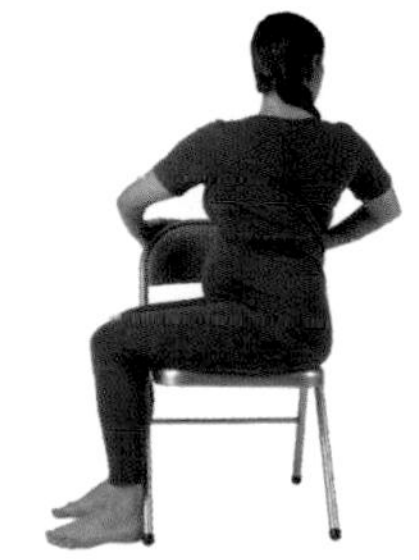

15 Bharadvajasana (on bolster with wall or on chair), *page 93*

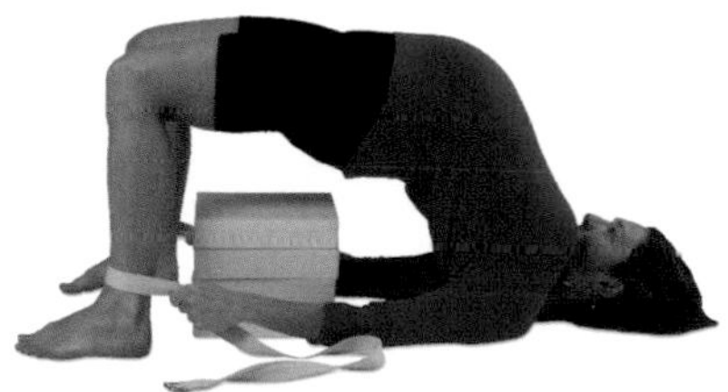

16 Chatushpadasana, *page 111*

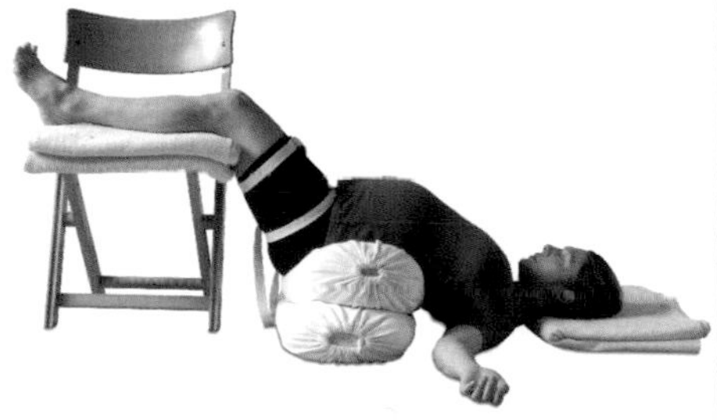

17 Viparita Karani (legs bent on chair), *page 113*

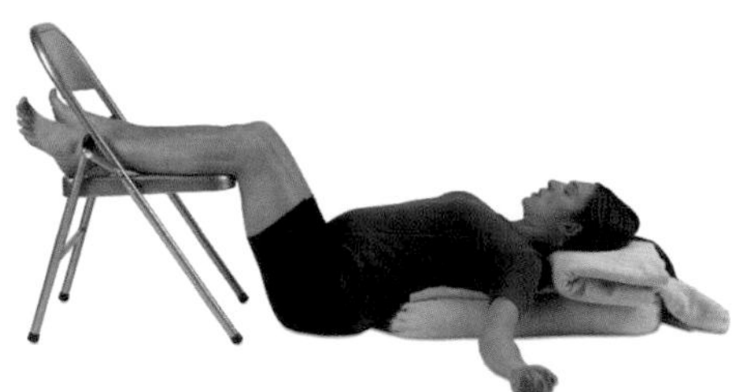

18 Shavasana (lower legs on chair), *page 138*

Chapter 4

Sequences of Asanas for Beginners

Classification of Asanas

The three trimesters of pregnancy refer to the following weeks:
1st trimester: weeks 1 to 16
2nd trimester: weeks 17 to 29
3rd trimester: weeks 30 to 40

Yoga asanas are classified according to the following considerations:

- The anatomic structure of the body
- The radius of movement and action of the body, specifically the spinal column
- How the asanas work on the body, mind, and soul

The asanas here are classified into nine categories, with pranayama appearing as the tenth.

The classification gives you a quick and useful reference tool for finding all the asanas and the trimesters in which they can be safely practiced; it does not, however, show the *order* in which they should be practiced.

The asanas were taken from these categories and brought into practice sequences by the authors. Sequencing is an art that takes experience and skill.

Standing Asanas
Uttishtha Sthiti

	1st Trimester	2nd Trimester	3rd Trimester
Tadasana		√	√
Urdhva Baddhanguliyasana in Tadasana		√	√
Pashchima Namaskarasana in Tadasana		√	√
Gomukhasana in Tadasana		√	√
Urdhva Hastasana		√	√
Utthita Hasta Padangushthasana 2 (to the side)		√	√
Utthita Trikonasana (wall/trestle)		√	√
Utthita Parshvakonasana (wall/trestle)		√	√
Parighasana		√	
Virabhadrasana 1 (wall/trestle)		√	√
Virabhadrasana 2 (wall/trestle)		√	√
Virabhadrasana 3 (wall/trestle)		√	√
Ardha Chandrasana (wall/trestle)		√	√
Parshvottanasana (wall)		√	√
Pashchima Namaskarasana in Parshvottanasana (concave back)		√	√
Prasarita Padottanasana		√	√
Ardha Uttanasana (wall/table)		√	√
Adho Mukha Shvanasana (supported)		√	√
Uttanasana (concave back)	√	√	√
Prasarita Padottanasana (concave back)	√	√	√

Standing asanas help strengthen the spine and widen the pelvis. When you're pregnant, take special care to stretch your spine without exerting pressure on your abdomen; that is, with precise alignment and full spinal extension.

Don't practice standing asanas if you've had miscarriages or have a disposition toward them because of a glandular problem. Please seek out the advice of an experienced Iyengar Yoga teacher.

Concentrate instead on the asanas in Chapter 3, including:
Janu Shirshasana, Concave Back (page 82)
Pashchimottanasana, Concave Back (page 87)
Baddha Konasana, Straight Back, Relief during Pregnancy (page 67), Shavasana (page 134)

◇

Sitting Asanas
Upavishtha Sthiti

	1st Trimester	2nd Trimester	3rd Trimester
Dandasana		√	√
Urdhva Hasta Dandasana		√	√
Baddha Konasana	√	√	√
Upavishtha Konasana (straight back)	√	√	√
Svastikasana	√	√	√
Parvatasana from Svastikasana	√	√	√
Virasana	√	√	√
Parvatasana from Virasana	√	√	√
Gomukhasana from Virasana	√	√	√

Forward Bends

Pashchima Pratana Sthiti

	1st Trimester	2nd Trimester	3rd Trimester
Adho Mukha Virasana	√	√	√
Maha Mudra		√	√
Urdhva Hasta and Urdhva Mukha Janu Shirshasana (concave back, lower chest lifted)	√	√	√
Urdhva Hasta and Urdhva Mukha Trianga Mukhaikapada Pashchimottanasana (concave back, lower chest lifted)	√	√	
Upavishtha Konasana (concave back)	√	√	√
Urdhva Hasta and Urdhva Mukha Pashchimottanasana (concave back, lower chest lifted)	√	√	√
Malasana (modified for labor, with ropes or sitting against wall)		√	√

Twists

Parivritta Sthiti

	1st Trimester	2nd Trimester	3rd Trimester
Bharadvajasana 1	√	√	√
Bharadvajasana (chair)	√	√	√
Parshva Svastikasana (chair) *	√	√	√
Parshva Padmasana (chair) *	√	√	√
Parshva Virasana (wall) *	√	√	√
Parshva Baddha Konasana (chair) *	√	√	√
Parshva Janu Shirshasana (chair) *	√	√	√

* If you have a history of miscarriage, avoid all Parshvas in your 1st trimester.

Inversions

Viparita Sthiti

	1st Trimester	2nd Trimester	3rd Trimester
Salamba Shirshasana (with teacher, preceded and followed by special sequence)	√	√	√
Salamba Sarvangasana (chair)	√	√	√
Ardha Halasana (chair)	√	√	√
Ardha Supta Konasana (2 chairs)		√	√
Setu Bandha Sarvangasana (bench or similar)	√	√	√
Chatushpadasana		√	√
Viparita Karani (legs bent on chair)	√	√	√
Viparita Karani (legs straight)		√	√

Asanas for Abdomen and Lumbar

Supta and Uttishtha Sthiti

	1st Trimester	2nd Trimester	3rd Trimester
Supta Padangushthasana 2 (to the side)	√	√	√
Utthita Hasta Padangushthasana 2 (to the side)		√	√

Back Bends
Purva Pratana Sthiti

	1st Trimester	2nd Trimester	3rd Trimester
Cross-bolsters	√	√	√
Bhujangasana (in ropes)		√	√
Bhujangasana (ropes, chair, and bolster)		√	√
Salamba Purvottanasana (trestle)		√	√
Salamba Purvottanasana		√	√
Dvi Pada Viparita Dandasana (fully supported, with Viparita Dandasana bench, L-shape)	√	√	√

Rope Asanas
Yoga Kurunta

	1st Trimester	2nd Trimester	3rd Trimester
Bhujangasana (in ropes)		√	√
Bhujangasana (ropes, chair, and bolster)		√	√
Ardha Uttanasana		√	√
Adho Mukha Shvanasana		√	√
Malasana (modified for labor)		√	√

Restorative Asanas
Vishranta Karaka Sthiti

	1st Trimester	2nd Trimester	3rd Trimester
Supta Virasana	√	√	√
Supta Baddha Konasana	√	√	√
Matsyasana	√	√	√
Supta Svastikasana	√	√	√
Salamba Purvottanasana		√	√
Cross-bolsters	√	√	√
Setu Bandha Sarvangasana (bench)	√	√	√
Viparita Karani (legs bent on chair)	√	√	√
Viparita Karani (legs straight)		√	√
Salamba Sarvangasana (chair)	√	√	√
Shavasana (bolster/s)	√	√	√
Shavasana (on bolster, legs on bolsters)	√	√	√

Pranayama
Breathing Techniques

	1st Trimester	2nd Trimester	3rd Trimester
Ujjayi 1 and 2, in Shavasana	√	√	√
Viloma Stage 1, in Shavasana	√	√	√
Viloma Stage 2, in Shavasana and sitting			√

Sequence for First Trimester and Throughout Pregnancy

Amid all the efforts to educate pregnant women on health, diet, and medical issues, scant attention has been paid to the benefits of Yoga for your own well-being and that of your baby.

One reason for this inattention could be concerns about safety. Iyengar Yoga, however, is especially safe, and in this book we give utmost consideration to this important issue.

Another factor that may cause you to hesitate about Yoga is fear of the poses themselves. For this reason, we've sequenced—and sometimes modified—the asanas for you, putting first not only the ones most suitable for beginners, but also those that will gradually increase your courage.

For example, you can start with the forward-bending asanas, which are done sitting down. The only way to conquer fear is by personal experience. Courage will come when fear is overcome. The forward bends help you gradually triumph over fear and build up courage.

Knowledge through Yoga, and the benefits of Yoga, can also only be attained by personal experience. You will only know what your capacity is to absorb these blessings by trying and experimenting. The simple sitting asanas mentioned above, with the forward extension of the spine, enable you to get a clear picture of your capabilities. Sitting down is more relaxing and less intimidating, especially when you're pregnant. The poses include Janu Shirshasana, Baddha Konasana, Supta Baddha Konasana, and Upavishtha Konasana.

Recommended Sequence

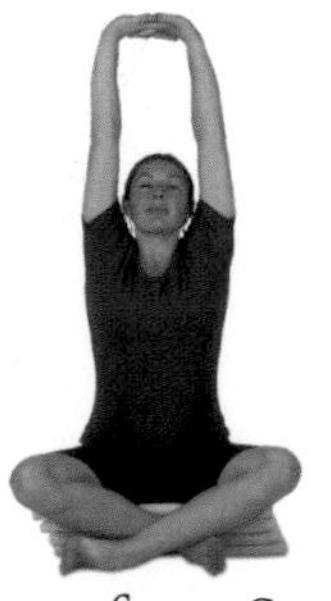

1 Parvatasana from Svastikasana (sitting on bolster), *page 74*

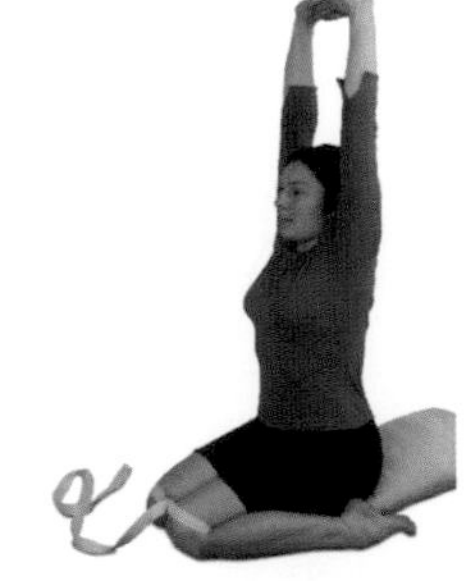

2 Parvatasana from Virasana (sitting on bolster), *page 74*

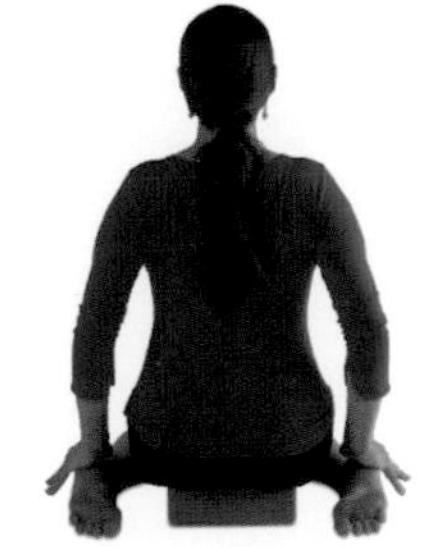

3 Virasana, *page 73*

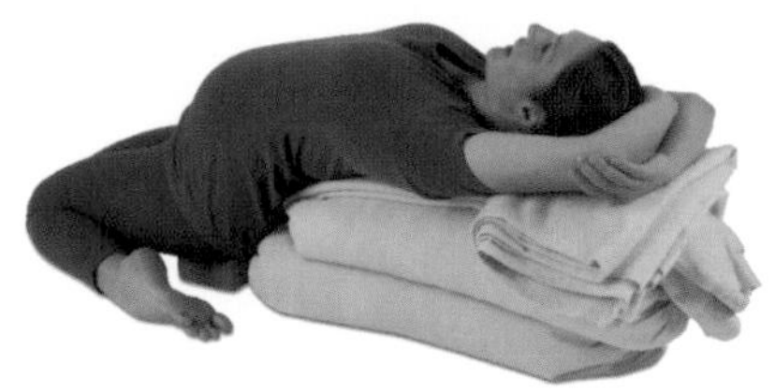

4 Supta Virasana (bolster/s), *page 130*

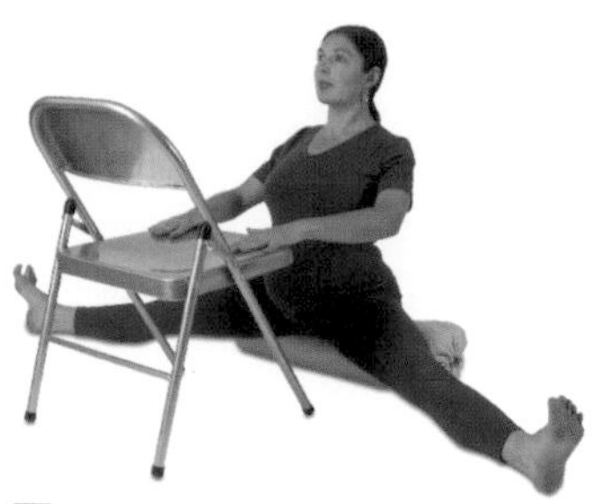

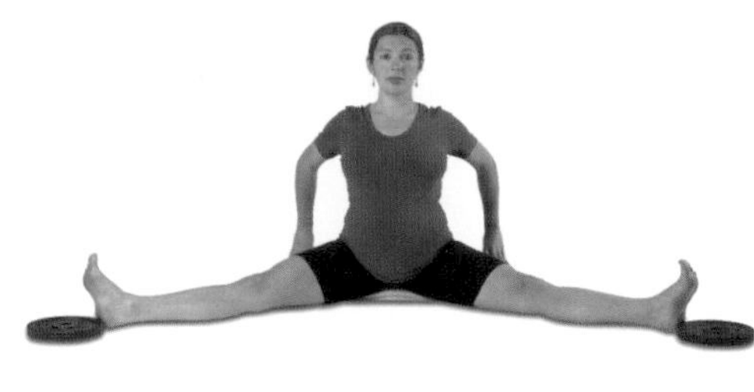

5 Upavishtha Konasana (sitting up), *page 71*

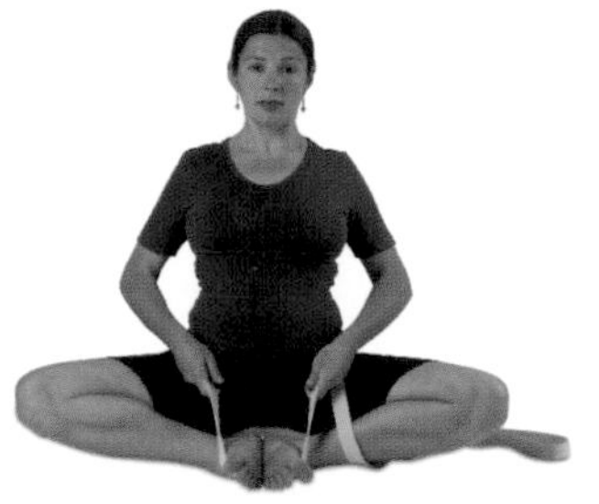

6 Baddha Konasana (straight back), *page 67*

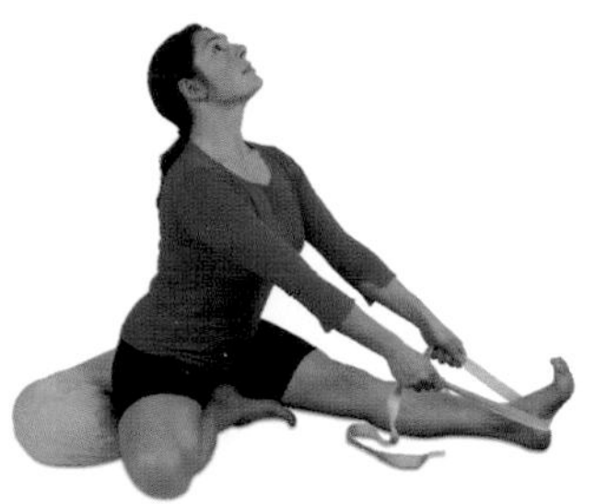

7 Janu Shirshasana (concave back, lower chest lifted), *page 83*

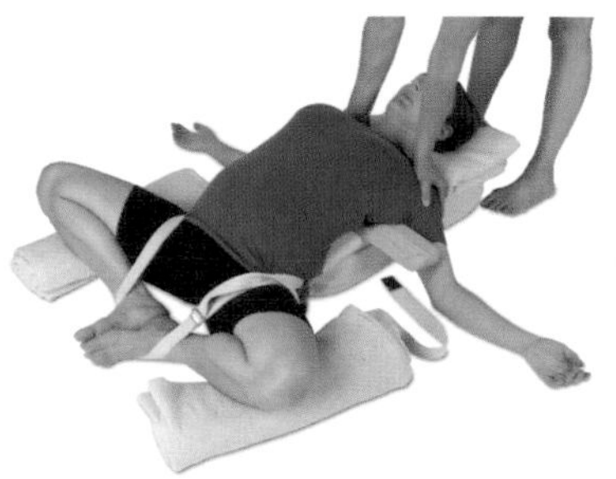

8 Supta Baddha Konasana (bolster lengthwise, slanted plank), *page 128*

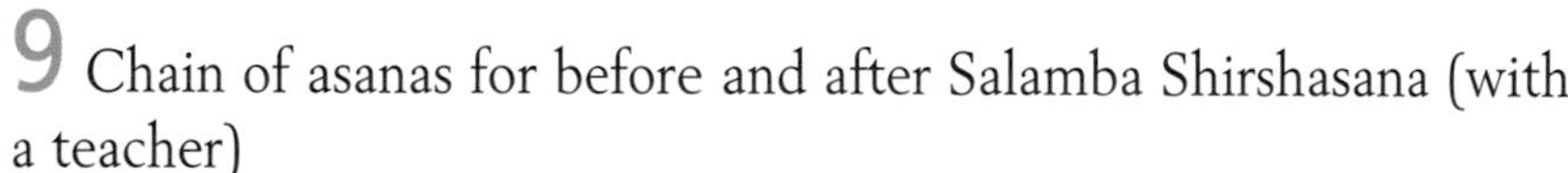

9 Chain of asanas for before and after Salamba Shirshasana (with a teacher)

Before: Maha Mudra, Adho Mukha Shvanasana, and Uttanasana (concave back)

After, reverse order: Uttanasana (concave back), Adho Mukha Shvanasana, and Maha Mudra.

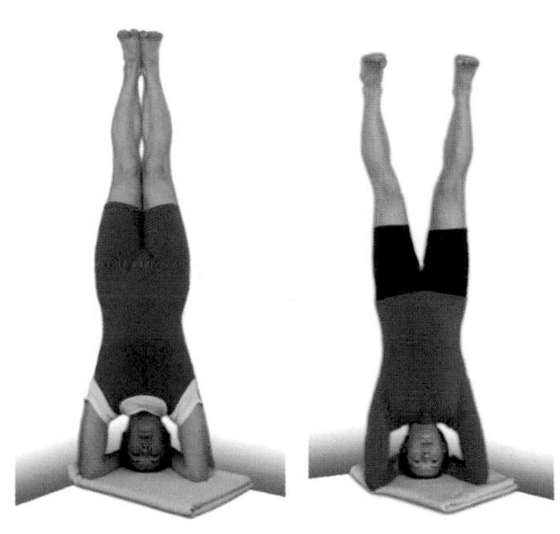

early pregnancy advanced pregnancy

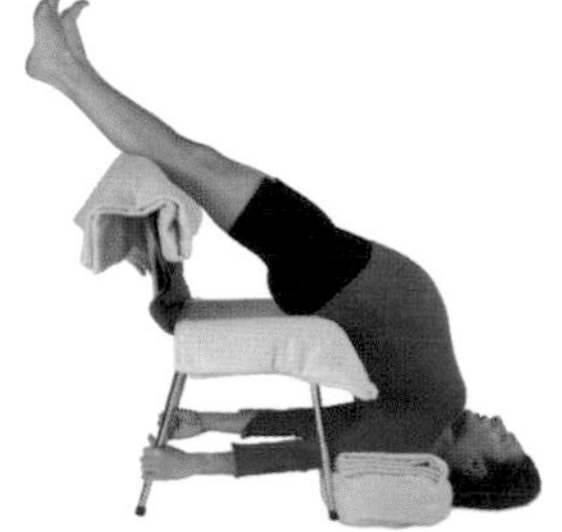

10 Salamba Sarvangasana (chair), *page 103*

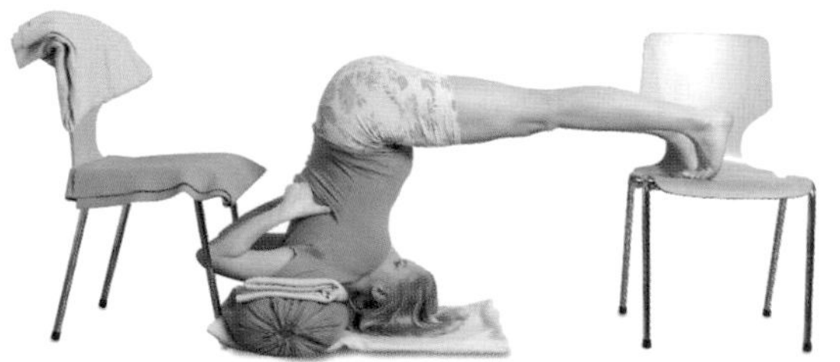

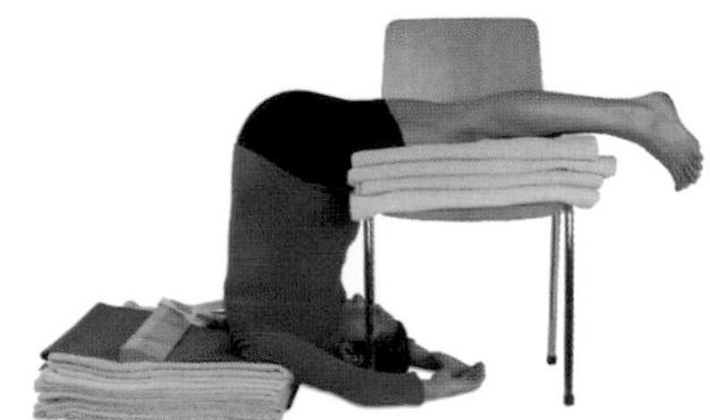

11 Ardha Halasana (chair), *pages 104 – 105*

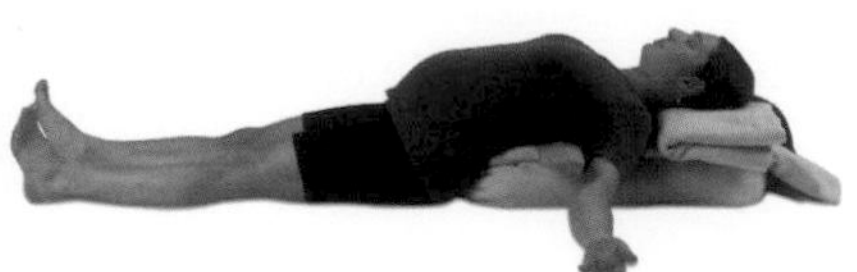

12 Shavasana (on bolster/s), at least twice a day for at least 10 – 15 minutes and whenever you feel like having a rest, *page 134*

13 Ujjayi Pranayama 1 and 2 (lying on bolster), *page 148*

These asanas widen and stretch both the space in the pelvis and the uterus. They ensure good blood circulation in the pelvis and enough space for the fetus: in the beginning, so it can settle, and later on, to avoid compression so that it can move freely. Together with the pranayama (pages 140 – 153), they soothe and quiet your nerves. You gain confidence, courage, strength, and energy.

Durations

- Janu Shirshasana: 30 seconds per side
- Parvatasana (with reversing the way you interlock your thumbs): 30 seconds each way
- Virasana: 1 to 2 minutes
- Rest of the poses: 5 minutes

Coming out of the pose

Maintain the space you have created while coming back.

Apart from the sequence above, we suggest that you see Part III, Chapter 9, Problems A – Z, and practice the asanas that help with:

- Spinal muscles, weakness of
- Abdomen, heaviness of
- Fatigue

Always stop earlier if you feel the need!

Sequences for the Second and Third Trimesters

Enhancing strength and inner balance
You can start these sequences in the second trimester and continue them throughout the third trimester as long as it is comfortable. You have made it through the first difficult months, and with your doctor's approval, can add some new poses.

This is a good time to begin the standing asanas. They help to strengthen the spine and widen the pelvis. Practice these with precise alignment and full extension of the spine, so that there is no pressure on your abdomen, but rather a lifting feeling from the pelvic floor.

Don't practice standing asanas if you've had miscarriages or have a disposition toward them because of a glandular problem. Please seek out the advice of an experienced Iyengar Yoga teacher.

Concentrate instead on the asanas in Chapter 3, including:
Janu Shirshasana, Concave Back (page 82)
Pashchimottanasana, Concave Back (page 87)
Baddha Konasana, Straight Back, Relief during Pregnancy (page 110)
Shavasana (page 134)

For more detailed descriptions of the asanas, and for modifications, see Chapter 3, "Instructions and Benefits."

Durations

- Asanas practiced on the right and left side: stay for 30 to 60 seconds per side
- Asanas that extend straight forward or backward (like Ardha Uttanasana or Chatushpadasana): 30 to 60 seconds
- Inversions (pages 96 – 114):
  - Salamba Sarvangasana: If you practice it without Ardha Halasana, stay in it 2 to 3 minutes longer than Salamba Shirshasana.
  - Ardha Halasana, Setu Bandha Sarvangasana, and Viparita Karani: up to 5 minutes
  - Rest of poses: 5 to 10 minutes
- Restorative Asanas (pages 126 – 139):
  - Shavasana: 15 minutes
  - Rest of poses: up to 5 minutes

HINT: There are too many asanas here to practice all at one time, so try alternating the sequences.

General Guidelines

- Always stretch your spine and keep it lifted.
- Never exert pressure on your abdomen, which also exerts pressure on the throat and thyroid.
- Don't invite hormonal disturbances by forcing yourself and relying on willpower; it's better to work on proper alignment with a soft abdomen and throat.
- Protect the growing life in your womb by not forcing out your breath, but letting it flow softly and smoothly.
- Don't jump into the standing asanas.
- Practice the back bends with the supports as indicated, to avoid weakening the inner lining of the uterus.
- Practice the twisting asanas as indicated, for the same reason as above.
- When you come back from an asana, always maintain your lift, extension, and expansion. Don't collapse or make jolting movements.

In addition, keep in mind the guidelines in Part II, Chapter 3, "The Beginning of Your Pregnancy."

Sequence 1: Widening and Stretching the Pelvis

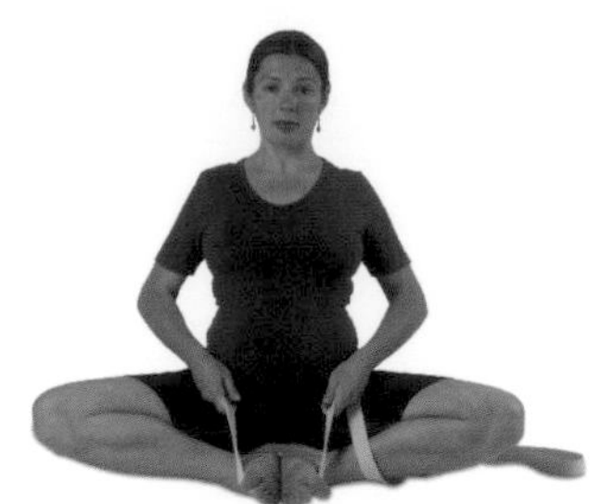

1 Baddha Konasana (straight back), *page 67*

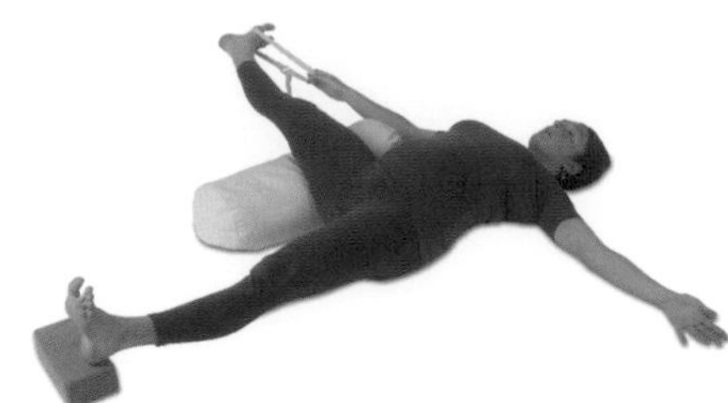

2 Supta Padangushthasana 2 (side stretch), *page 115*

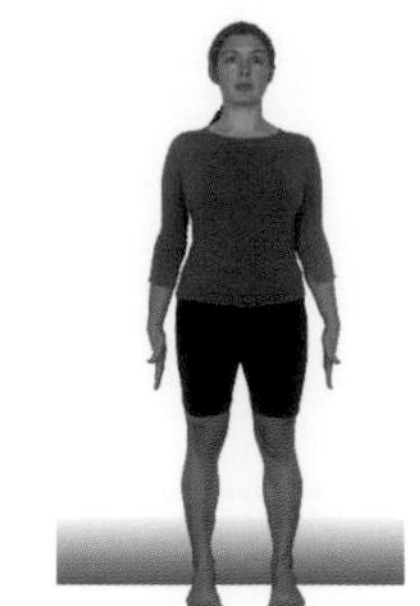

3 Tadasana, *page 32*

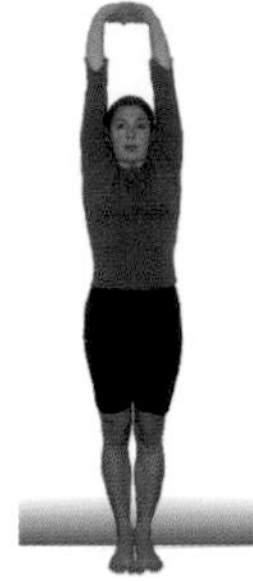

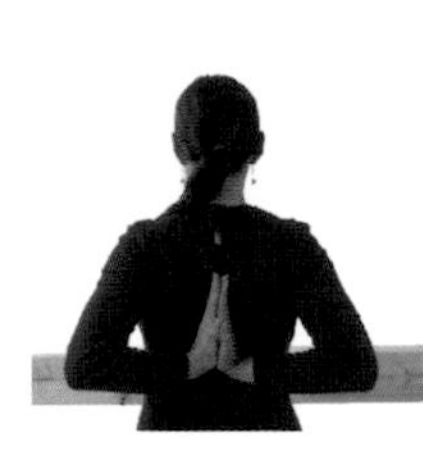

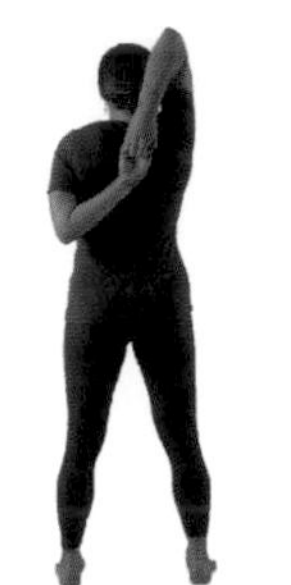

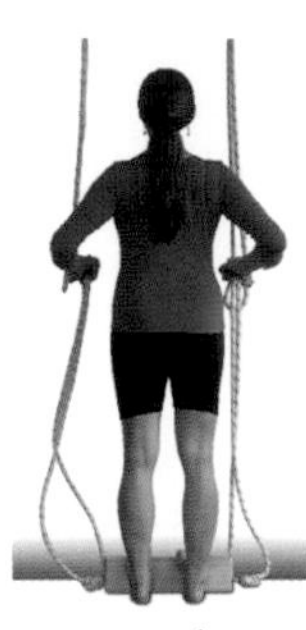

4 Urdhva Baddhanguliyasana, *page 34*, Pashchima Namaskarasana, *page 36*, Gomukhasana in Tadasana, *page 37*, and Tadasana (with wall and quarter-round block), *page 33*

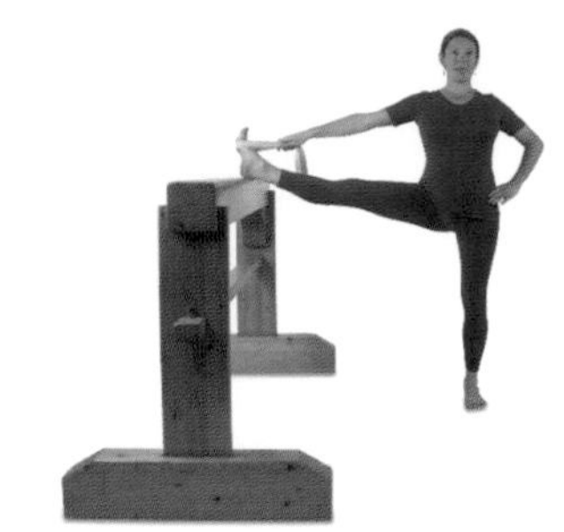

5 Utthita Hasta Padangushthasana 2 (side stretch), *page 117*

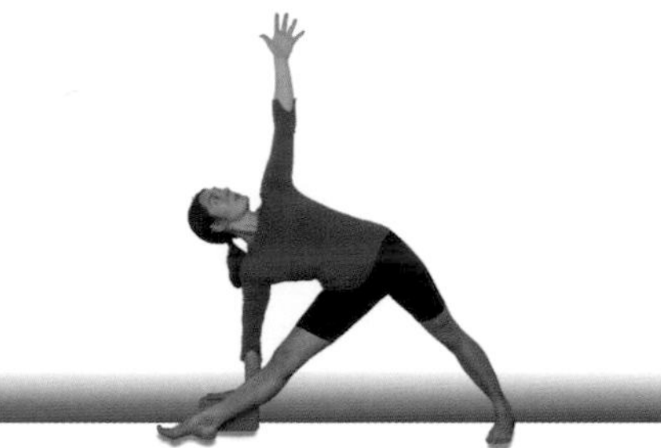

6 Utthita Trikonasana, *page 39*

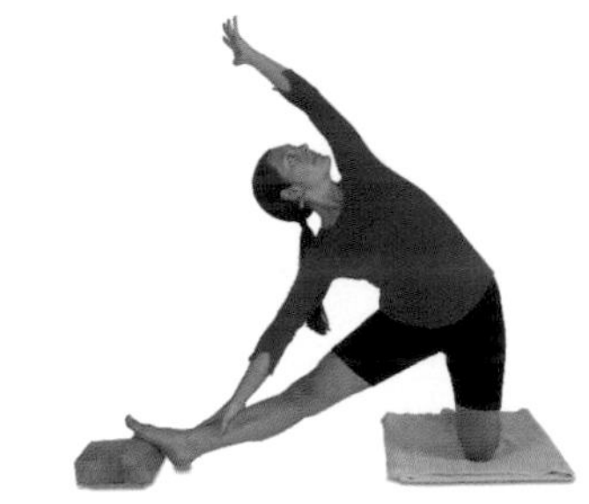

7 Parighasana, *page 44*

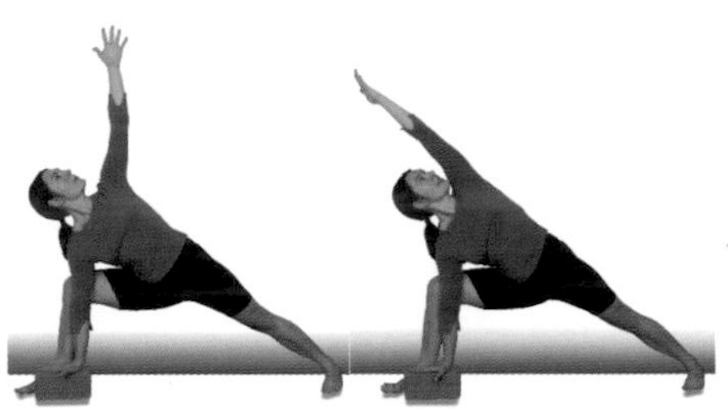

8 Utthita Parshvakonasana, *page 41*

Note

Always start the standing poses from Tadasana. When you finish the pose, come back to Tadasana. If you feel tired, rest in Ardha Uttanasana.

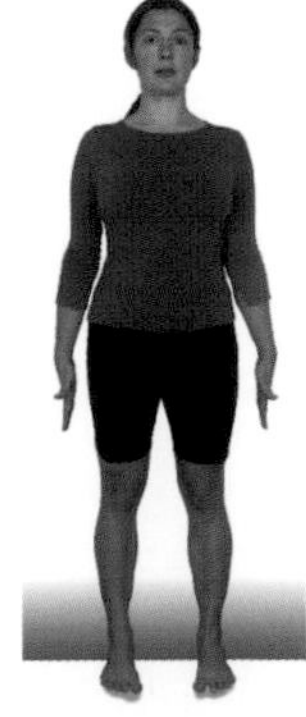

Tadasana

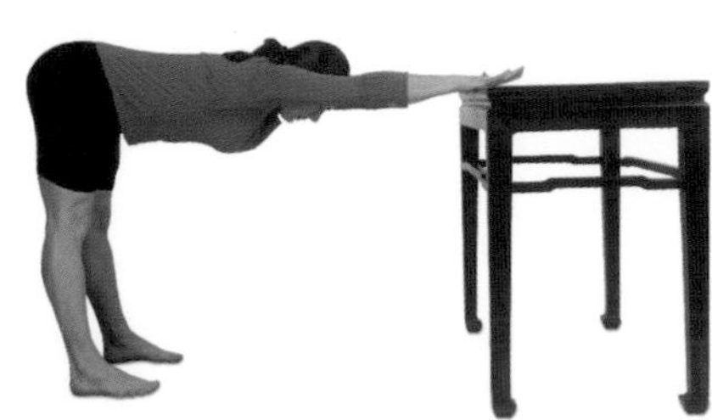

Ardha Uttanasana

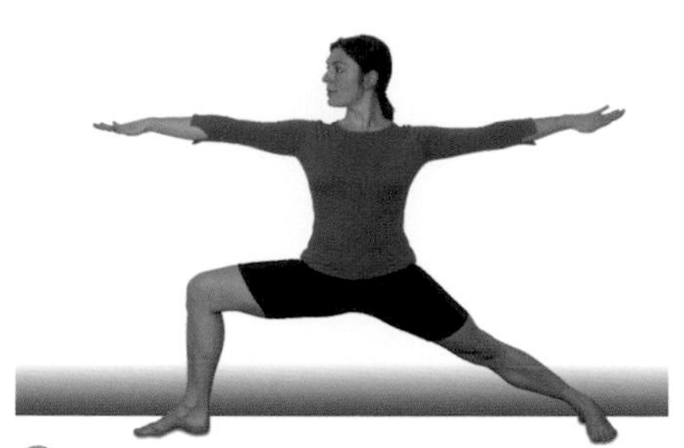

9 Virabhadrasana 2, *page 42*

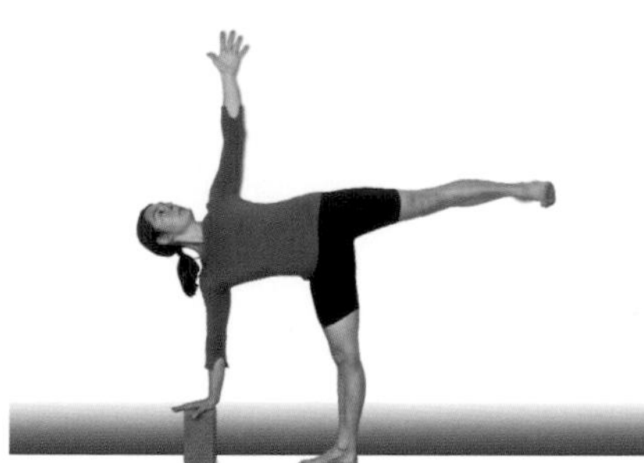

10 Ardha Chandrasana, *page 45*

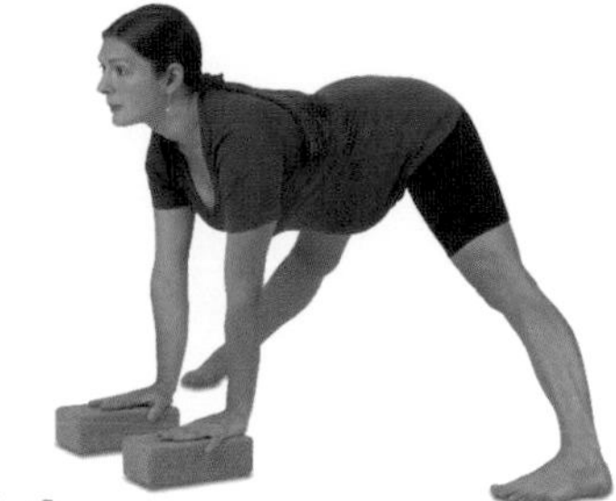

11 Prasarita Padottanasana, *page 56*

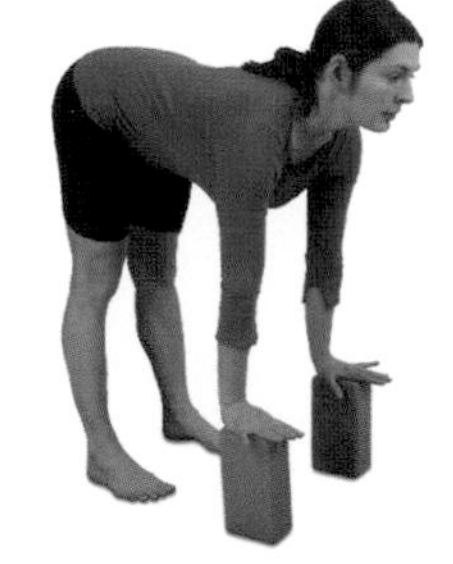

12 Ardha Uttanasana, *page 60*

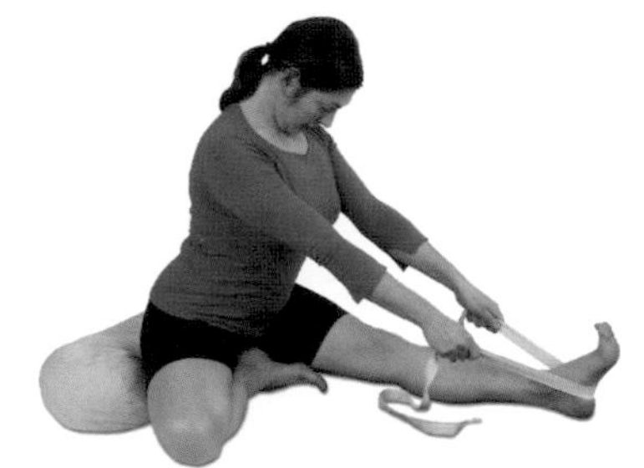

13 Maha Mudra, *page 80*

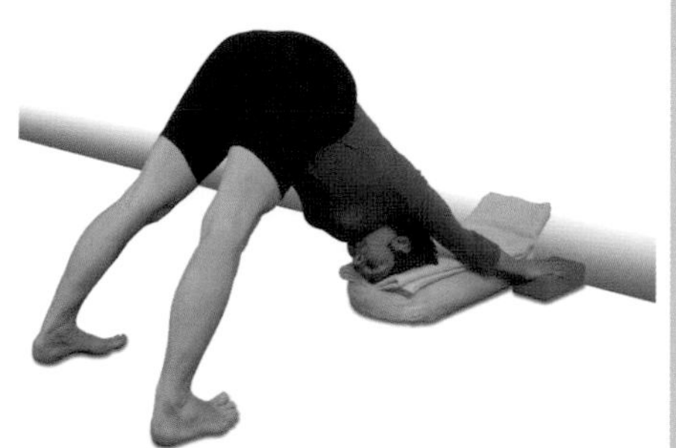

14 Adho Mukha Shvanasana, *page 62*

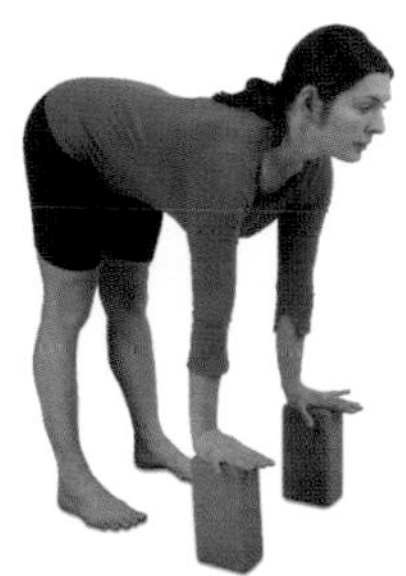

15 Uttanasana (concave back), *page 213*

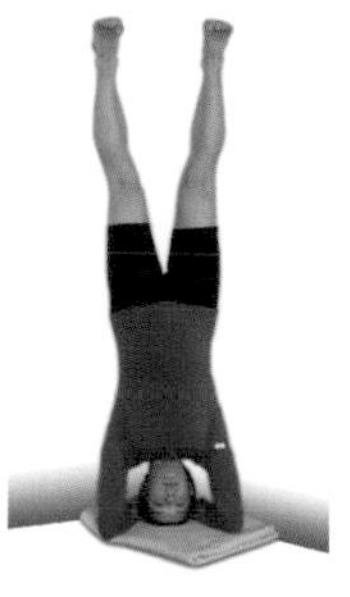

16 Salamba Shirshasana (with wall and teacher), *page 99*

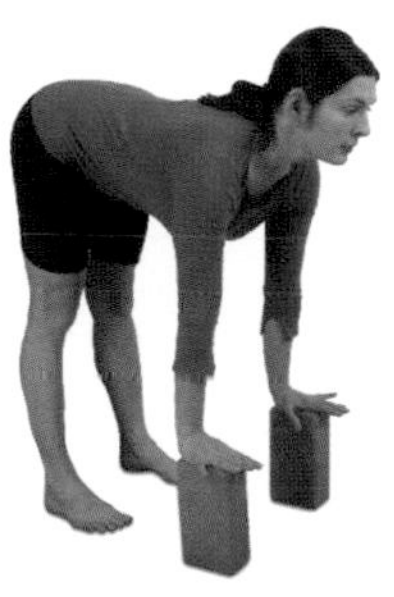

17 Uttanasana (concave back), *page 213*

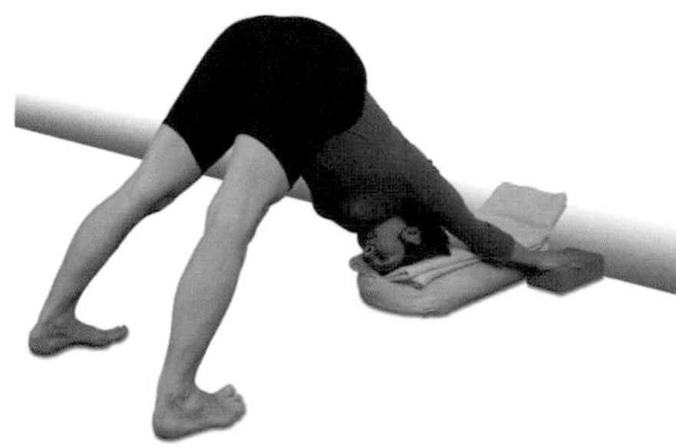

18 Adho Mukha Shvanasana, *page 62*

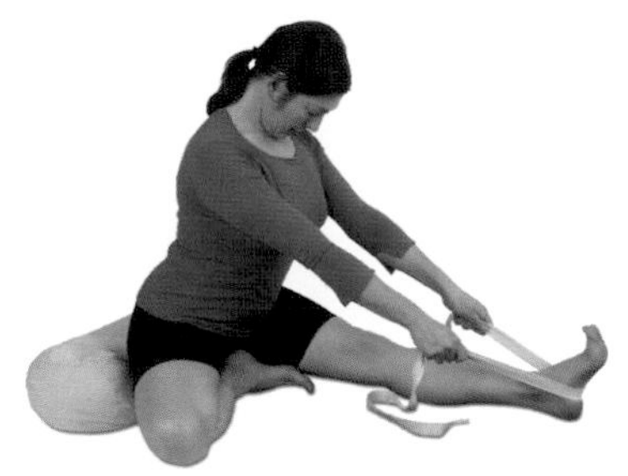

19 Maha Mudra, *page 80*

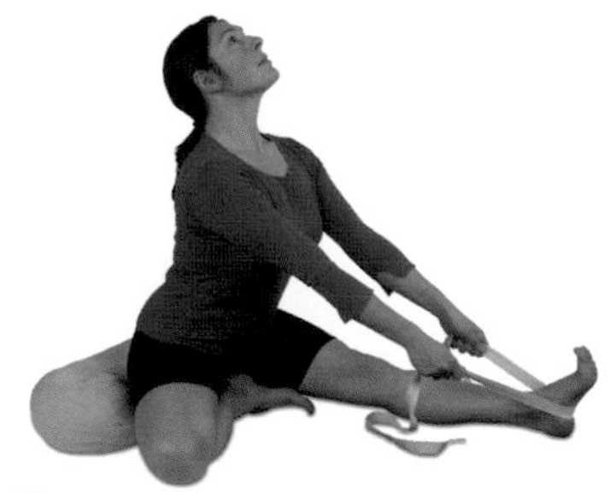

20 Janu Shirshasana (concave back), *page 83*

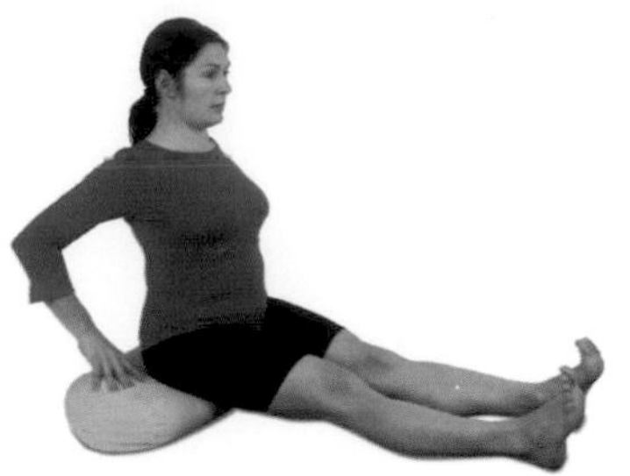

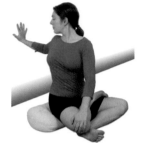

21 Dandasana, *page 65*

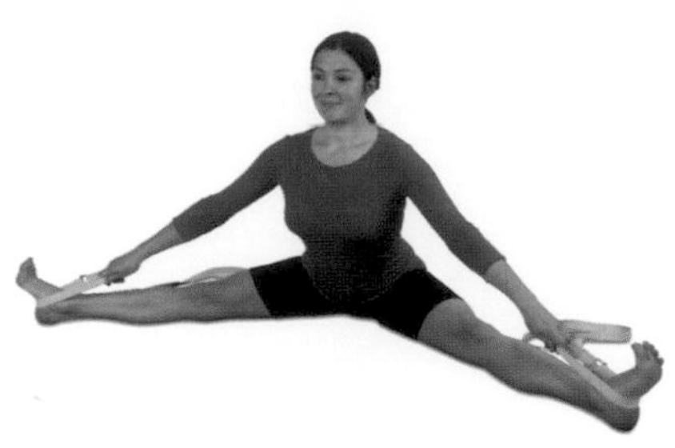

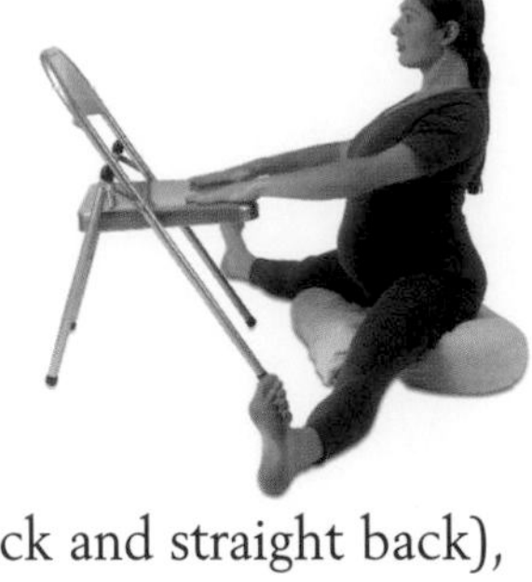

22 Upavishtha Konasana (concave back and straight back), *pages 85 – 86*

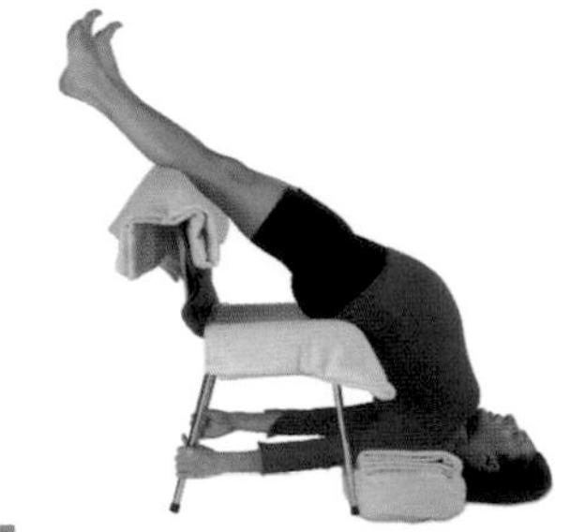

23 Parshva Svastikasana or Ardha Padmasana/full Padmasana (twisting, with wall), *page 94*

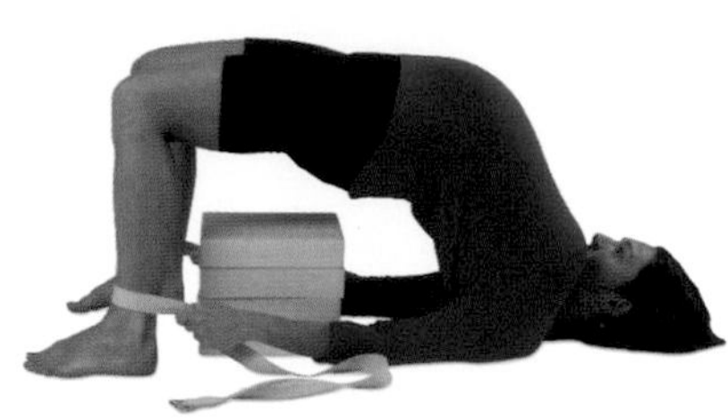

24 Salamba Sarvangasana (chair), *page 103*

25 Chatushpadasana, *page 111*

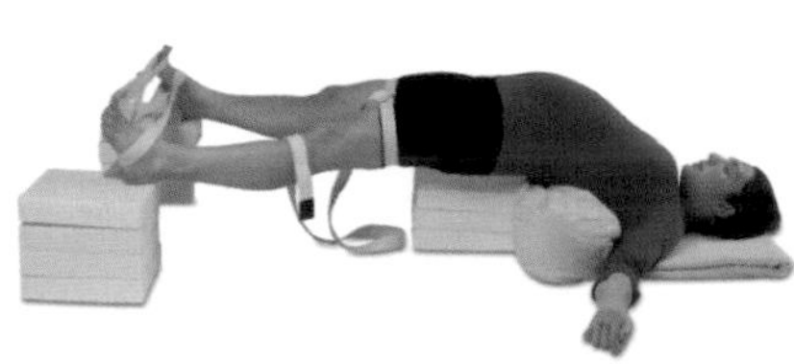

26 Setu Bandha Sarvangasana, *page 108*

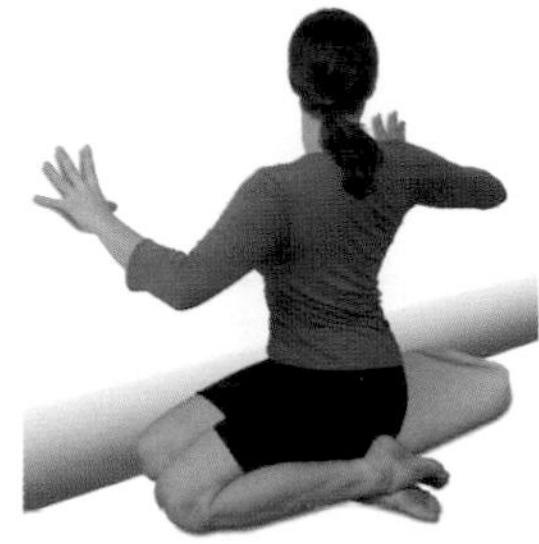

27 Bharadvajasana (chair or bolster), *page 93*

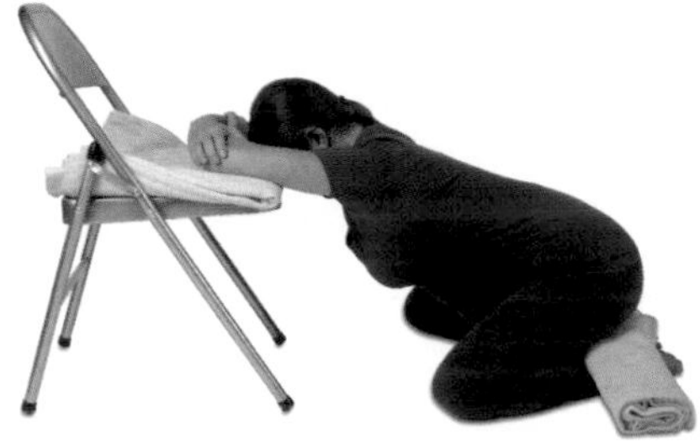

28 Adho Mukha Virasana, *page 76*

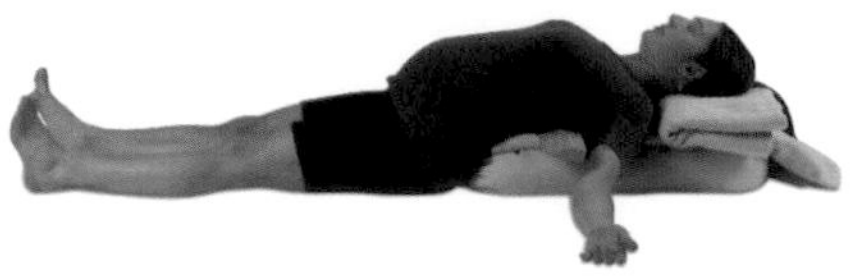

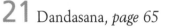

29 Shavasana (bolster/s), *page 134*

30 Ujjayi Pranayama 1, *page 148*

Sequence 2: Stretching the Sides of the Body

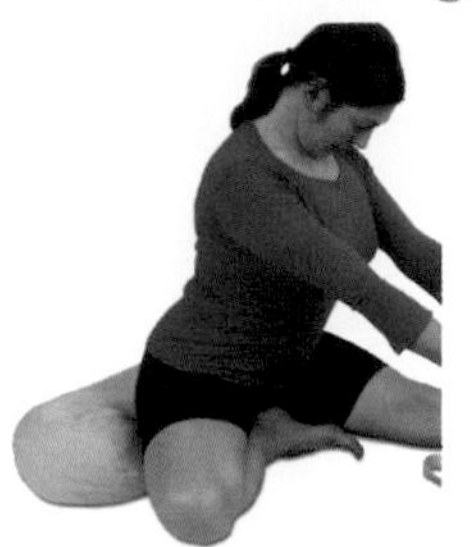

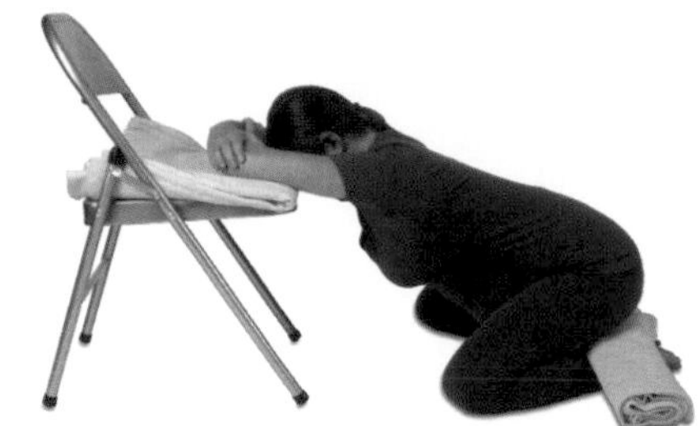

1 Adho Mukha Virasana, *page 76*

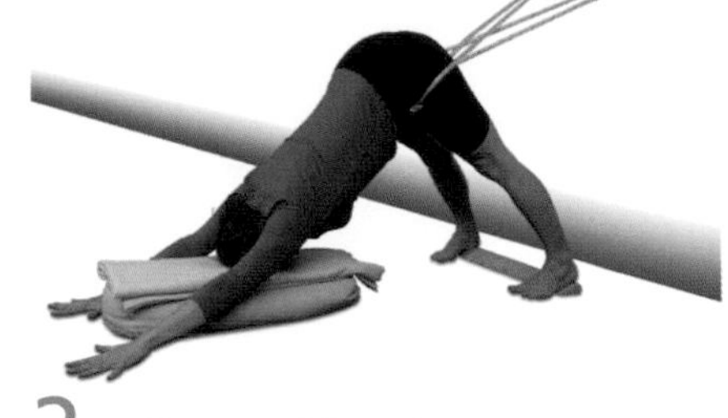

2 Adho Mukha Shvanasana (ropes), *page 125*

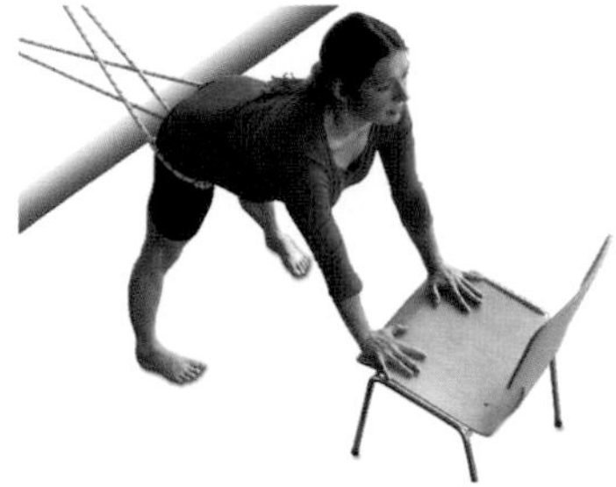

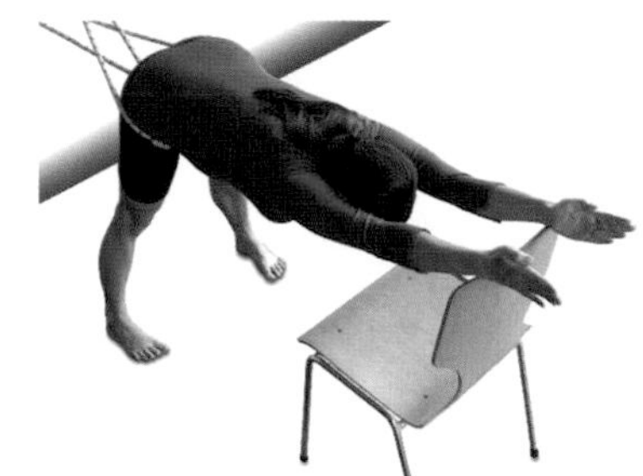

3 Uttanasana (with ropes and chair), *page 124*

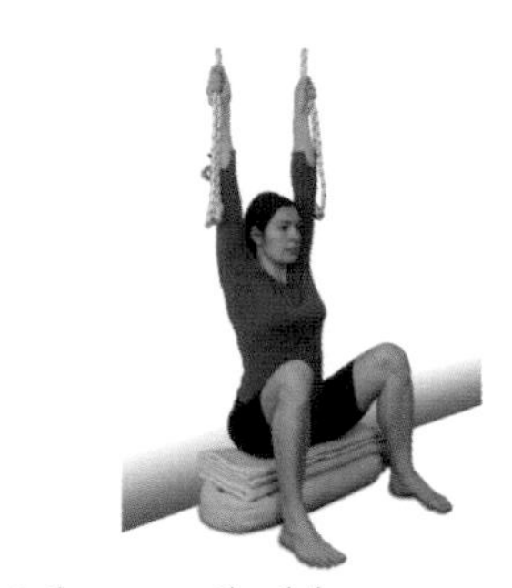

4 Malasana (holding ropes), *page 77*

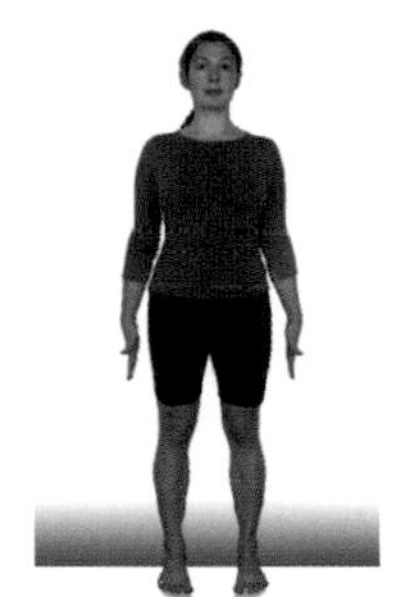

5 Tadasana, *page 32*

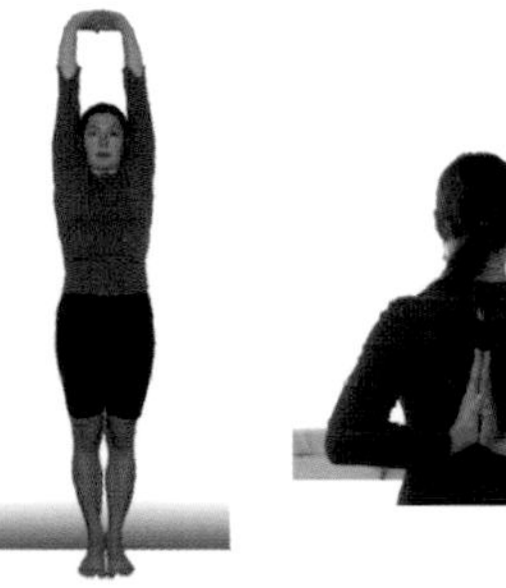

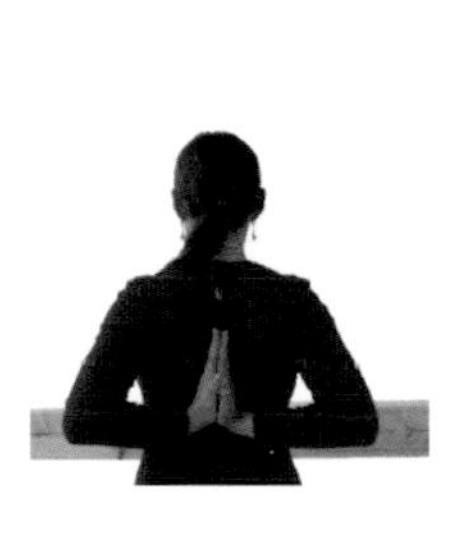

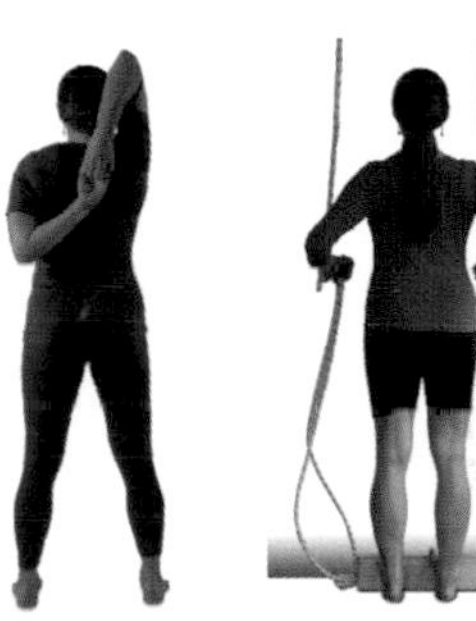

6 Urdhva Baddhanguliyasana, *page 34*, Pashchima Namaskarasana, *page 36*, Gomukhasana in Tadasana, *page 37*, and Tadasana (with wall and quarter-round block), *page 33*

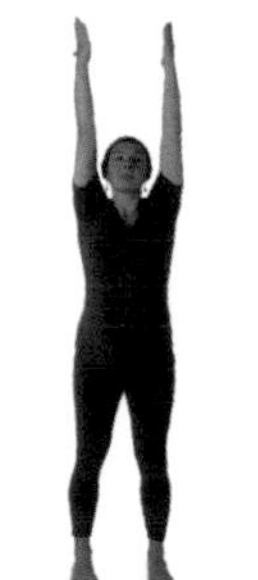

7 Urdhva Hastasana, *page 35*

Note

Always start the standing poses from Tadasana. When you finish the pose, come back to Tadasana. If you feel tired, rest in Ardha Uttanasana.

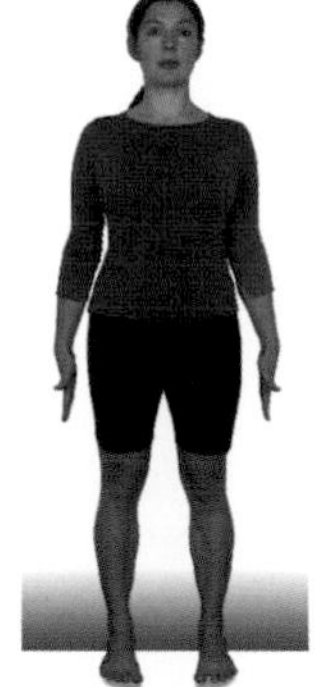

Tadasana

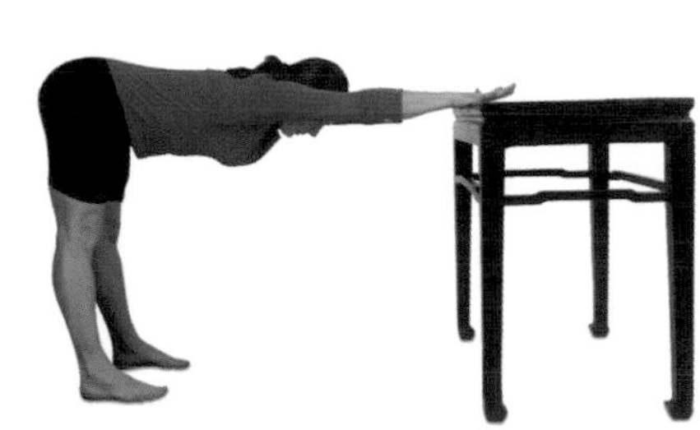

Ardha Uttanasana

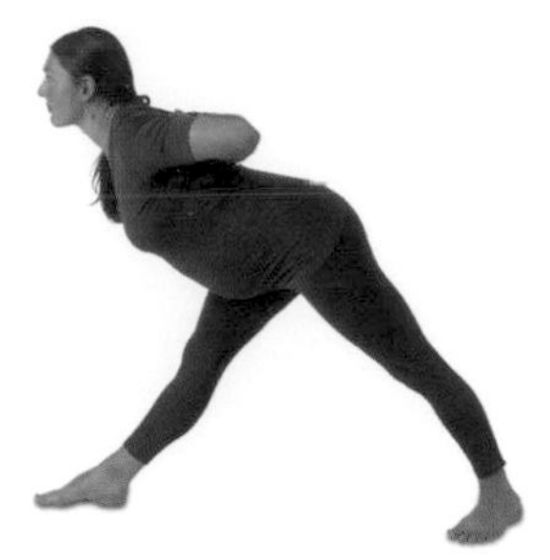

8 Pashchima Namaskarasana in Parshvottanasana, *page 50*

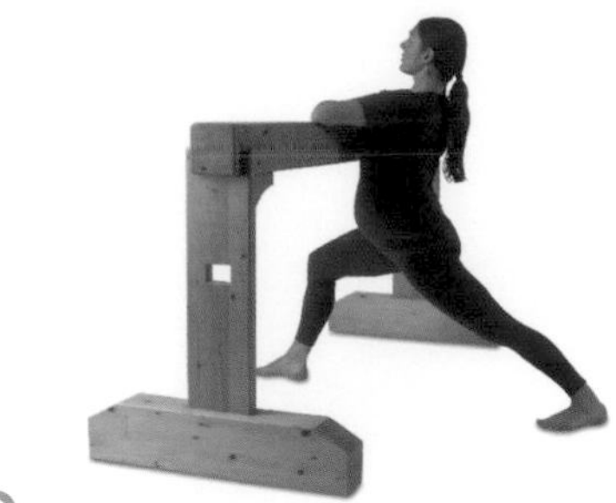

9 Virabhadrasana 1, *page 53*

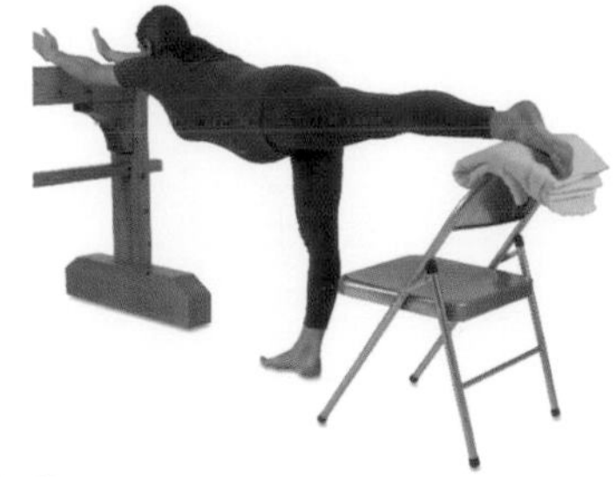

10 Virabhadrasana 3, *page 54*

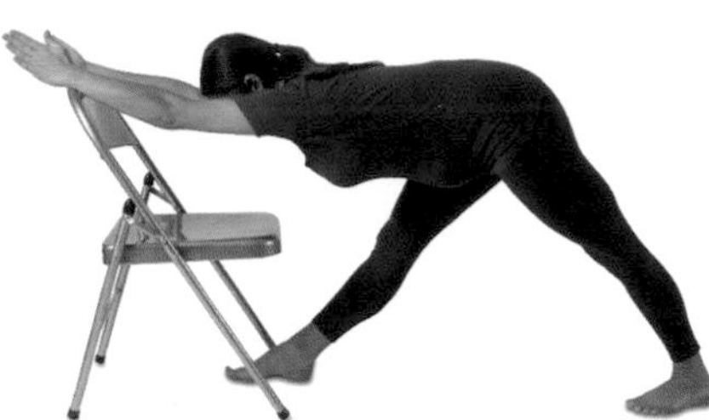

11 Parshvottanasana, hands on support , *page 51*

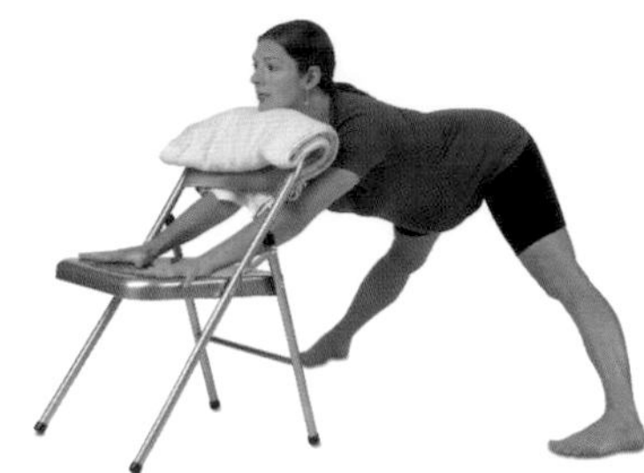

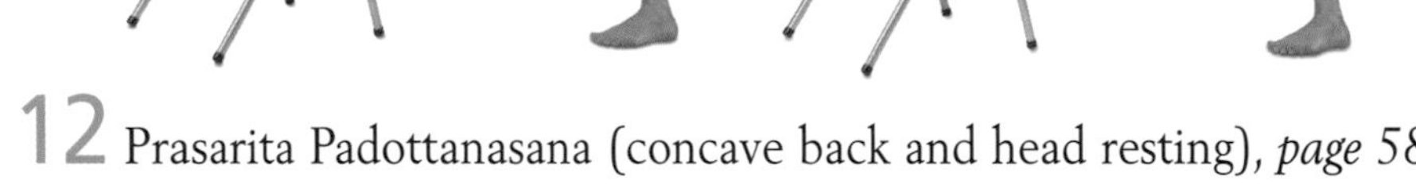

12 Prasarita Padottanasana (concave back and head resting), *page 58*

13 If you practice Salamba Shirshasana with a teacher, add:

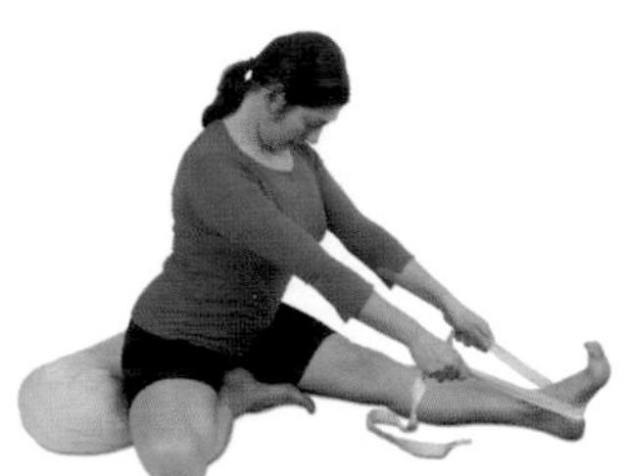

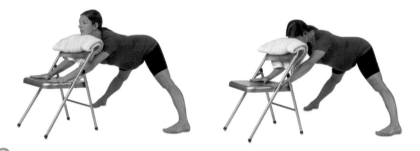

Maha Mudra, *page 80*

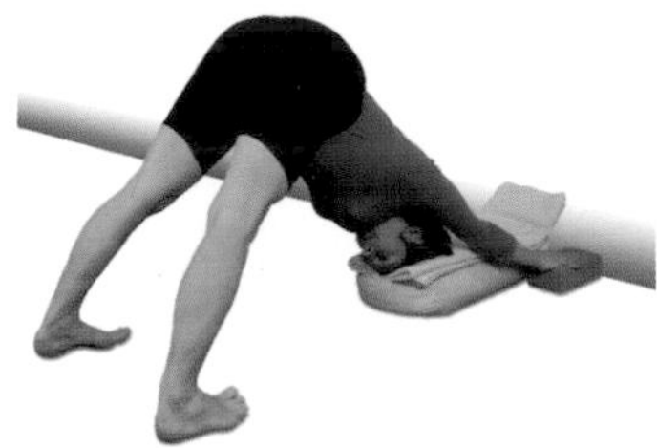

Adho Mukha Shvanasana, *page 62*

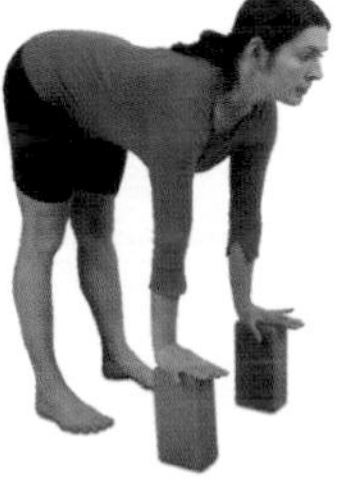

Uttanasana (concave back), *page 213*

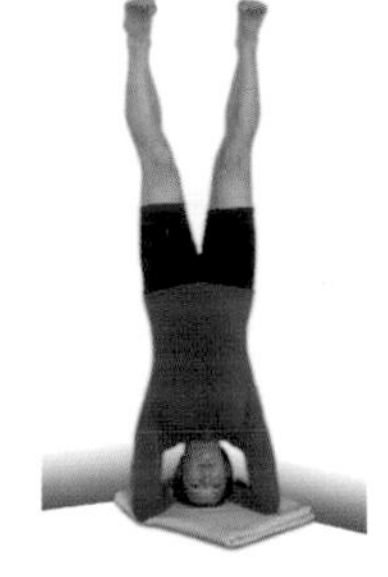

Salamba Shirshasana (with wall and teacher), *page 99*

Reverse sequence following Shirshasana:

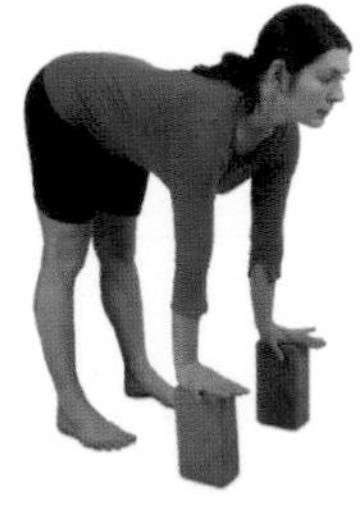

Uttanasana (concave back), *page 213*

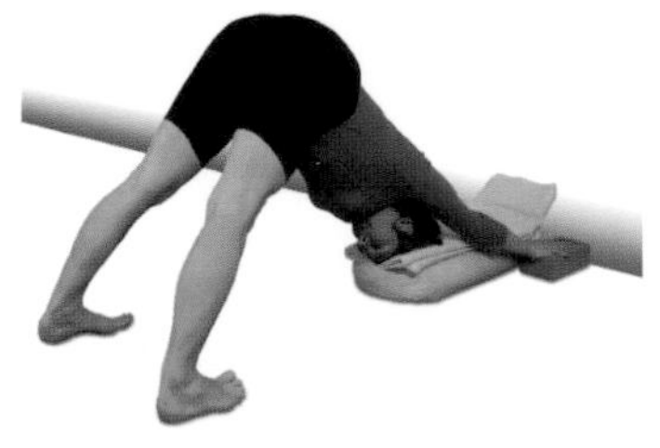

Adho Mukha Shvanasana, *page 62*

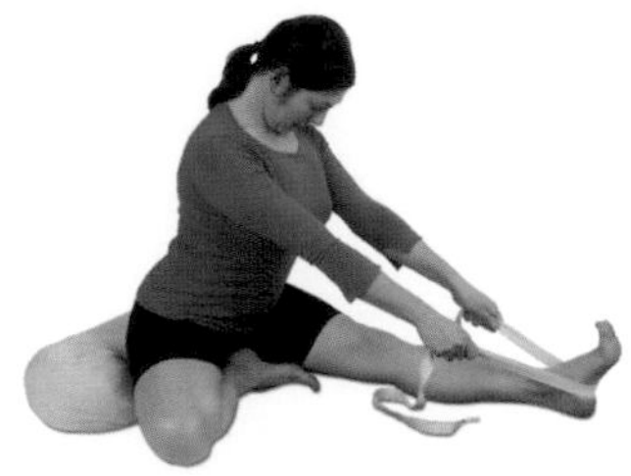

Maha Mudra, *page 80*

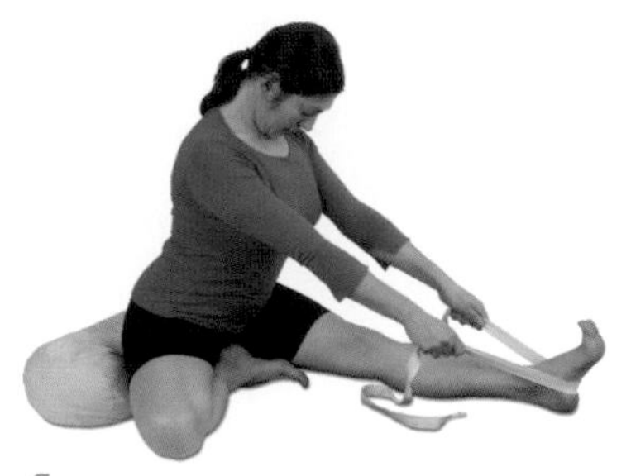

14 Maha Mudra (if you didn't do the Shirshasana sequence), *page 80*

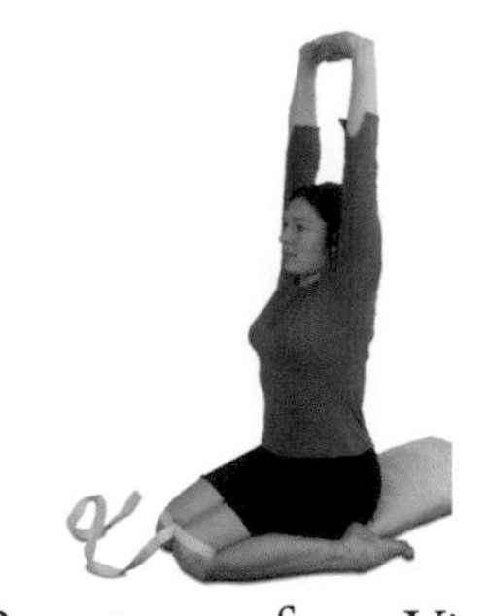

15 Parvatasana from Virasana, *page 74*

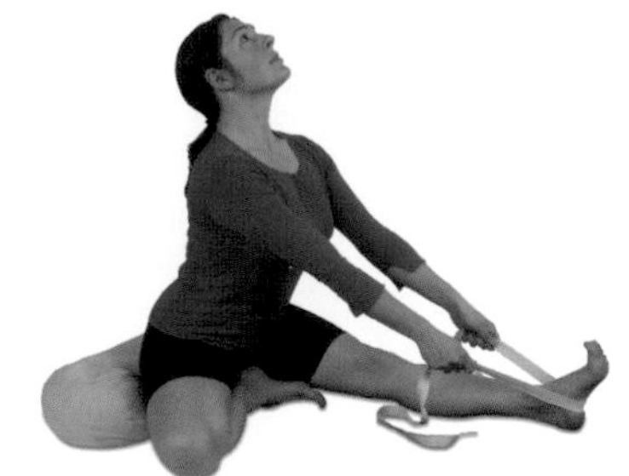

16 Janu Shirshasana (concave back), *page 83*

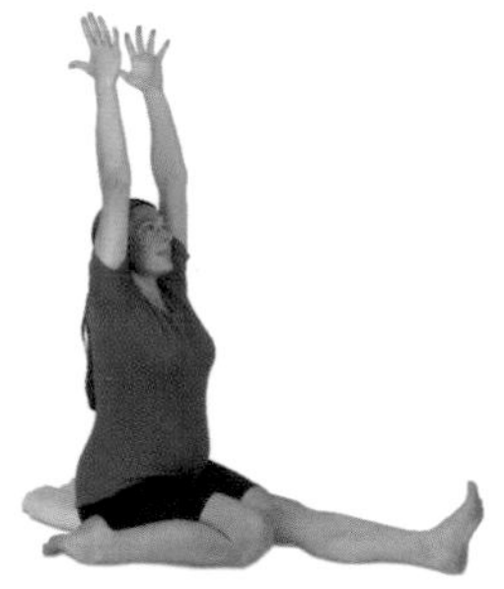

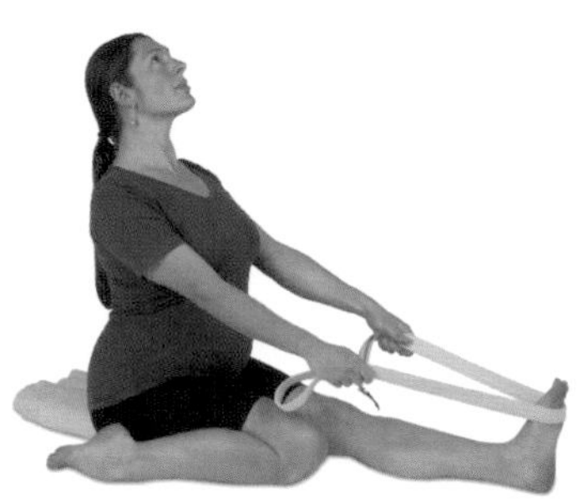

17 Trianga Mukhaikapada Pashchimottanasana (concave back), not in 3rd trimester, *pages 89 – 90*

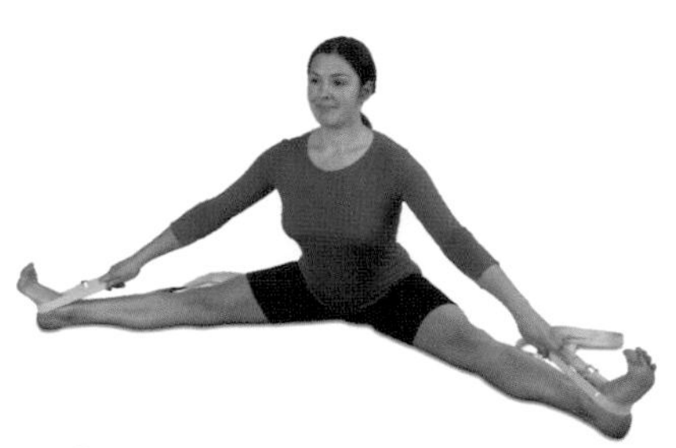

18 Upavishtha Konasana (concave back and straight back), *pages 71 and 85*

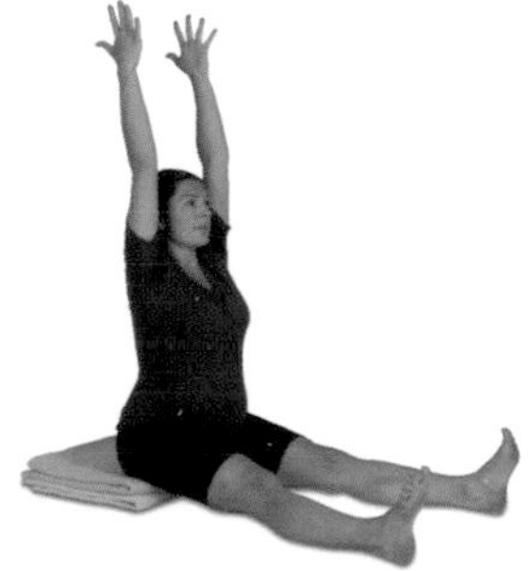

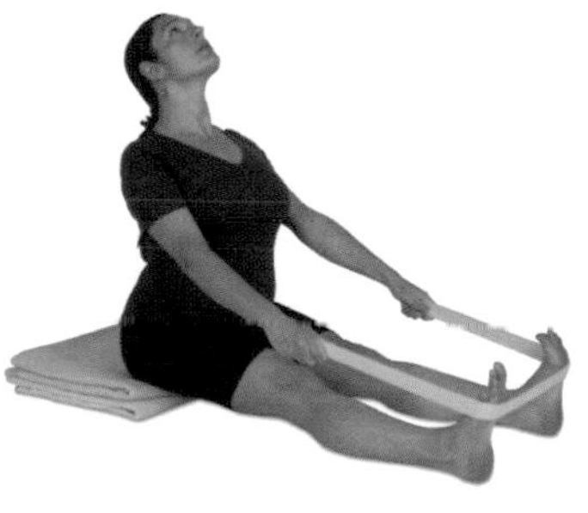

19 Pashchimottanasana (concave back, lower chest lifted), *pages 87 – 88*

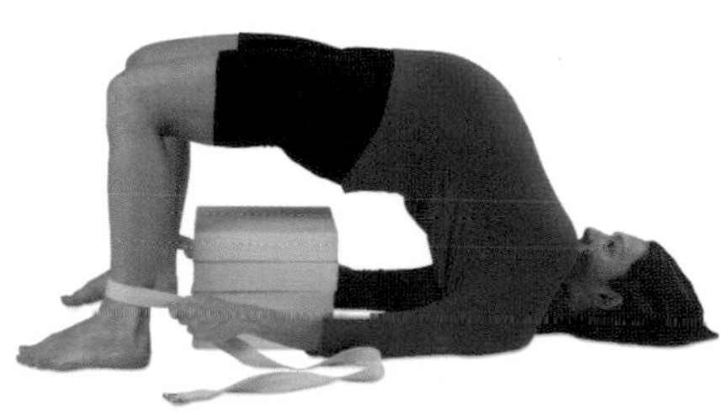

20 Chatushpadasana, *page 111*

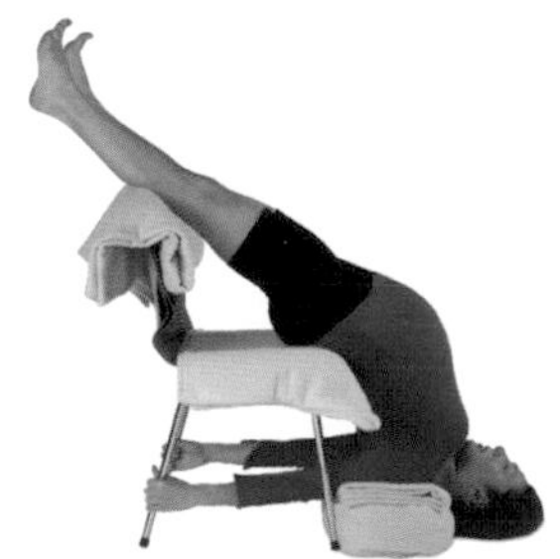

21 Sarvangasana (chair), *page 103*

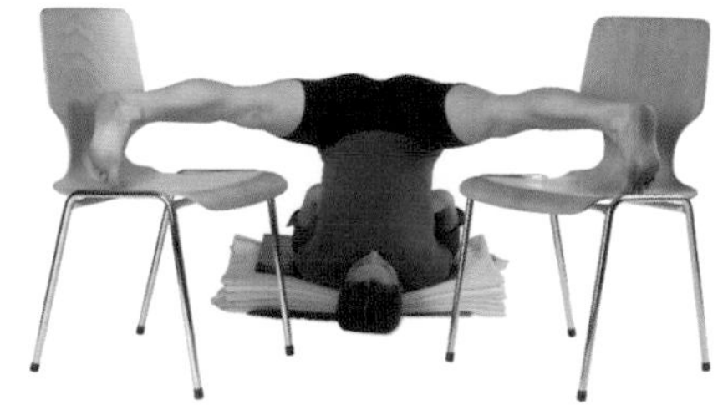

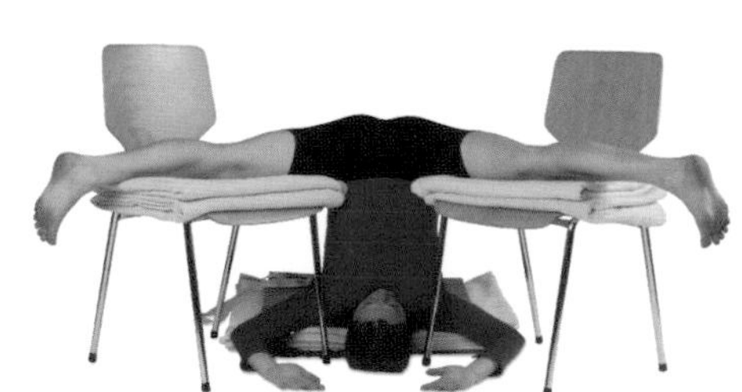

22 Supta Konasana (2 chairs), *page 106*

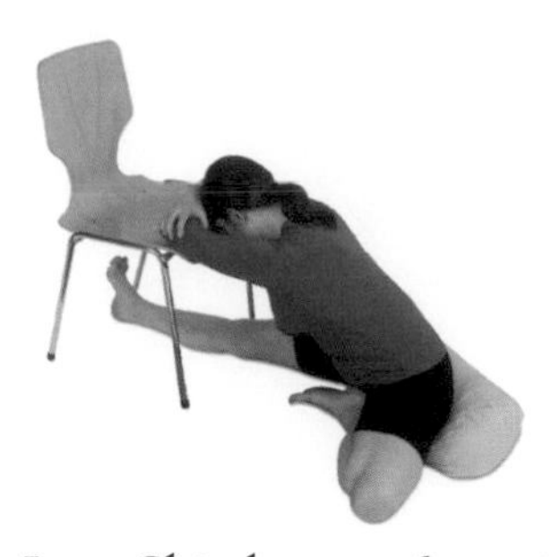

23 Janu Shirshasana (twisting with chair), *page 95*

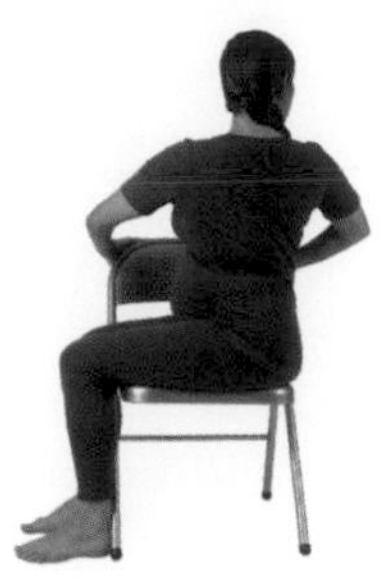

24 Bharadvajasana (bolster or chair), *page 93*

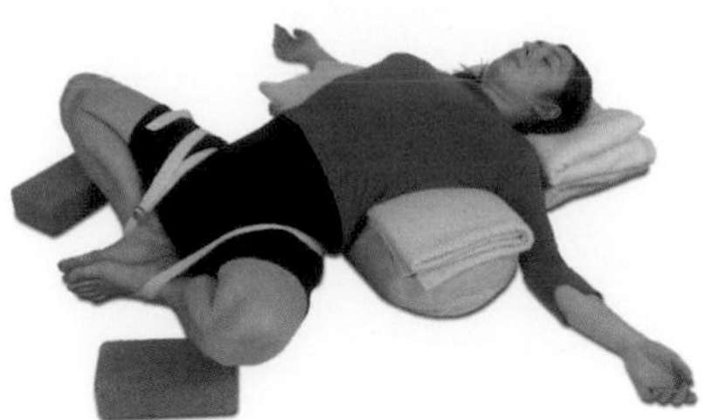

25 Supta Baddha Konasana (bolster crosswise), *page 128*

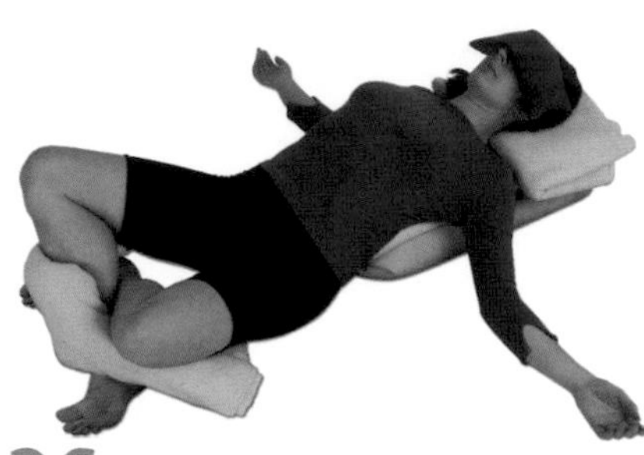

26 Shavasana (bolster length-wise), *page 131*

27 Pranayama, *page 188*

Sequence 3: Bending Backward

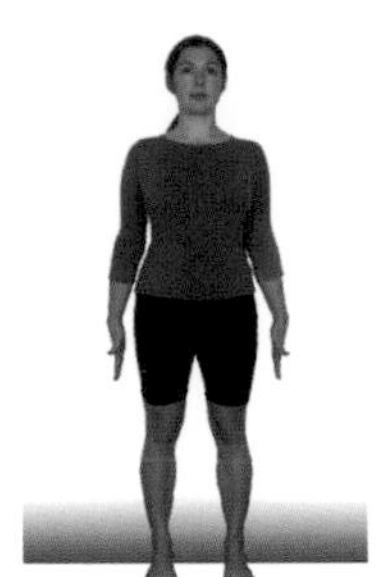

1 Tadasana, *page 32*

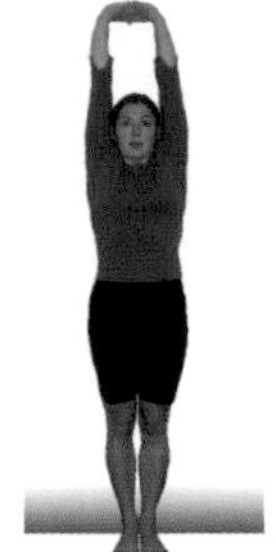

2 Urdhva Baddhanguliyasana in Tadasana, *page 34*

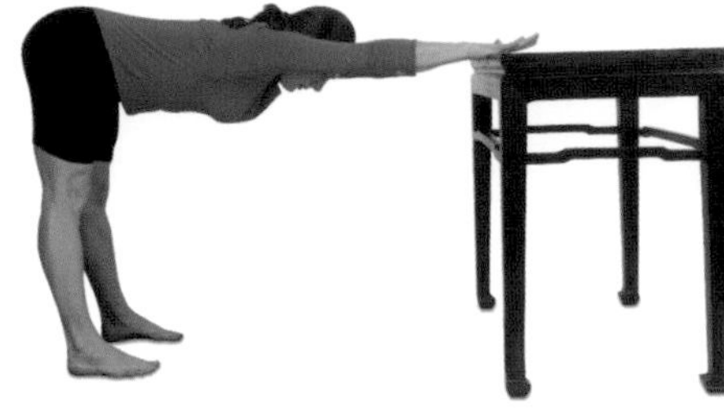

3 Ardha Uttanasana, *page 60*

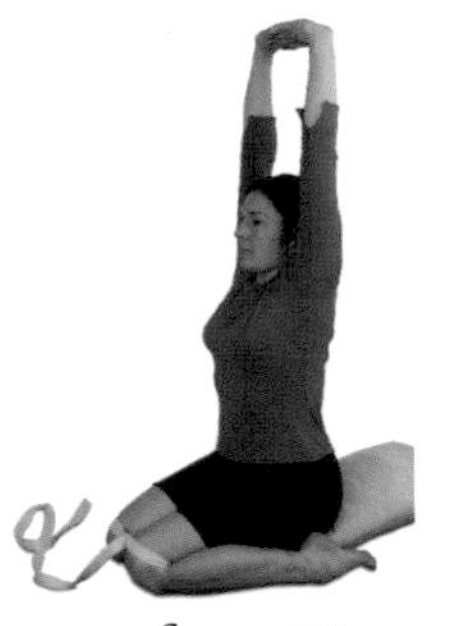

4 Parvatasana from Virasana, *page 74*

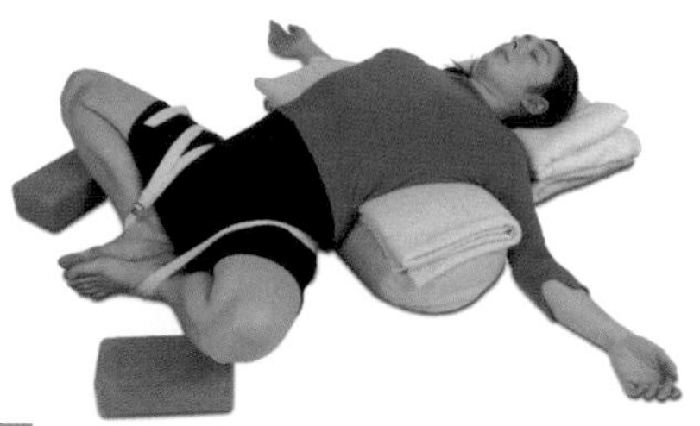

5 Supta Baddha Konasana (bolster crosswise for breastbone lift), *page 128*

6 If you practice Salamba Shirshasana with a teacher, add:

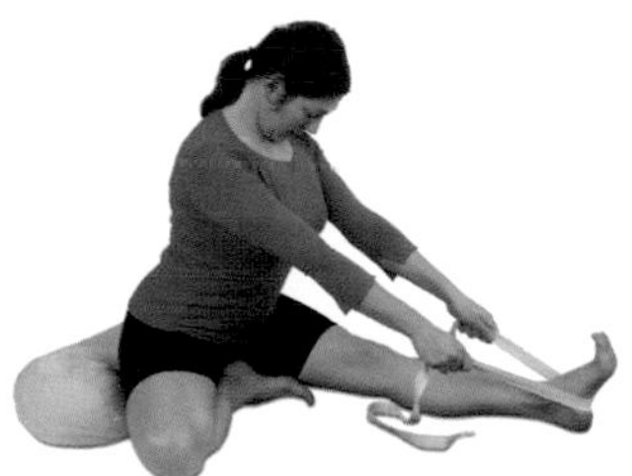

Maha Mudra, *page 80*

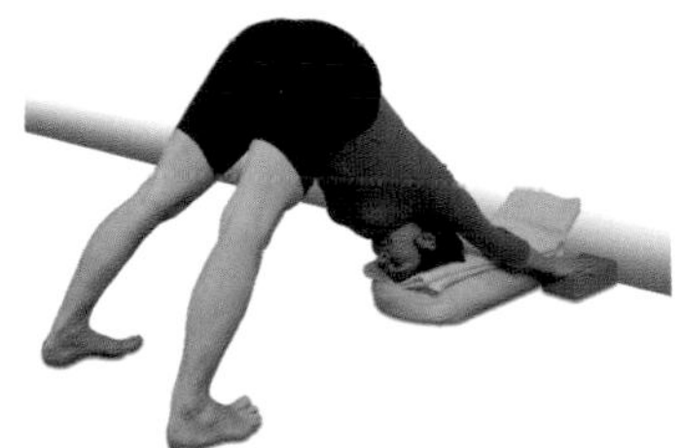

Adho Mukha Shvanasana, *page 62*

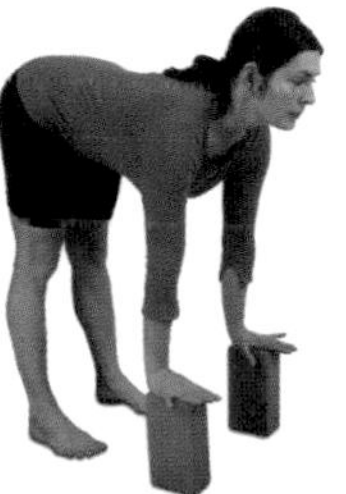

Uttanasana (concave back), *page 213*

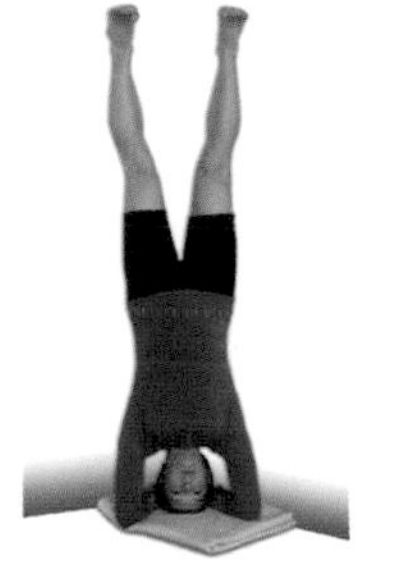

Salamba Shirshasana (with wall and teacher), *page 99*

Reverse sequence following Shirshasana:

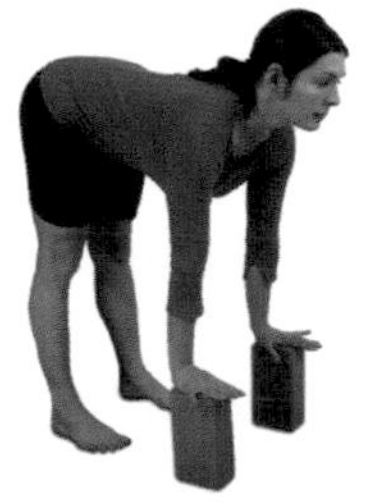

Uttanasana (concave back), *page 213*

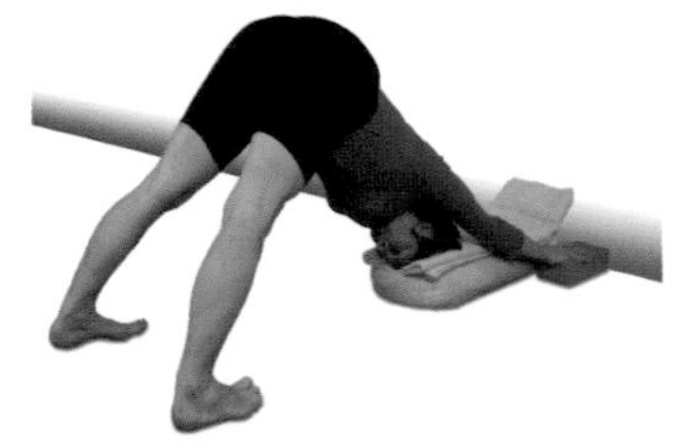

Adho Mukha Shvanasana, *page 62*

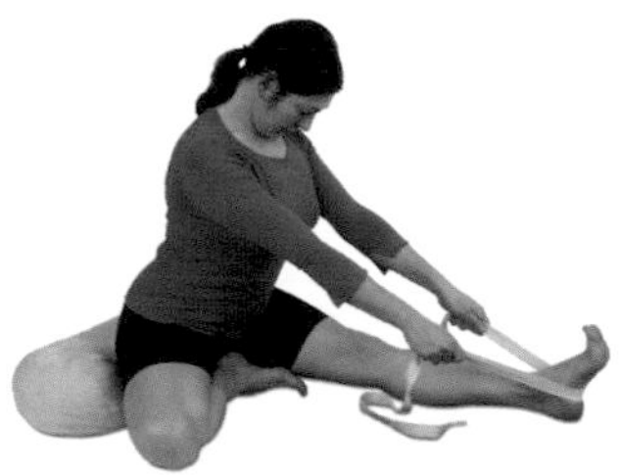

Maha Mudra, *page 80*

Sequence 4: Restorative Program

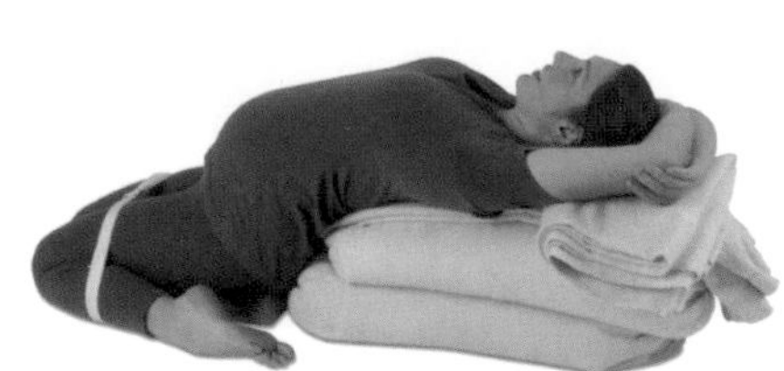

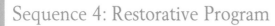

1 Supta Virasana (bolster/s), *page 129*

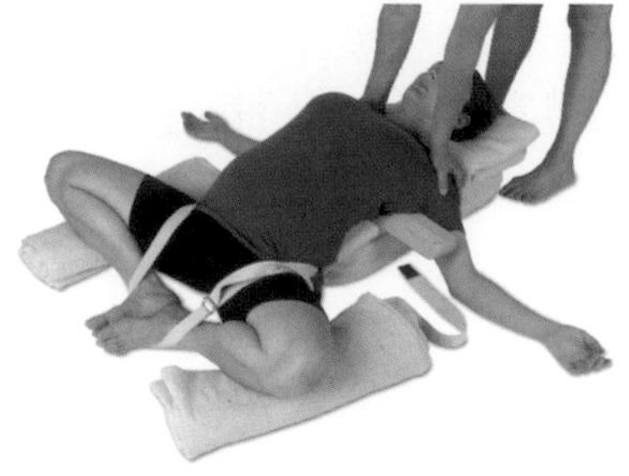

2 Supta Baddha Konasana (bolster lengthwise, slanted plank), *page 128*

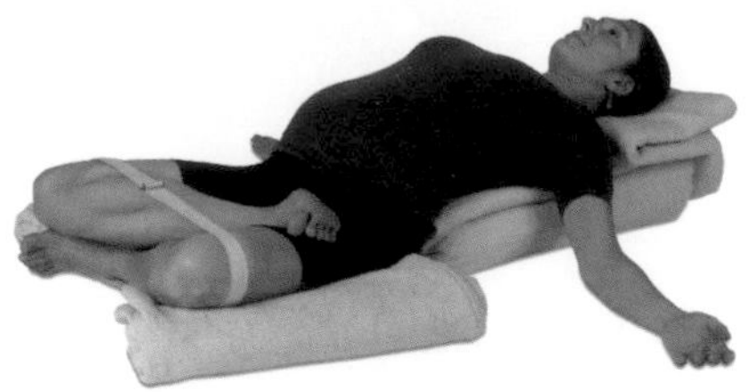

3 Matsyasana (bolster/s), *page 131*

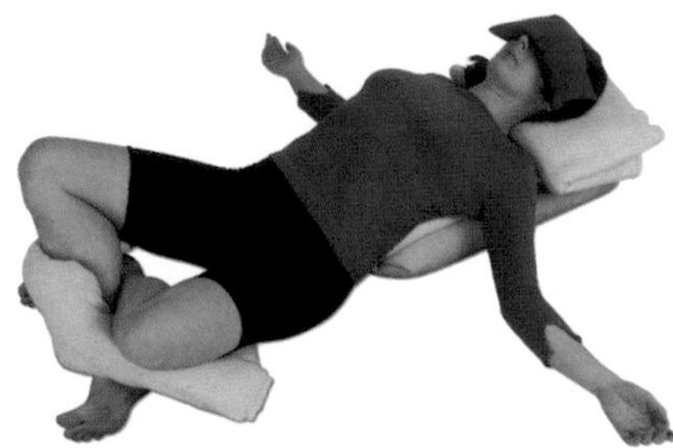

4 Supta Svastikasana (bolster/s), *page 131*

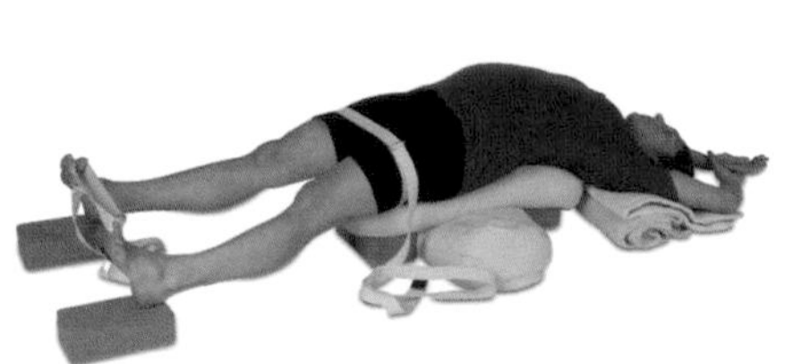

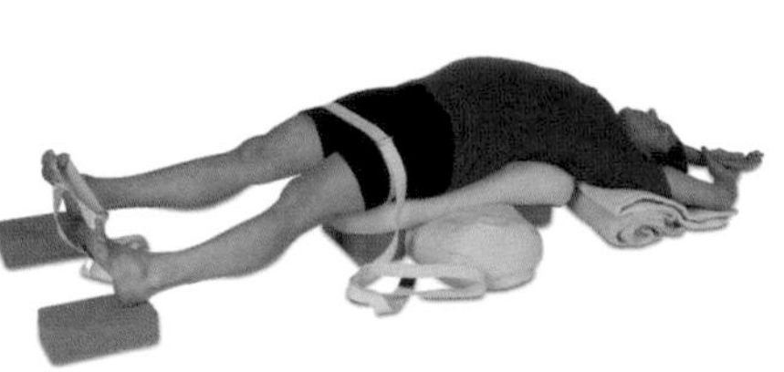

5 Cross-bolsters (passive back bend), *page 118*

and/or

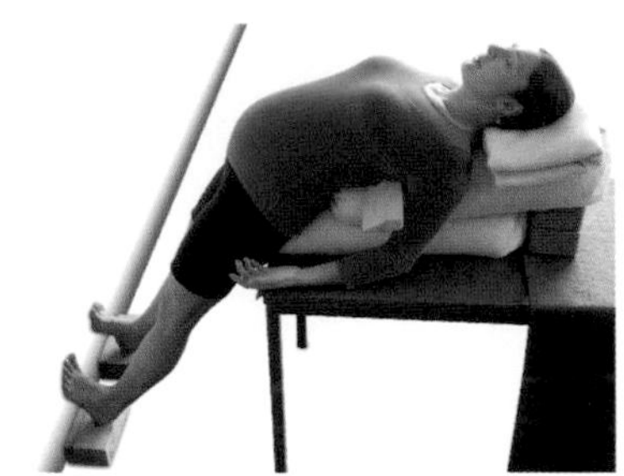

Salamba Purvottanasana, *page 133*

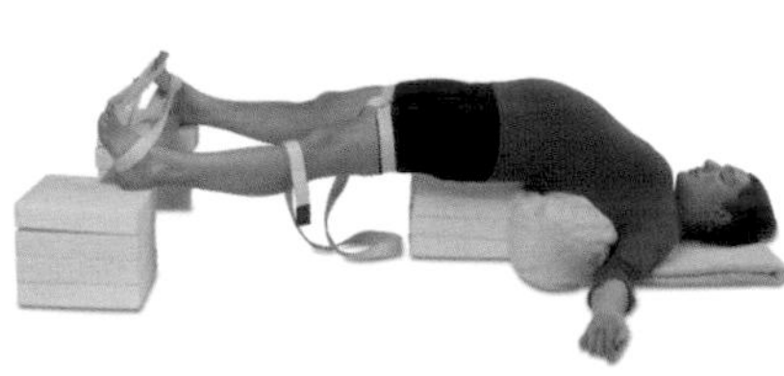

6 Setu Bandha Sarvangasana, *page 108*

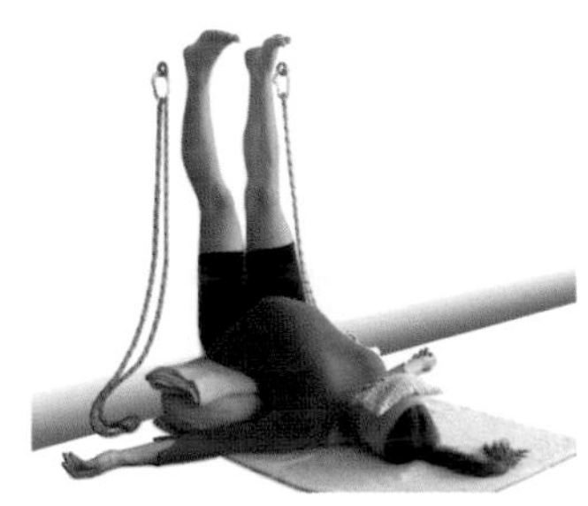

7 Viparita Karani, *page 114*

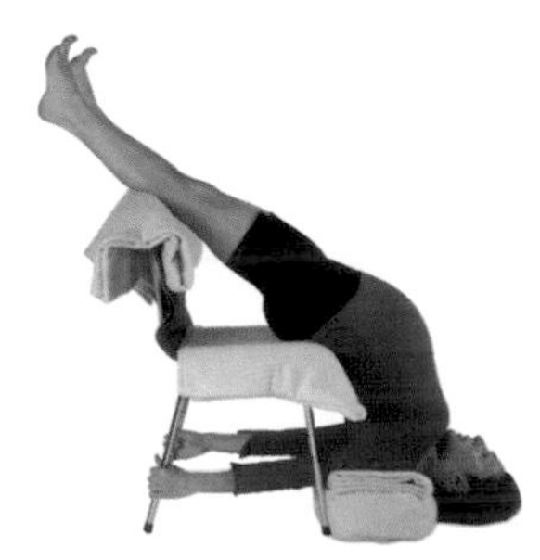

8 Salamba Sarvangasana (chair), *page 103*

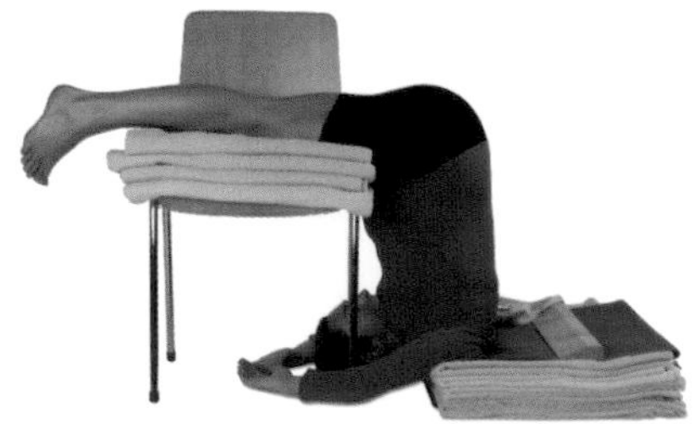

9 Ardha Halasana (thighs resting on chair), *page 105*

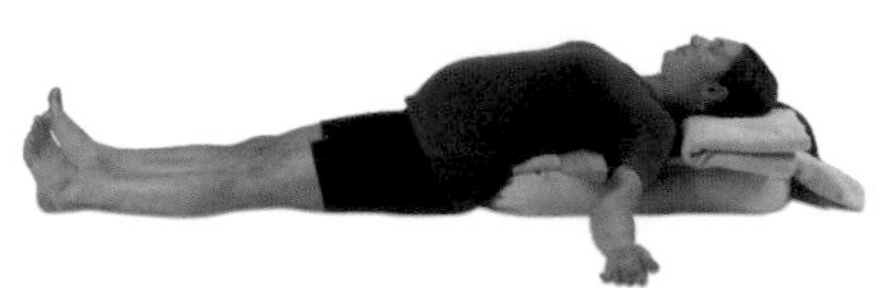

10 Shavasana (bolster/s), *page 134*

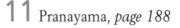

11 Pranayama, *page 188*

Sequence for Third Trimester, Preparing for Delivery

During your last trimester, you can add the sequences for the third trimester. You might want to try practicing the sequences for the 2nd trimester and the one below on alternating days.

At this point in your pregnancy, it's important to practice according to your needs. For example, if your abdomen is placing too much pressure in the inverted poses like Shirshasana or Sarvangasana, then just stop them; there is no need to force yourself and summon the willpower to continue.

When you feel tired, practice the restorative asanas in this chapter, Sequence 4.

General Guidelines

- Always stretch your spine and keep it lifted.
- Never exert pressure on your abdomen, which also exerts pressure on the throat and thyroid.
- Don't invite hormonal disturbances by forcing yourself and relying on willpower; it's better to work on proper alignment with a soft abdomen and throat.
- Don't jump into the standing asanas.
- Protect the growing life in your womb by not forcing out your breath, but letting it flow softly and smoothly.
- Always pay attention to your chest; keep it open to increase your courage and breathing capacity, which will lessen your tension.

In addition, keep in mind the guidelines found in "The Beginning of Your Pregnancy," page 154.

The asanas below will widen the pelvic floor and help prepare you for your delivery.

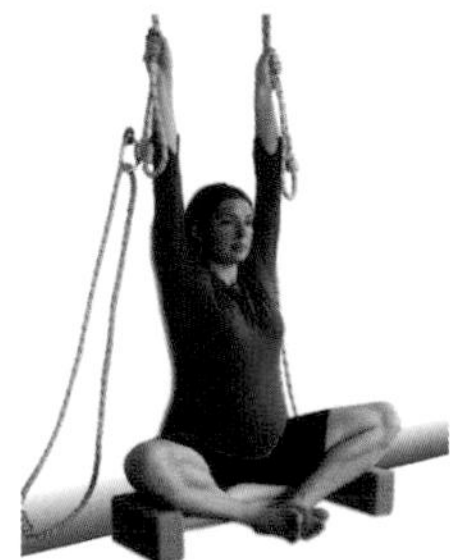

1 Baddha Konasana (straight back), *page 69*
Widens the pelvic floor and diaphragm, and relaxes the sacroiliac area, creating space for deeper breathing

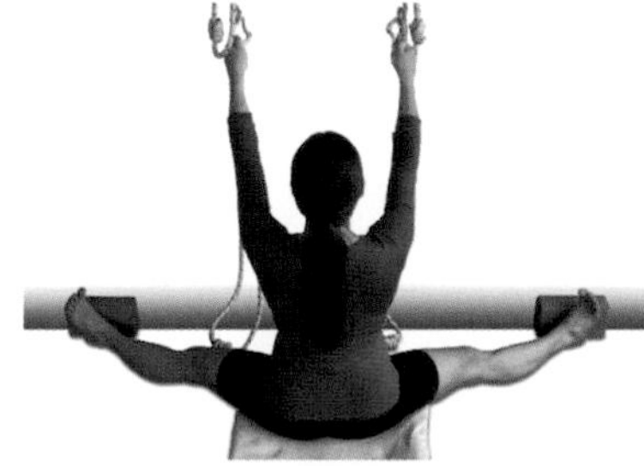

2 Upavishtha Konasana, *page 71*
Widens the pelvic floor and diaphragm, and relaxes the sacroiliac area, creating space for deeper breathing

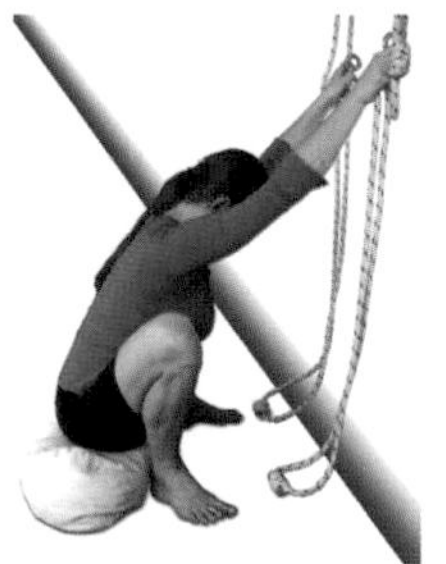

3 Malasana (with ropes), *page 77*
Prepares for labor and delivery

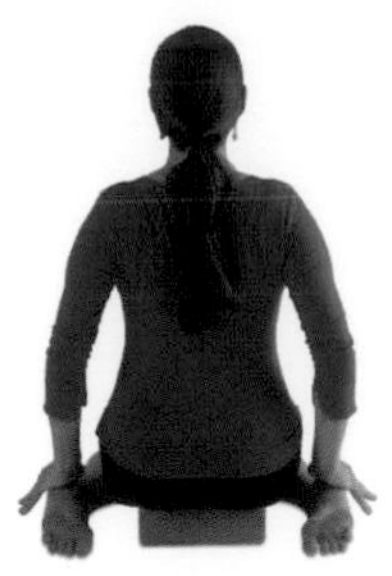

4 Virasana, *page 73*. Relaxes the pelvis and deepens breathing

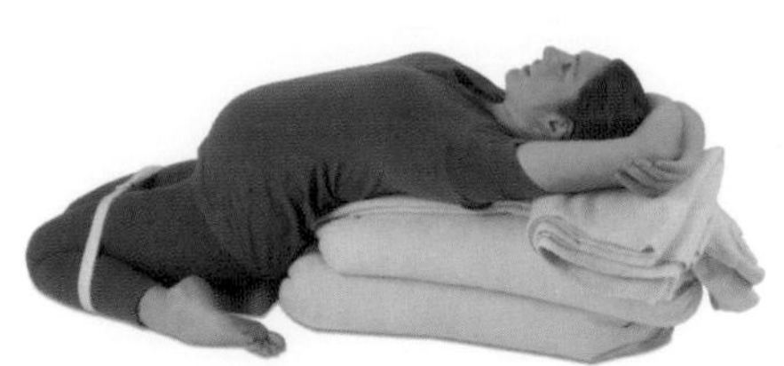

5 Supta Virasana, *page 129*

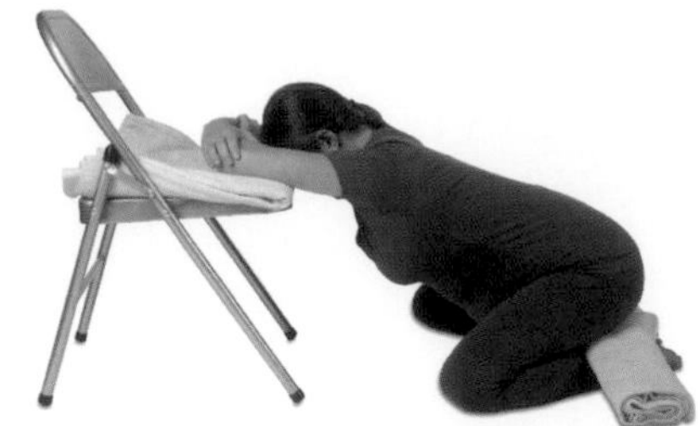

6 Adho Mukha Virasana, *page 76*. Prepares for labor and deep breathing into the pelvis itself

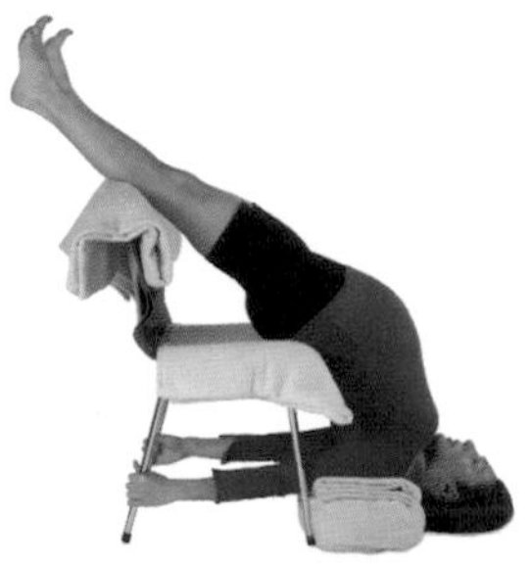

7 Salamba Sarvangasana (chair), *page 103*. Aligns the pelvis and improves glandular function

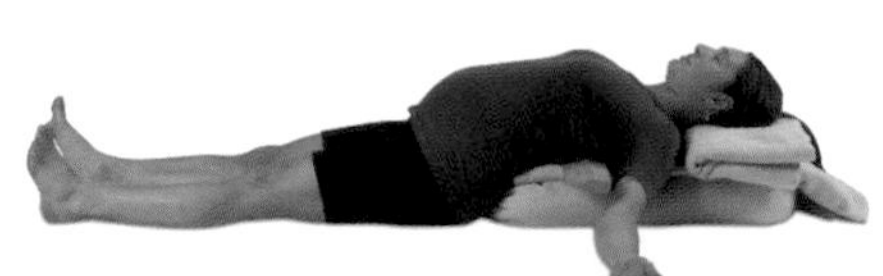

8 Shavasana (bolster/s), *page 134*

Pranayama

You can practice pranayama separately, in the morning or in the evening at bedtime, page 140.

Concentrate on Ujjayi Pranayama 2 and especially on Viloma Pranayama Stage 2. Develop your ability to exhale in stages and hold your breath in between, thus elongating the process of exhaling. This is the technique for the birth itself, when you softly push your baby down to the pelvic floor.

Start these pranayama in a supine position on a bolster. Later on, after four to five weeks, you can do them in an upright position, sitting on a bolster with your back against the wall (pages 140 – 153.)

Durations

- Salamba Sarvangasana (chair): 5 to 10 minutes
- Shavasana (well supported): 15 minutes
- Rest of the poses: up to 5 minutes

Coming out of the pose

Maintain the space that the asana created.

CHAPTER 5

SEQUENCES OF ASANAS FOR ADVANCED STUDENTS

Classification of Asanas

The three trimesters of pregnancy refer to the following weeks:
1st trimester: weeks 1 to 16
2nd trimester: weeks 17 to 29
3rd trimester: weeks 30 to 40

How do you know whether you're an advanced student? If the following applies to you:

- Before your pregnancy, you practiced Yoga for five or six years with a teacher.
- You've also worked on your own.
- You're fully familiar with full arm balances, head balances, and similar poses.

Even if that describes you, *your pregnancy is not the time to try something new!*
Practice and develop the asanas you already know, and you'll reap their benefits while taking full responsibility for yourself and your baby.

We would like to emphasize that all the sequences and techniques that appear in this chapter are for *advanced students only*.

Yoga asanas are classified according to the following considerations:

- The anatomic structure of the body
- The radius of movement and action of the body, specifically the spinal column
- How the asanas work on the body, mind, and soul

The asanas here are classified into nine categories, with pranayama appearing as the tenth. The classification gives you a quick and useful reference tool for finding all the asanas and the trimesters in which they can be safely practiced; it does not, however, show the *order* in which they should be practiced.

The asanas were taken from these categories and brought into practice sequences by the authors.

Standing Asanas
Uttishtha Sthiti

Standing asanas help strengthen the spine and widen the pelvis. Practice these with precise alignment and full extension of the spine, so that there is no pressure on your abdomen, but rather a lifting feeling from the pelvic floor.

Don't practice standing asanas if you've had miscarriages or have a disposition toward them because of a glandular problem. Please seek out the advice of an experienced Iyengar Yoga teacher.

Concentrate instead on the asanas in Chapter 3, including:
Janu Shirshasana, Concave Back, page 82
Pashchimottanasana, Concave Back, page 87
Baddha Konasana, Straight Back, Relief during Pregnancy, page 67
Shavasana, page 134

	1st Trimester	2nd Trimester	3rd Trimester
Tadasana	√	√	√
Urdhva Baddhanguliyasana in Tadasana	√	√	√
Pashchima Namaskarasana in Tadasana	√	√	√
Gomukhasana in Tadasana	√	√	√
Urdhva Hastasana	√	√	√
Utthita Hasta Padangushthasana 2 (side)	√	√	√
Utthita Trikonasana (wall/trestle)	√	√	√
Utthita Parshvakonasana (wall/trestle)	√	√	√
Parighasana	√	√	
Virabhadrasana 1 (wall/trestle)		√	√
Virabhadrasana 2 (against wall)	√	√	√
Virabhadrasana 3 (wall/trestle)		√	√
Ardha Chandrasana (wall/trestle)	√	√	√
Parshvottanasana	√	√	√
Pashchima in Parshvottanasana (concave back)	√	√	√
Prasarita Padottanasana	√	√	√
Uttanasana (concave back, feet together)	√		
Uttanasana (legs spread, concave back, hands on support)	√	√	√
Ardha Uttanasana	√	√	√
Adho Mukha Shvanasana	√	√	√

Sitting Asanas
Upavishtha Sthiti

	1st Trimester	2nd Trimester	3rd Trimester
Dandasana		√	√
Urdhva Hasta Dandasana		√	√
Baddha Konasana (straight back)	√	√	√
Upavishtha Konasana (straight back)	√	√	√
Svastikasana	√	√	√
Parvatasana from Svastikasana	√	√	√
Virasana	√	√	√
Parvatasana from Virasana	√	√	√
Gomukhasana from Virasana	√	√	√

Forward Bends
Pashchima Pratana Sthiti

	1st Trimester	2nd Trimester	3rd Trimester
Adho Mukha Virasana	√	√	√
Maha Mudra	√	√	√
Urdhva Hasta Janu Shirshasana and Urdhva Mukha Janu Shirshasana (concave back, lower chest lifted)	√	√	√
Urdhva Hasta Trianga Mukhaikapada Pashchimottanasana and Urdhva Mukha Trianga Mukhaikapada Pashchimottanasana (concave back, lower chest lifted)	√	√	
Upavishtha Konasana (concave back, lower chest lifted)	√	√	√
Urdhva Hasta Pashchimottanasana and Urdhva Mukha Pashchimottanasana (concave back, lower chest lifted)	√	√	√
Malasana (modified for labor, with ropes or sitting against wall)		√	√

Twists
Parivritta Sthiti

	1st Trimester	2nd Trimester	3rd Trimester
Bharadvajasana 1	√	√	√
Bharadvajasana (chair)	√	√	√
Parshva Svastikasana (chair)	√	√	√
Parshva Padmasana (chair/wall)	√	√	√
Parshva Virasana (wall)	√	√	√
Parshva Baddha Konasana (chair/wall)	√	√	√
Parshva Janu Shirshasana (chair)	√	√	√

Inversions
Viparita Sthiti

	1st Trimester	2nd Trimester	3rd Trimester
Adho Mukha Vrikshasana		√	√
Pichcha Mayurasana		√	√
Salamba Shirshasana *Remember to precede Salamba Shirshasana with:* *Maha Mudra* *Adho Mukha Shvanasana* *Uttanasana (concave back)* *And follow it with:* *Uttanasana (concave back)* *Adho Mukha Shvanasana* *Maha Mudra*	√	√	√
Salamba Shirshasana variations against the wall: Parshva Shirshasana		√	√
Eka Pada Shirshasana		√	√
Parshvaikapada Shirshasana		√	√
Upavishtha Konasana in Shirshasana (also called Prasarita Pada Shirshasana)	√	√	√
Baddha Konasana in Shirshasana	√	√	√
Shirshasana (wall ropes)		√	√
Salamba Sarvangasana	√	√	√
Niralamba Sarvangasana (toes on wall)	√	√	√
And its variations: Ardha Eka Pada Sarvangasana	√	√	√
Ardha Parshvaikapada Sarvangasana		√	√
Upavishtha Konasana in Sarvangasana (also called Prasarita Pada Sarvangasana)	√	√	√
Baddha Konasana in Sarvangasana	√	√	√
Ardha Halasana (chair)	√	√	√
Ardha Supta Konasana (2 chairs)	√	√	√
Setu Bandha Sarvangasana	√	√	√
Chatushpadasana		√	√

Asanas for Abdomen and Lumbar
Supta and Uttishtha Sthiti

	1st Trimester	2nd Trimester	3rd Trimester
Supta Padangushthasana 2 (to the side)	√	√	√
Utthita Hasta Padangushthasana 2 (to the side)		√	√

Back Bends
Purva Pratana Sthiti

	1st Trimester	2nd Trimester	3rd Trimester
Cross-bolsters	√	√	√
Bhujangasana (in ropes)		√	√
Bhujangasana (ropes, chair, and bolster)		√	√
Salamba Purvottanasana (trestle)		√	√
Urdhva Dhanurasana with chair, wall, and props		√	√
Salamba Purvottanasana		√	√
Dvi Pada Viparita Dandasana: (with Viparita Dandasana bench, chair, fully supported, L-shape)	√	√	√
Dvi Pada Viparita Dandasana with 2 chairs, L-shape		√	√

Rope Asanas
Yoga Kurunta

	1st Trimester	2nd Trimester	3rd Trimester
Shirshasana (wall ropes)		√	√
Adho Mukha Vrikshasana		√	√
Bhujangasana (ropes)		√	√
Bhujangasana (ropes, chair, and bolster)		√	√
Ardha Uttanasana	√	√	√
Adho Mukha Shvanasana	√	√	√
Malasana (modified for labor)		√	√

Restorative Asanas
Vishranta Karaka Sthiti

	1st Trimester	2nd Trimester	3rd Trimester
Supta Virasana	√	√	√
Supta Baddha Konasana	√	√	√
Matsyasana	√	√	√
Supta Svastikasana	√	√	√
Salamba Purvottanasana		√	√
Cross-bolsters	√	√	√
Setu Bandha Sarvangasana	√	√	√
Viparita Karani (legs bent on chair)	√	√	√
Viparita Karani		√	√
Salamba Sarvangasana (chair)	√	√	√
Shavasana (bolster/s)	√	√	√
Shavasana (bolster, legs on bolsters)	√	√	√

Breathing Techniques
Pranayama

	1st Trimester	2nd Trimester	3rd Trimester
Ujjayi 1, 2 (sitting and in Shavasana)	√	√	√
Viloma 1, 2 (sitting and in Shavasana)	√	√	√

Sequence for First Trimester

Enhancing Strength and Inner Balance
Standing poses help strengthen your spine and widen your pelvis. Practice these with precise alignment and full extension of the spine, so that there is no pressure on your abdomen, but rather a lifting feeling from the pelvic floor.

Don't practice standing asanas if you've had miscarriages or have a disposition toward them because of a glandular problem. Please seek out the advice of an experienced Iyengar Yoga teacher.

Concentrate instead on the asanas from Chapter 3 including:
Janu Shirshasana, Concave Back (page 82)
Pashchimottanasana, Concave Back (page 87)
Baddha Konasana, Straight Back, Relief during Pregnancy (page 67)
Shavasana (page 134)

More Information
For the sequence recommended for throughout pregnancy, see Chapter 4, page 172.

For help with problems, see Chapter 2, "Preparing for Pregnancy," page14

For detailed descriptions and modifications of the asanas, see Chapter 3, "Instructions and Benefits," page 31, and the rest of this chapter.

General Guidelines

- Always stretch your spine and keep it lifted.
- Never exert pressure on your abdomen, which also exerts pressure on the throat and thyroid.
- Don't invite hormonal disturbances by forcing yourself and relying on willpower; it's better to work on proper alignment with a soft abdomen and throat.
- Don't jump into the standing asanas.
- Protect the growing life in your womb by not forcing out your breath, but letting it flow softly and smoothly.
- Practice the back bends with the supports indicated in Chapter 3, from page 118, to avoid weakening the inner lining of the uterus.
- Practice the twisting asanas as indicated in Chapter 3, from page 91, for the same reason as above.
- When you come back from an asana, always maintain your lift, extension, and expansion. Don't collapse or make jolting movements.

Durations

- Asanas practiced on the right and left side: stay for 30 to 60 seconds per side
- Asanas that extend straight forward or backward (like Uttanasana or Chatushpadasana): 30 to 60 seconds
- Inversions (pages 96 – 114):
  - Salamba Sarvangasana: If you practice it without Ardha Halasana, stay in it 2 to 3 minutes longer than Salamba Shirshasana.
  - Ardha Halasana, Setu Bandha Sarvangasana, and Viparita Karani: up to 5 minutes
  - Rest of poses: 5 to 10 minutes
- Restorative Asanas (pages 126 – 139):
  - Shavasana: 15 minutes
  - Rest of poses: up to 5 minutes

Recommended Sequence

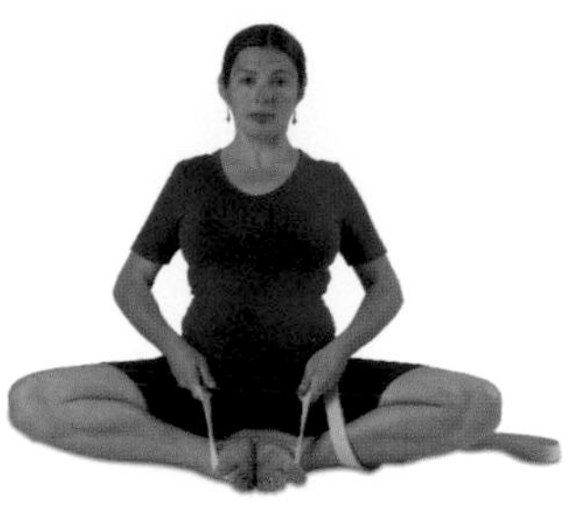

1 Baddha Konasana (straight back), *page 67*

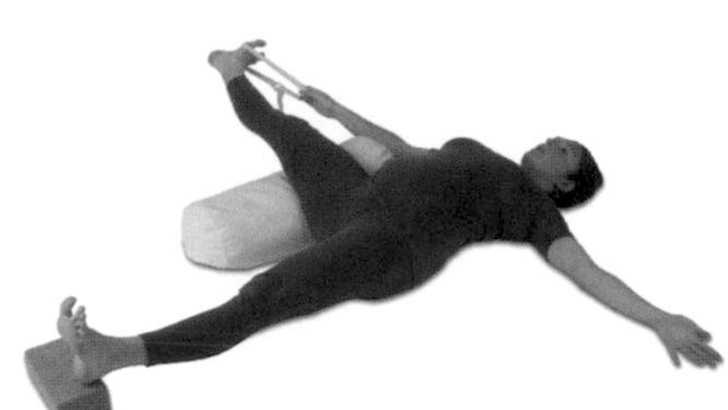

2 Supta Padangushthasana 2 (side stretch), *page 115*

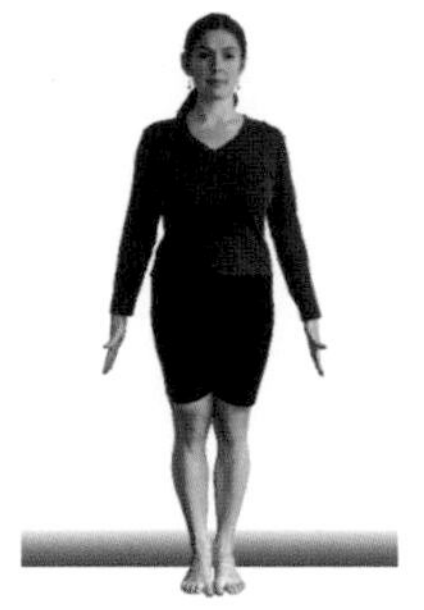

3 Tadasana, *page 32*

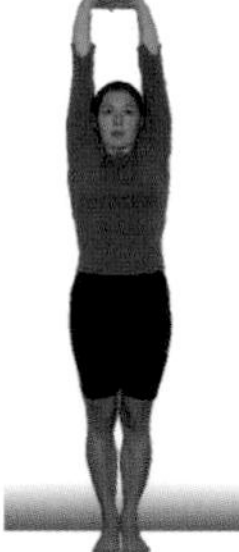

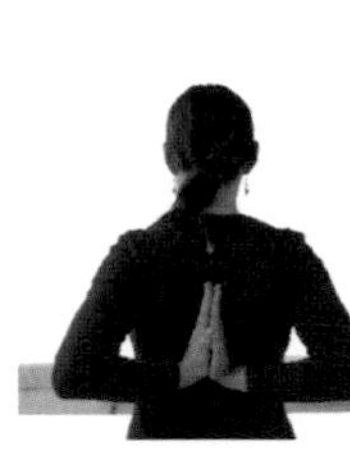

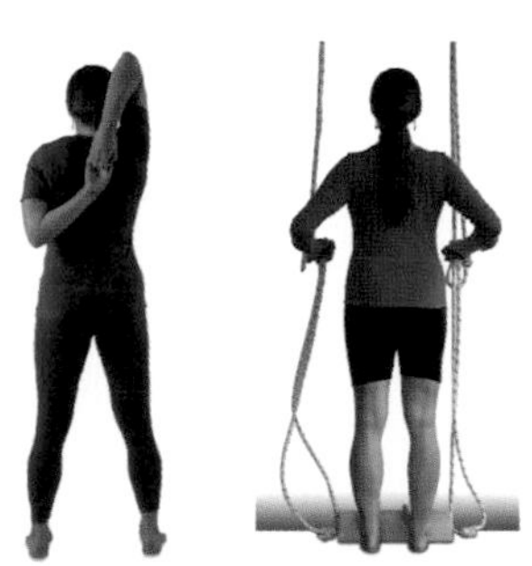

4 Urdhva Baddhanguliyasana, *page 34*, Pashchima Namaskarasana, *page 36*, Gomukhasana in Tadasana, *page 37*, and Tadasana (heels down), *page 33*

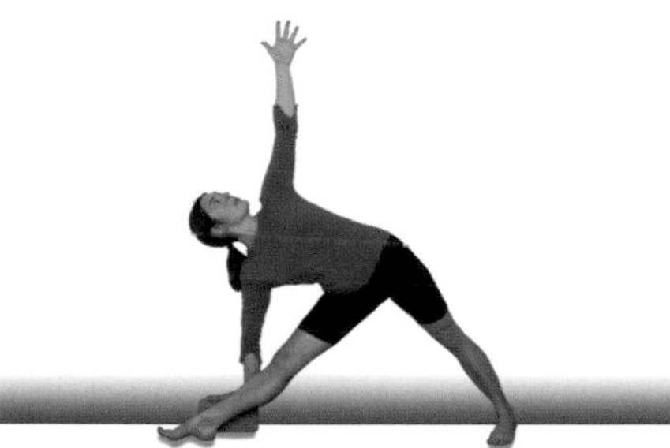

5 Utthita Trikonasana, *page 39*

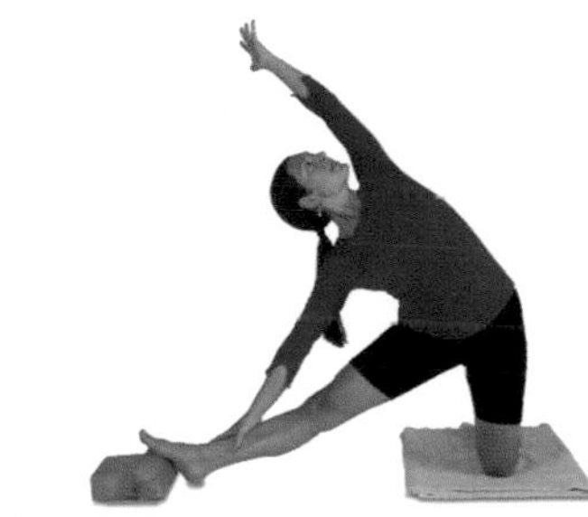

6 Parighasana, *page 44*

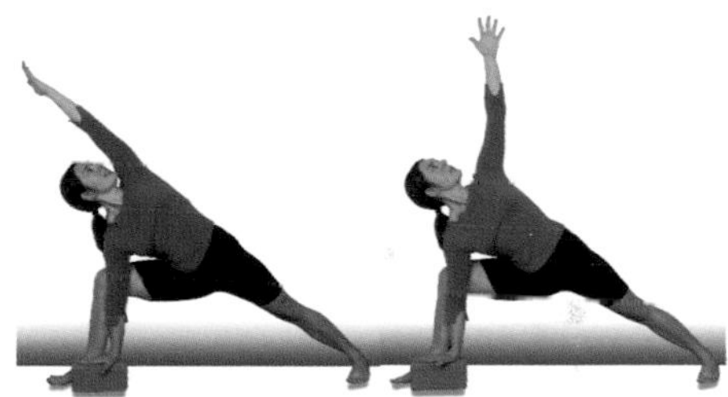

7 Utthita Parshvakonasana, *pages 40 – 41*

Note

Always start the standing poses from Tadasana. When you finish the pose, come back to Tadasana. If you feel tired, rest in Ardha Uttanasana.

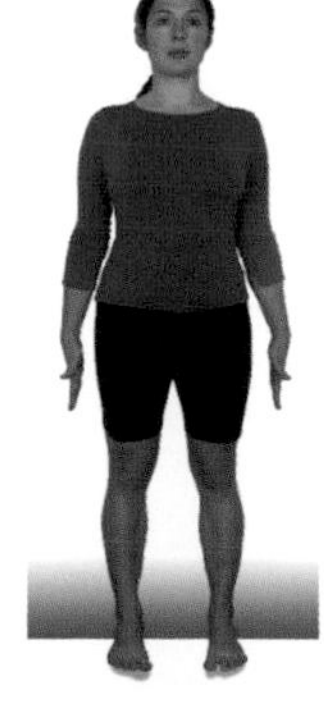

Tadasana

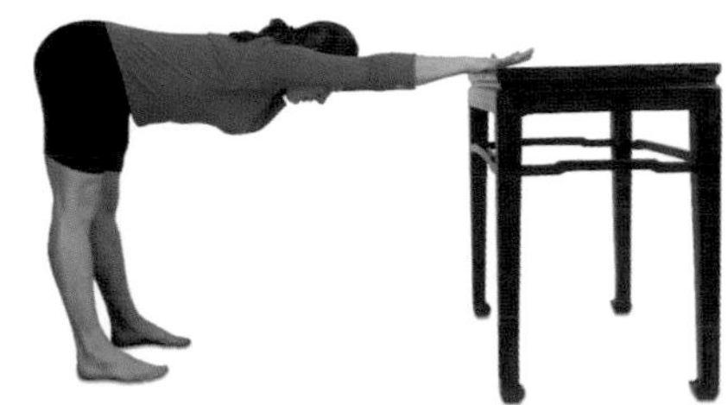

Ardha Uttanasana

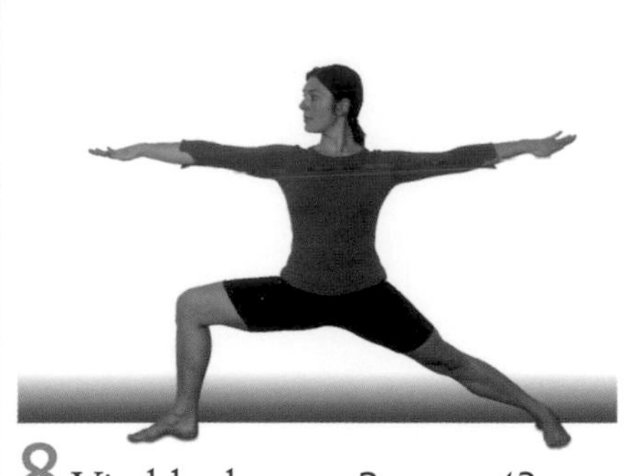
8 Virabhadrasana 2, *page 42*

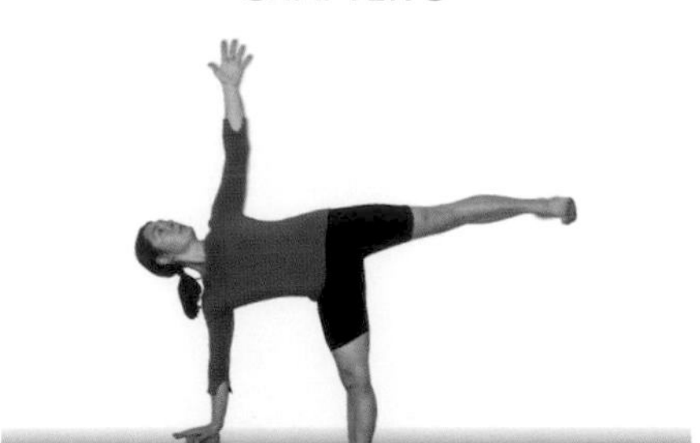
9 Ardha Chandrasana, *page 48*

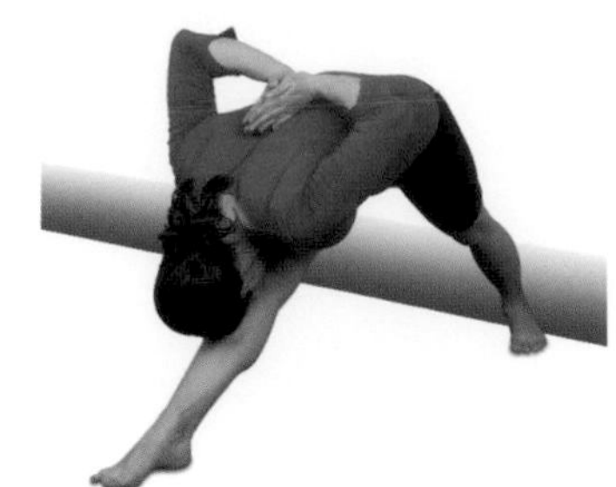
10 Parshvottanasana, *page 287*

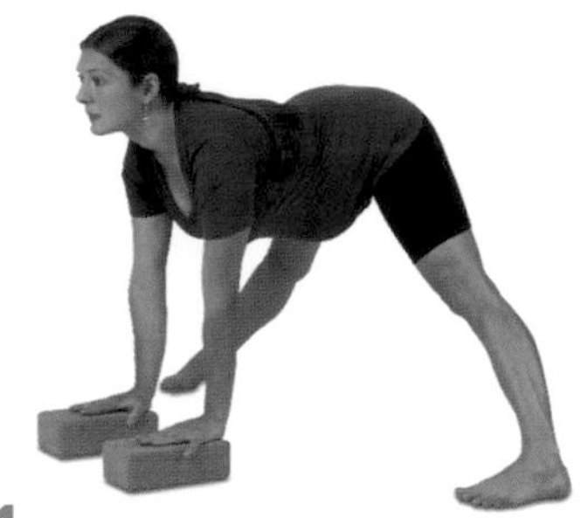
11 Prasarita Padottanasana, *page 56*

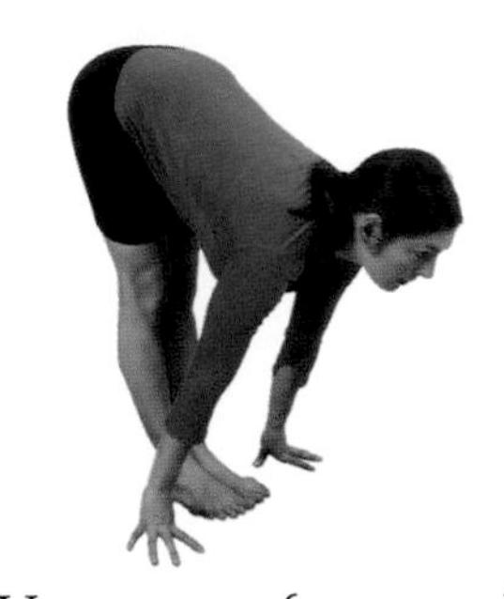
12 Uttanasana (concave back), *page 213*

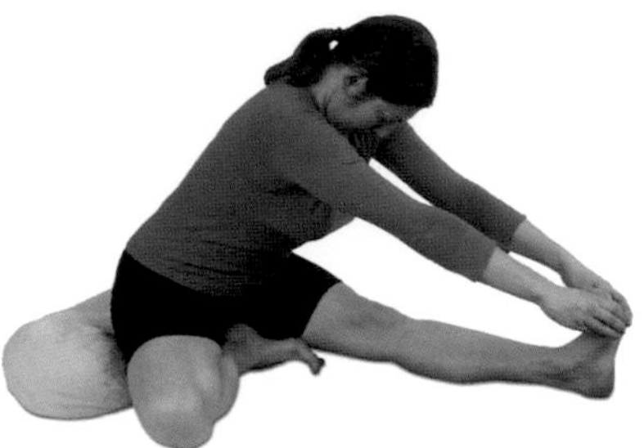
13 Maha Mudra, *page 216*

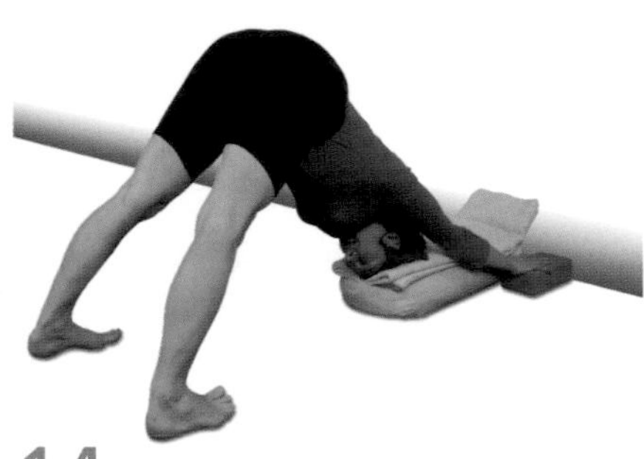
14 Adho Mukha Shvanasana, *page 62*

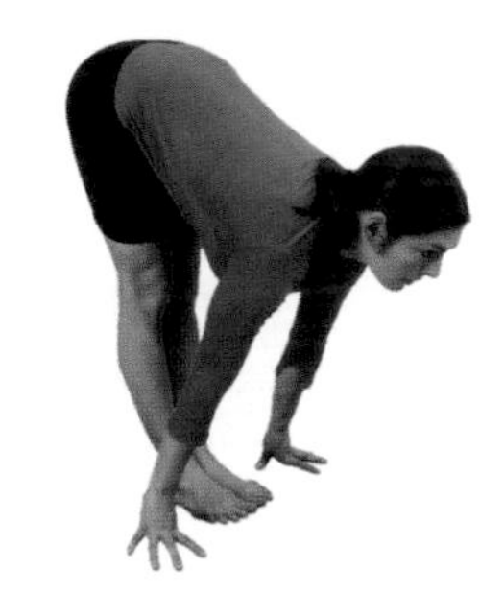
15 Uttanasana (concave back), *page 213*

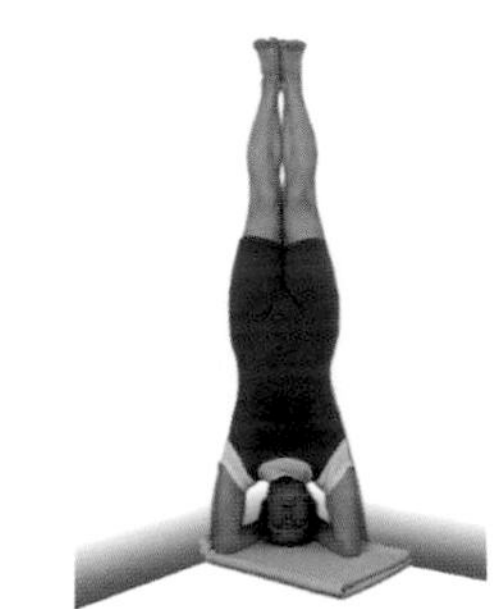
16 Salamba Shirshasana (feet together), *page 99*

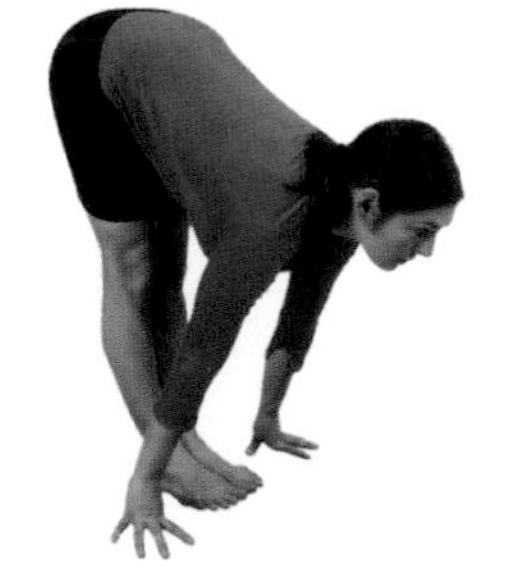
17 Uttanasana (concave back), *page 213*

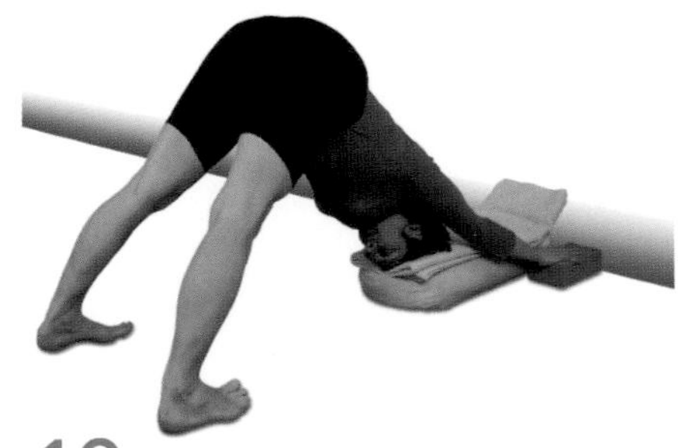
18 Adho Mukha Shvanasana, *page 62*

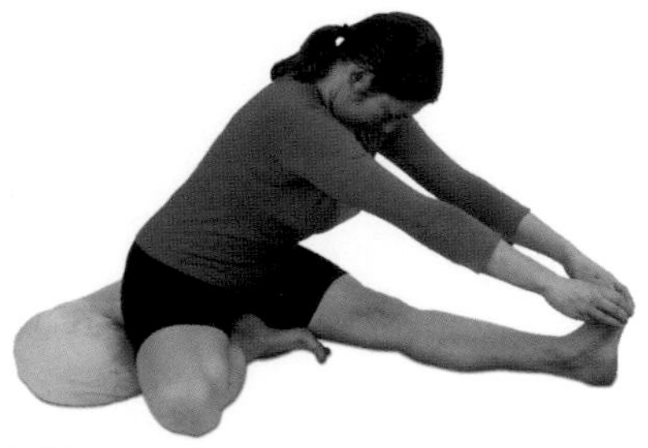
19 Maha Mudra, *page 216*

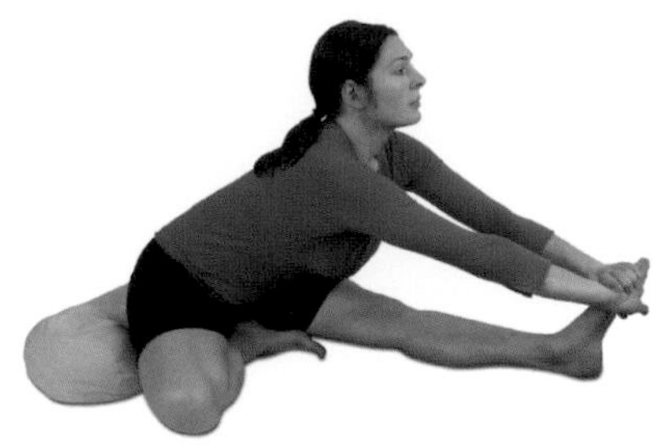

20 Janu Shirshasana (concave back), *page 217*

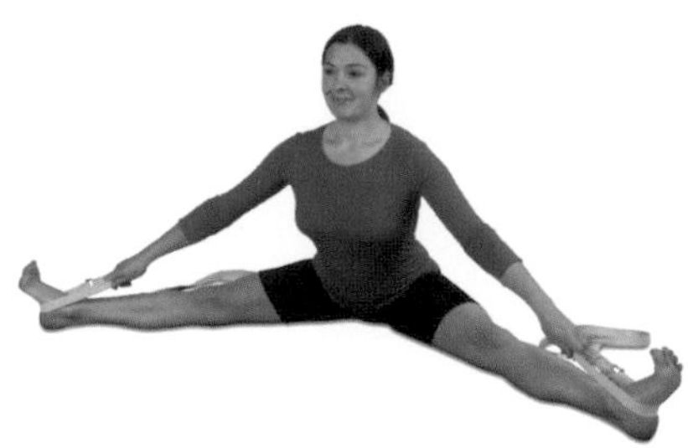

21 Upavishtha Konasana (concave back, gripping toes), *page 85*

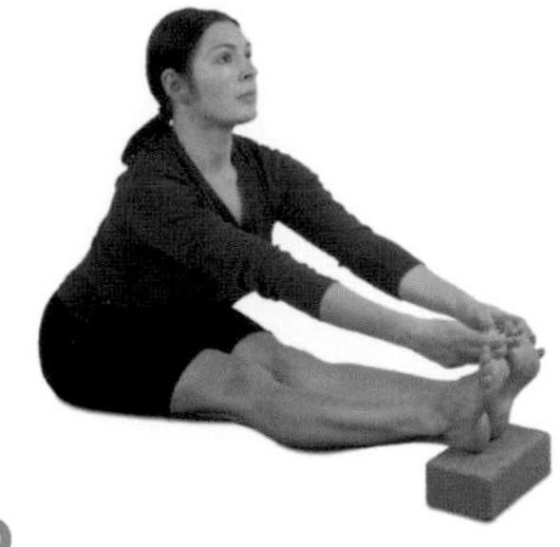

22 Pashchimottanasana, (concave back, heels on block), *page 308*

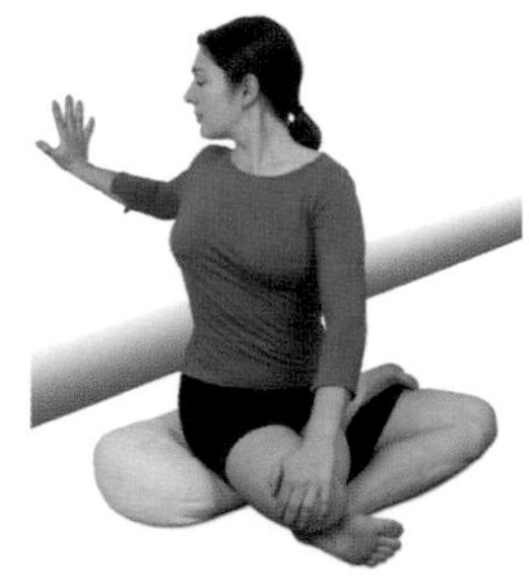

23 Parshva Svastikasana or Ardha Padmasana/full Padmasana (twisting with wall), *page 94*

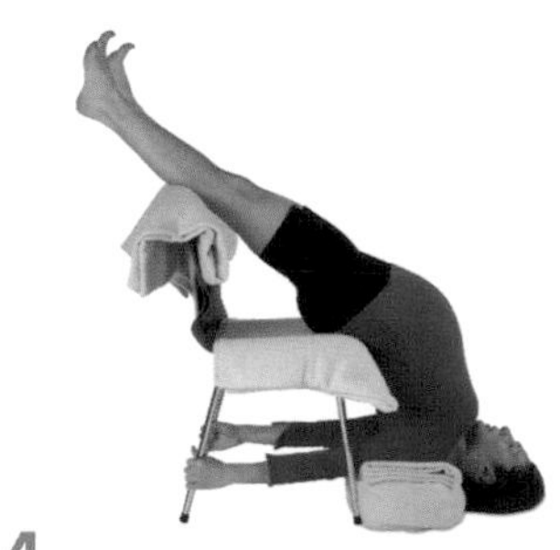

24 Salamba Sarvangasana (chair), *page 103*

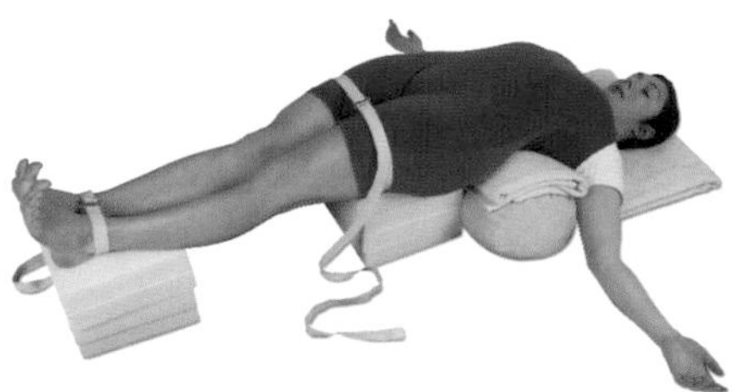

25 Setu Bandha Sarvangasana, *page 108*

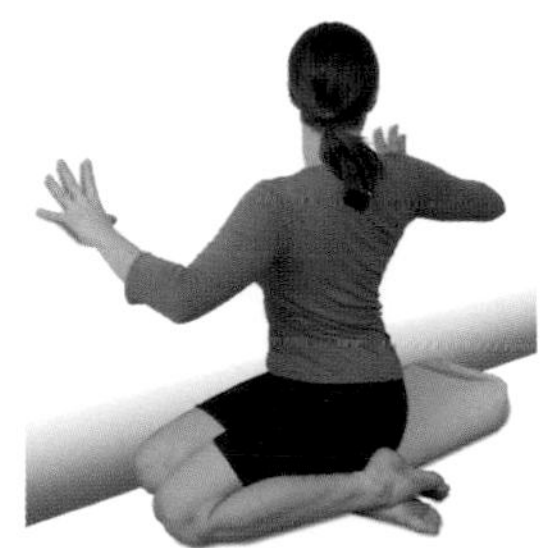

26 Bharadvajasana (chair or bolster), *page 93*

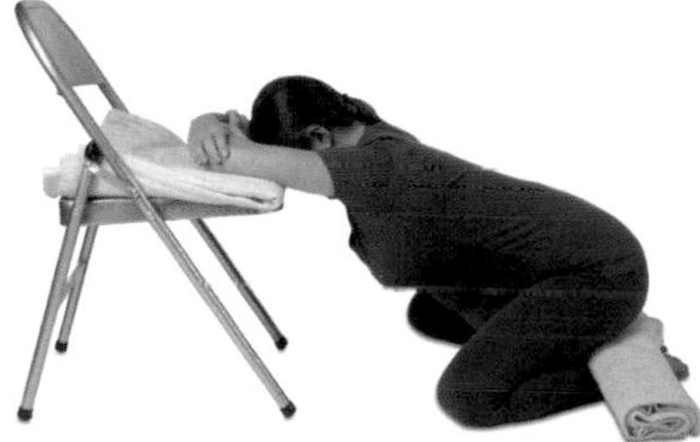

27 Adho Mukha Virasana, *page 76*

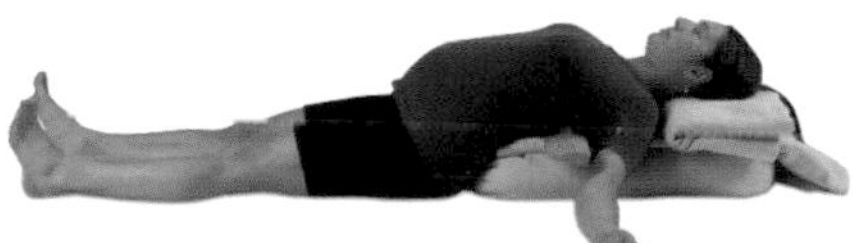

28 Shavasana (bolster/s), *page 134*

29 Ujjayi Pranayama 1, *page 148*

CHAPTER 5

Sequences for Second and Third Trimesters

Sequence 1: Widening and Stretching the Pelvis

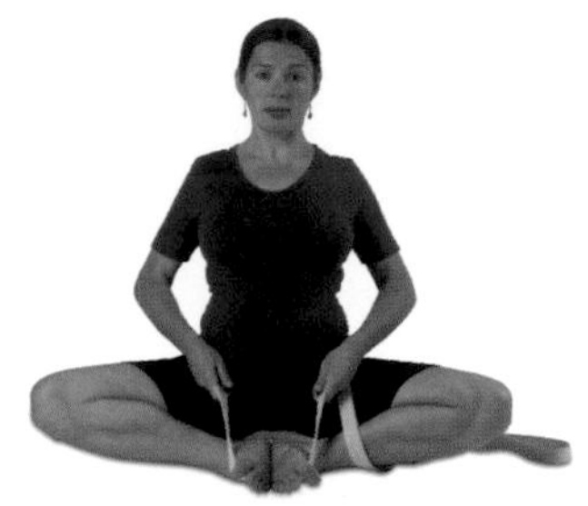

1 Baddha Konasana (straight back), *page 67*

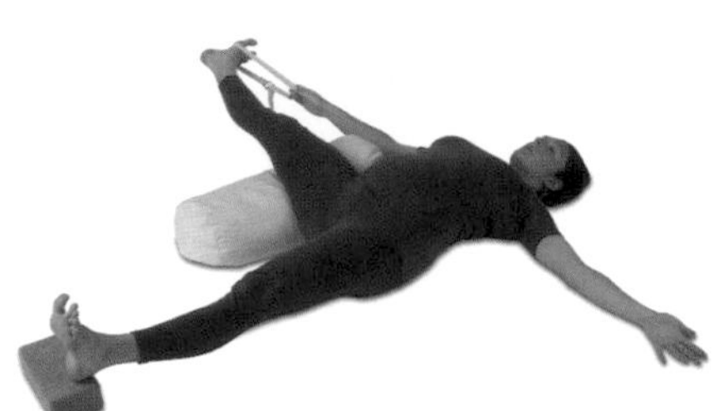

2 Supta Padangushthasana 2 (side stretch), *page 115*

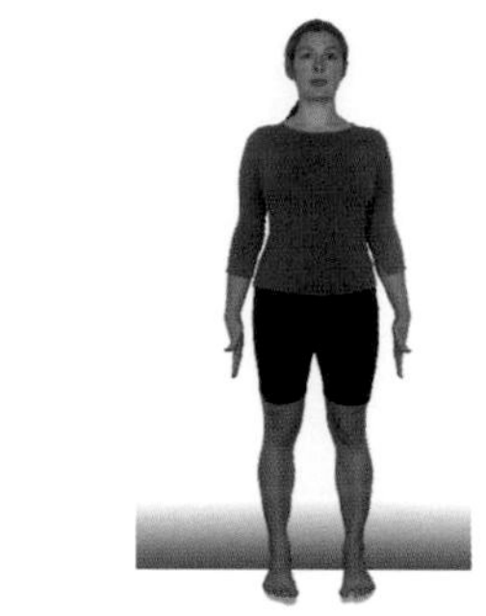

3 Tadasana, *page 32*

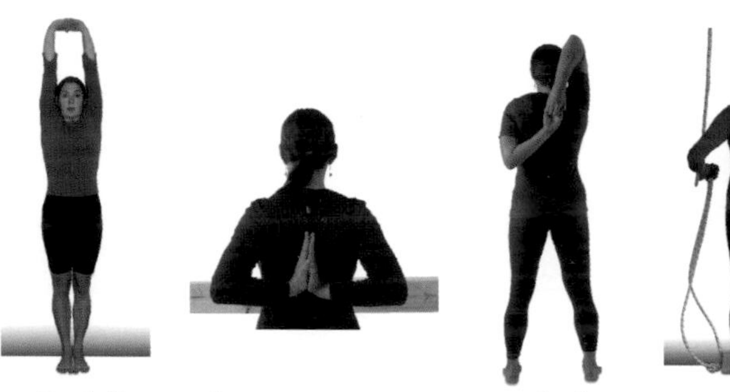

4 Urdhva Baddhanguliyasana, *page 34*, Pashchima Namaskarasana, *page 36*, Gomukhasana in Tadasana, *page 37*, and Tadasana (heels down), *page 33*

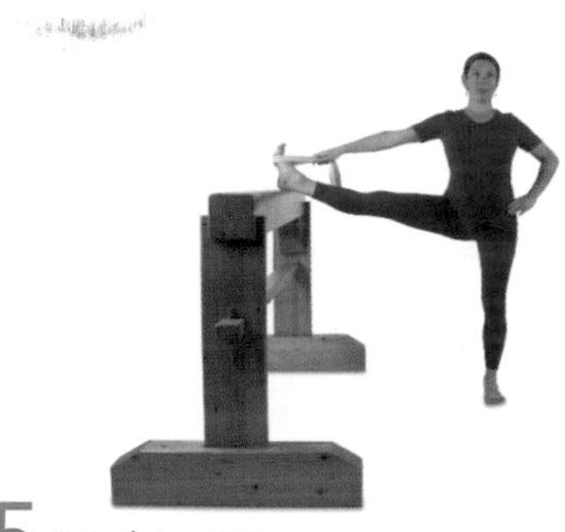

5 Utthita Hasta Padangushthasana 2 (side stretch), *page 117*

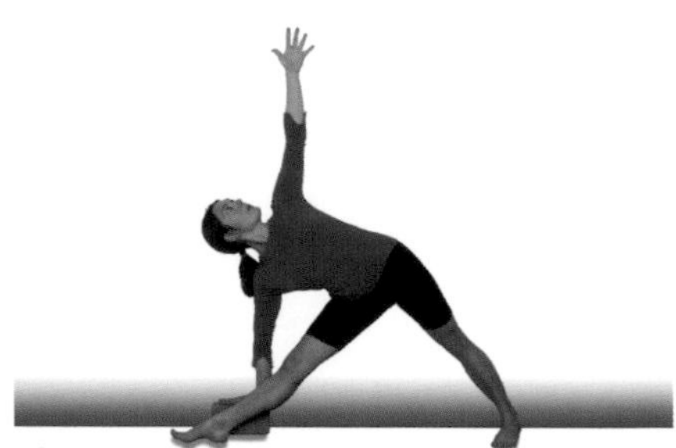

6 Utthita Trikonasana, *page 39*

Note

Always start the standing poses from Tadasana. When you finish the pose, come back to Tadasana. If you feel tired, rest in Ardha Uttanasana.

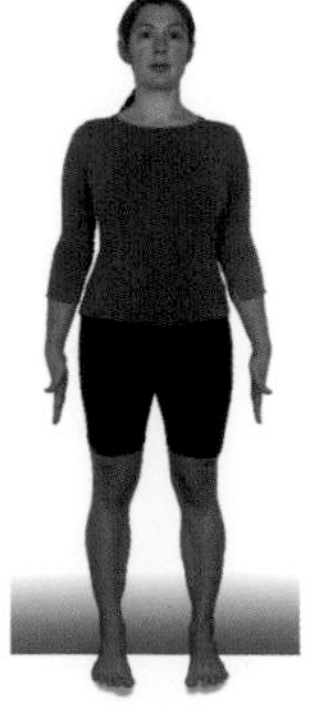

Tadasana

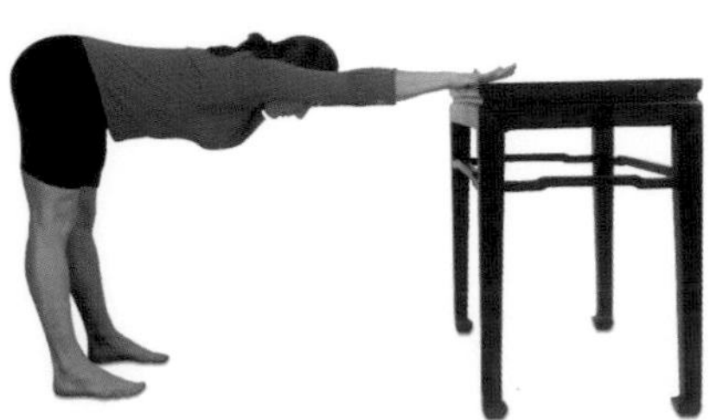

Ardha Uttanasana

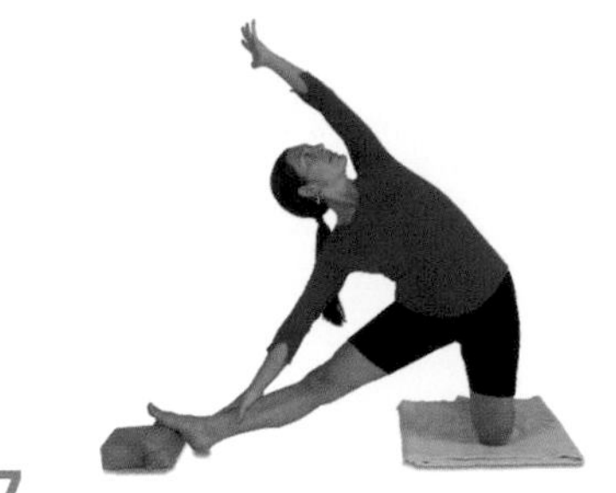

7 Parighasana, *page 44*

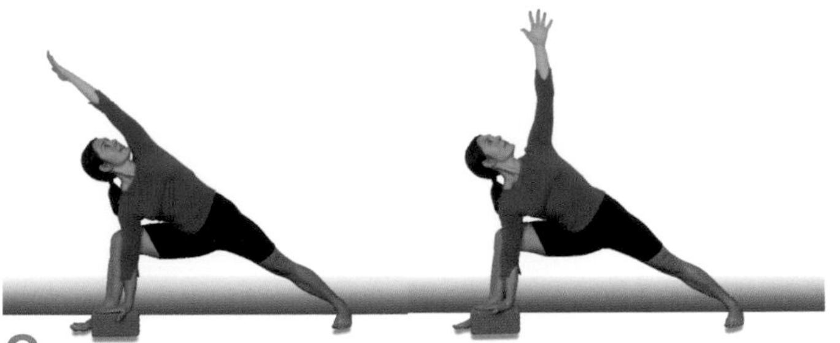

8 Utthita Parshvakonasana, *pages 40 – 41*

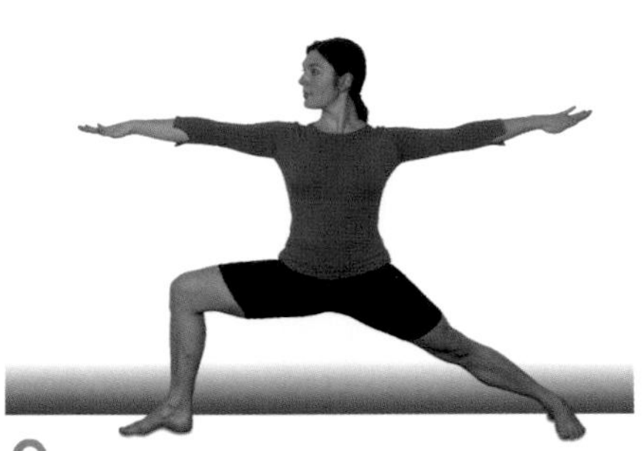

9 Virabhadrasana 2, *page 42*

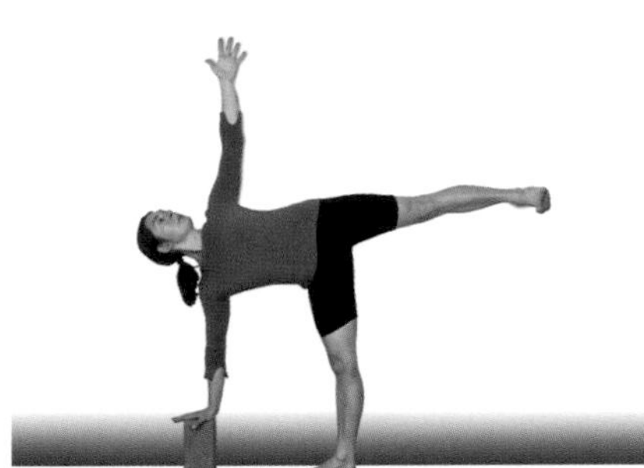

10 Ardha Chandrasana, *page 45*

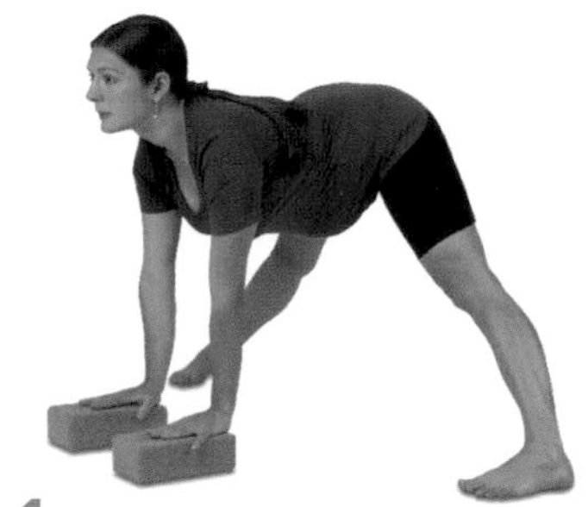

11 Prasarita Padottanasana, *page 56*

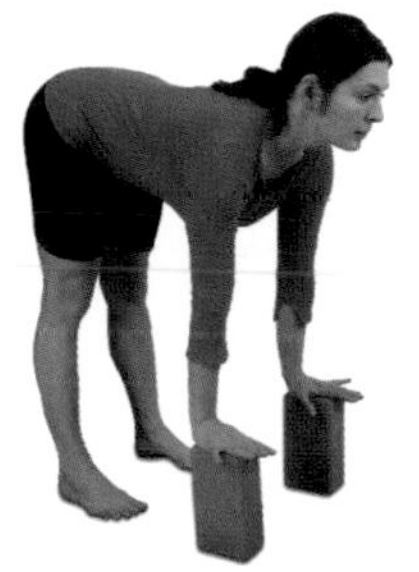

12 Uttanasana (concave back), *page 213*

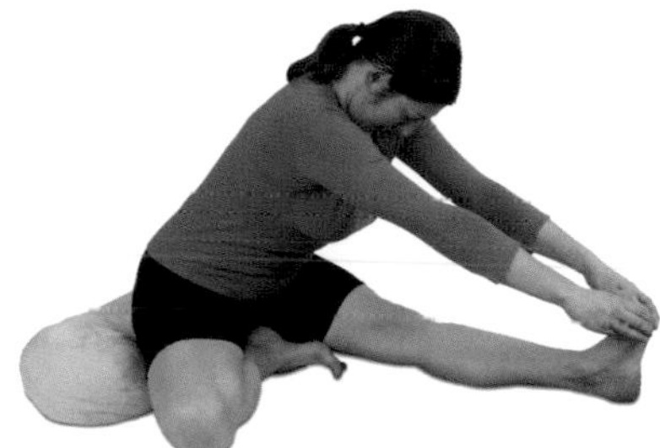

13 Maha Mudra, *page 216*

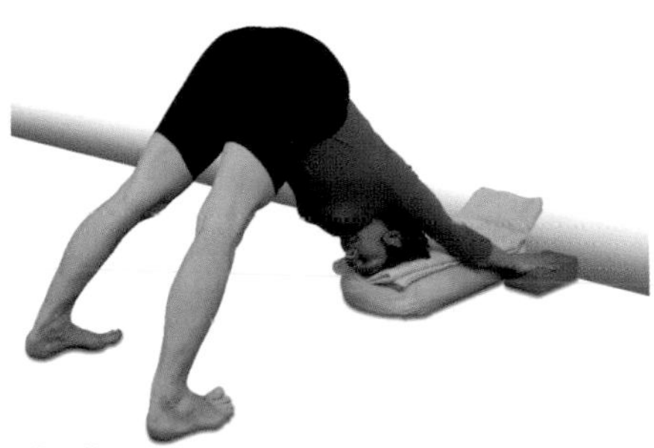

14 Adho Mukha Shvanasana, *page 62*

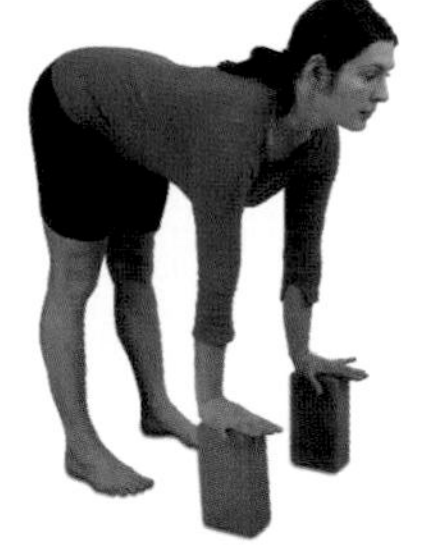

15 Uttanasana (concave back), *page 213*

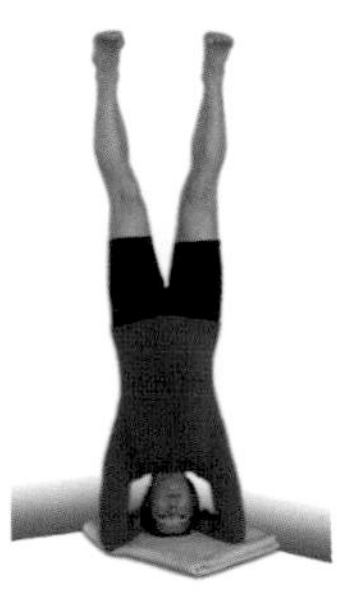

16 Salamba Shirshasana (wall), *page 99*

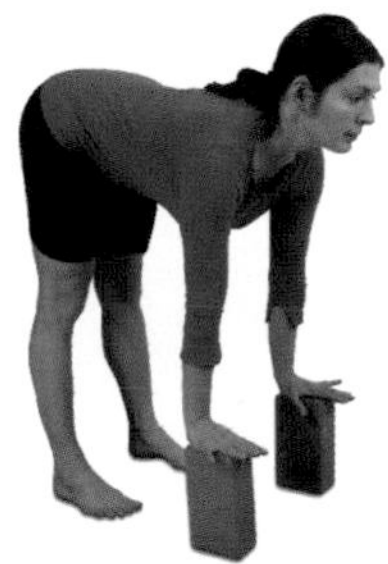

17 Uttanasana (concave back), *page 213*

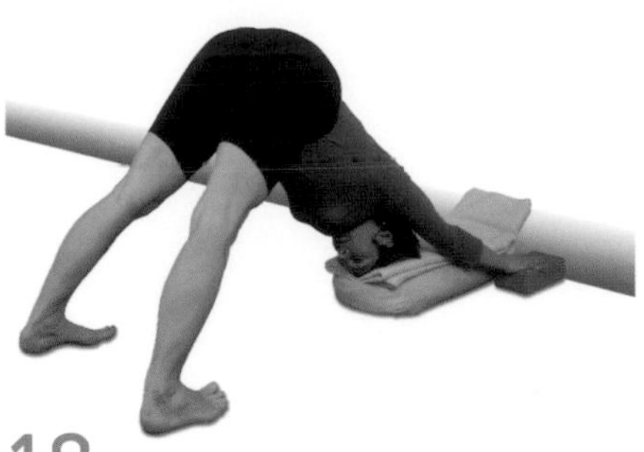

18 Adho Mukha Shvanasana, *page 62*

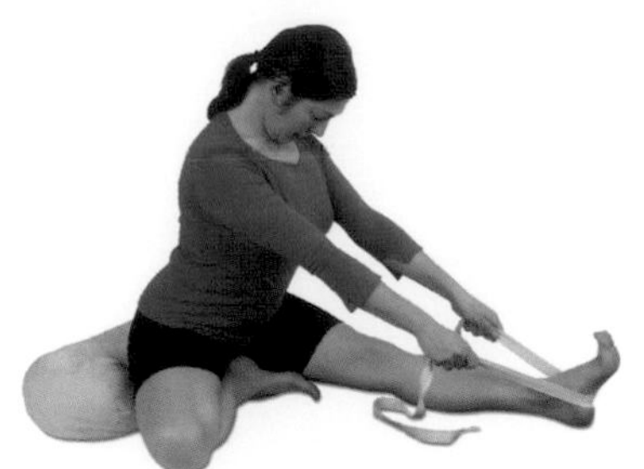

19 Maha Mudra, *page 80*

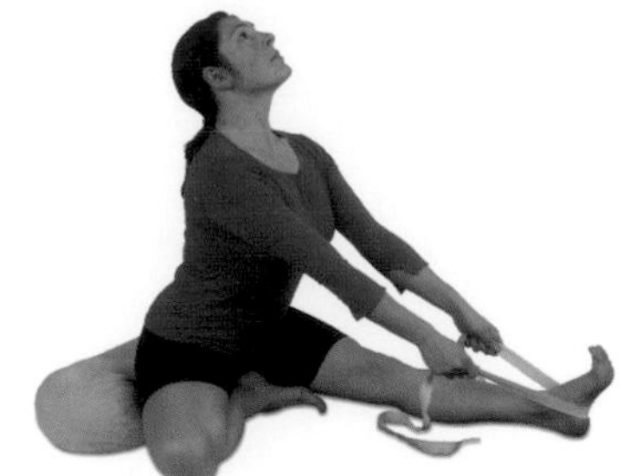

20 Janu Shirshasana (concave back), *page 83*

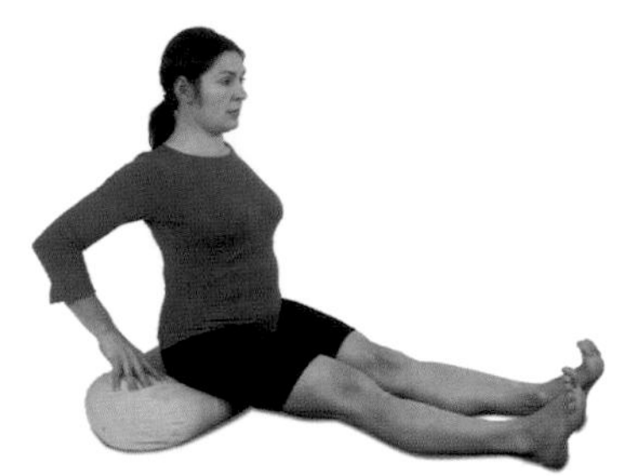

21 Dandasana, *page 65*

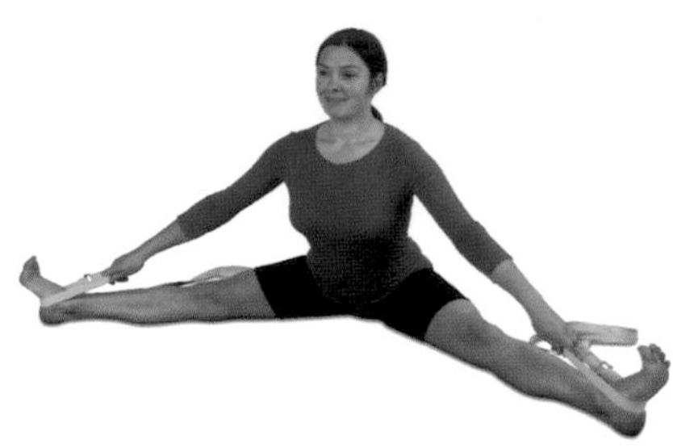

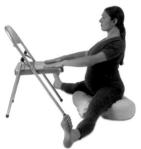

22 Upavishtha Konasana (concave back) and straight, *pages 85 and 86*

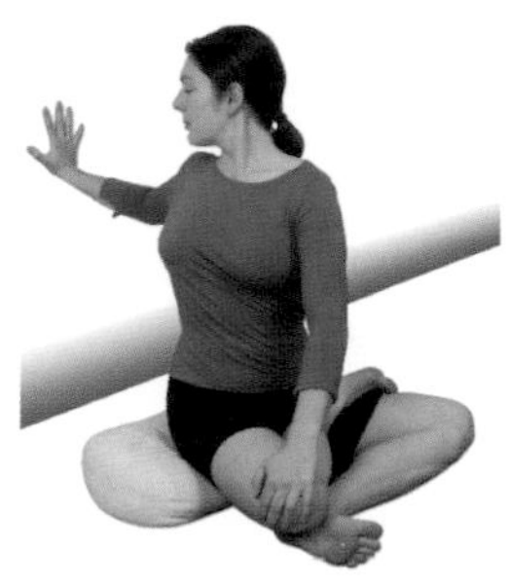

23 Parshva Svastikasana or Ardha Padmasana/full Padmasana (twisting with wall), *page 94*

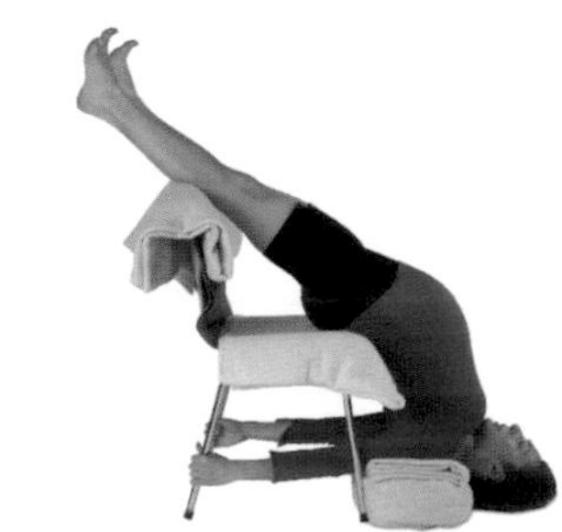

24 Salamba Sarvangasana (chair), *page 103*

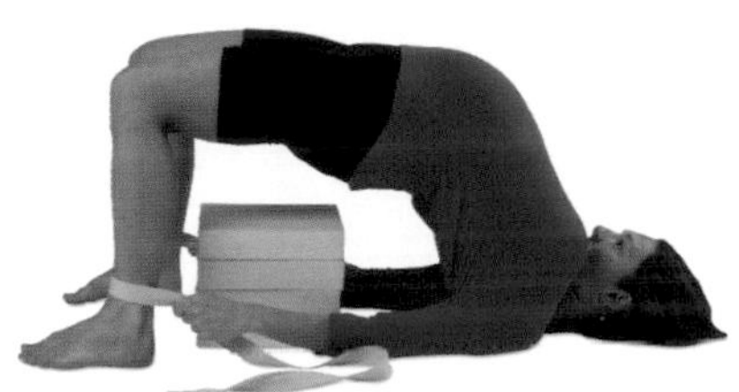

25 Chatushpadasana, *page 111*

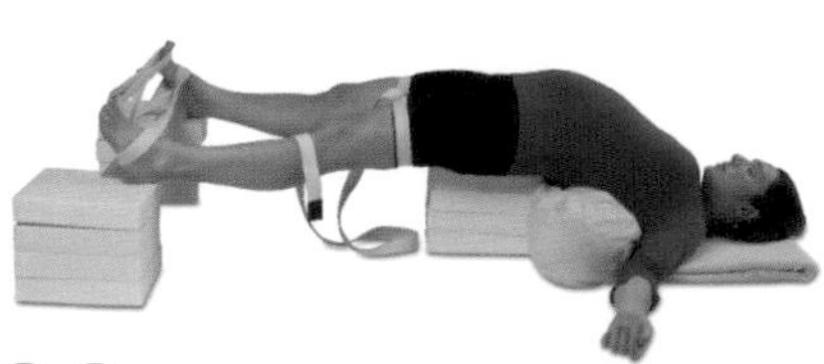

26 Setu Bandha Sarvangasana, *pages 108 – 109*

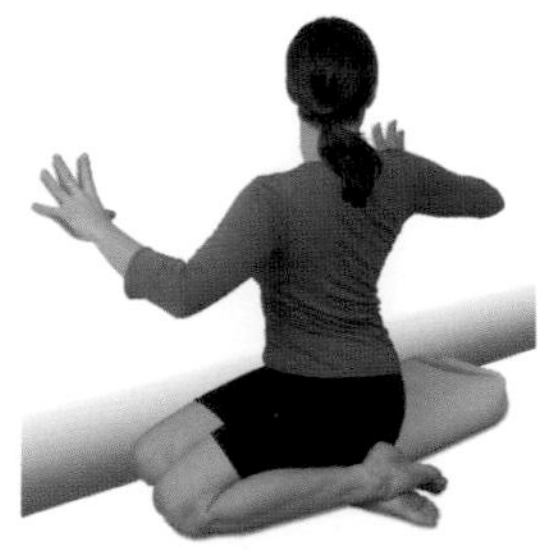

27 Bharadvajasana (chair or bolster), *page 93*

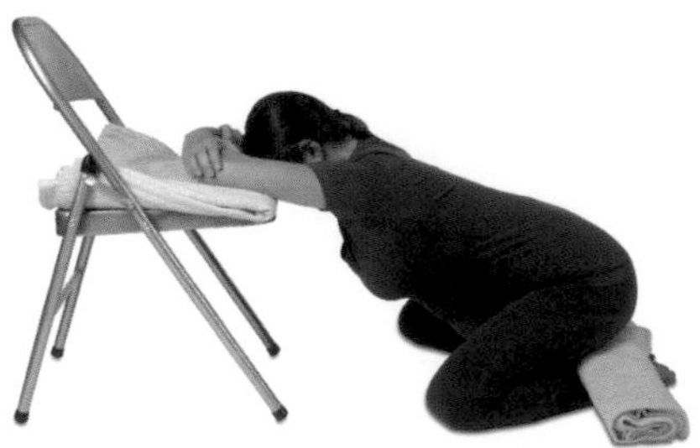

28 Adho Mukha Virasana, *page 76*

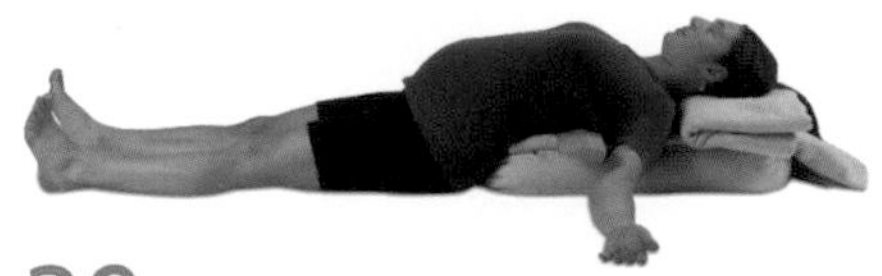

29 Shavasana (bolster/s), *page 134*

30 Ujjayi Pranayama 1 (bolster) and Viloma Pranayama Stage 1 (sitting), *page 148*

Sequence 2: Stretching the Sides of the Body

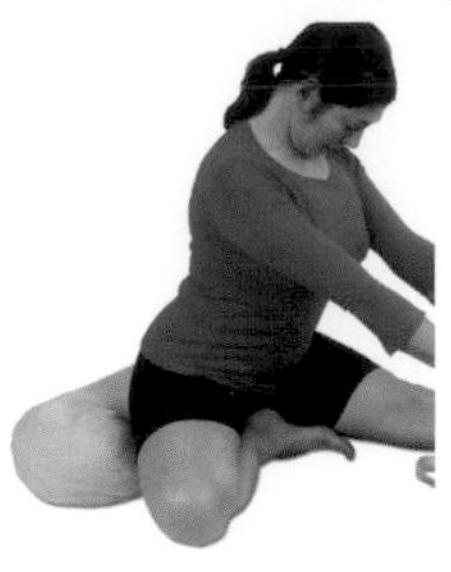

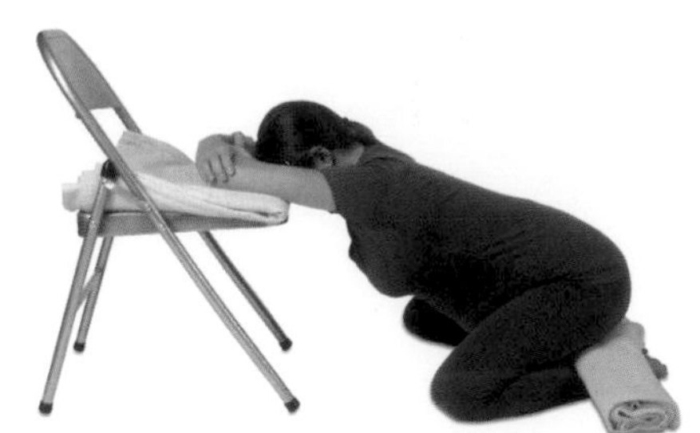

1 Adho Mukha Virasana, *page 76*

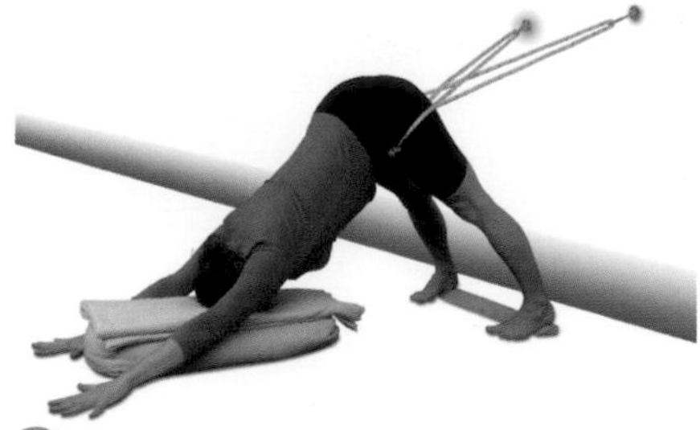

2 Adho Mukha Shvanasana (ropes), *page 63*

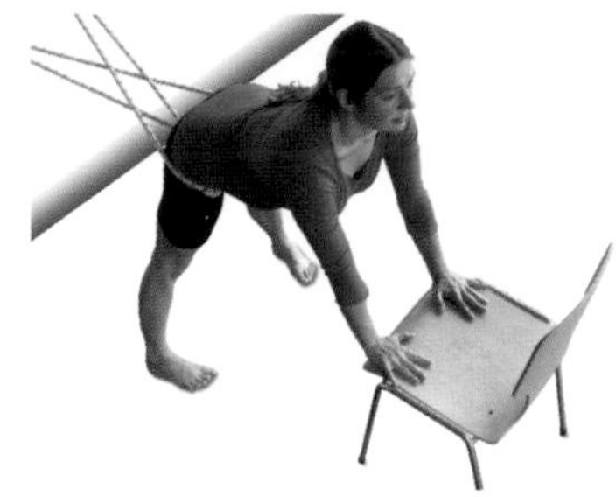

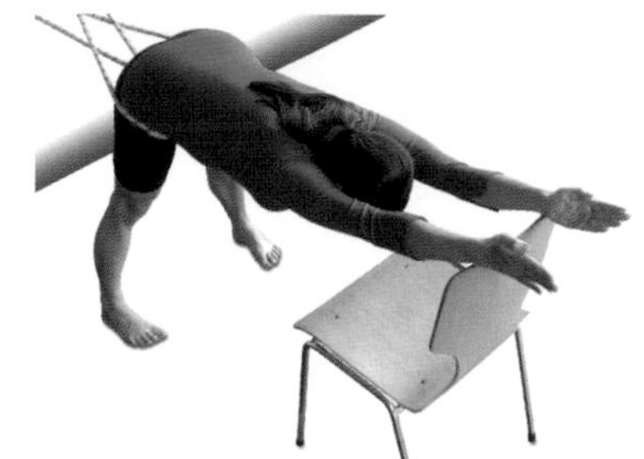

3 Ardha Uttanasana (ropes and chair, concave back), *page 124*

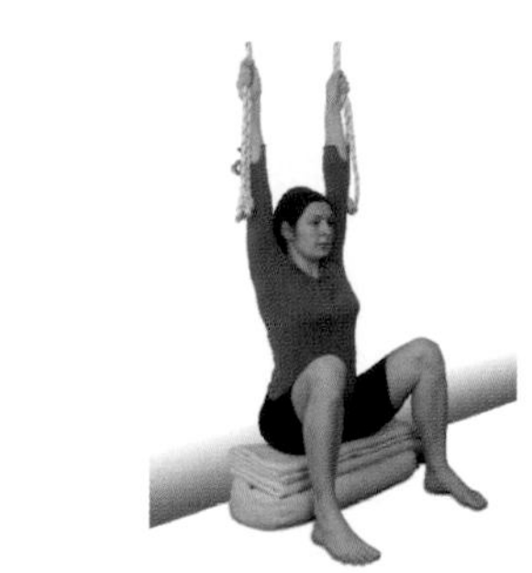

4 Malasana (holding ropes), *page 77*

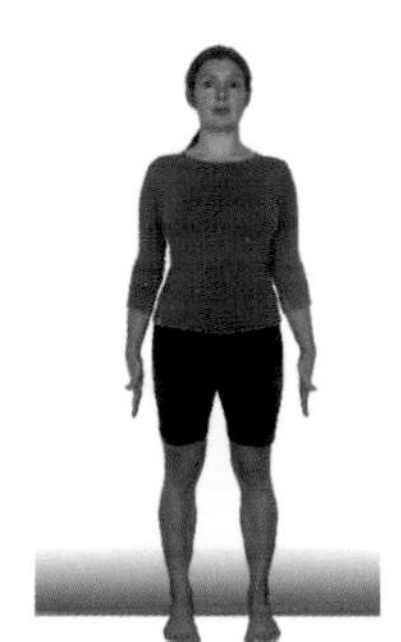

5 Tadasana, *page 32*

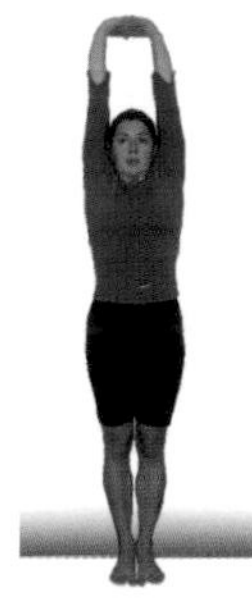

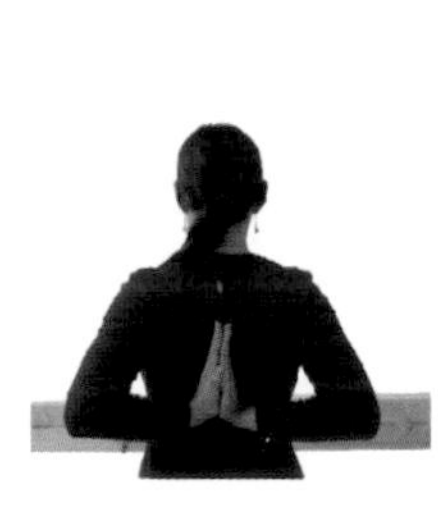

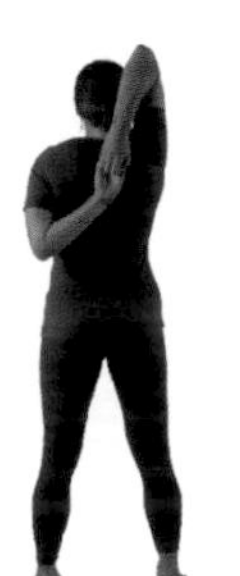

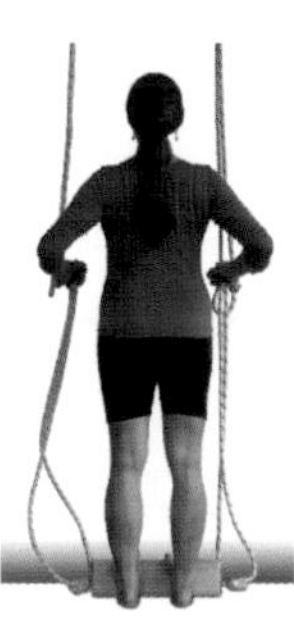

6 Urdhva Baddhanguliyasana, *page 34*, Pashchima Namaskarasana, *page 36*, Gomukhasana in Tadasana, *page 37*, and Tadasana (heels down), *page 33*

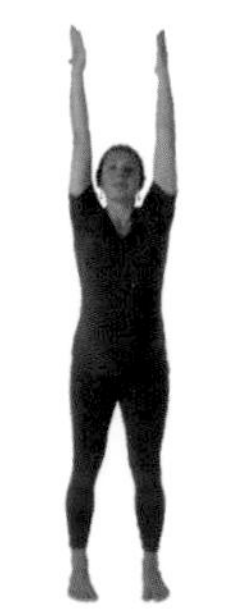

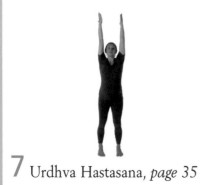

7 Urdhva Hastasana, *page 35*

Note

Always start the standing poses from Tadasana. When you finish the pose, come back to Tadasana. If you feel tired, rest in Ardha Uttanasana.

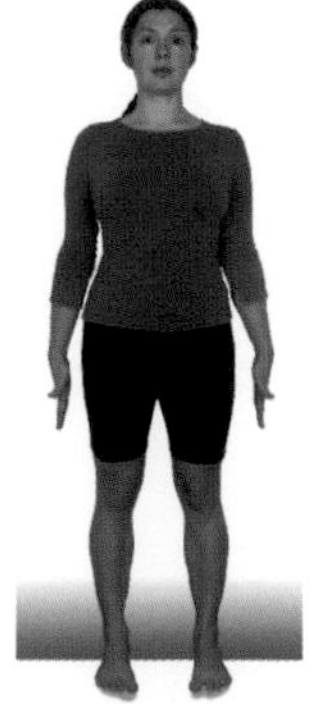

Tadasana

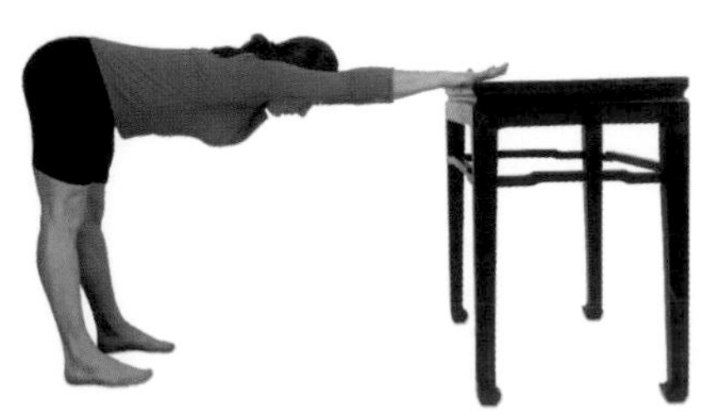

Ardha Uttanasana

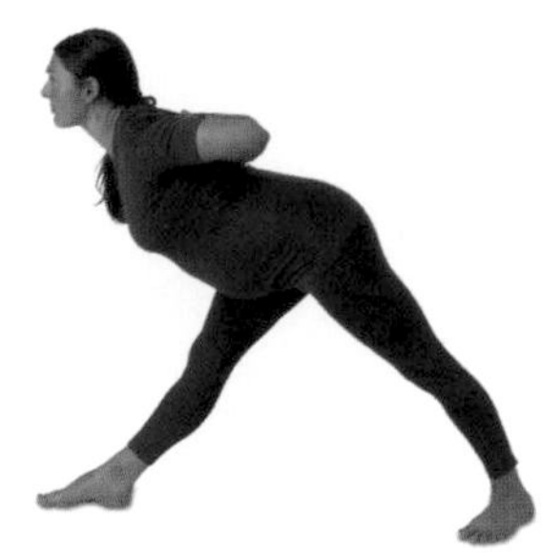

8 Pashchima Namaskarasana in Parshvottanasana, *page 50*

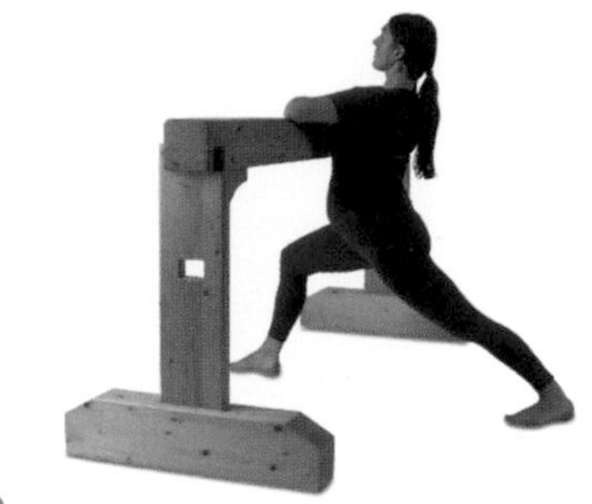

9 Virabhadrasana 1, *page 53*

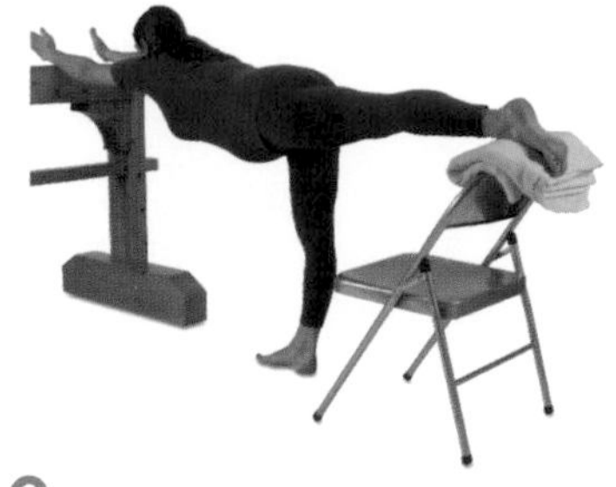

10 Virabhadrasana 3, *page 54*

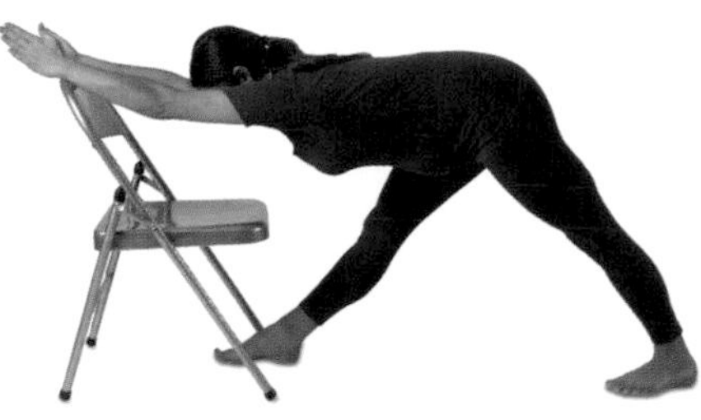

11 Parshvottanasana, *page 51*

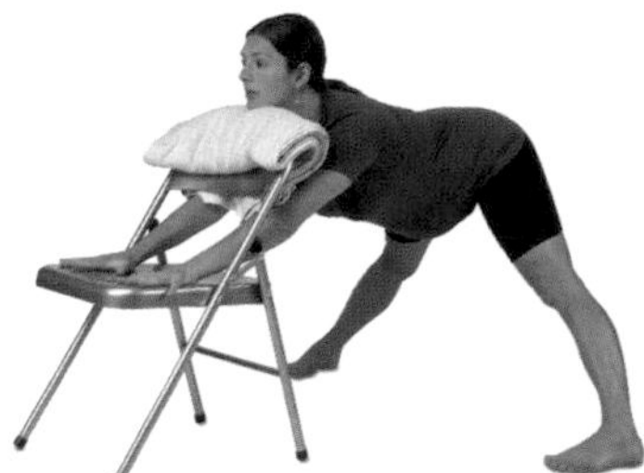

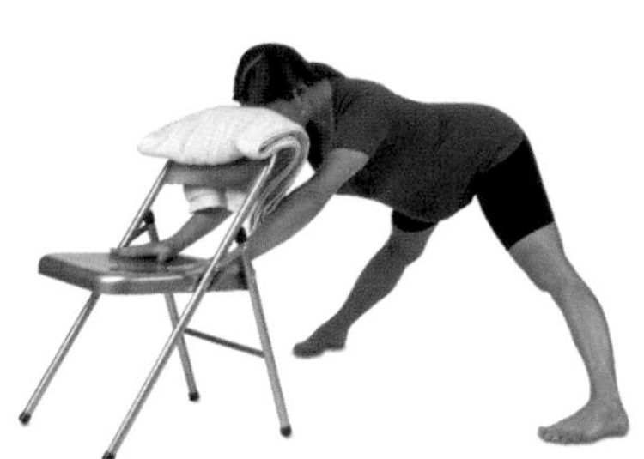

12 Prasarita Padottanasana (concave back and head resting), *page 58*

13 If you practice Salamba Shirshasana add:

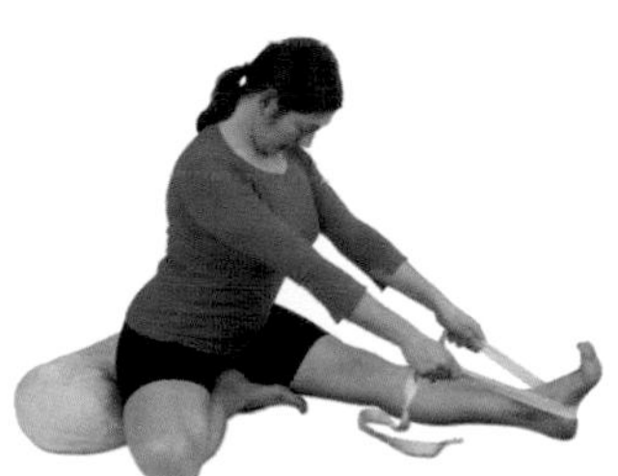

Maha Mudra, *page 80*

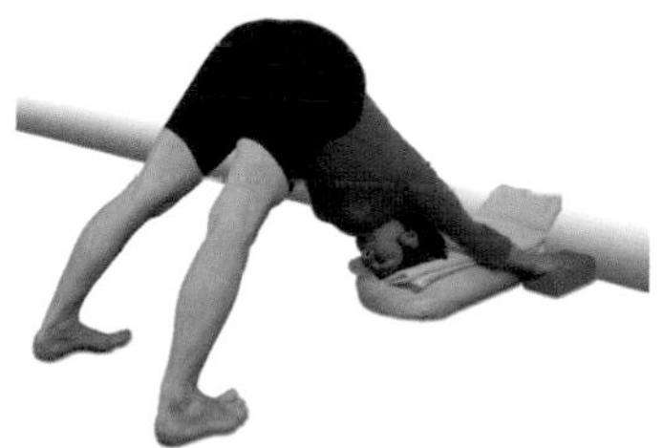

Adho Mukha Shvanasana, *page 62*

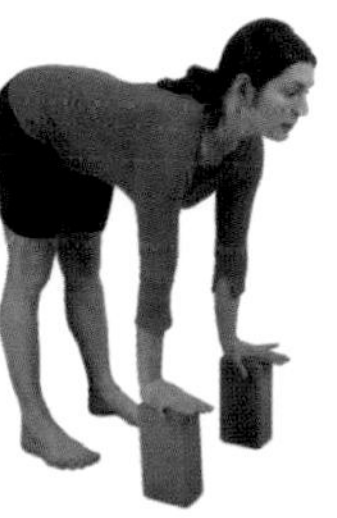

Uttanasana (concave back), *page 213*

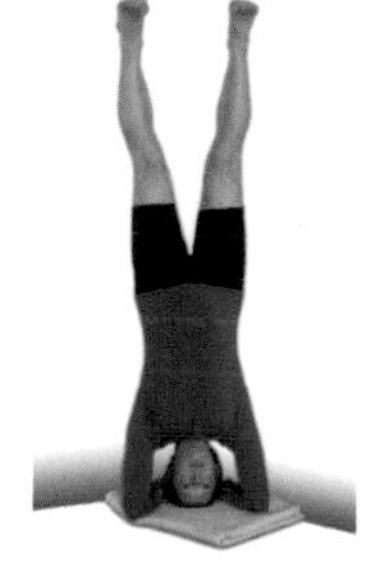

Salamba Shirshasana (with wall and teacher), *page 99*

Reverse sequence following Shirshasana:

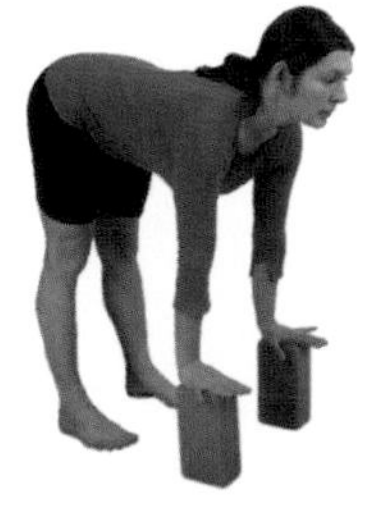

Uttanasana (concave back), *page 213*

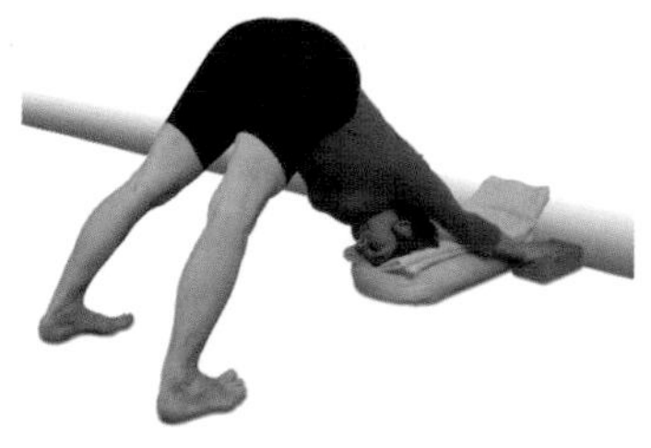

Adho Mukha Shvanasana, *page 62*

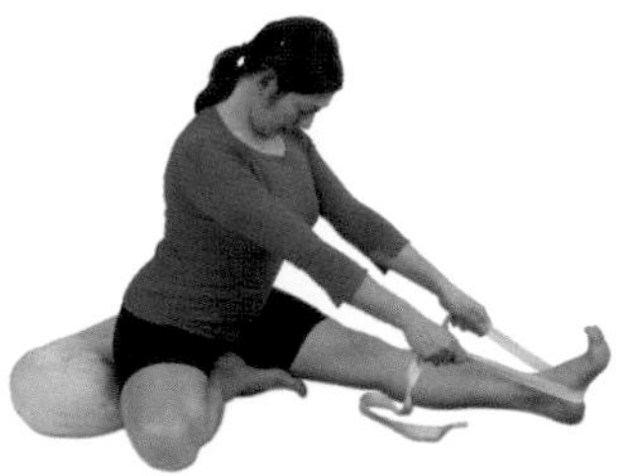

Maha Mudra, *page 80*

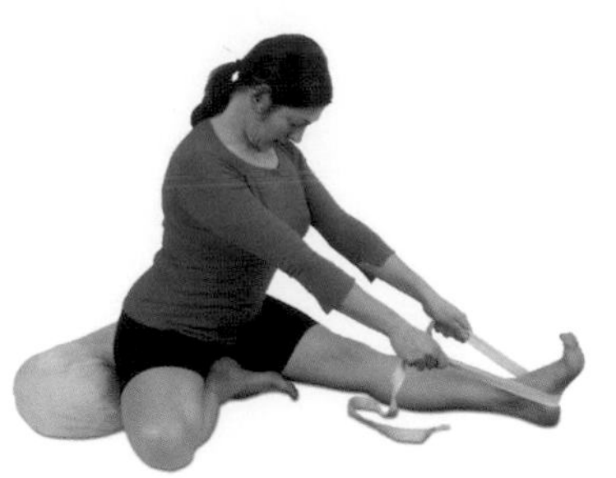

14 Maha Mudra (if you didn't do the Shirshasana sequence), *page 80*

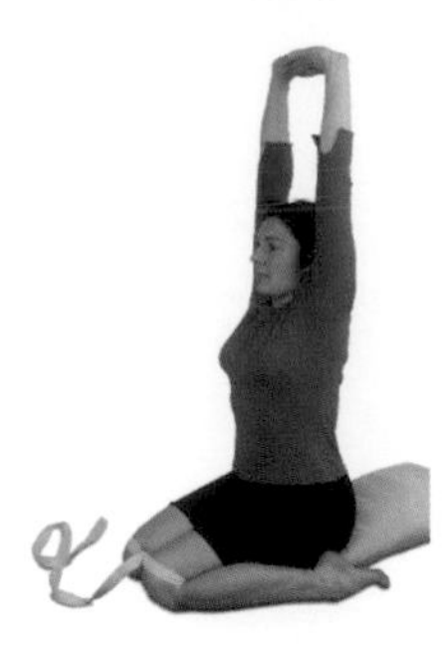

15 Parvatasana from Virasana, *page 74*

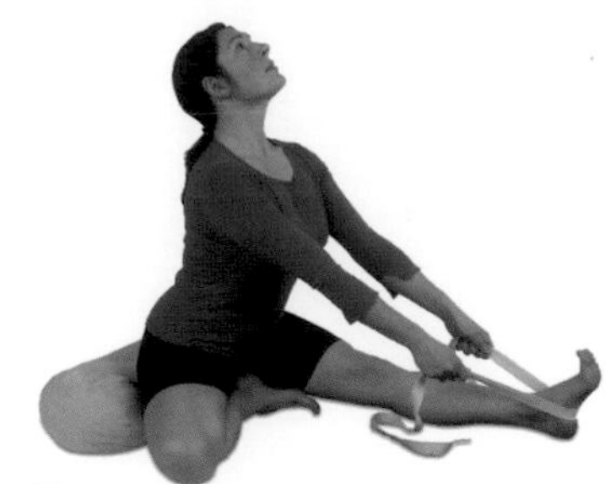

16 Janu Shirshasana (concave back), *page 83*

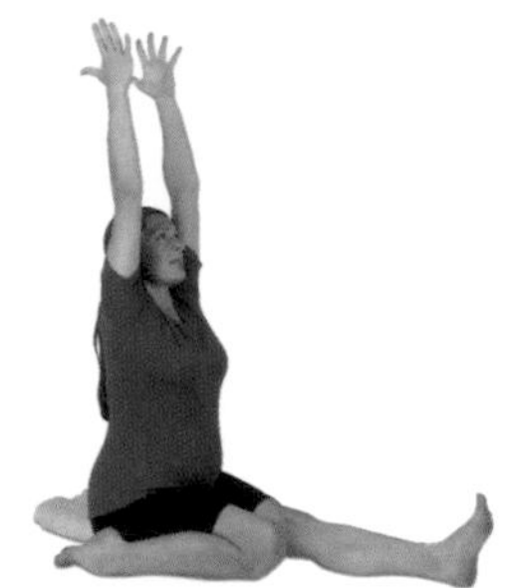

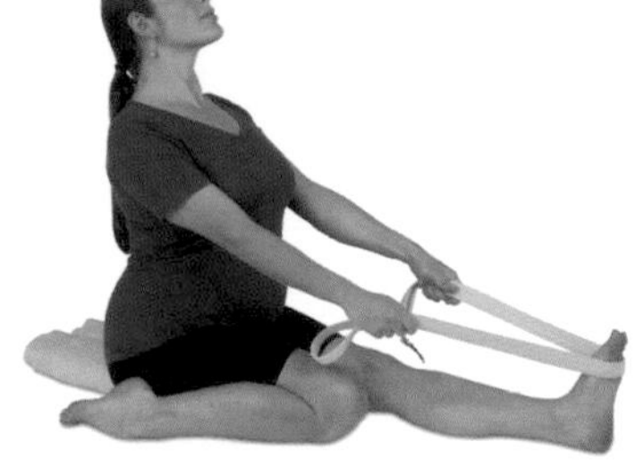

17 Trianga Mukhaikapada Pashchimottanasana (concave back), *pages 89 – 90*

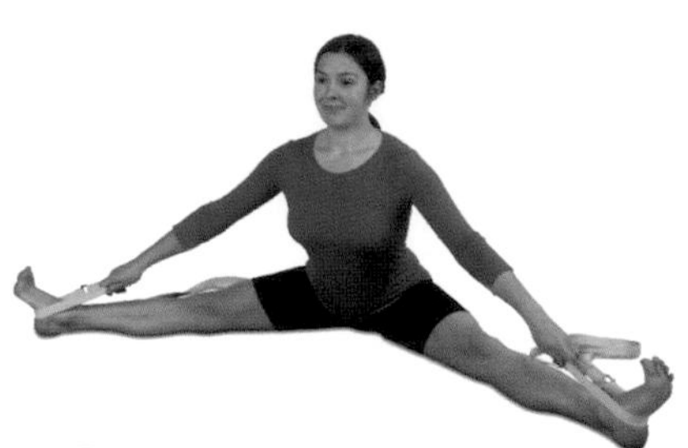

18 Upavishtha Konasana (straight back, gripping feet), *page 85*

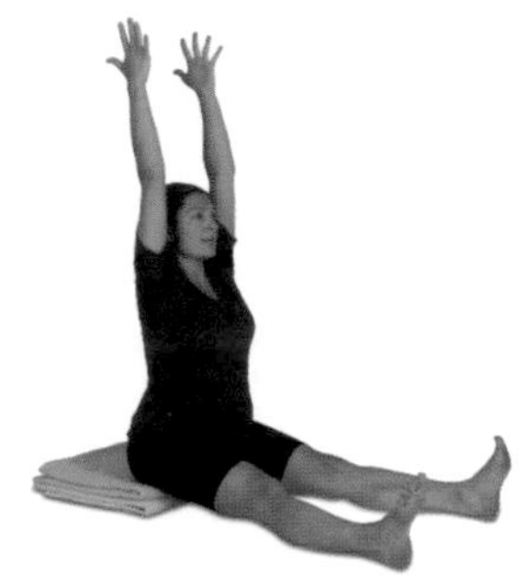

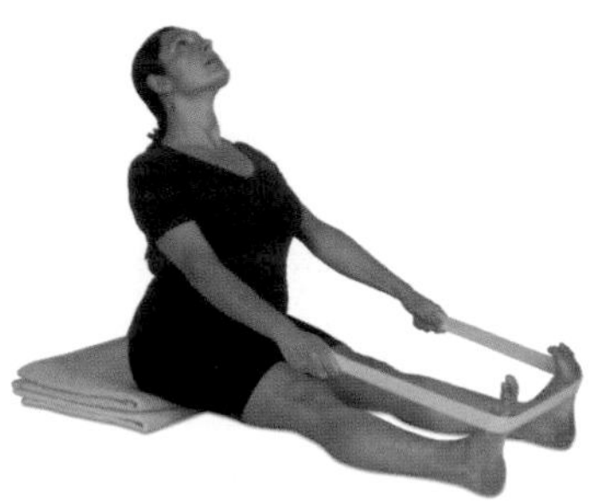

19 Pashchimottanasana (concave back), *pages 87 – 90*

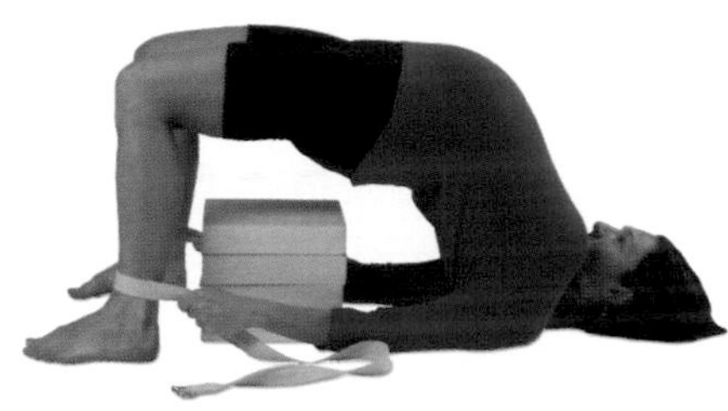

20 Chatushpadasana, *page 111*

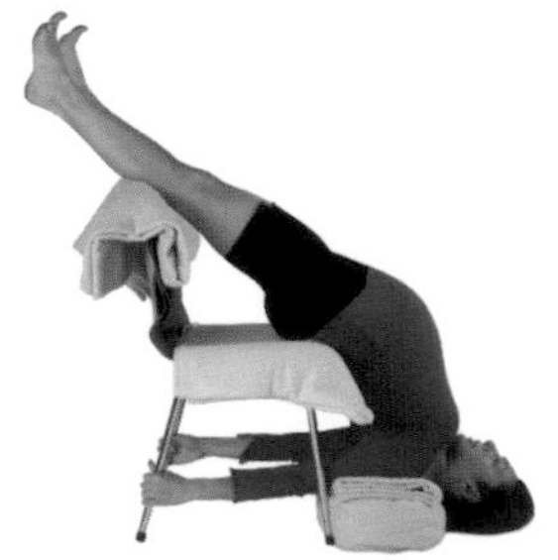

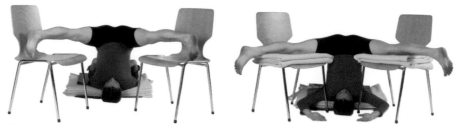

21 Salamba Sarvangasana (chair), *page 103*

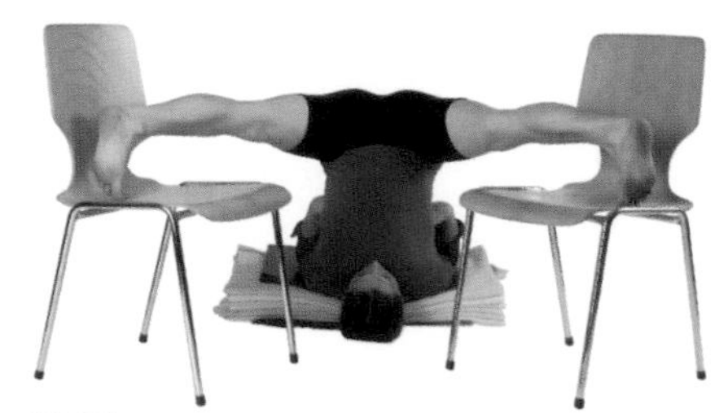

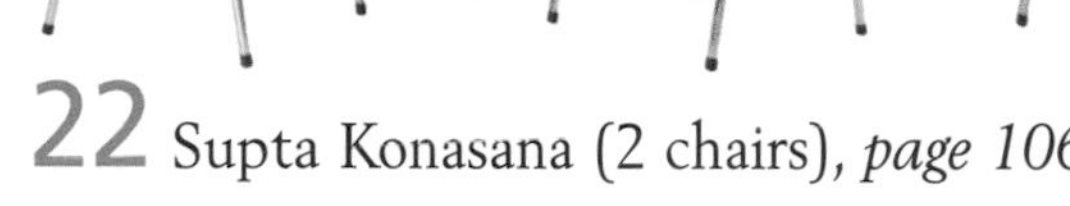

22 Supta Konasana (2 chairs), *page 106*

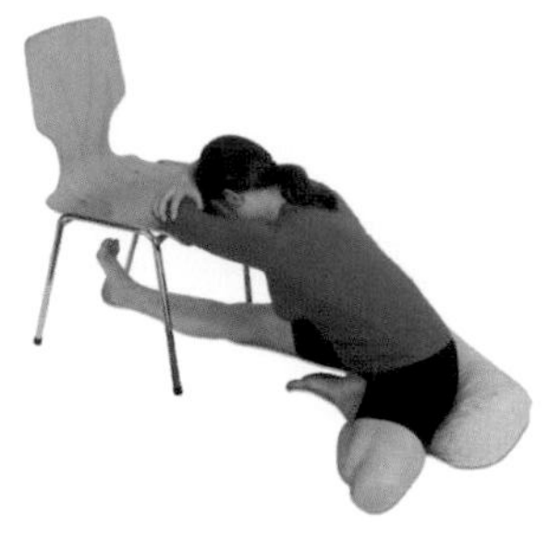

23 Parshva Janu Shirshasana (twisting with chair), *page 95*

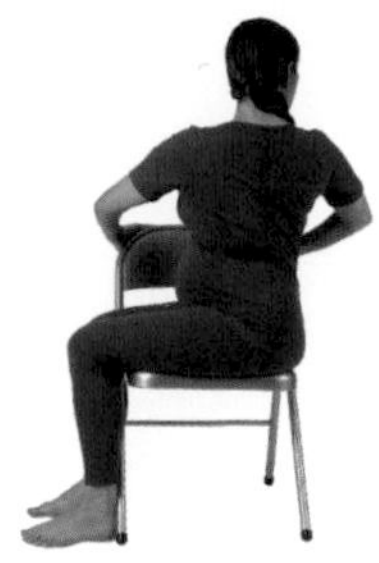

24 Bharadvajasana (bolster or chair), *page 93*

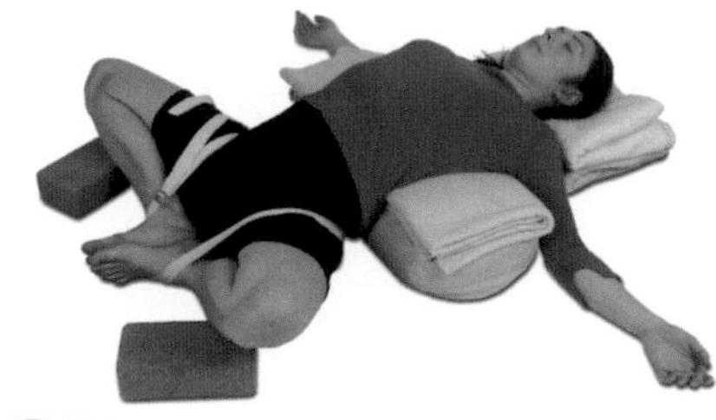

25 Supta Baddha Konasana (bolster crosswise), *page 128*

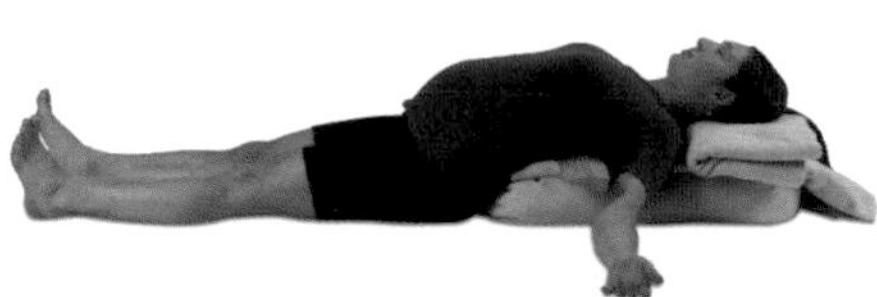

26 Shavasana (bolster lengthwise), *page 134*

27 Viloma Pranayama Stage 1 (lying on bolster) and Viloma Pranayama Stage 2 (sitting), *pages 151 – 153*

Sequence 3: Bending Backward

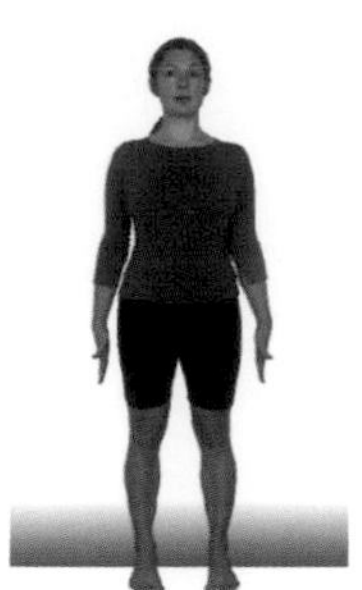

1 Tadasana, *page 32*

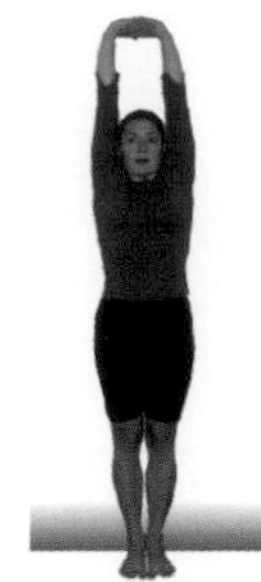

2 Urdhva Baddhanguliyasana in Tadasana (practice with feet apart), *page 34*

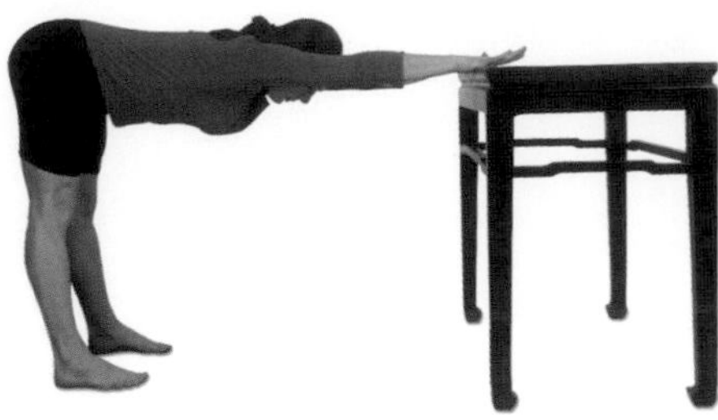

3 Ardha Uttanasana, *page 60*

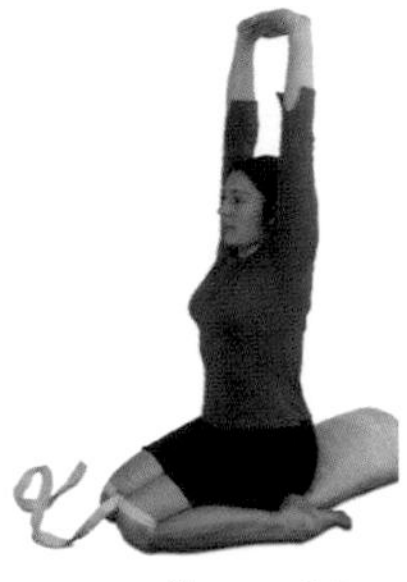

4 Parvatasana from Virasana, *page 74*

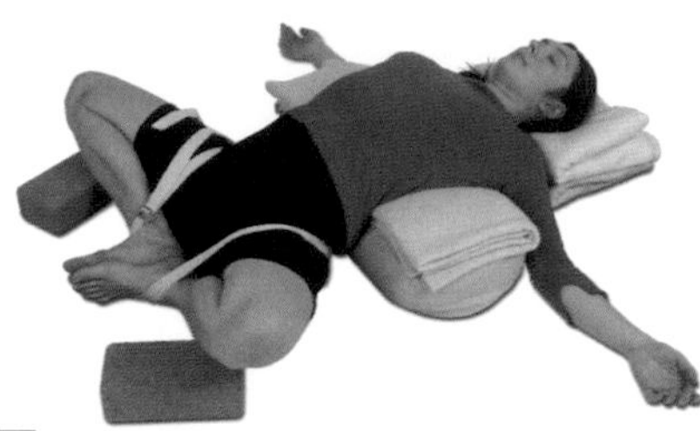

5 Supta Baddha Konasana (bolster crosswise for breastbone lift), *page 128*

6 If you practice Salamba Shirshasana add:

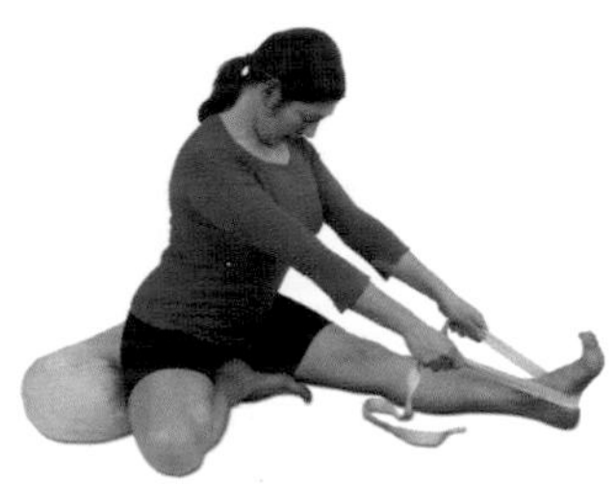

Maha Mudra, *page 80*

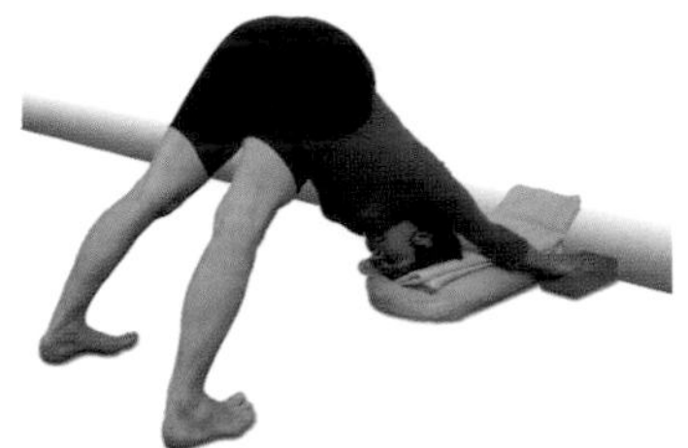

Adho Mukha Shvanasana, *page 62*

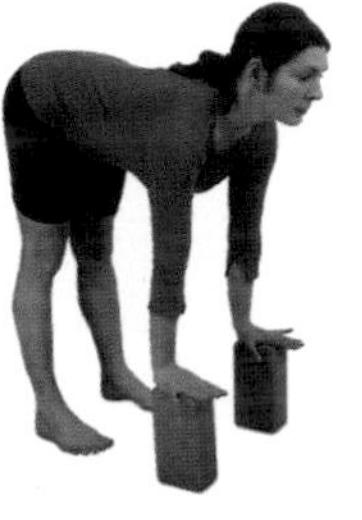

Uttanasana (concave back), *page 213*

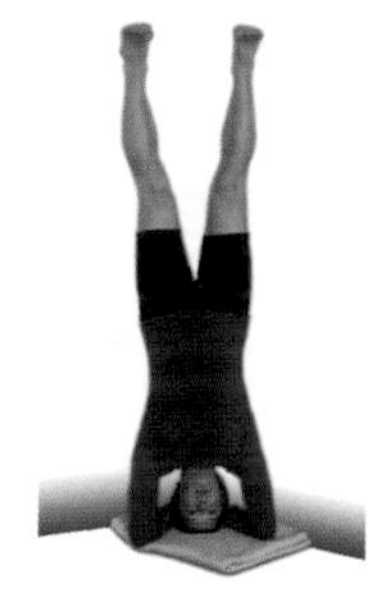

Salamba Shirshasana (with wall), *page 99*

Reverse sequence following Shirshasana:

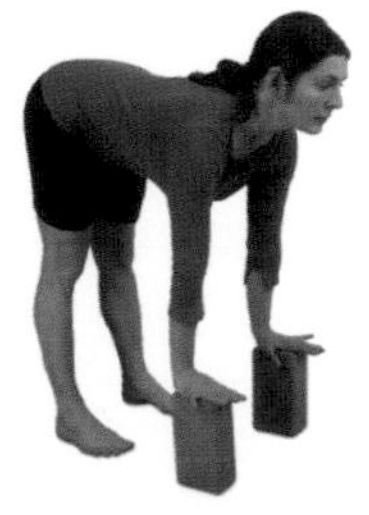

Uttanasana (concave back), *page 213*

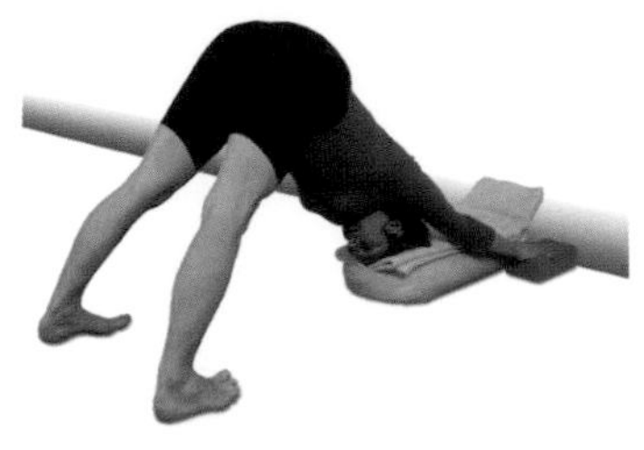

Adho Mukha Shvanasana, *page 62*

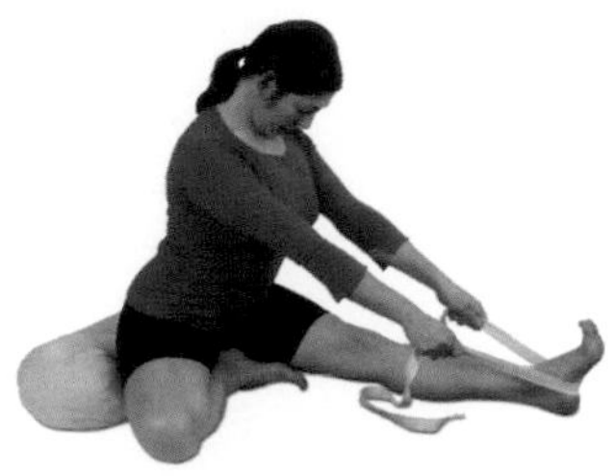

Maha Mudra, *page 80*

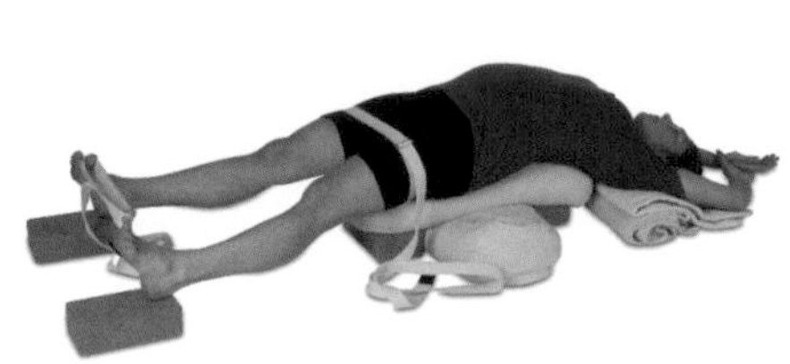

7 Cross-bolsters (passive back bend), *page 118*

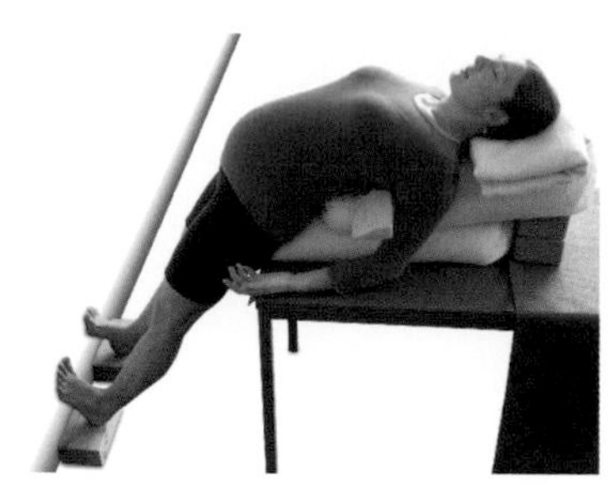

8 Salamba Purvottanasana, *page 133*

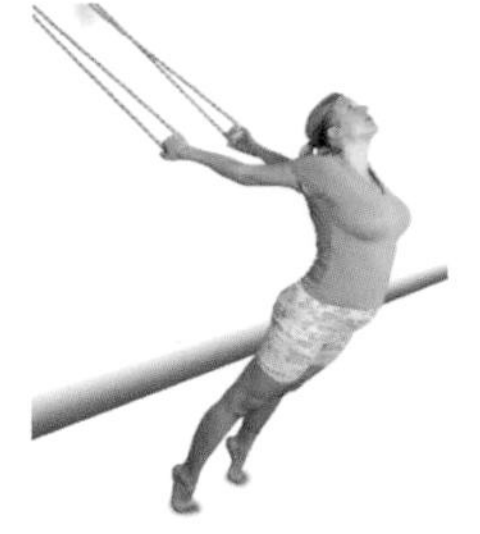

9 Bhujangasana (ropes), *page 119*

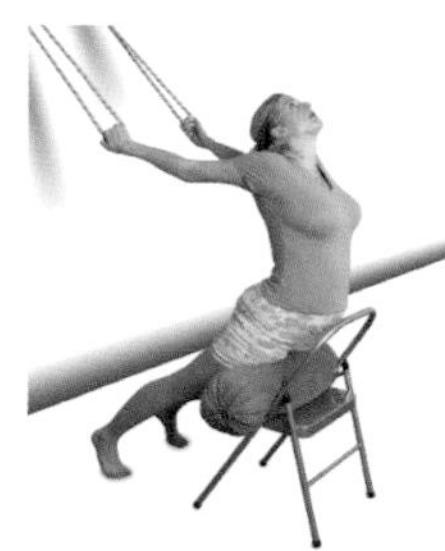

10 Bhujangasana (ropes and chair), *page 120*

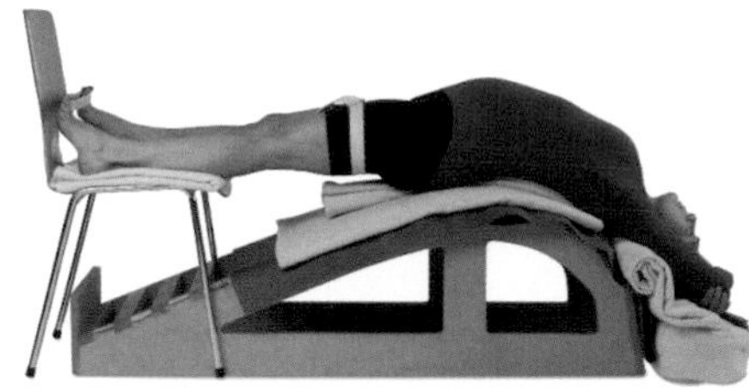

11 Dvi Pada Viparita Dandasana (fully supported, L-shape, on Viparita Dandasana bench), *page 123*

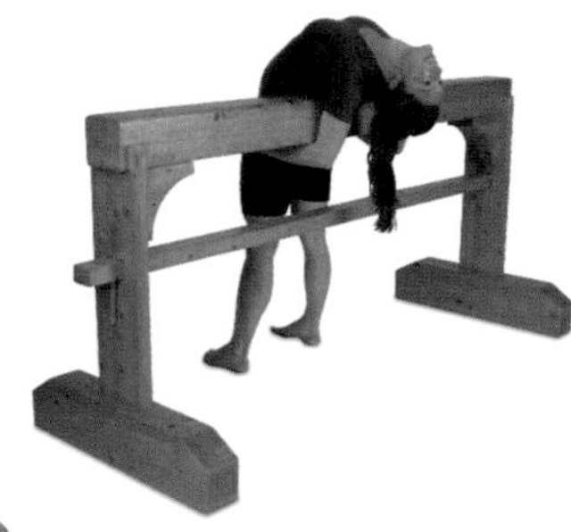

12 Salamba Purvottanasana (trestle), *page 121*

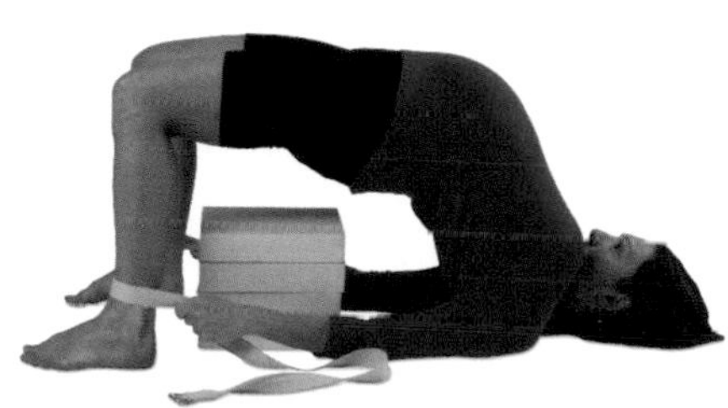

13 Chatushpadasana, *page 111*

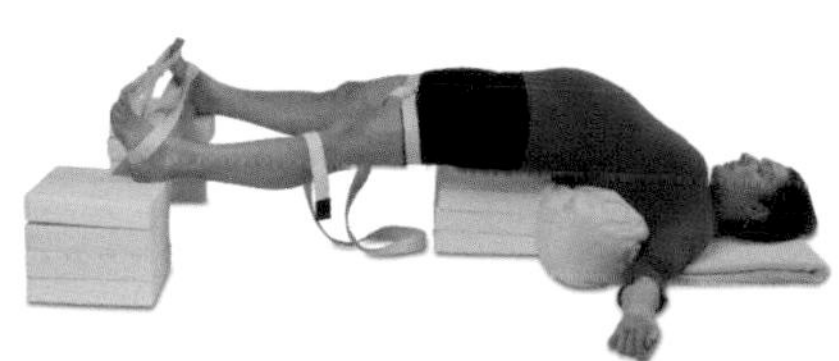

14 Setu Bandha Sarvangasana, *page 108*

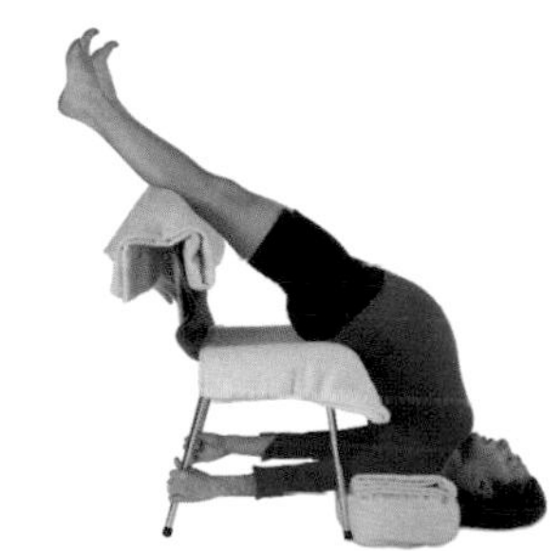

15 Salamba Sarvangasana (chair), *page 103*

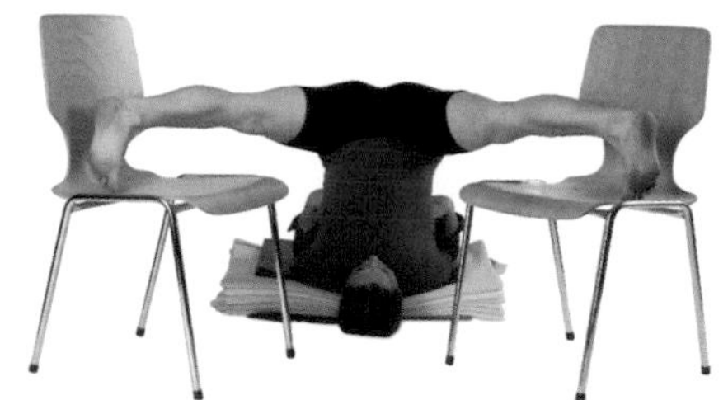

16 Supta Konasana (2 chairs), *page 106*

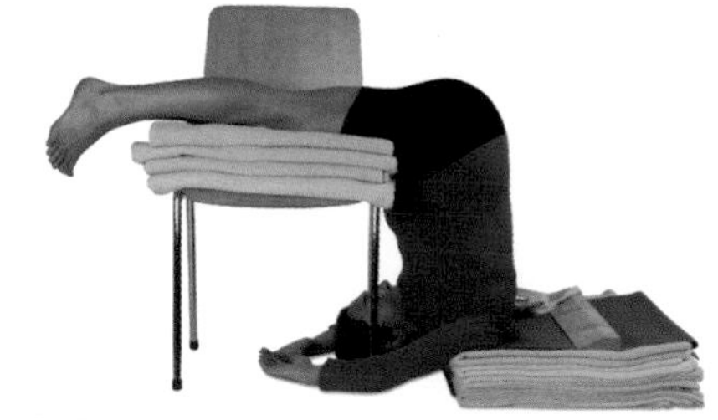

17 Ardha Halasana (thighs resting on chair), *page 105*

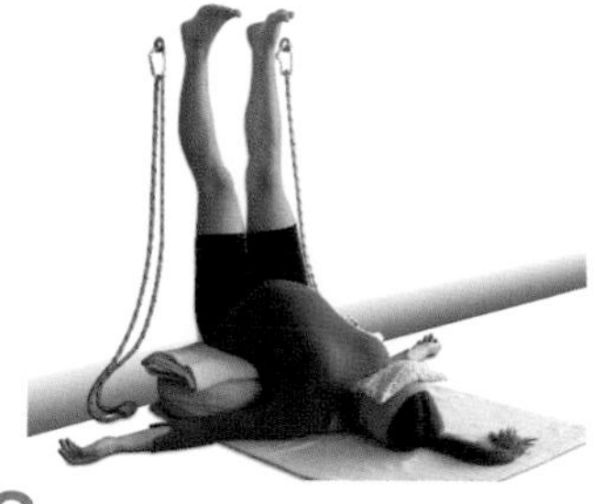

18 Viparita Karani, *page 114*

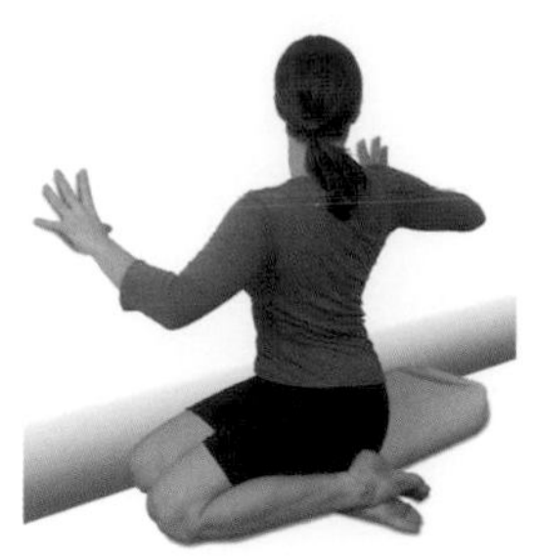

19 Bharadvajasana 1, *page 93*

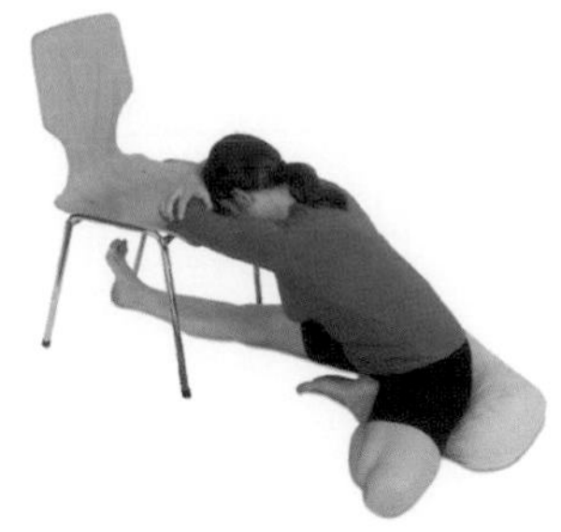

20 Parshva Janu Shirshasana (twisting with chair), *page 95*

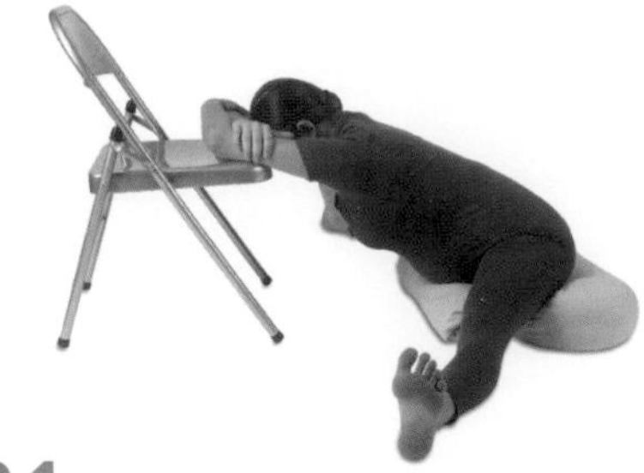

21 Upavishtha Konasana (head resting on chair), *page 86*

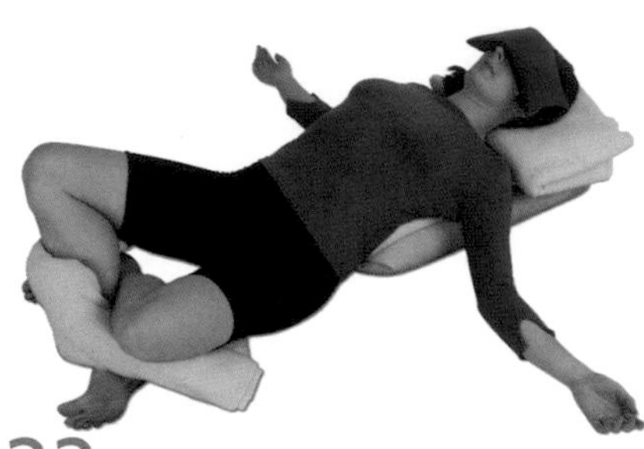

22 Supta Svastikasana (bolster/s), *page 131*

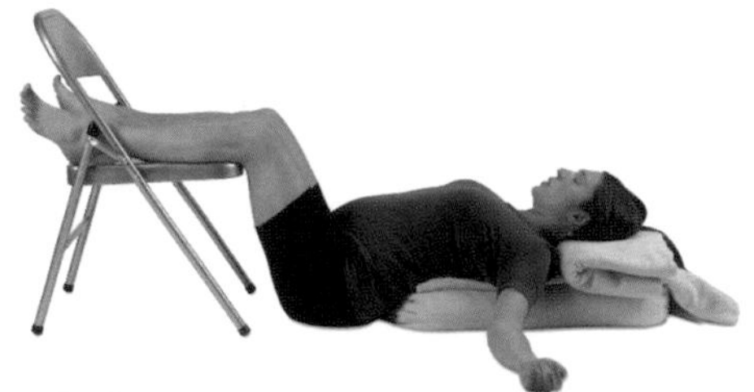

23 Shavasana (bolster/s), *page 138*

24 Viloma Pranayama Stage 1 (lying on bolster), *page 151*, and Ujjayi Pranayama 2 (sitting with bolster), *pages 149 – 150*

Sequence 4: Restorative Program

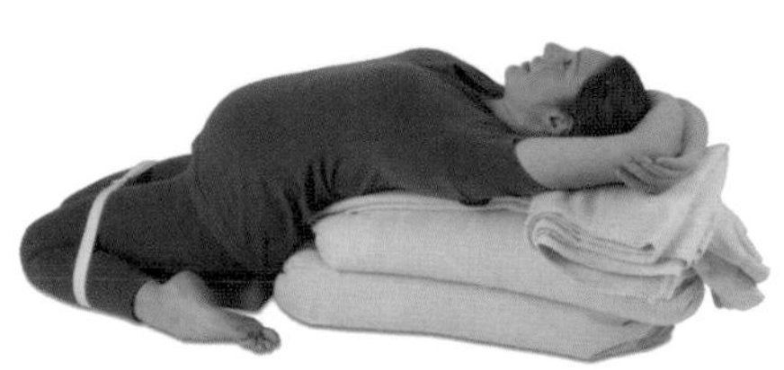

1 Supta Virasana (bolster/s), *page 129*

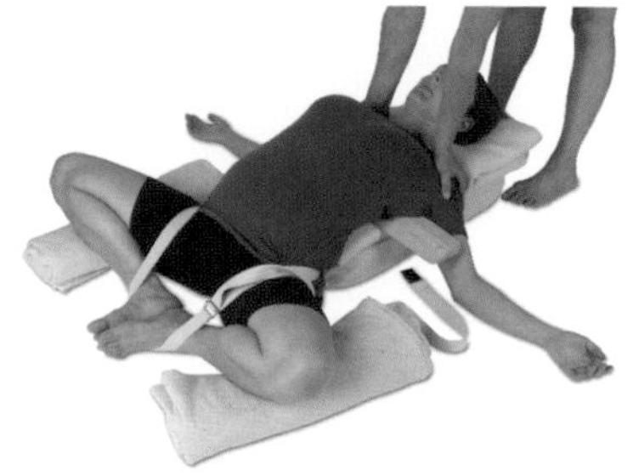

2 Supta Baddha Konasana (bolster lengthwise, slanted plank), *page 127*

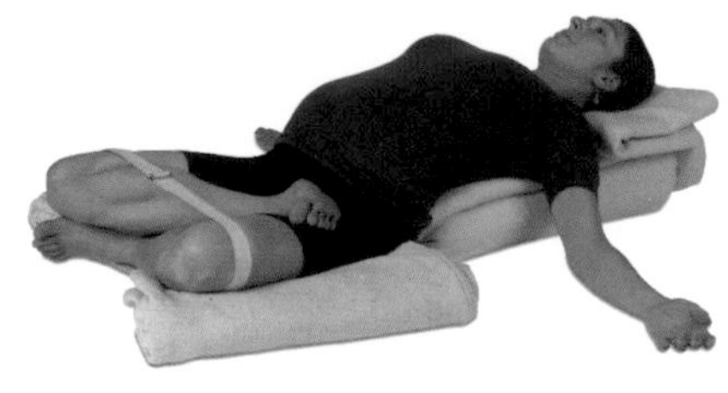

3 Matsyasana (bolster/s), *page 131*

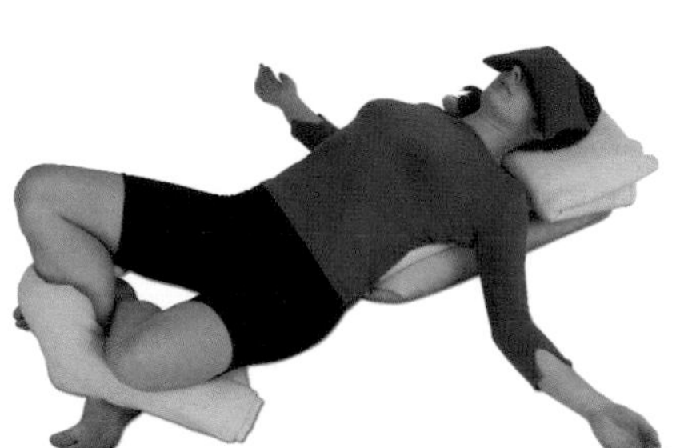

4 Supta Svastikasana (bolster/s), *page 131*

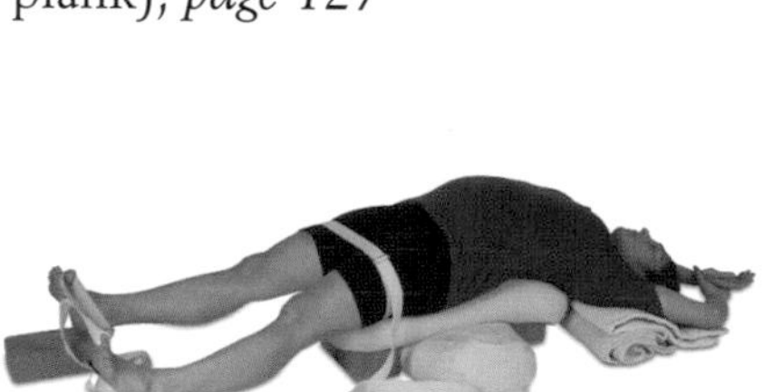

5 Cross-bolsters (passive back bend), *page 118*

and/or

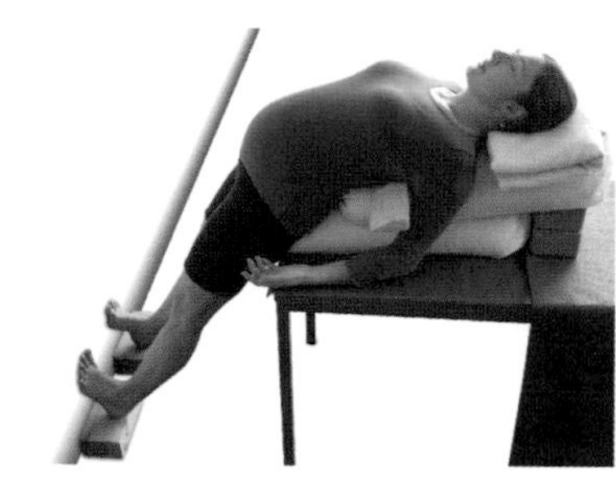

Salamba Purvottanasana, *page 133*

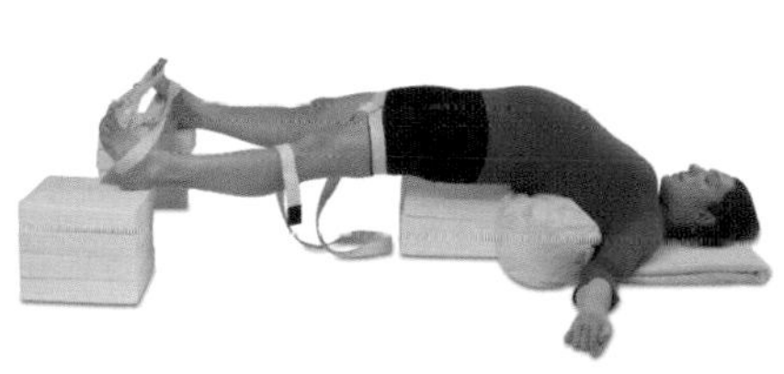

6 Setu Bandha Sarvangasana, *page 108*

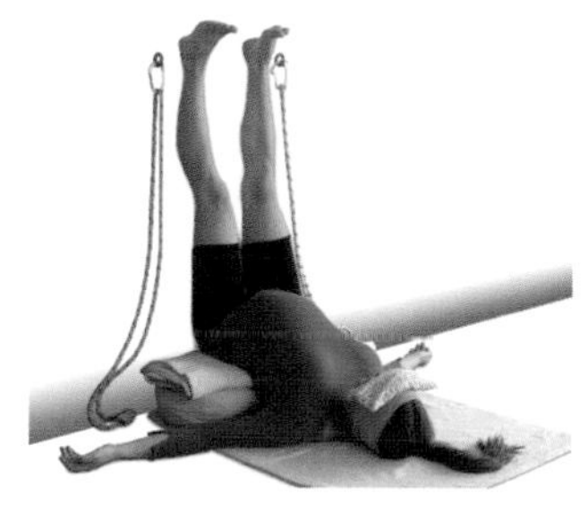

7 Viparita Karani, *page 114*

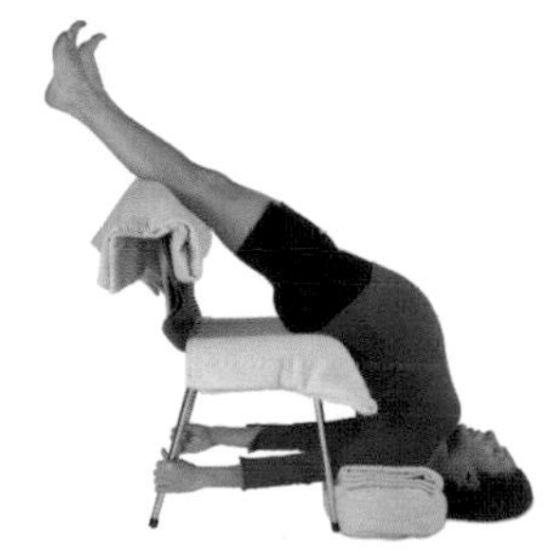

8 Salamba Sarvangasana (chair), *page 103*

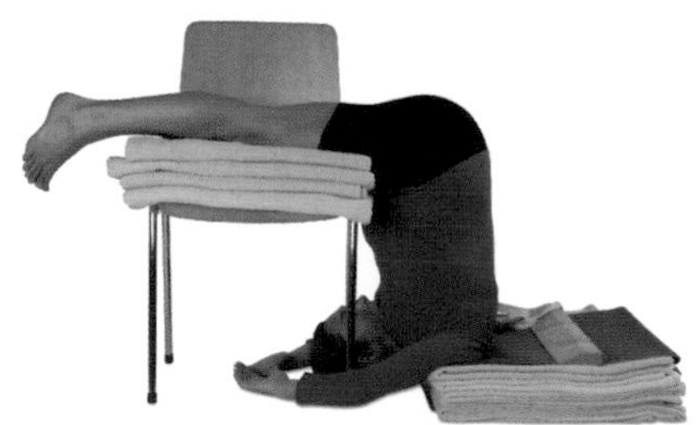

9 Ardha Halasana (thighs resting on chair), *page 105*

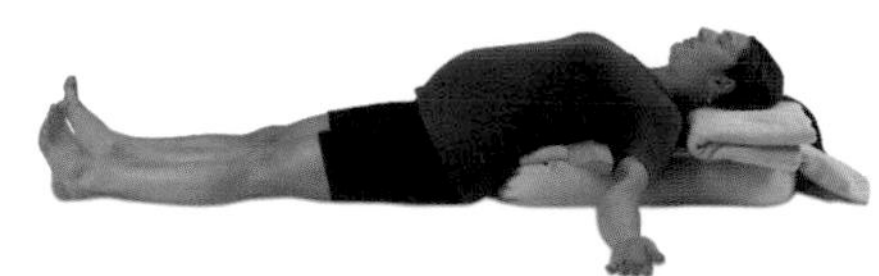

10 Shavasana (bolster/s), *page 134*

Note

You can practice the pranayama separately, in the morning or in the evening at bedtime. (See next page.)

Pranayama

Practice the first sequence followed by the second sequence, and then return to the first one again, and so on.

If you prefer, you can always practice pranayama while lying down, until you feel ready to begin practicing sitting up.

1st Sequence

1st day: Ujjayi Pranayama 1 in Shavasana with Viloma Stage 1, sitting
2nd day: Viloma Stage 1 in Shavasana with Viloma Stage 2, sitting
3rd day: Viloma Stage 1 in Shavasana with Ujjayi Pranayama 2, sitting

2nd Sequence

1st day: Ujjayi Pranayama 1 in Shavasana with Ujjayi Pranayama 2, sitting
2nd day: Viloma Stage 2 in Shavasana with Viloma Stage I, sitting
3rd day: Viloma Stage 2, in Shavasana and sitting

Advanced Asanas

Add these asanas according to your own capability, understanding, knowledge, and state of health. Perform them in any order that suits your practice best; they do not appear here in any prescribed sequence.

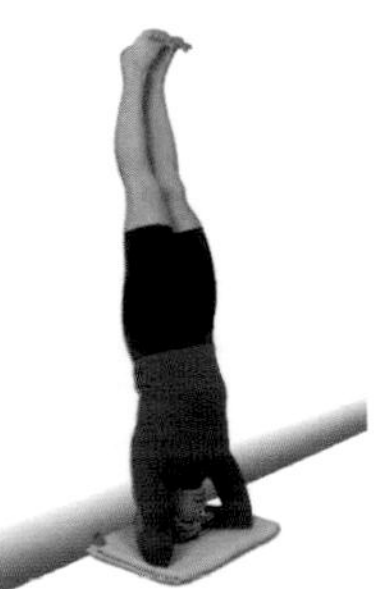

1 Salamba Shirshasana (against the wall) *page 99*

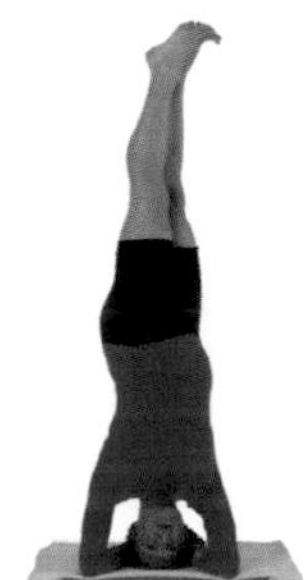

2 Parshva Shirshasana, *page 230*

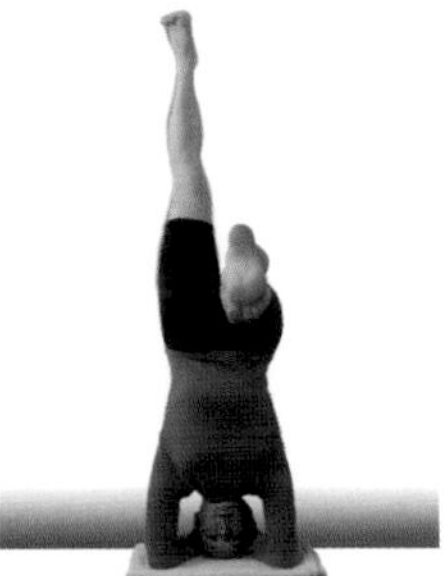

3 Ardha Eka Pada Shirshasana, *page 231*

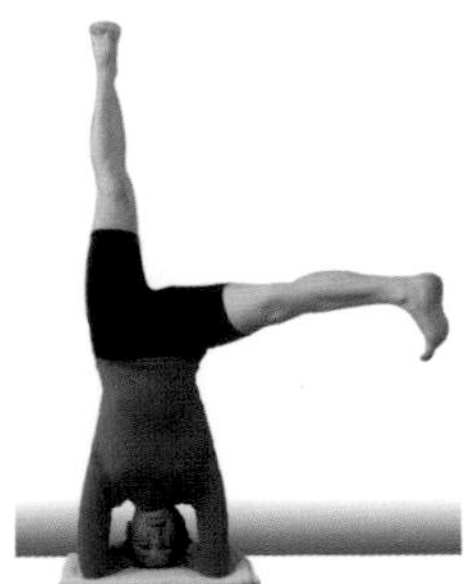

4 Ardha Parshvaikapada Shirshasana, *page 232*

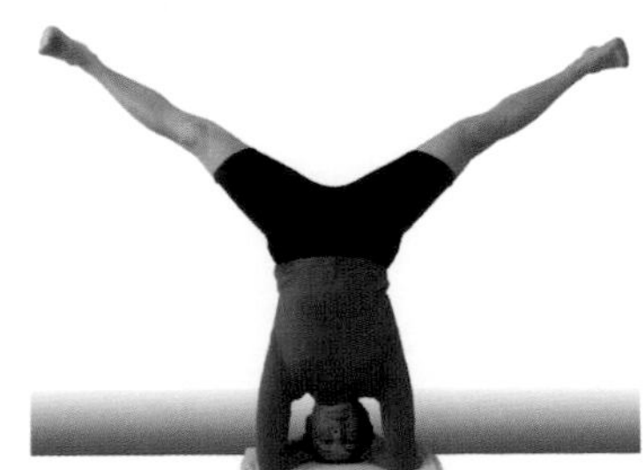

5 Upavishtha Konasana in Shirshasana, *page 233*

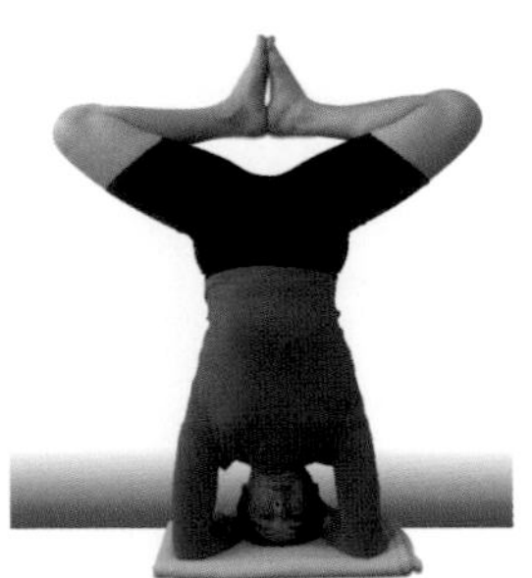

6 Baddha Konasana in Shirshasana, *page 234*

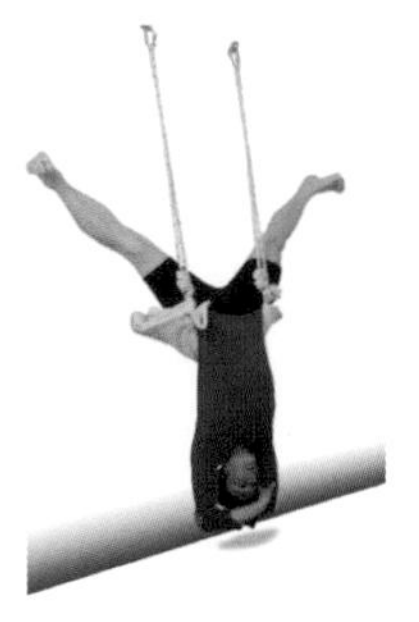

7 Shirshasana (wall ropes), *page 240*

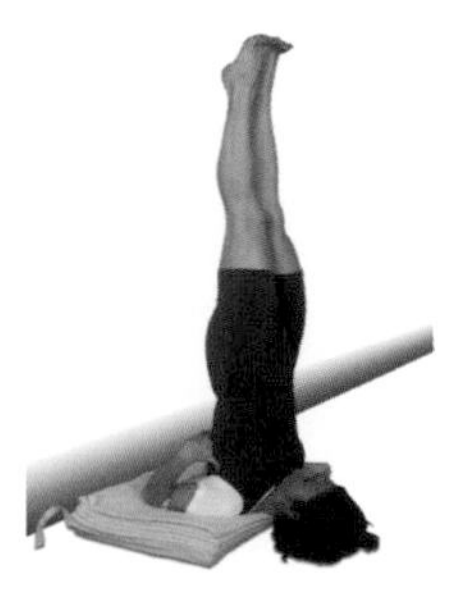

8 Salamba Sarvangasana, from the Wall, *page 326*
or From Ardha Halasana (toes on table), *page 332*

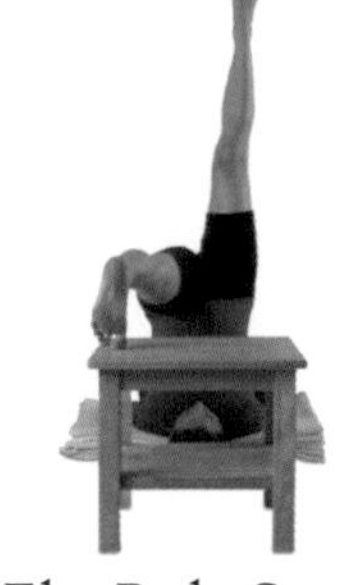

9 Ardha Eka Pada Sarvangasana, *page 222*

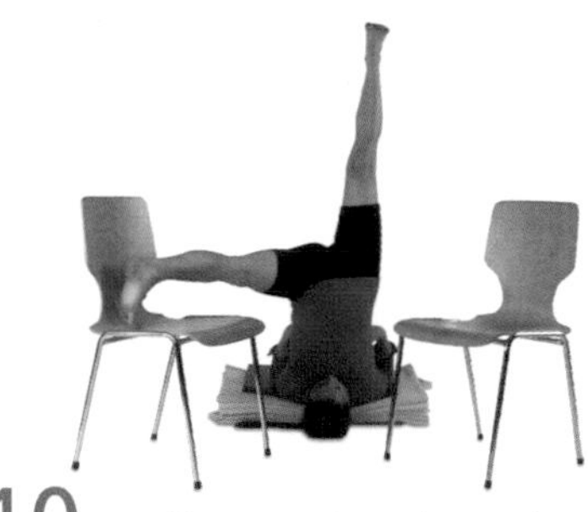

10 Ardha Parshvaikapada Sarvangasana, *page 223*

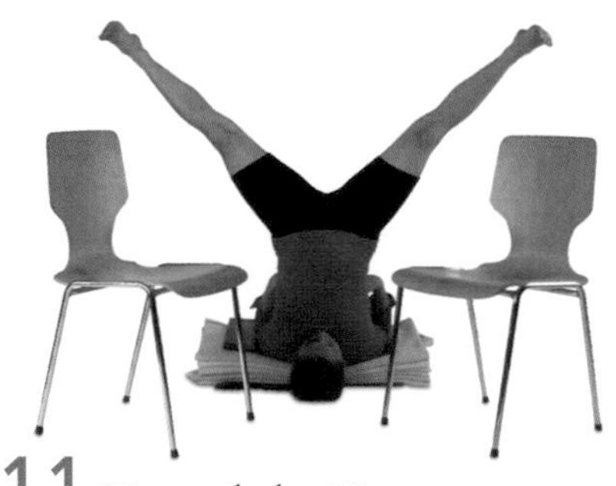

11 Upavishtha Konasana in Sarvangasana, *page 224*

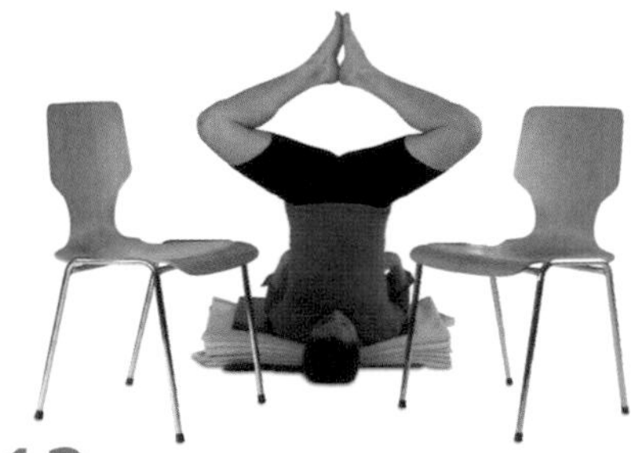

12 Baddha Konasana in Sarvangasana, *page 225*

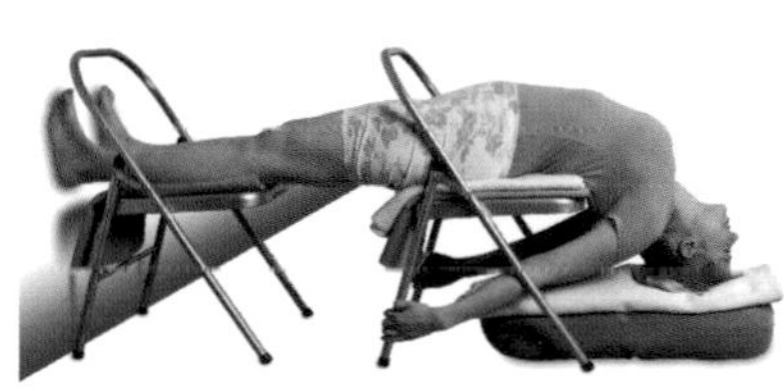

13 Dvi Pada Viparita Dandasana (with 2 chairs), *page 237*

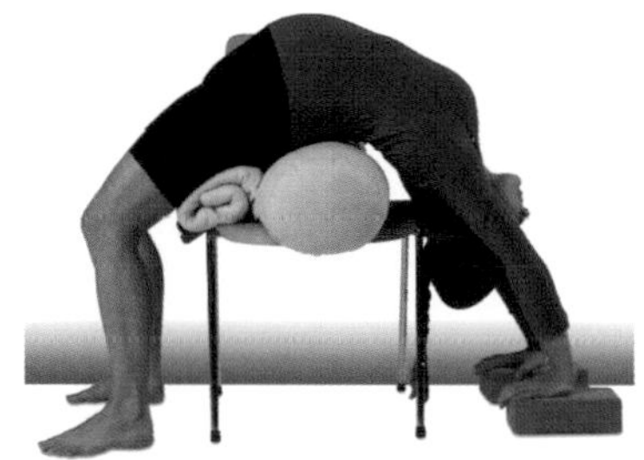

14 Urdhva Dhanurasana (chair, blocks, and wall), *page 239*

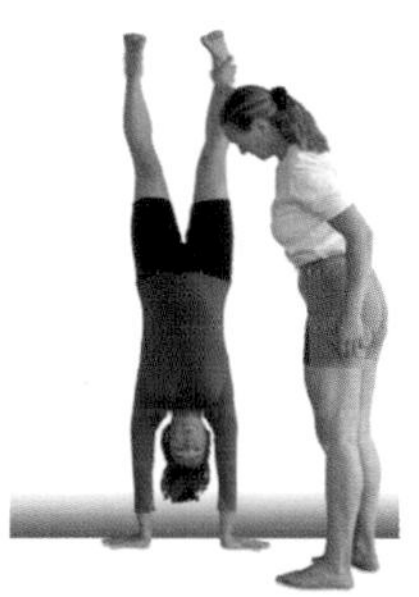

15 Adho Mukha Vrikshasana (wall and helper), *page 226*

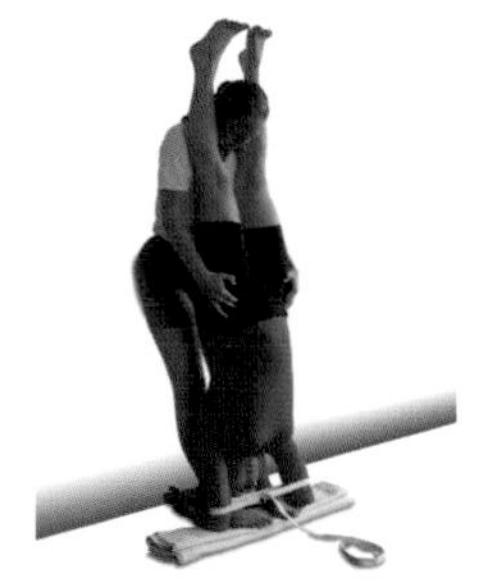

16 Pichcha Mayurasana (wall and helper), *page 228*

Note

You can practice the pranayama separately, in the morning or in the evening at bedtime, *page 210*.

Chapter 5

Sequence for Third Trimester, Preparing for Delivery

See Part II, Chapter 4, page 187, "Sequence for the Third Trimester, Preparing for Delivery"

Instructions and Benefits

Be sure to follow the "General Rules" and "Cautions" sections in Chapter 3, pages 28 – 30.

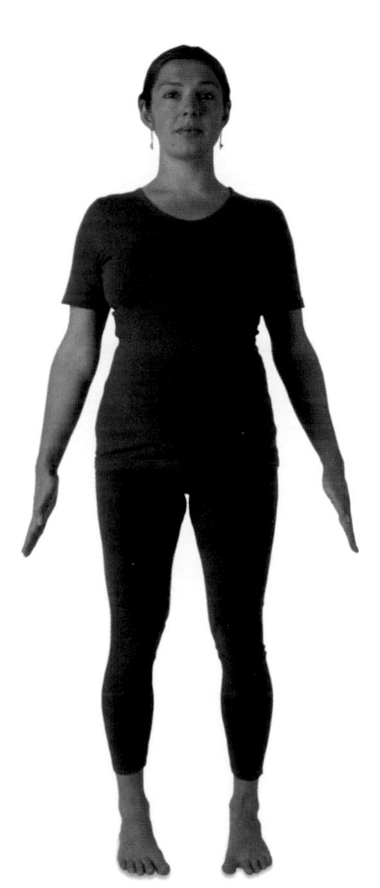

Standing Asanas
Uttishtha Sthiti

Follow the instructions as in Chapter 3 with the following notes:

- Virabhadrasana 1 and 3: Don't practice these in the first trimester.
- Tadasana: Practice with your feet together in the first trimester.

Uttanasana
Intense forward stretch pose

1st trimester: yes
2nd trimester: no
3rd trimester: no

This is the third of the asanas in the chain for before and after Shirshasana.

The technique below is modified for your first trimester only; it must be modified further for advancing pregnancy.

1 Stand in Tadasana (page 32).

2 Tighten your knees, stretch both legs, and lift both arms in Urdhva Baddhanguliyasana in Tadasana (page 34). Loosen your grip and stretch your arms up towards the ceiling in Urdhva Hastasana (page 35), palms facing forward. Take one or two breaths.

3 Extend your spine, exhale, and bend your torso forward.

4 Rest your palms on the floor by the sides of your feet. Stretch your torso forward by keeping your head up and your spine concave. Take one or two breaths.

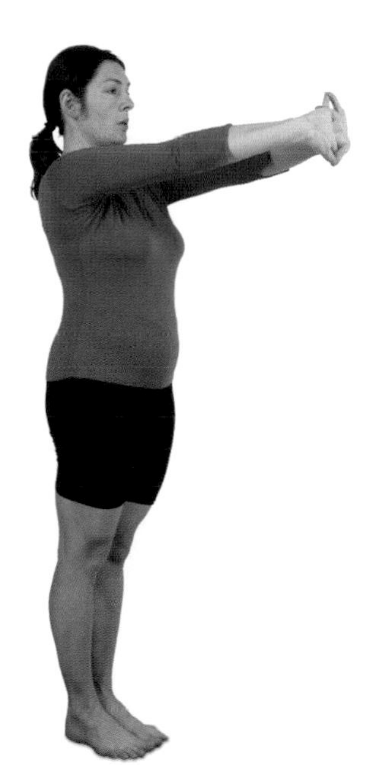

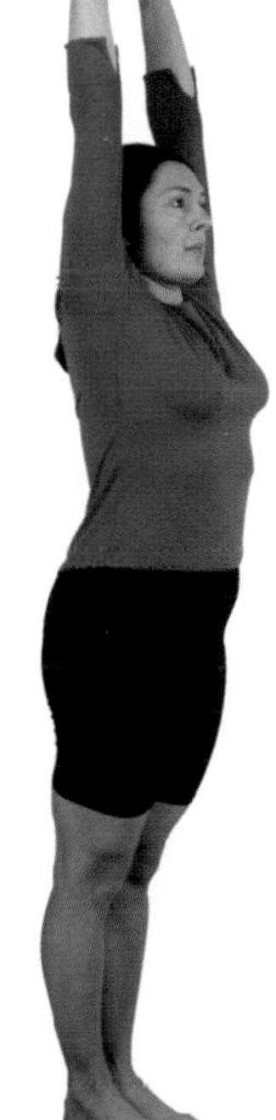

CHECK YOURSELF
> *Extend your bottom ribs and the back of your torso. Make sure your back is concave. Lift your abdomen and the front of your torso.*
> *Extend the sides of your torso.*
> *Inhale, maintain the space in your sides and chest, and come back to Tadasana.*

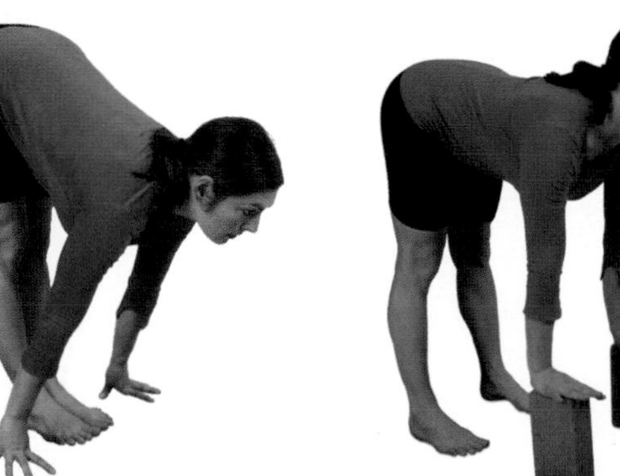

Modify with advancing pregnancy

Adho Mukha Shvanasana
Downward-facing dog pose

1st trimester: yes
2nd trimester: yes
3rd trimester: yes

This asana is the second in the chain of asanas to be performed before Shirshasana, coming after Maha Mudra. It is important in the chain because it is designed to do away with fatigue.

Adho means "downward," *mukha* means "face," and *shvana* means "dog." This asana resembles a dog stretching with its head down.

You can practice the asana with or without the wall ropes shown in the photo.

As your pregnancy progresses and your abdomen gets heavier, you may find that this asana puts too much pressure on your hands. In this case, we suggest that you try the modifications found in Chapter 3, page 62.

1 Stand in Tadasana (page 32).

2 Exhale and come down to Uttanasana (page 213).

3 Place your palms on the floor next to and in line with the sides of your feet.

4 Bend your knees and place your legs 4 to 4$^1/_2$ feet back, one by one. Keep your hands and feet 1 to 1$^1/_2$ feet apart. Spread your palms and extend your fingers. Keep your feet parallel and extend your toes.

Note
As your pregnancy advances, you should keep your feet farther apart.

5 Stretch your thighs backward and pull your kneecaps in. Put your heels on the floor or onto a slanted plank. Take one or two breaths.

6 Exhale, stretch your arms and legs, and push your thighs back. Move your torso towards your legs.

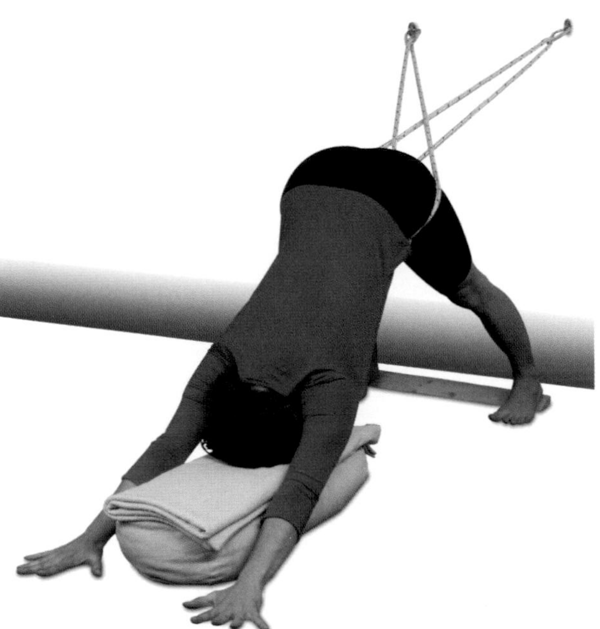

7 Press your heels into the floor and place the crown of your head on the floor, or on a bolster.

8 Remain in this final position for 15 to 20 seconds, breathing normally.

Coming out of the pose
Maintaining the space in your spine and the strength in your arms and legs, inhale, lift your head off the ground, bring your feet near your palms, and come to Tadasana.

CHECK YOURSELF
> *Don't bend your knees.*
> *Tuck your shoulder blades in and broaden your chest.*
> *Lock your elbows.*
> *Pressurize and extend your index fingers and thumbs.*
> *Keep your outer feet parallel.*
> *Keep your inner ankles lifted.*
> *Stretch your inner thighs and inner knees back.*
> *Relax your diaphragm and throat.*

Sitting Asanas
Upavishtha Sthiti

Follow the instructions as in Chapter 3, pages 64 – 75, with the following note:

- Dandasana and Urdhva Hasta Dandasana: Don't practice these in the first trimester for longer than five seconds. Just use them to go from one sitting pose to the next or to change sides.

Forward Bends
Pashchima Pratana Sthiti

For detailed descriptions of the forward bend asanas that don't appear below, see Chapter 3, pages 76 – 90.

Maha Mudra
The great seal pose

1st trimester: yes
2nd trimester: yes
3rd trimester: yes

Maha Mudra is a mudra in Janu Shirshasana. This asana is the first in the chain to be performed before Shirshasana (and after it in reverse order). The asana chain is intended to strengthen the spine for Shirshasana.

What is Maha Mudra?
Maha means "great" or "noble," and *mudra* means "lock," "seal," or "the act of sealing or closing." In this pose, the main openings of the body are sealed. One leg is bent near the lower abdomen, and the other is stretched out. The straightened foot is held with the palms or a belt, and the spine is raised by keeping the head down, thereby closing the throat, anus, and vagina—sealing the body at both the ends.

The spine and the abdomen are lifted by gripping and pulling the foot, which gives the spine a firm support and helps it in its upward stretch.

Maha Mudra practices lifting the spine with support and controlling the contraction of the abdominal organs.

1 Sit in Dandasana (page 64).

2 Keep your left leg straight, bend your right knee, place the outer sides of your thigh and calf on the floor, and bring your heel close to the perineum. Your bent leg should be at a right angle to the extended one.

3 Extend your arms and hook your left big toe with the thumbs and the index and middle fingers of both hands.

4 Straighten both arms at the elbows.

5 Grip your toe well to lift up your torso and extend your spine (*see "Help" below*). Raise your torso further by maintaining your grip and pressing your thighs to the floor.

6 Lower your head from the nape of your neck until your chin rests in the notch between your collarbones.

7 Relax your head and forehead. Don't constrict your throat while you lower your head.

Here, what is known as Jalandhara Bandha occurs. *Jalan* means "net," and *bandha* means "bondage" or "binding." In Jalandhara Bandha, the neck and the throat are contracted and the chin rests in the notch between the collarbones.

During the practice of asanas, mudras, or pranayama, the brain is made to bow down, reducing its dominance over the practitioner. This provides for a state of neutrality and makes breathing quiet and subtle.

CHECK YOURSELF

- *Exhale all the air in your lungs and then inhale fully. Lift your abdomen from its base to the diaphragm and stretch your spine upward.*
- *Remain in this final position for 3 to 5 seconds, holding your breath.*
- *Keep your chest expanded.*
- *Relax your eyes, forehead, tongue, and facial muscles.*
- *Don't tilt your body to one side.*
- *Increase the grip on your toe or foot to extend your spine.*
- *While exhaling, relax the abdominal tension without dropping your spine.*
- *Inhalation, retention, and exhalation complete one cycle; perform 5 to 8 cycles.*
- *After completing the cycles, raise your head, open your eyes, straighten your right leg, and come to Dandasana.*
- *Repeat the technique by keeping your right leg straight and bending your left knee.*
- *The retention of breath should be equal on both sides.*

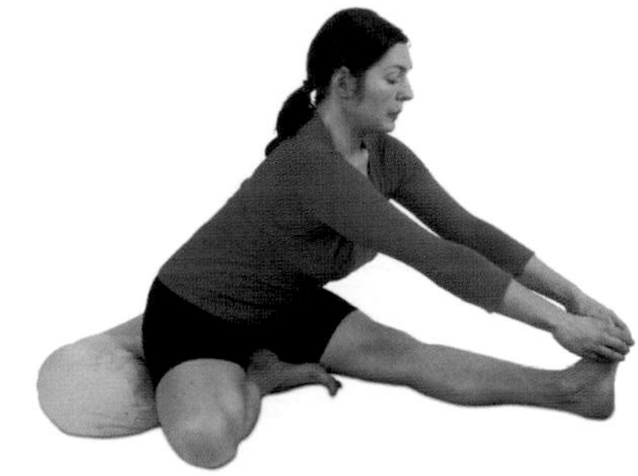

1st trimester advanced students

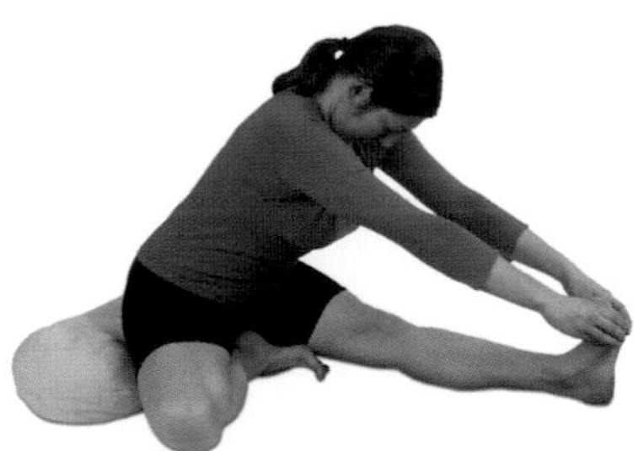

Help

In your first trimester, you should be able to grip your big toe. If you can't, then practice as in the second and third trimesters as shown in Chapter 3, page 79.

Janu Shirshasana

Head on knee pose, concave back

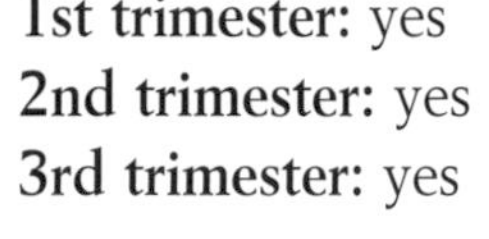

1st trimester: yes
2nd trimester: yes
3rd trimester: yes

1st Trimester

- Grip your foot with your hands and follow the details as given in Maha Mudra, pages 215 – 216, and in Chapter 3, pages 82 – 83.
- Your torso and leg should be at a 45° angle.

2nd and 3rd Trimesters

With the growth of the fetus, adjust the practice as in Chapter 3, pages 82 – 83.

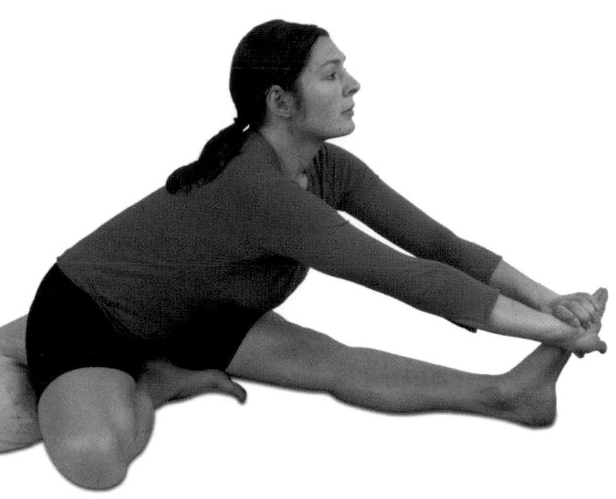

Pashchimottanasana

Intense west stretch pose, concave back

1st trimester: yes
2nd trimester: yes
3rd trimester: yes

Follow the instructions in Chapter 3, pages 87 – 88, with the following notes:

Benefits

See page 87

From the 14th week onward, you should keep your legs apart and:

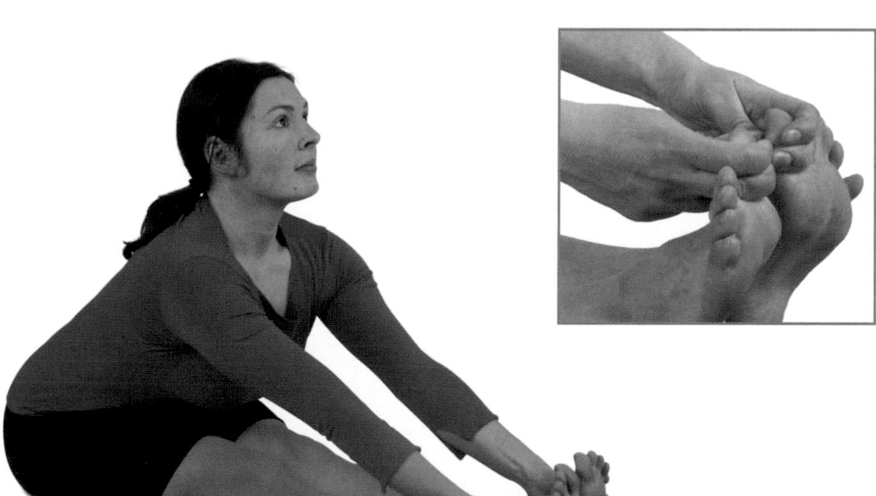

- Grip the outer edges of your feet

or

- Grip your big toes

Trianga Mukhaikapada Pashchimottanasana

Three limbs intense west stretch pose, concave back

1st trimester: yes
2nd trimester: yes
3rd trimester: no

Follow the instructions in Chapter 3, pages 89 – 90, with the following note: In the first trimester, grip the outer and inner edges of your feet with your hands.

Benefits

See page 89

Twists

Parivritta Sthiti

Follow the instructions in Chapter 3, pages 91 – 95, with the following note:

Because you're an advanced student, you can practice the twisting asanas in the first trimester.

Inversions

Viparita Sthiti

Salamba Sarvangasana

Shoulderstand pose

1st trimester: yes
2nd trimester: yes
3rd trimester: yes

Benefits

See page 103

Starting from the Wall and/or Chair

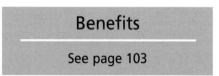

1 Have a belt ready in your right hand.

2 Lie flat on your back with your shoulders on the support and with your legs bent. Stretch your arms alongside your body. Keep your shoulders down and move them away from your head. Keep your palms facing down. Your head and neck should be in line with your spine. Stay in this position for a while, breathing normally.

3 Exhale, either go from the wall to the chair with straight legs to the chair (2nd and 3rd trimester) or go directly to the chair (1st trimester), and then bend your knees towards your chest, and put your toes on the chair.

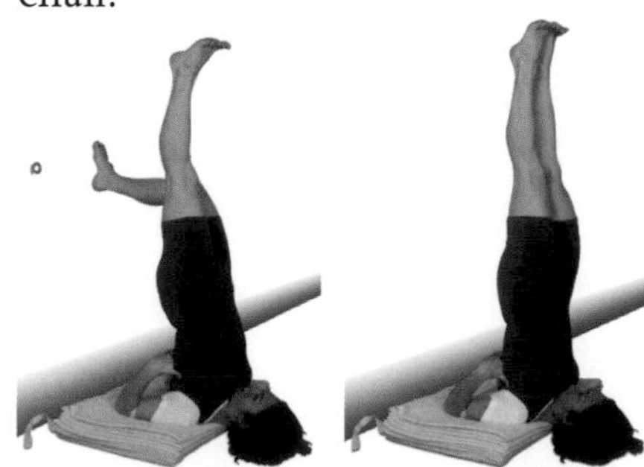

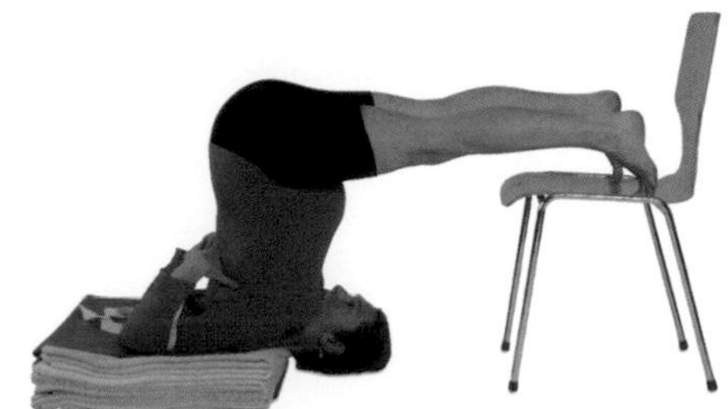

4 Press your hands down, and with a slight swing, raise your buttocks, waist, and hips. While stretching your knees, support your back with your hands and raise your torso. Take a breath.

5 Roll your shoulders away from your ears, extend your arms away from your shoulders, and bend your elbows and put a belt around them.

6 Once more, extend your arms, bend them, and press your hands into your back, lifting the sides of your torso upward. Keep your palms on your back with your thumbs pointing towards the front of your body and your fingers pointing towards your spine.

7 Lift one leg after the other up into Salamba Sarvangasana and tighten your leg and buttock muscles, so that your lumbar region (lower back) and tailbone remain tucked in. Straighten your legs towards the ceiling.

8 Stay in this final position for 5 minutes with normal breathing, and observe the following points:

- Press your palms and fingers into your back to straighten your whole body from armpits to toes.
- Don't allow your elbows to spread outward; keep them in as much as possible using the belt.
- Keep your shoulders back and away from the direction of your head. Move your upper arms towards each other.
- When you lift your body up, the top of your breastbone should touch your chin in Jalandhara Bandha. You should not choke, however; if you cough when lifting or lowering your body, it indicates pressure on the throat. Don't try to touch your chin to your breastbone; the action should be the reverse: Lift your chest in such a way that your breastbone touches your chin. Otherwise, the benefits of Sarvangasana are lost.
- If your chest is not properly lifted, you'll have difficulty breathing. If this happens, raise the support for your shoulders.
- Don't turn your head sideways to ease your breathing; broaden your chest and raise your torso.

Coming out of the pose

1 Exhale, slowly take your feet down one by one onto the chair, remove the belt, press your hands into your back, and gradually slide your buttocks and back downward without jerking your spine.

2 When you reach the floor, release your hands from your back, take your buttocks down to the floor, and straighten your legs.

Special Instructions

- For safety, first arrange your props, such as chairs and 3 or 4 blankets or other support. Start either from the wall or from Ardha Halasana.
- You can practice with a chair, as in the technique below, or independently.
- You can start from the floor during your first trimester, but only if you're sure it's completely safe.

End of the 2nd Trimester, 3rd Trimester

Keep your feet slightly apart, with the toes turning inward and the heels outward, in order to give more space to the abdomen.

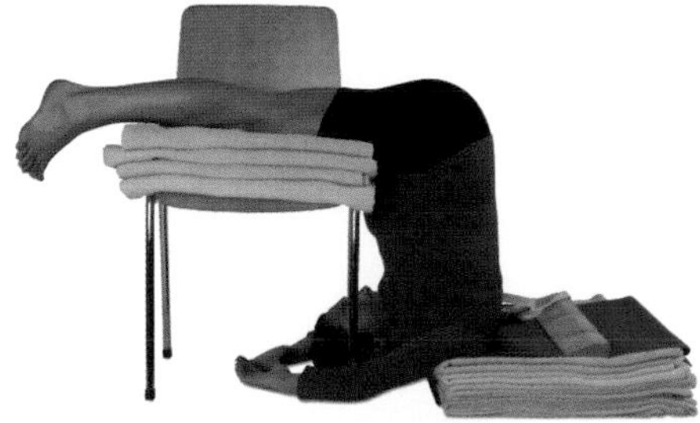

Help

If you can't press your elbows down, have a slanting plank or a rolled mat/blanket for under your elbows.

Variations of Salamba Sarvangasana

Ardha Halasana, the Plough

Half plough pose

Start in Salamba Sarvangasana with steps 1 to 3 (page 218), to the point where your toes are on the chair.

Continue:

1 Keeping your shins, knees, and thighs lifted, lift your spine and the sides of your torso.

2 Keep your arms stretched over your head or extended backward, or hold the edge of the blanket and press your arms down to raise your torso.

3 Stay for 3 to 5 minutes, breathing normally.

Coming out of the pose

1 Place your hands on your back, bend your knees, and move your buttocks back.

2 Lift your feet off the chair and carefully slide down.

1st trimester: yes
2nd trimester: yes
3rd trimester: yes (as long as comfortable)

Benefits

- Alleviates headaches and fatigue
- Soothes the brain and nerves
- Relieves hot flashes
- Helps treat menstrual and urinary disorders
- Reduces arthritis and stiffness of the shoulders and arms

Restorative Variation

Take a complete rest in this position with your upper and lower legs fully supported on the chair.

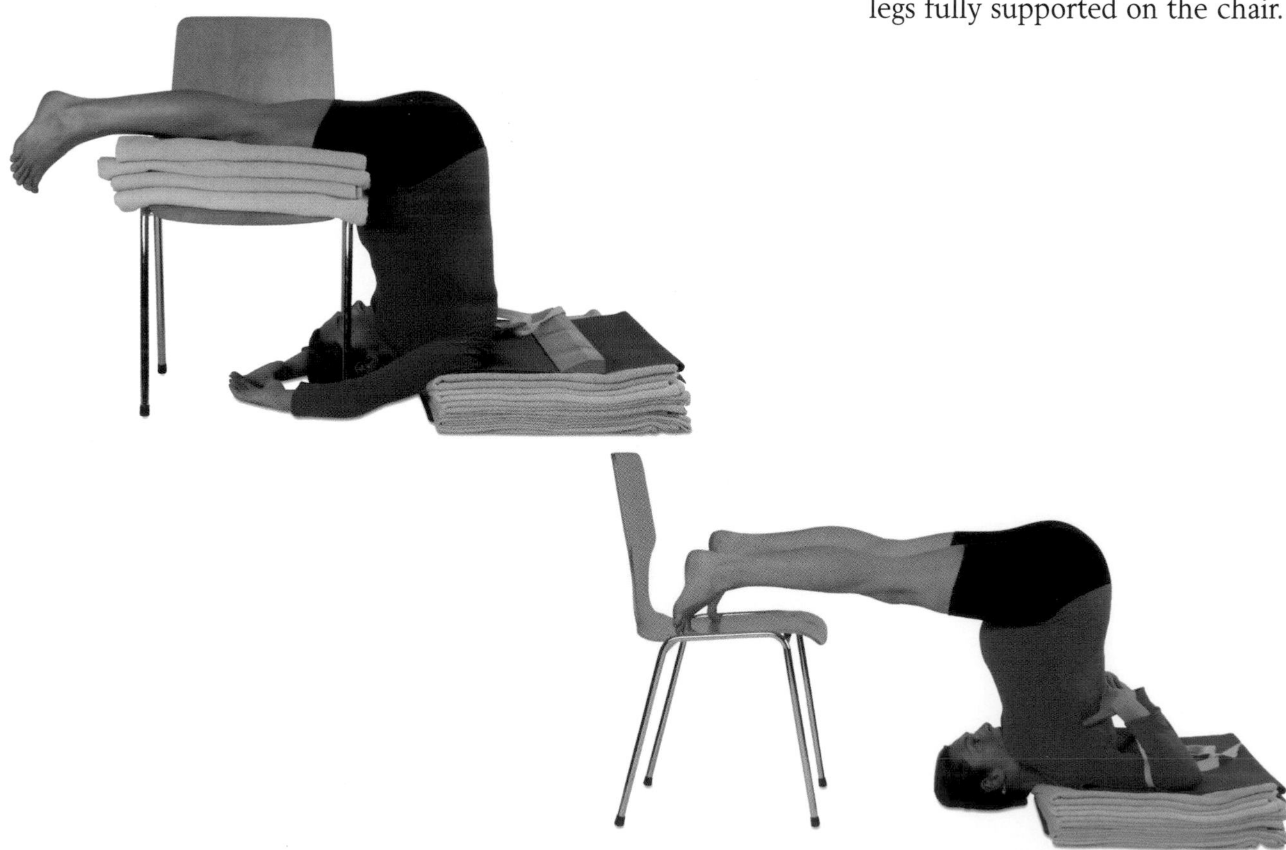

Ardha Supta Konasana

Half reclined angle pose

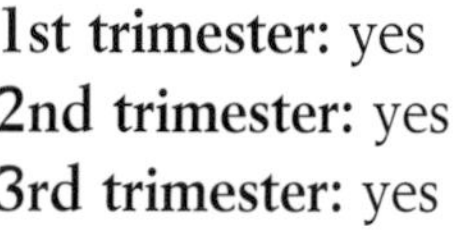

1st trimester: yes
2nd trimester: yes
3rd trimester: yes

Start in Salamba Sarvangasana (page 218) with steps 1 to 3, to the point where your toes are on the two chairs.

Continue:

1 Keeping your shins, knees, and thighs lifted, lift your spine and the sides of your torso.

2 Keep your arms stretched over your head or extended backward, or hold the edge of the blanket and press your arms down to raise your torso.

3 Stay for 3 to 5 minutes, breathing normally, and observing the following points:

- Keep your chest lifted.
- Raise your back and buttocks with the help of your hands on your back.
- Continue widening your legs further as your flexibility increases.
- Your feet should remain perpendicular to the floor and should not drop to the sides.

4 For maximum benefit, try to remain the entire 5 minutes.

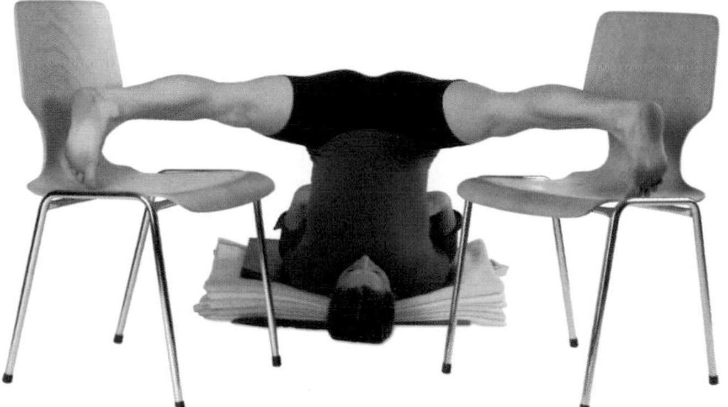

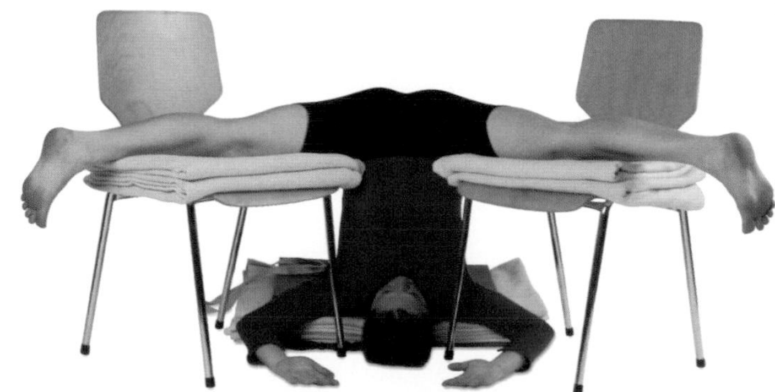

Benefits

Great help in treating kidney problems

Removes pain and heaviness in the uterus and corrects its position

Checks menstrual flow and vaginal discharge

Widens the pelvis

Coming out of the pose

1 Place your hands on your back, bend your knees, and bring your buttocks back.

2 Lift your feet off the chair and carefully slide down.

Restorative Variation

Take a complete rest in this position with your upper and lower legs fully supported on the chairs.

Ardha Eka Pada Sarvangasana
Half one-legged shoulderstand pose

1st trimester: yes
2nd trimester: yes
3rd trimester: yes (as long as it is comfortable)

Benefits

Relieves pain in the small of the back

Tones the back muscles

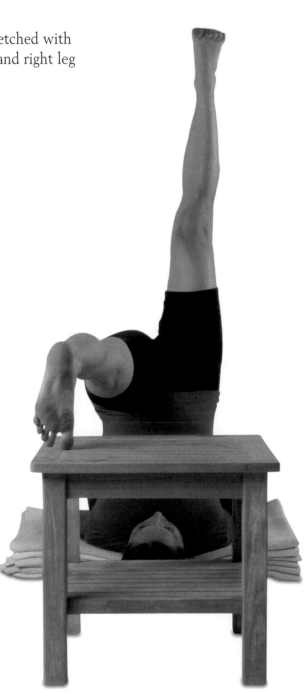

1 Begin in Sarvangasana (page 218).

2 Exhale and lower your right leg parallel to the floor. You can use a chair for your toes.

3 Keep both legs stretched with your left leg upward and right leg downward.

4 Stay in this final position for 10 to 15 seconds with normal breathing, observing the following points:

- Stretch your left leg from the groin upward.
- Pull your left knee and keep it taut.
- Your left foot should stay in line with your head and not tilt forward.
- Keep your chest expanded and your shoulder blades tucked in.

5 Exhale, lift your right leg, and come to Sarvangasana. Take one or two breaths.

6 Repeat the asana on the other side.

Ardha Parshvaika Pada Sarvangasana
Half side one foot shoulderstand pose

1st trimester: no
2nd trimester: yes
3rd trimester: yes (as long as it is comfortable)

1 Begin in Sarvangasana (page 218).

2 Exhale and bring your left leg sideways to the left, as much as possible in line with your left shoulder and parallel to the floor. Place your toes on a stool or chair, or if you feel strong enough, keep your leg parallel to the floor.

3 Stay in this position for 10 to 15 seconds, breathing normally and observing the following points:
- Keep your right leg upright and stretch it from the groin; don't allow it to sway to the right.
- Don't bend your left knee.
- Lift your waist and tighten your buttocks up.
- Don't allow your left buttock to sag.

4 Exhale, raise your left leg to Sarvangasana, and place it near your right leg. Stay in Sarvangasana and take a few breaths.

5 Repeat the asana on the other side. From there, maintain the lift and come back to Sarvangasana.

Benefits
Circulates blood in the pelvic organs, which keeps them toned and healthy
Relieves backache
Alleviates tailbone pain

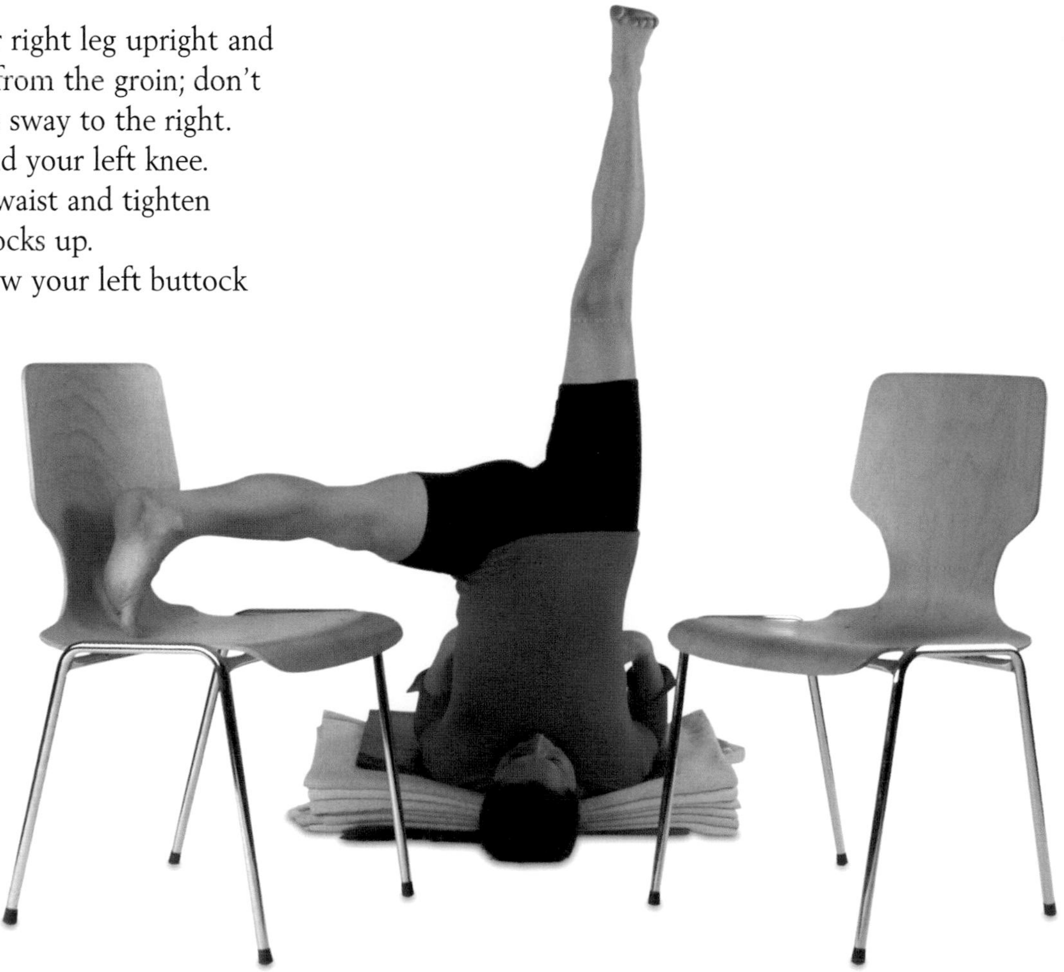

Upavishtha and Baddha Konasana in Sarvangasana

These two asanas can be practiced throughout your pregnancy and remain wonderfully helpful up to the last days.

Upavishtha Konasana in Sarvangasana (also called Prasarita Pada Sarvangasana)

Upward angle shoulderstand pose

1st trimester: yes
2nd trimester: yes
3rd trimester: yes

Kona means "corner" or "angle." In this asana, the legs are spread in an upward movement.

1 Begin in Sarvangasana (page 218) and spread your legs apart from the groin.

2 Tighten your thighs and lift your buttock muscles, extending your legs towards your feet. Stretch the back of your torso and spine. Don't bend your knees. Keep your toes in line with your knees and stretch them.

3 Stay in this final position for 15 to 20 seconds, breathing normally.

4 Proceed directly to the next asana.

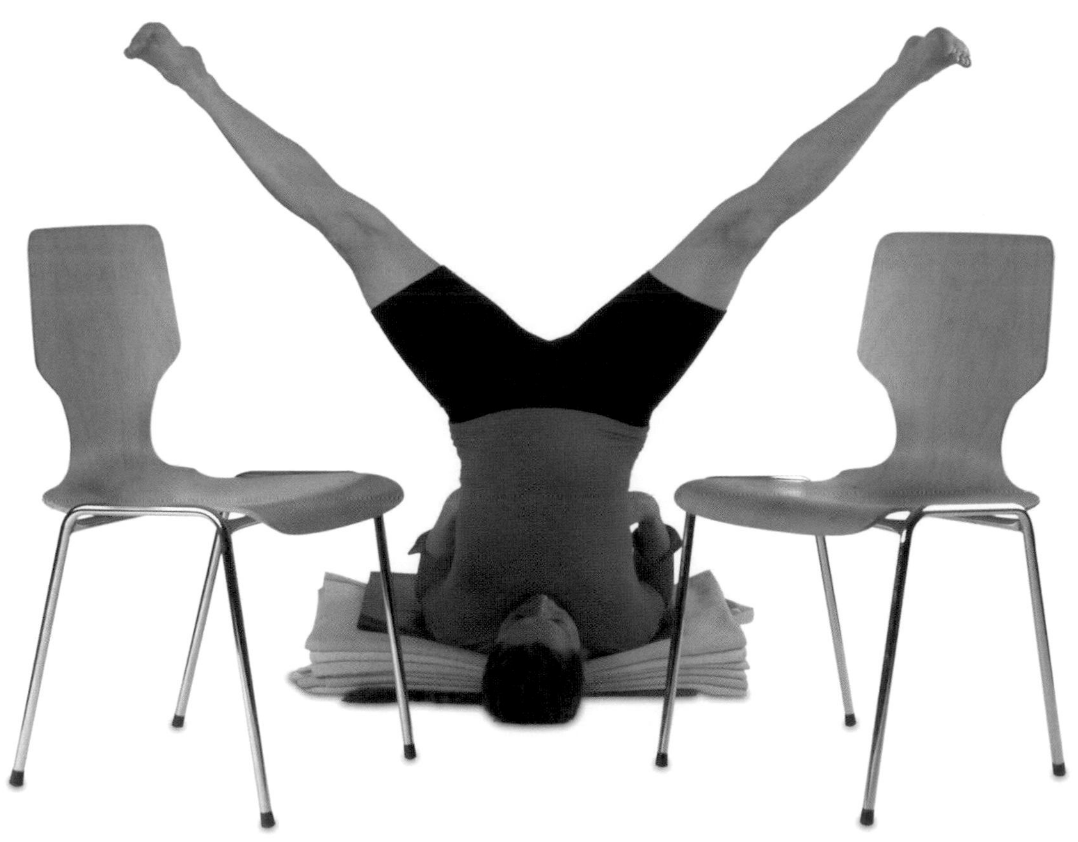

Baddha Konasana in Sarvangasana
Bound angle shoulderstand pose

1st trimester: yes
2nd trimester: yes
3rd trimester: yes

Baddha means "caught" or "restrained." In this asana, the knees are bent outward and the feet are together.

1 Bend your legs, spreading your knees outward and bringing your feet together with the soles, heels, and toes as in Namaste.

2 Breathing normally, remain in this final position for 15 to 20 seconds, observing the following points:
- Keep your knees wide apart.
- Press your soles firmly together.
- Keep your hips up.

3 Spread your legs to Upavishtha Konasana and close them to Sarvangasana.

Benefits

These two asanas are a gift to women. They give: reduced discharge, and after pregnancy, regulated menstrual flow

Invaluable help with urinary disorders

A healthy stretch to the groin and thighs

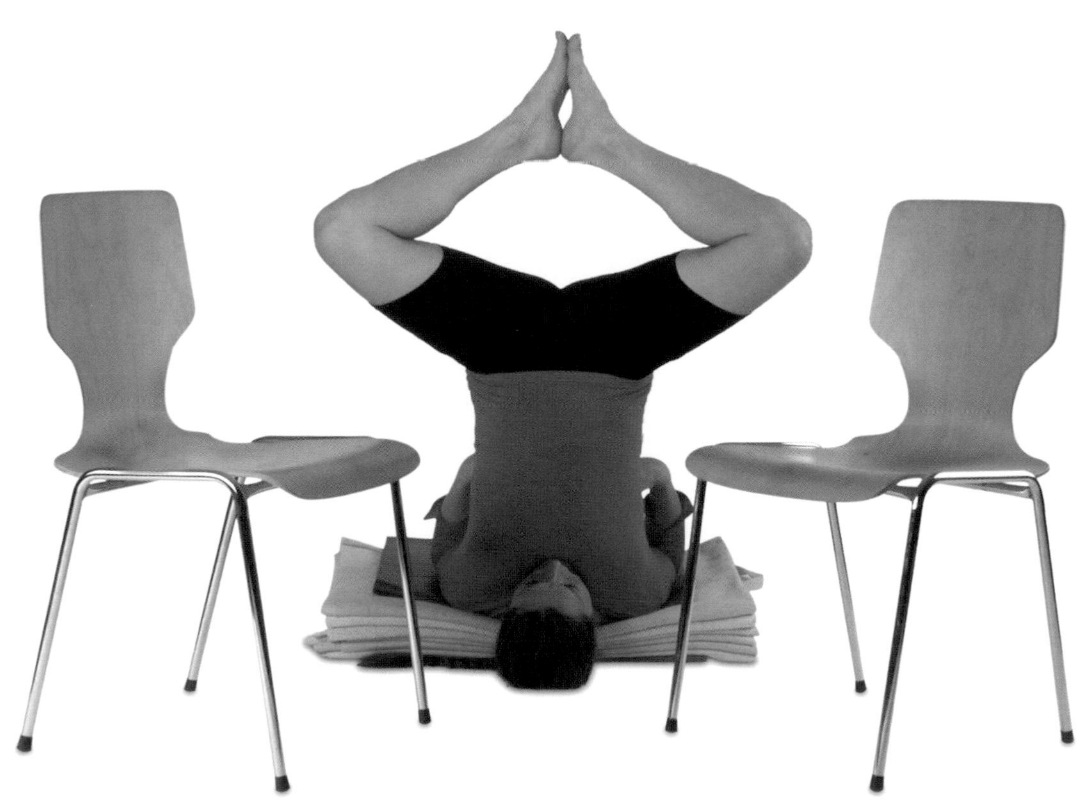

Adho Mukha Vrikshasana, with Teacher/Helper

Downward-facing handstand pose

In this asana, be sure not to jump.

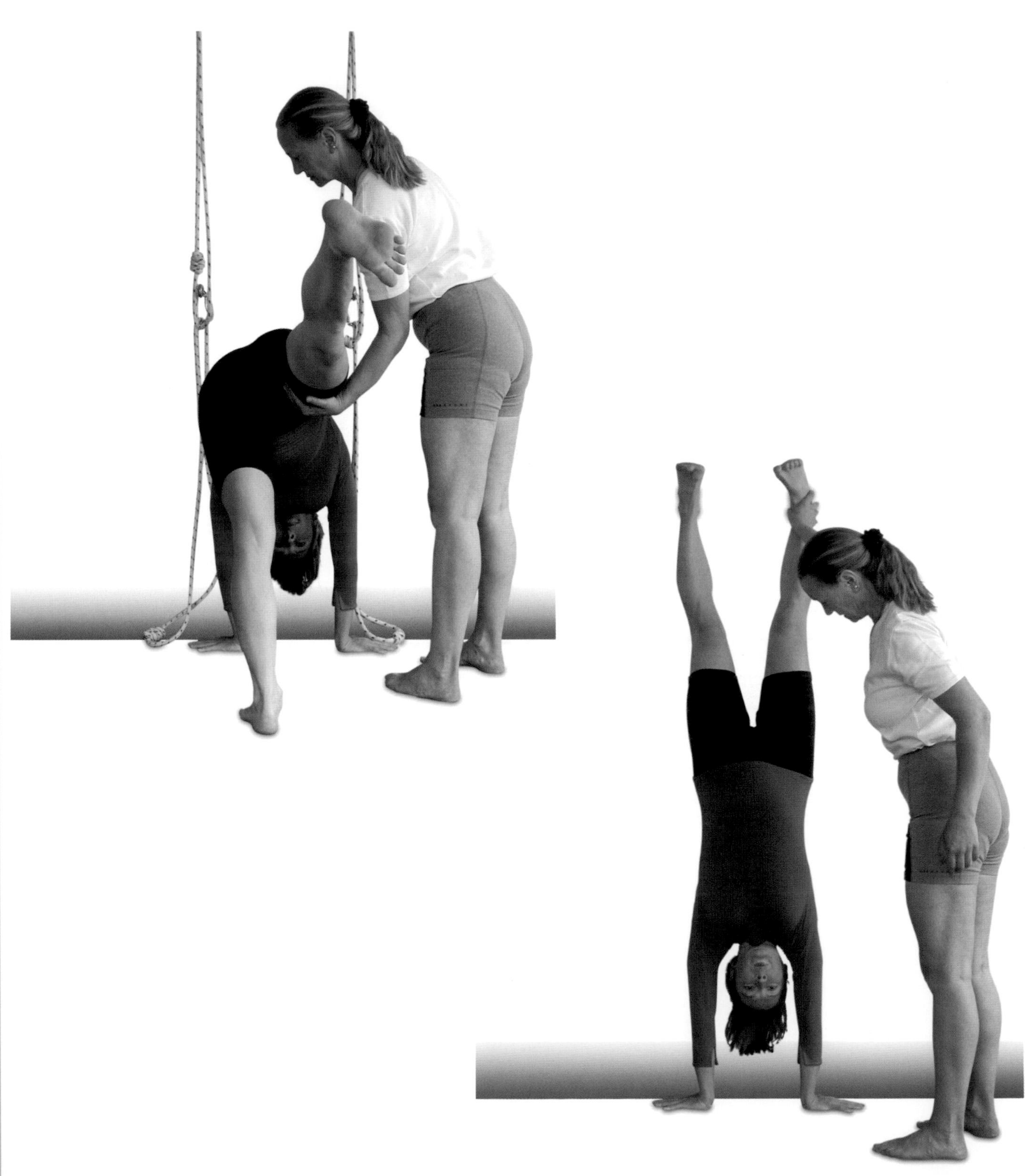

Adho Mukha Vrikshasana, with Ropes
Downward-facing handstand pose

With rope support, you can do this asana almost independently. Measure the length of the wall ropes and the distance to the floor to make sure that you can easily reach the floor and push up. Take care that your hips do not slip from the rope.

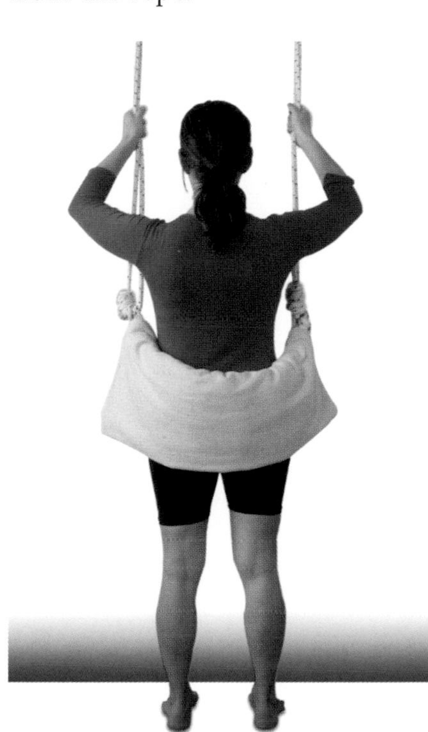

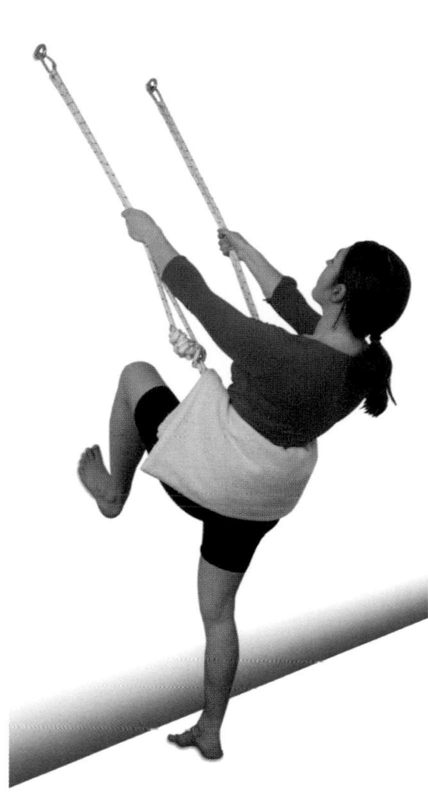

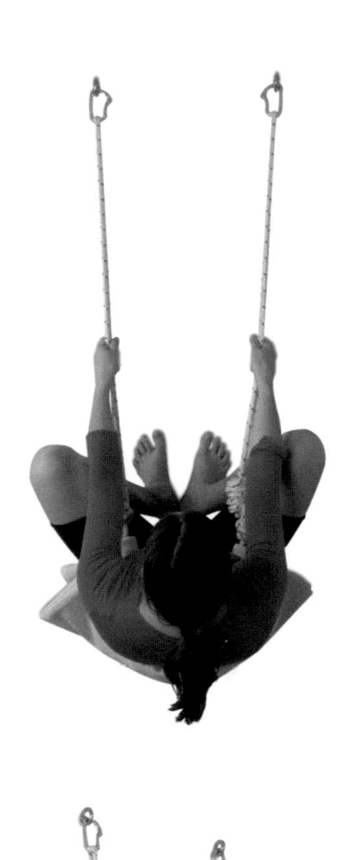

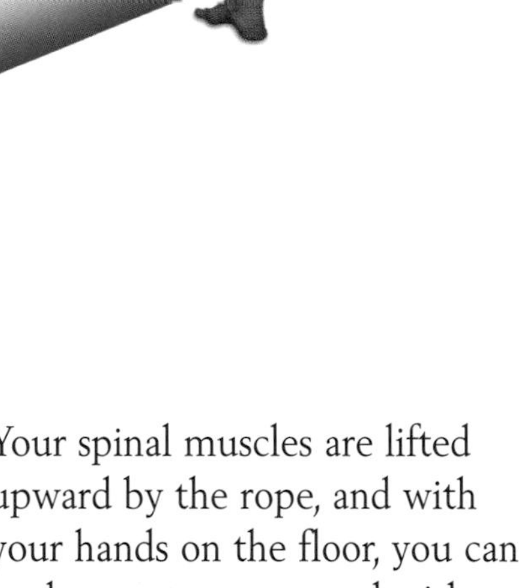

Your spinal muscles are lifted upward by the rope, and with your hands on the floor, you can push your torso upward without bearing too much weight.

Coming out of the pose
By reversing the way you entered it.

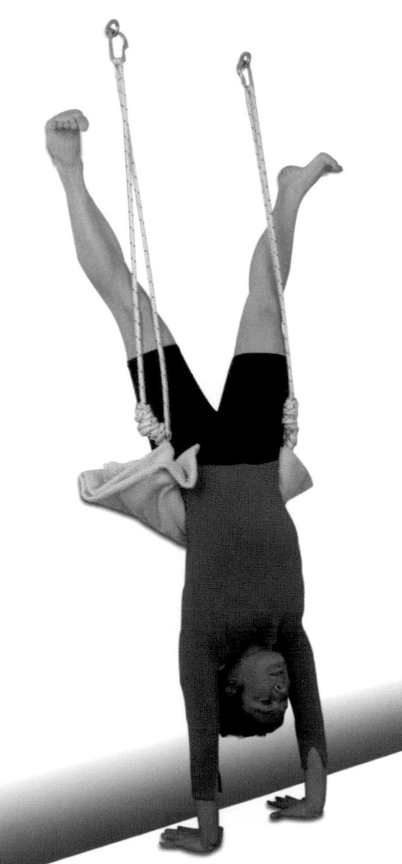

Pichcha Mayurasana, with Teacher/Helper

Forearm balance pose

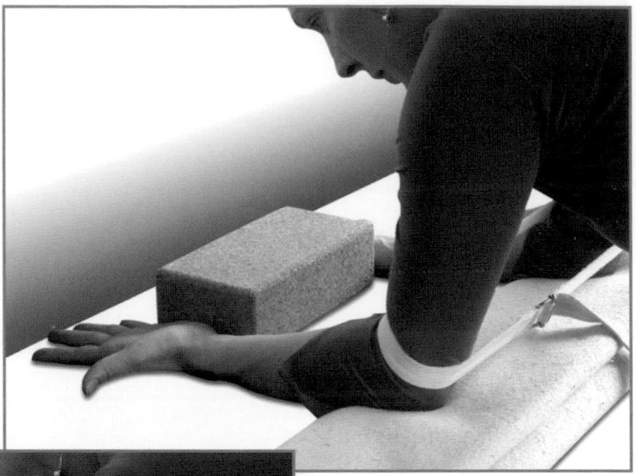

Practice this asana only with a teacher or helper, to make sure that you **do not jump at all!**

Pichcha means "tail" or "feather", *Mayur* means "peacock".

Have a block for your hands, a belt for your elbows and a support for them such as a rolled sticky mat or slanted plank, and a sticky mat for your lower arms.

Turn your hands and open your palms so that they face the ceiling. This opens your chest.

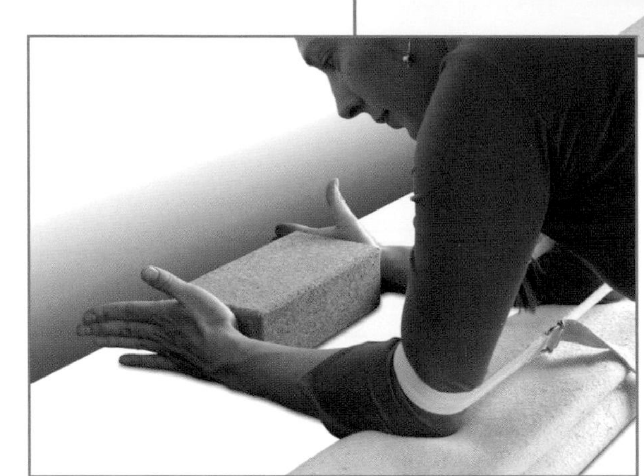

Maintain the wideness of your chest, turn your palms, and hold the block with your wrists and palms.

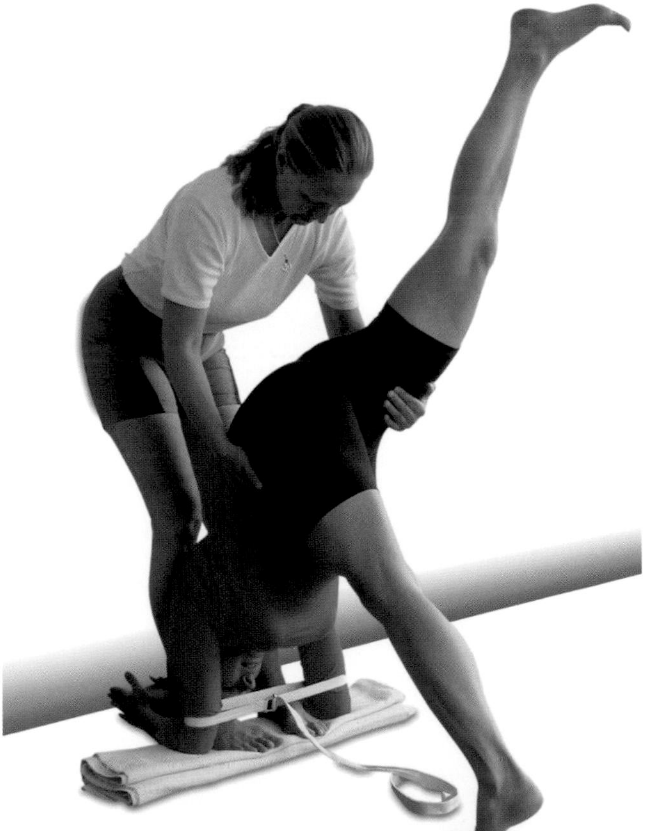

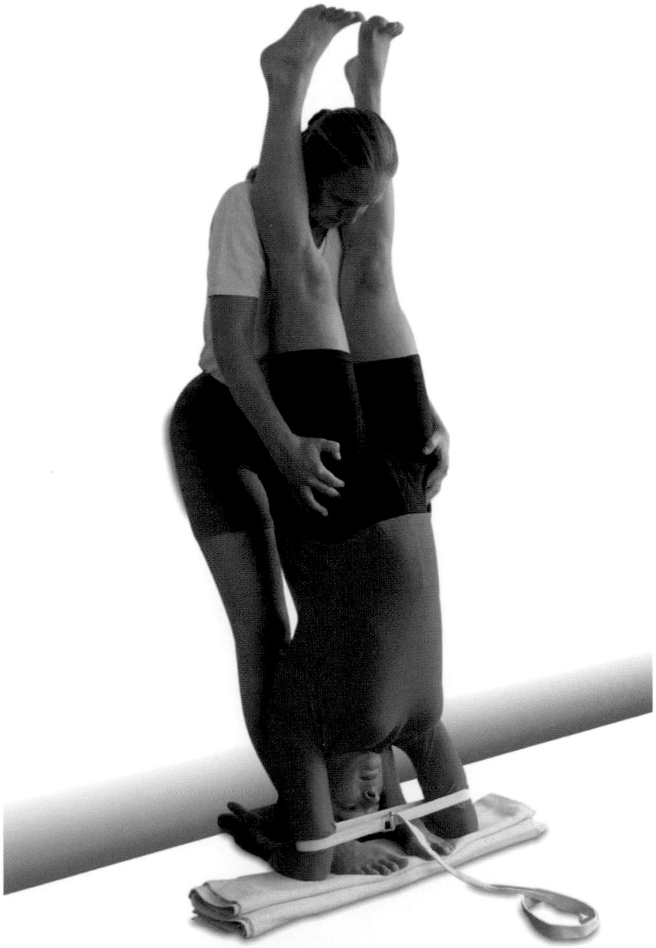

Salamba Shirshasana
Headstand pose

The description of Salamba Shirshasana in Chapter 3, page 97, explains how you can practice at the intersection of two walls. If you are confident and experienced enough, however, you can do it without props: lift your back and put your legs up in a bent position, or lift your straight legs one after the other and maintain your balance. Don't lift both straight legs at the same time from Urdhva Dandasana.

As you perform Shirshasana, keep your lumbar spine in an ascended state. You're likely to take it in because of the weight of your abdomen, so be sure to bring it back out, which keeps your abdominal muscles soft. This also ensures that the muscles below the pelvic girdle don't get inflated or tightened. Keep your torso lifted, so that your spinal muscles don't collapse.

Remember to perform the chain for before and after Salamba Shirshasana:

- Before: Maha Mudra, Adho Mukha Shvanasana, and Uttanasana (concave back)
- After, reverse order: Uttanasana, Adho Mukha Shvanasana, and Maha Mudra

1st Trimester

Your legs can be held up together. In fact, this is beneficial at this stage of your pregnancy because it helps build up strength in the muscles.

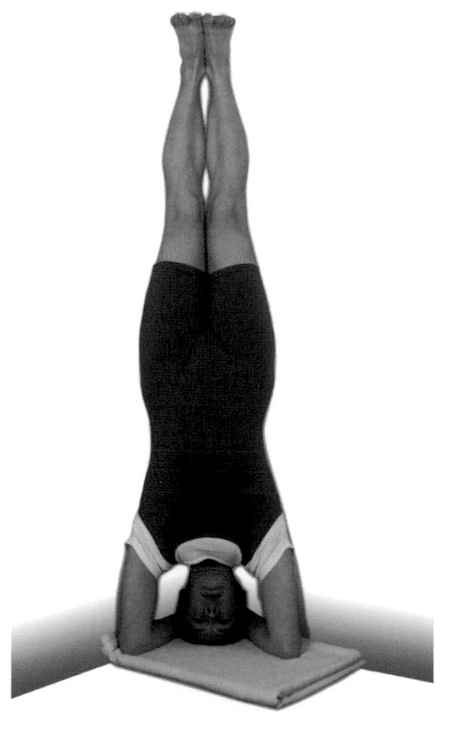

2nd Trimester

As the fetus grows, you should vary the positioning of your legs: keep your toes together and your heels apart. This helps hold the thighs together and helps support the waist muscles in ascending.

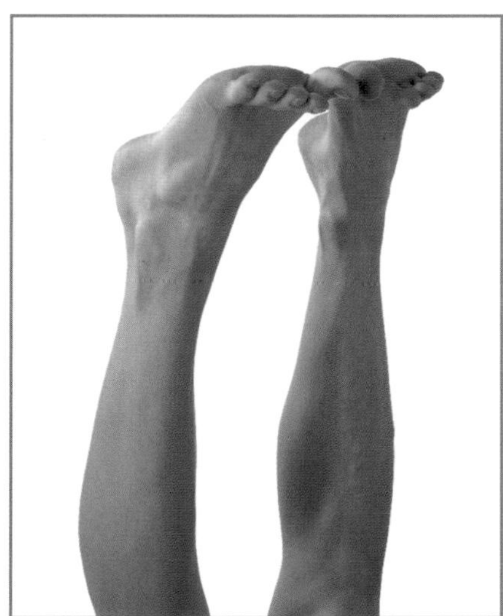

3rd Trimester

You may find that you need to keep your thighs apart, too. Don't forget to keep your toes in and your heels apart as in the second trimester. This lets the outer thigh muscles roll inward, keeping the groin soft. Be sure that you keep your thighs lifted and ascending, to lessen the weight on your abdomen.

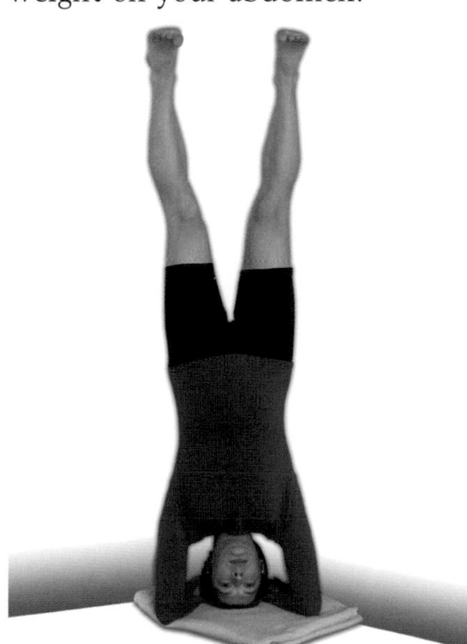

NOTE

With this positioning of your legs the descent of the placenta is stopped and the mouth of the uterus is kept closed.

Variations of Salamba Shirshasana

1st trimester: no
2nd trimester: yes
3rd trimester: yes

If you feel confident enough, you can continue your practice of Shirshasana with the variations below. All of these variations, in addition to their many other benefits, help to ease your delivery.

Parshva Shirshasana
Lateral headstand pose

1st trimester: no
2nd trimester: yes
3rd trimester: yes

Parshva means "side" or "flank." For more confidence and safety, practice this asana against a wall.

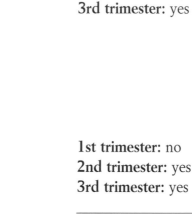

1 Begin in Shirshasana (page 229). Exhale and turn your torso to the right. Don't move your head, neck, or arms.

2 Stay in this final position for 10 to 15 seconds, breathing normally, and observing the following points:

- Your body should revolve on its own axis and stay perpendicular to the floor when it turns; it should not tilt.
- Turn the left side of your torso more and more to the right, so that the right side revolves backward and the outer edge of your right foot touches the wall.
- Turn your body to the right from your hips to your feet, lifting your floating ribs.
- Keep your right leg and right buttock firm.
- Lift your shoulders and tuck in your shoulder blades.

3 Exhale, tighten your hip muscles, come to Shirshasana, turn to the left side, and come back to Shirshasana.

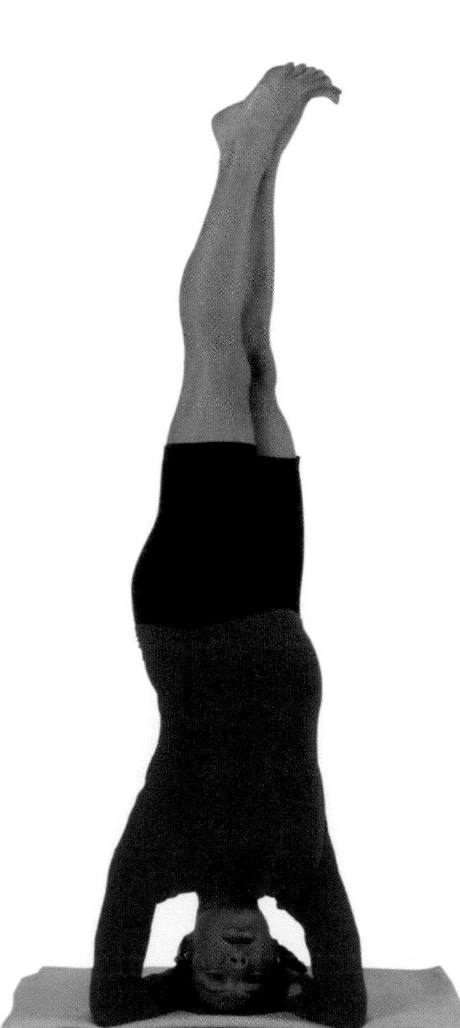

Benefits

- Strengthens the spine
- Relieves lower back pain
- Relieves bloated abdomen and constipation

Ardha Eka Pada Shirshasana
Half one-legged headstand pose

1st trimester: no
2nd trimester: yes
3rd trimester: yes

Benefits
Strengthens the spine, back, and abdomen
Aids digestion
Lessens feelings of heaviness

In this variation, you'll balance with one leg in Shirshasana and one leg down. Practice with your upper heel hooked on the wall.

1 Begin in Shirshasana (page 229). Stretch your legs from the hip joint upward and keep them firm. Keep your torso lifted.

2 Hook your left heel on the wall, exhale, and lower your right leg to a 90° angle, parallel to the floor. Extend your soles.

3 Stay in this final position for 10 to 15 seconds, breathing normally. Because your upper heel is hooked on the wall, you'll be able to avoid:
- Bending your torso
- Shifting your balance
- The right side of your torso moving forward and the left side backward, causing your pelvis to tilt
- Dropping your collarbone
- Contracting your neck muscles

4 Inhale, lift your leg up, and change sides.

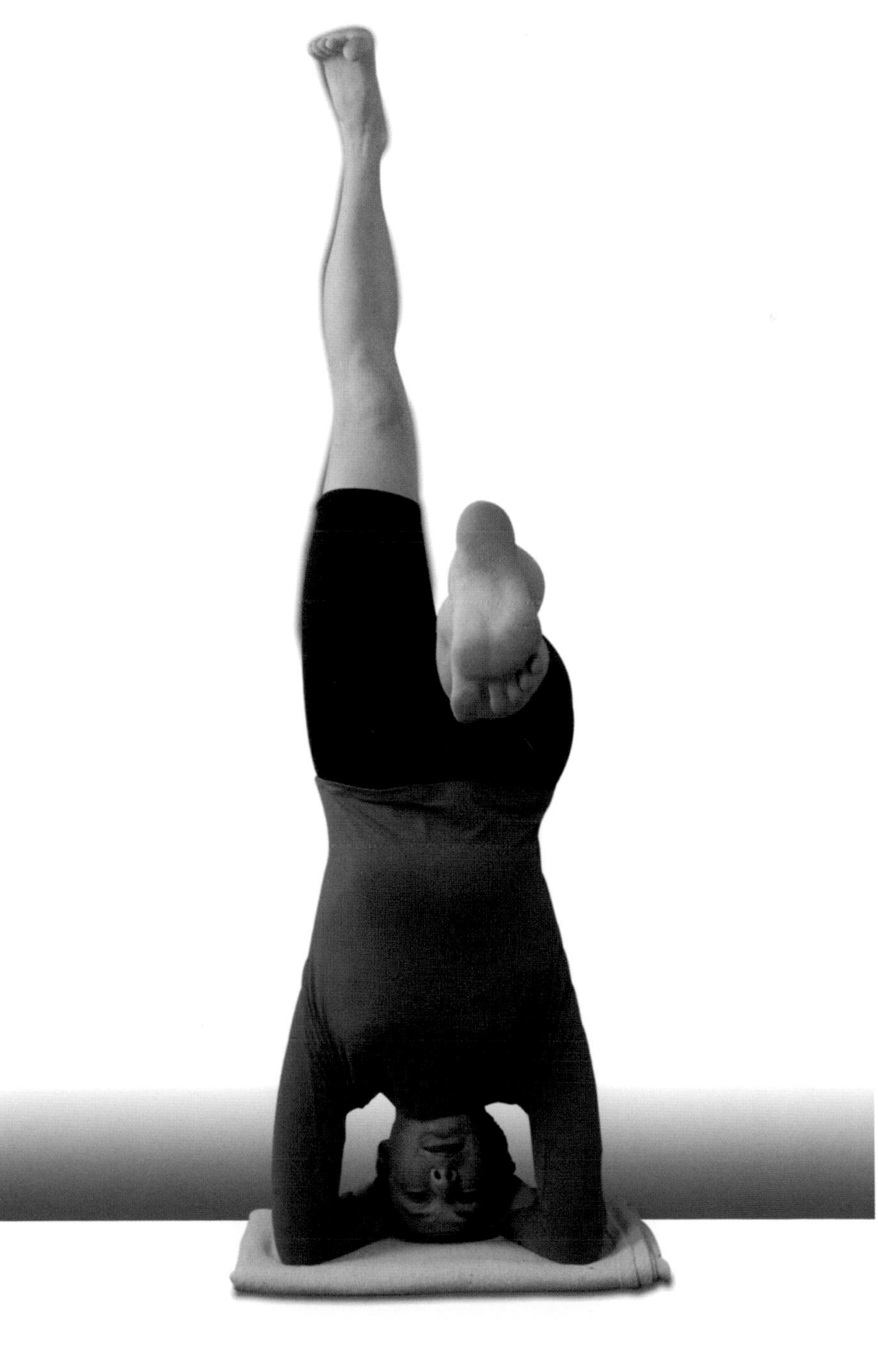

Ardha Parshvaikapada Shirshasana
Half sideways headstand pose

1st trimester: no
2nd trimester: yes
3rd trimester: yes

Benefits

Strengthens the spine and abdomen

Strengthens and activates the intestines

In this variation, one leg is lowered sideways in line with your shoulder.
For more confidence and safety, and to avoid a shift in balance, practice against the wall.

1 Begin in Shirshasana (page 229) and keep your legs firm. Hook your left heel on the wall and turn your right hip joint to the right so that your thigh-bone, knee, ankle, and foot turn to the right.

2 Exhale and lower your right leg sideways to a 90° angle, parallel to the floor and in line with your right ear.

3 Retain this final position for 10 to 15 seconds, breathing normally and observing the following points:
- Hook your upper heel on the wall to remain in the center.
- Don't bend your knees.
- Don't contract the back of the right side of your torso.
- Lift your right floating rib.
- Don't throw your body weight onto your right foot. If you find your eight off-balance, align the outer hip and outer heel of your left leg.

4 Exhale and raise your right leg to Shirshasana.

5 Repeat the asana on the left side and come back to Shirshasana.

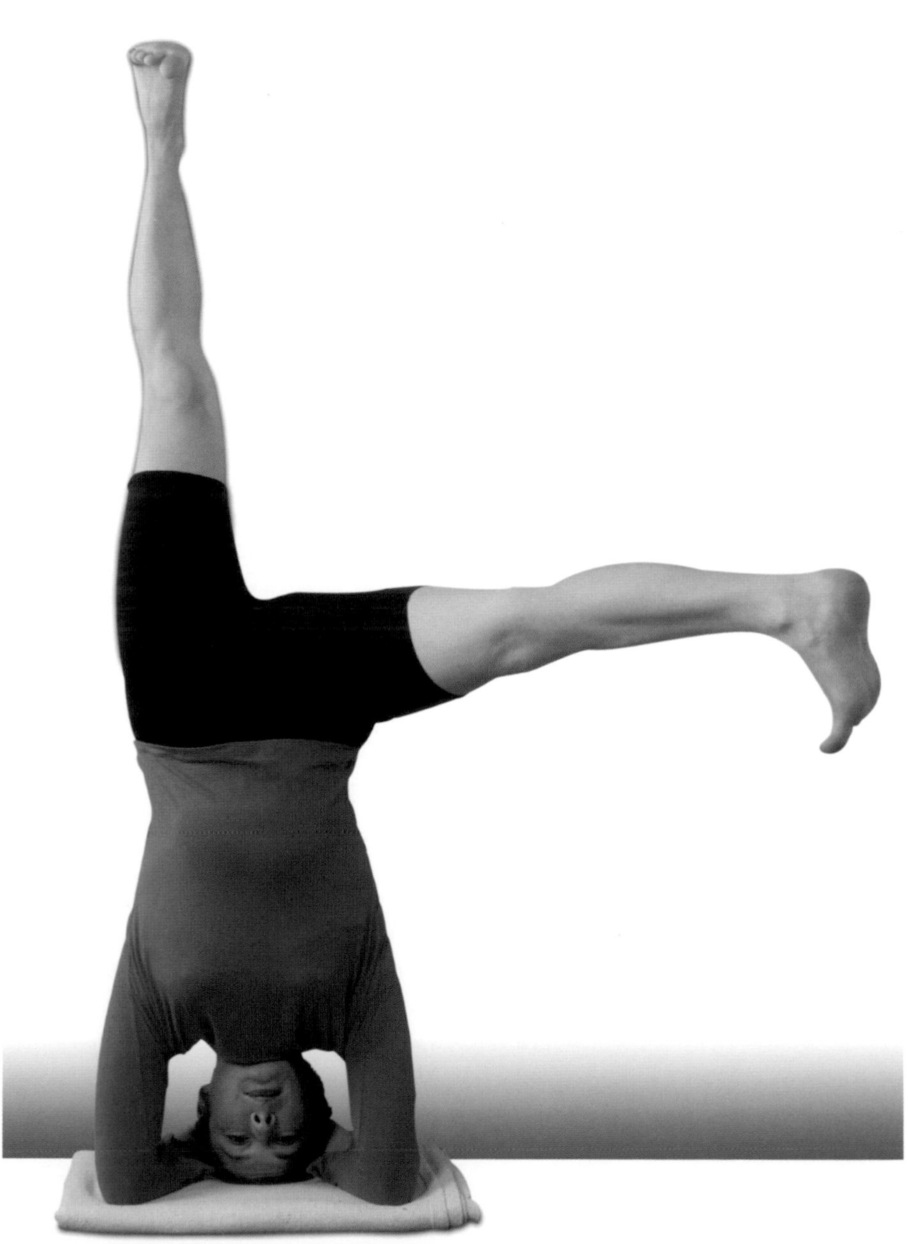

Upavishtha Konasana in Shirshasana (also called Prasarita Pada Shirshasana)
Upward angle headstand pose

1st trimester: no
2nd trimester: yes
3rd trimester: yes

Kona means "corner" or "angle." In this asana, the legs are spread as in Prasarita Padasana, but in an upward stretch.

This asana and Baddha Konasana in Shirshasana below are the highlights of the Shirshasana variations because of the wide range of benefits they provide during your pregnancy—right up to the last day.

For more confidence and safety, practice against the wall.

1 Begin in Shirshasana (page 229). Spread your legs apart from the groin and hook your heels on the wall.

2 Tighten your muscles inward, extending your legs towards your feet. Stretch your back and spine. Don't bend your knees. Keep your toes in line with your knees and stretch them.

3 Stay in this final position for 15 to 20 seconds, breathing normally.

4 Proceed directly to the next asana.

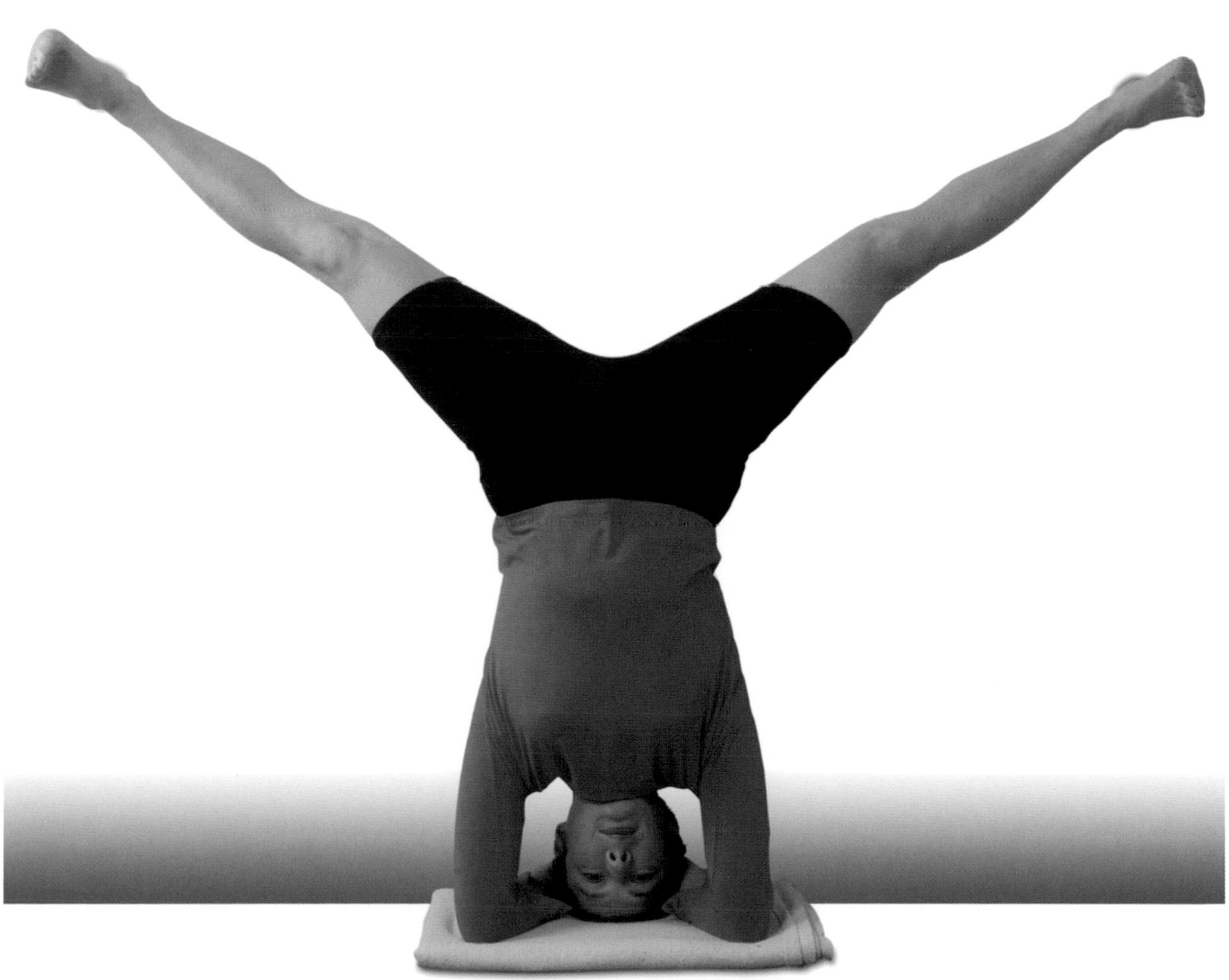

Baddha Konasana in Shirshasana
Bound angle headstand pose

1st trimester: no
2nd trimester: yes
3rd trimester: yes

Baddha means "caught" or "restrained." In this asana, the knees are bent outward and the feet are together.

Continue practicing against the wall, as you did before.

1 Bend your legs, spreading your knees outward and bringing your feet together with the soles, heels, and toes as in Namaste. Place the outer edges of your feet on the wall.

2 Breathing normally, remain in this final position for 15 to 20 seconds, observing the following points:
- Keep your knees wide apart.
- Press your soles firmly against each other.
- Keep your hips up.

3 Spread your legs to Upavishtha Konasana and close them to Shirshasana.

Benefits

These two asanas are a gift to women. They give: reduced discharge, and after pregnancy, regulated menstrual flow

Invaluable help with urinary disorders

A healthy stretch to the groin and thighs

As do all the variations, an easier delivery

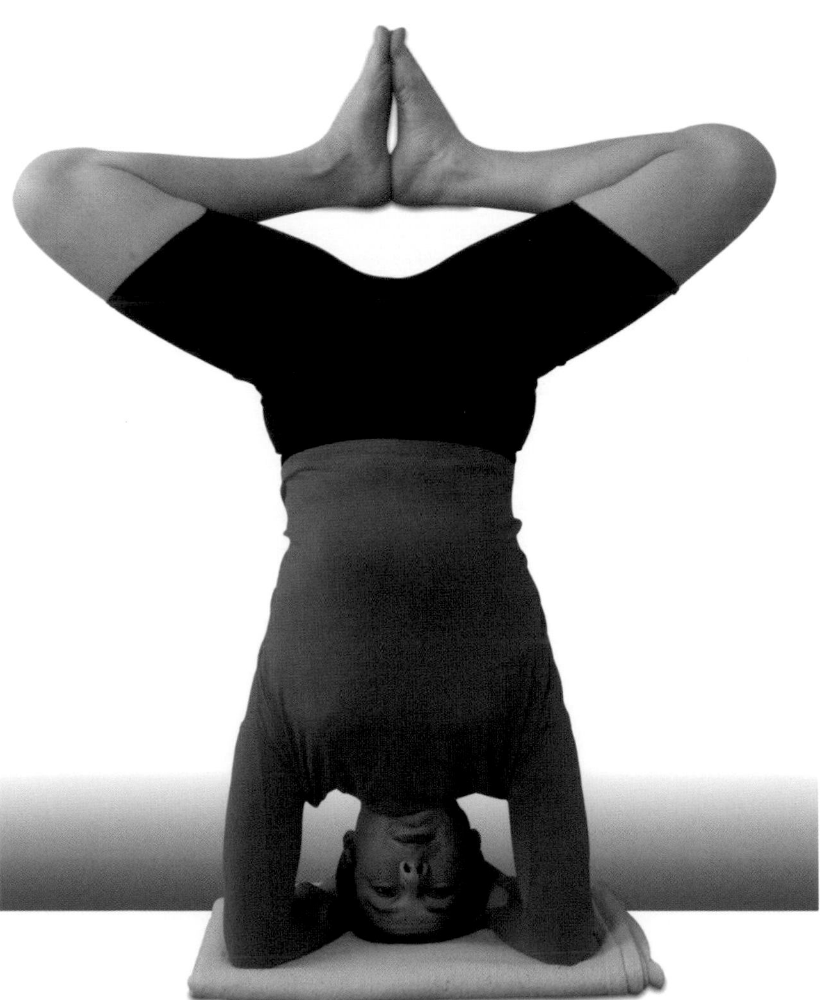

Shirshasana with Wall Ropes, see also page 240.

Asanas for Abdomen and Lumbar

Supta and Uttishtha Sthiti

Supta Padangushthasana 2

Reclining big toe 2 pose

1st trimester: yes
2nd trimester: yes
3rd trimester: yes

(For a detailed description, see page 115)

Utthita Hasta Padangushthasana 2, Extending to the Side

Standing big toe 2 pose

1st trimester: no (even advanced students)
2nd trimester: yes
3rd trimester: yes

(For a detailed description, see page 116)

◇

Back Bends

Purva Pratana Sthiti

The backward-extending asanas in the pages ahead are for your second and third trimesters only.

We recommend that you also perform some of the back bends in Chapter 3, page 118, to tone yourself up.

Dvi Pada Viparita Dandasana

Two-legged inverted staff pose

1st trimester: yes
2nd trimester: yes
3rd trimester: yes

In this asana, the back is completely arched, supported on the one hand by the crown of the head and the forearms, and on the other by the feet. As a result, you have to hold yourself with almost no support, and indeed, under normal conditions, this asana is performed without props. But when you're pregnant, you need to fully support your back.

We recommend, therefore, the modified version with props that appears here. Even this variation, however, is *only* for those who learned the asana before their pregnancy, and will not find it difficult.

The chest expansion in this asana brings about a feeling of happiness. Practiced in this modified technique, it is particularly helpful if you are

Benefits
Brings about a feeling of happiness
Builds self-confidence
Eliminates anxiety
Improves respiration and circulation

depressed, weak, or overly sensitive or emotional; it builds self-confidence and eliminates anxiety.

Practice this asana with a teacher if you are not familiar with it.

The backward spinal arch in this asana is a movement that rarely occurs among everyday movements; most household or other jobs involve bending your spine forward.

This pose counters the constant forward bending with a backward bend. The extension of the frontal spine caused by the backward bend creates space and thus freedom for the diaphragm to move.

Because the asana is performed with the lumbar (lower) spine and the buttocks well supported, your torso gets a full extension without strain on the spinal muscles. This lessens the load on the abdomen, bringing about improvement in crucial body functions such as respiration and circulation.

You can perform the asana in either of the two following ways:

Technique 1

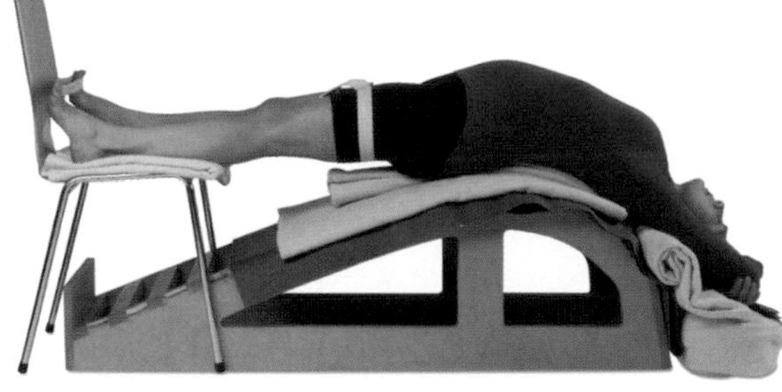

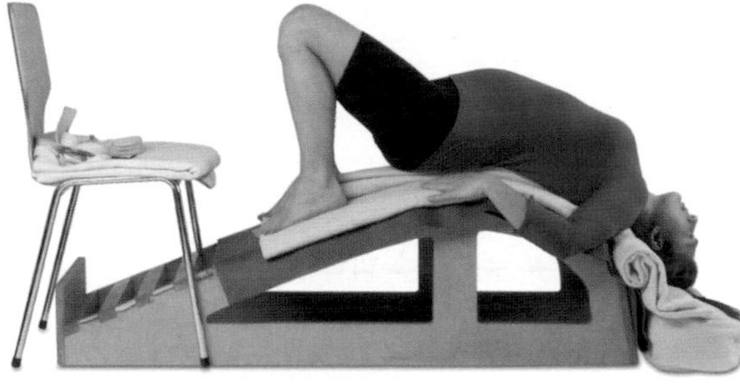

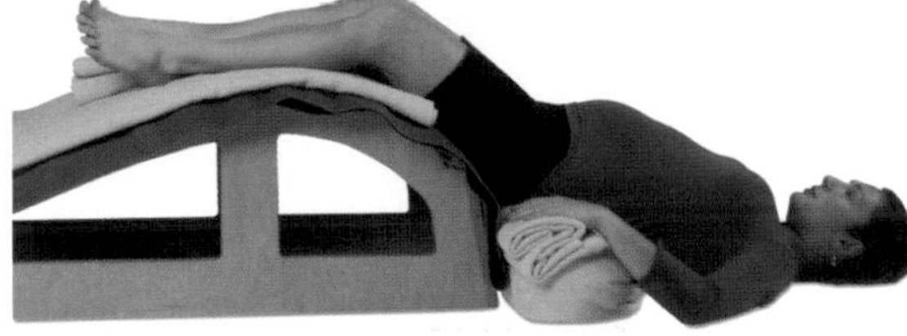

1 Prepare a Viparita Dandasana bench and one or two chairs. Have a belt for your legs, a folded blanket on the edge of the bench to protect your back, a bolster or folded blankets for your head, and a rolled blanket for your neck.

2 Sit on the bench, tie the belt around your legs, hold the edge of the bench, and slowly slide down until your head reaches the bolster or folded blankets below. Place your feet on the chair either closed (first trimester), or hip-wide (from the second trimester), and extend your legs.

3 Put your arms over your head and grip your elbows or keep the arms relaxed on the floor.

4 Broaden your chest.

5 Stay in this position for 3 to 5 minutes, breathing normally and observing the following points:
- Your chest should not cave in.
- Your head should not remain in a suspended state.
- Keep your face relaxed.

Special Instructions

- Perform this asana **only** with props, and **only** if you are already very familiar with it.
- The asana must be done after Salamba Shirshasana and the chain of asanas that go with it.
- Don't practice this asana if you suffer from high blood pressure during pregnancy.
- Going into the pose is difficult, so you need some amount of skill to perform it. Once you're in the pose, however, you can relax and enjoy its soothing and exhilarating effects.
- You can avoid any strain by understanding how to go into the pose.

Coming out of the pose

Exhale, release your arms, bend your knees, lower your torso to the floor, and lie flat on your back.

If you don't have a low bench or bed, you can do the asana as follows:

Technique 2

1 Bend your legs, and place your feet to the left and right of the chair or support, and grip the backrest.

2 Slide your buttocks and pelvis slightly down towards your feet. Lift your head off the support, grip the front legs of the chair, and lift your torso up. Sit upright and relax.

3 Keep your feet up on the second stool.

4 Make sure you have a bolster or blankets in place to rest the crown of your head.

5 Exhale and bend slightly backward, resting your back on the blankets on the stool. Slide forward slowly and smoothly, so that the crown of your head is brought to rest on the bolster or blankets. The backward movement of your spine should be more of a lying back and sliding motion than a bending one. You can do this because your back and spine are fully supported. Your dorsal and lumbar regions (mid and lower back) achieve their curvature on the chair. With your buttocks fully supported, you won't feel any fear.

6 Grip the back legs of the chair or rest your arms as in Technique 1.

CHECK YOURSELF

- *Your lumbar region should curve on the edge of the stool.*
- *Your buttocks should be on the stool and not left suspended.*
- *Your feet should be held up by the stool.*
- *Don't hold your breath.*
- *Broaden your chest.*
- *Go into and come out of the asana smoothly; don't fall into it or jump out of it abruptly.*

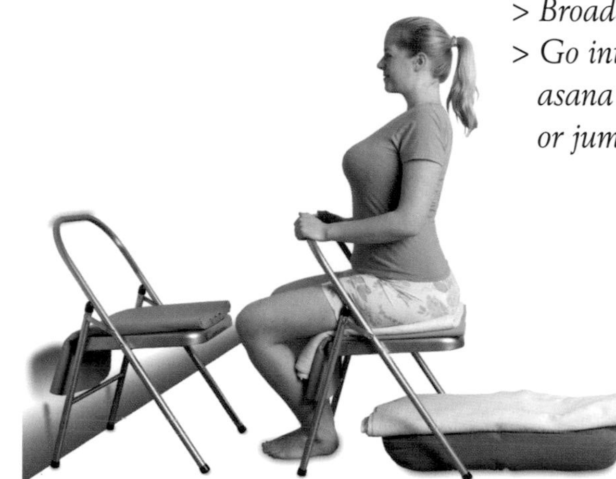

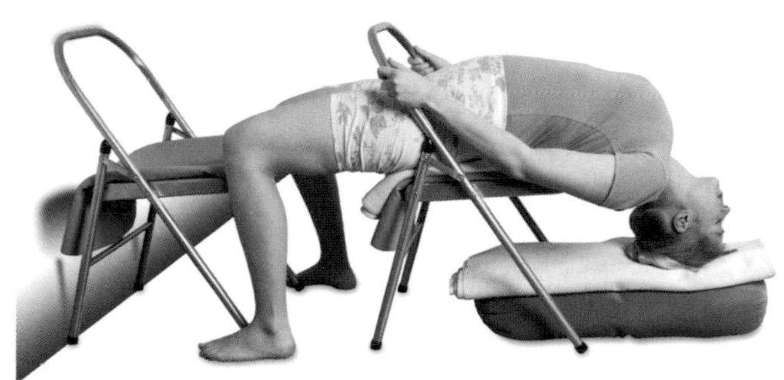

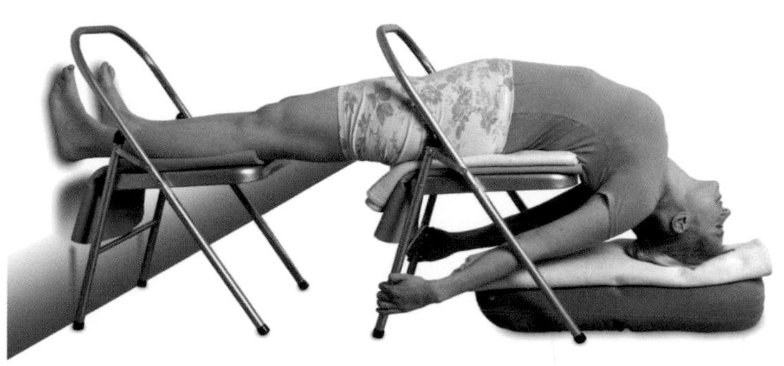

Coming out of the pose

Exhale, bend your knees, and bring your feet back to the floor. Slide your buttocks backward in the direction of your feet, until your buttocks are on the edge of the chair. Grip the backrest, lift your torso, inhale, and come back to a sitting position.

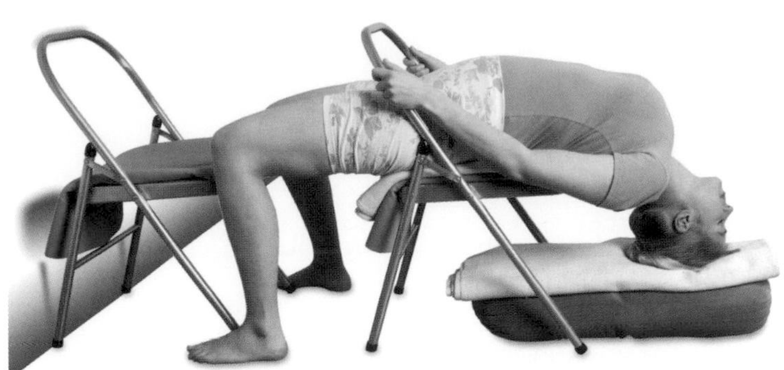

- Go into and come out of the asana smoothly; don't fall into it or jump out of it abruptly.

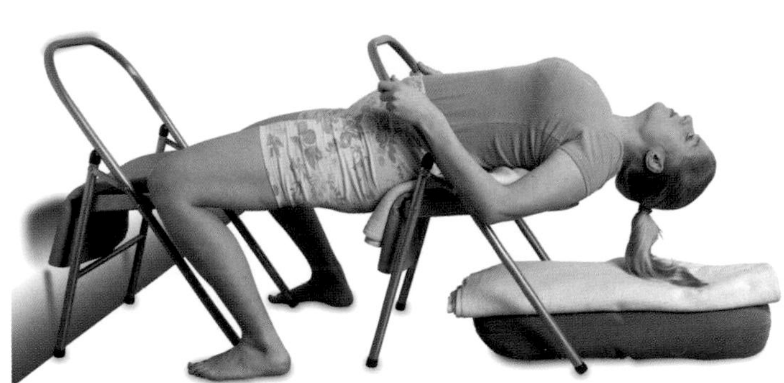

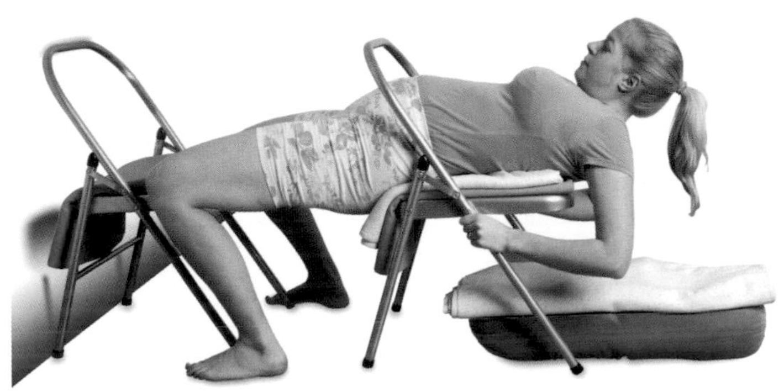

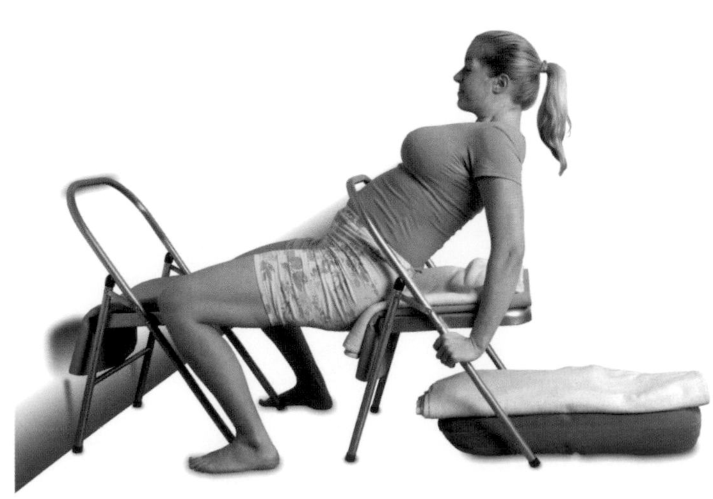

Urdhva Dhanurasana, with Wall, Chair, and Blocks

Upward-facing bow pose

1st trimester: no
2nd trimester: yes
3rd trimester: yes

As with the previous asana, you should practice this one only if you were familiar with it before your pregnancy, and only fully supported by the suggested props.

1 Place a sticky mat on the seat of a chair, a crosswise bolster on the mat, and a crosswise rolled blanket in front of the bolster. Put 2 blocks or a similar support for your hands behind the chair, against a wall.

2 Sit on the blanket and place your feet 1 to $1^1/_2$ feet apart on the floor, with the outer edges of your feet parallel. Extend your soles from your heels towards the balls of your toes. Keep your outer knees facing the ceiling.

3 Gripping the backrest of the chair with one hand and the seat with the other, bend your knees, lift your buttocks slightly away from the blanket, and bring them down away from your waist towards the back of your knees.

4 Slowly bring your spine, vertebra by vertebra, down onto the bolster. Extend your spine towards your head, lift your breastbone, expand your chest, and pull your shoulder blades into your ribs.

5 Stretch your arms above your head and stay there for 10 to 15 seconds, bringing your lower back ribs and shoulder blades deeper into your body.

6 Press your palms on the blocks and the bottoms of your feet evenly on the floor. Exhale, lift your thighs, buttocks, and back from the bolster, push your shoulder blades in, and broaden your chest and ribs.

7 Stay for a couple of seconds, breathing normally. Exhale, slowly lower your pelvis, and bring your thighs, buttocks, and back onto the support.

8 To come up, lower your buttocks and lower back a little bit more towards your feet, grip the backrest and seat of the chair, inhale, and lift your breastbone and head.

9 Repeat if you like.

Benefits

Gives a feeling of happiness and other benefits like those of Viparita Dandasana.

(For more back bends, see also instructions and benefits, page 118, and Bhujangasana with Ropes and Bhujangasana with Ropes, Chair, and Bolster, pages 119 and 120.)

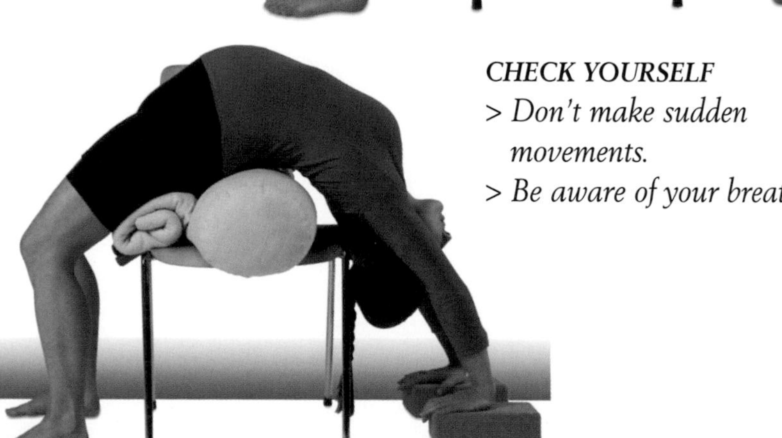

CHECK YOURSELF
> Don't make sudden movements.
> Be aware of your breathing.

Rope Asanas

Yoga Kurunta

Shirshasana, with Wall Ropes

Headstand pose

1st trimester: no
2nd trimester: yes
3rd trimester: yes

This passive way of practicing Shirshasana is well known to most students of Iyengar Yoga.
Come out of the pose by reversing the way you entered it.

(For all other rope asanas, see Chapter 3, *pages 124 – 125)*

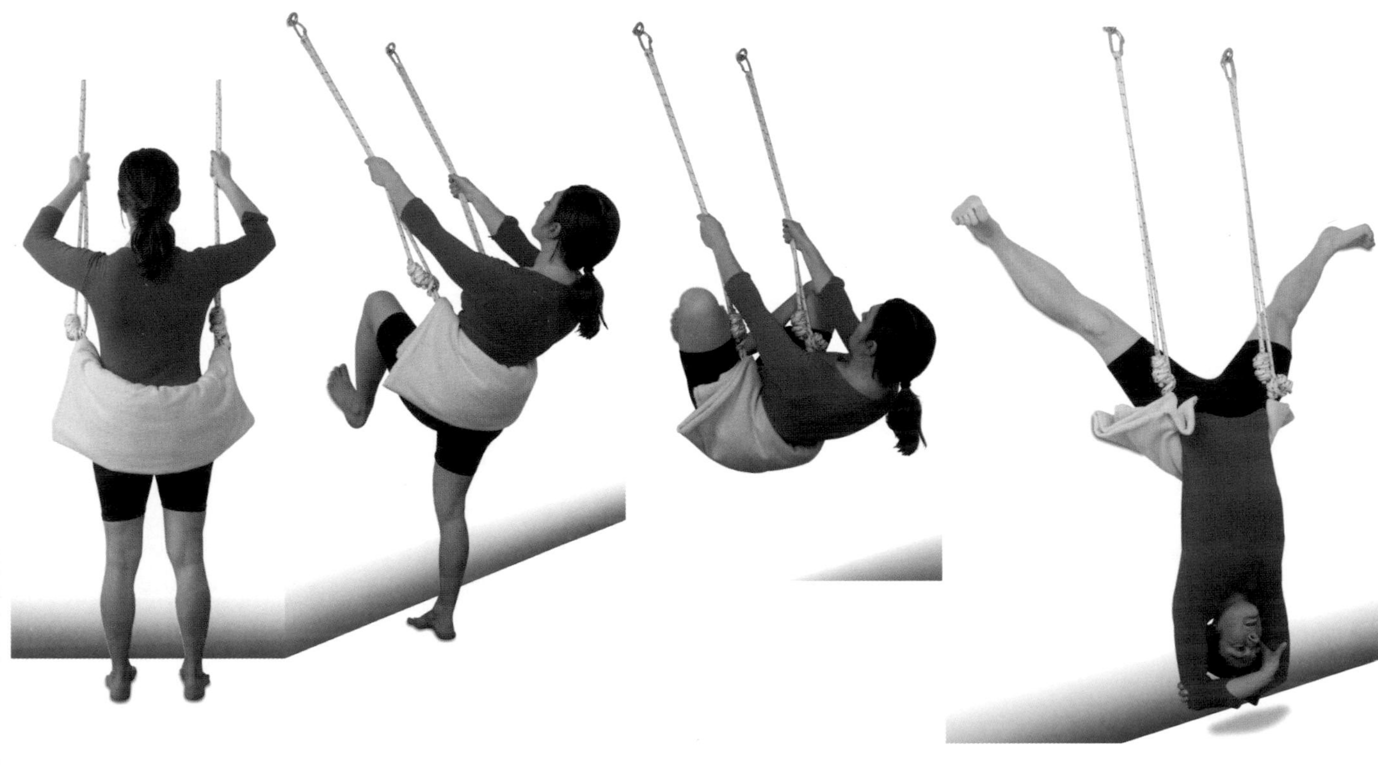

◇

Restorative Asanas

Vishranta Karaka Sthiti

(see Chapter 3, *pages 126 – 139)*

◇

Pranayama

Breathing Techniques

(see Chapter 3, *pages 140 – 153)*

CHAPTER 6

DELIVERY

Practicing Yoga during your pregnancy is good for your health, and also gives you confidence for your delivery. That's why we have dealt throughout this book with the psychological effects. Regular practice of asanas creates a climate of self-assurance and removes the clouds of doubt. Pranayama brings about moral support from within.

Labor pains are natural; they signify that the various muscles, particularly the muscles of the uterus, are contracting in order to expel the baby. The yogasanas you practiced during pregnancy have strengthened your uterine muscles, so that they can function efficiently during delivery.

Baddha Konasana and Upavishtha Konasana are especially beneficial, as they help broaden the pelvic area and dilate the cervix. Pranayama strengthens the nerves to enable you to breathe calmly in the periods between the contractions, which is essential for easy delivery.

When you're at the point of delivery, remain at ease and wait calmly. The baby will come when it is ready to be born. Anxiety can tighten your muscles, create nervous tension, and affect your delivery.

Your Yoga training can help you relax during labor and make the pain more bearable. Keep in mind that more than the actual pain, it is your imagination of pain that is disturbing you. As soon as you've begun labor with the preliminary contractions, concentrate on proper breathing. If you have practiced pranayama regularly, then you have felt the freedom and flow of energy it creates in the body.

Although it's hard during labor to think about controlling and using your breath, remember that free, deep, and wide breathing will make you more comfortable. Try to feel as though every cell is breathing, and that this breath is reaching every nook and corner of your body. You want to break the rigidity of mind and body you may be experiencing, which creates tension that slows down labor and makes it more painful.

Your child has decided to enter the outer world. You have prepared yourself and your unborn baby well, and now you can look forward to this unique event in your womanhood, your parenthood, and the life of your child.

There are three main stages of delivery. In stage 1, contractions begin and the cervix dilates. In stage 2, the pushing and birthing stage, the baby is born. Stage 3 includes the after-birth processes, including the expulsion of the placenta.

Asanas for Breathing during Contractions (Stage 1)

The first contractions will start to gently open the passage for the baby to go through, and the cervix will slowly shorten. Afterwards, the cervix will open in contractions lasting 35 to 50 seconds, coming at intervals of 4 to 10 minutes.

During the first stage of labor, you can practice just one of these positions, or you can alternate among them. Find the rhythm that's right for you.

• Baddha Konasana

(page 69)

Widens the pelvic floor and diaphragm and relaxes the sacroiliac area, creating space for deeper breathing

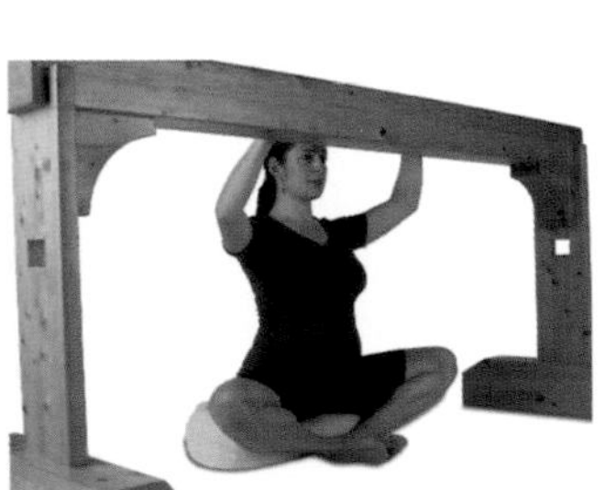

with trestle

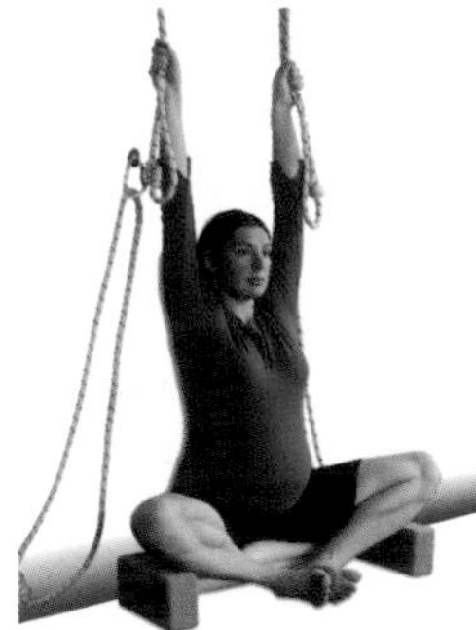

with wall ropes

• Upavishtha Konasana

(page 71)

Similar effects to Baddha Konasana

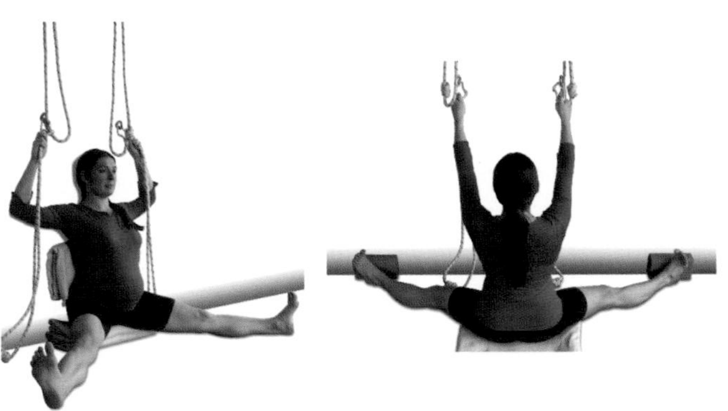

• Malasana

(pages 77 – 78)

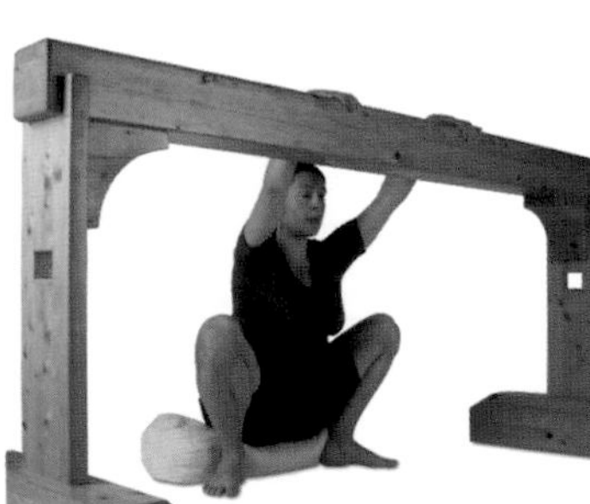

with trestle

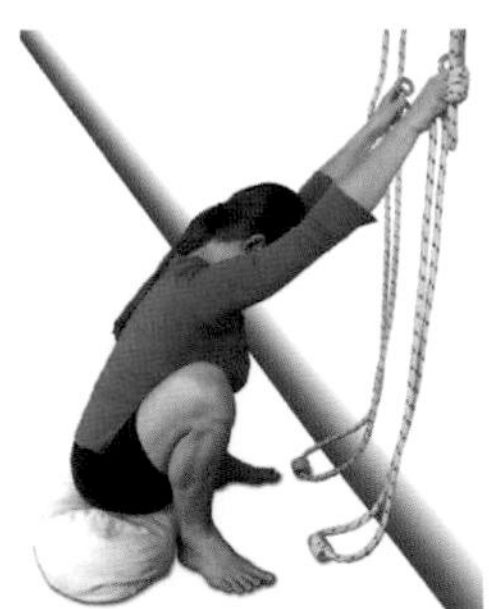

with wall ropes

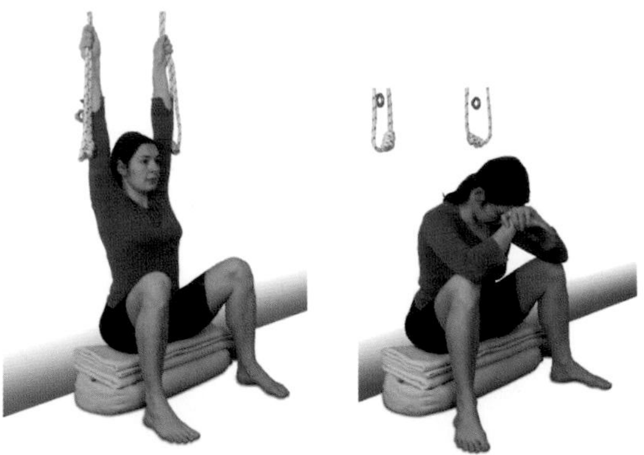

with wall ropes and back against the wall

• Adho Mukha Virasana

(page 76)

For deep breathing, especially into the pelvis itself

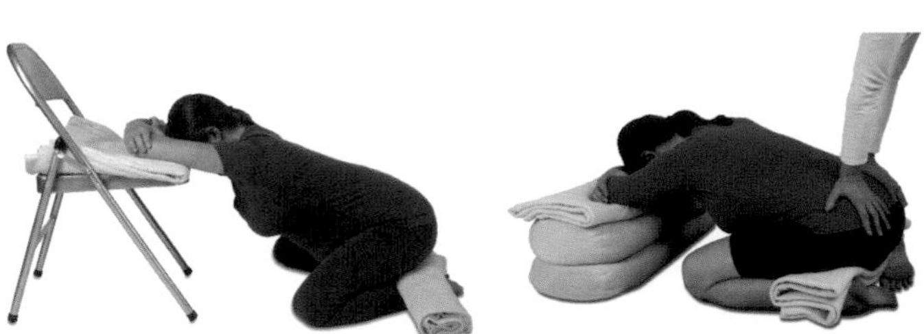

squatting pose

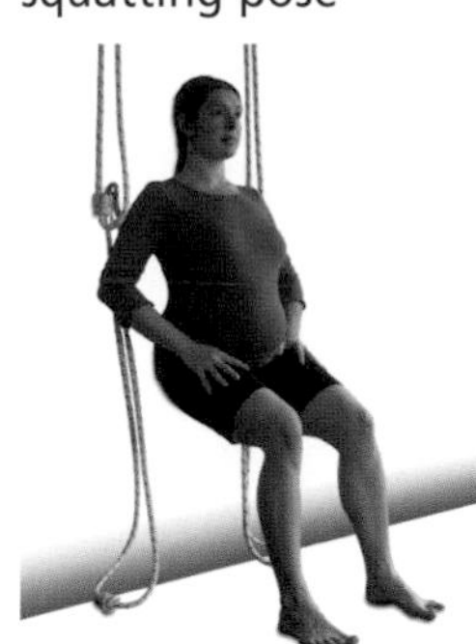

With the back against the wall, similar to Utkatasana (page 278). You can also use wall ropes, if they are available.

If You Feel Tired: Shavasana and its Variations

• When you feel tired and have to lie down, you can lie in Shavasana with bolsters at your back.

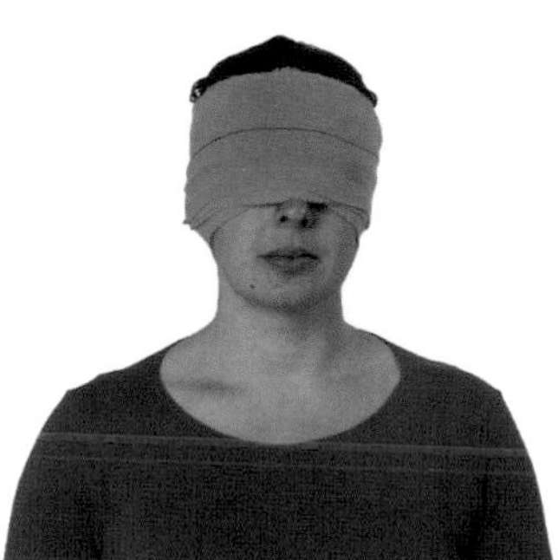

with eye bandage

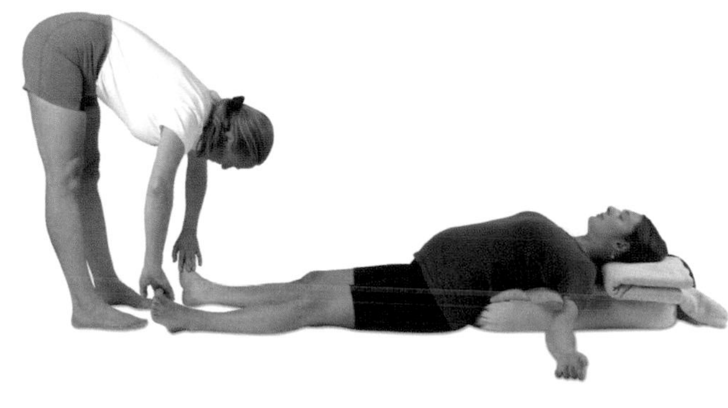

• For more comfort, you can lie on your right side. If the baby is pressing on the inferior vena cava (lower vein that leads to the heart), lie on your left side to take the pressure off the vein.

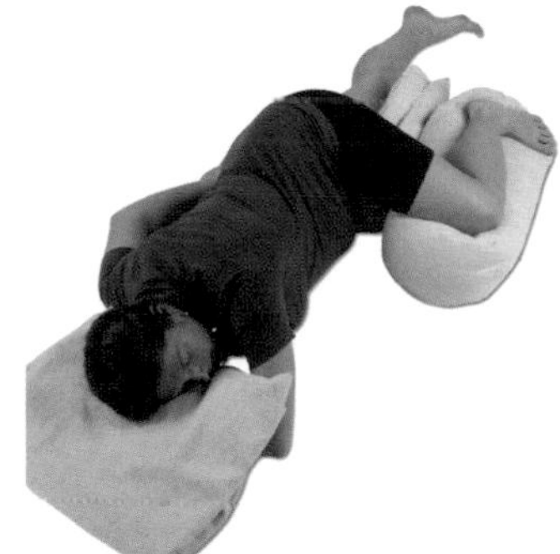

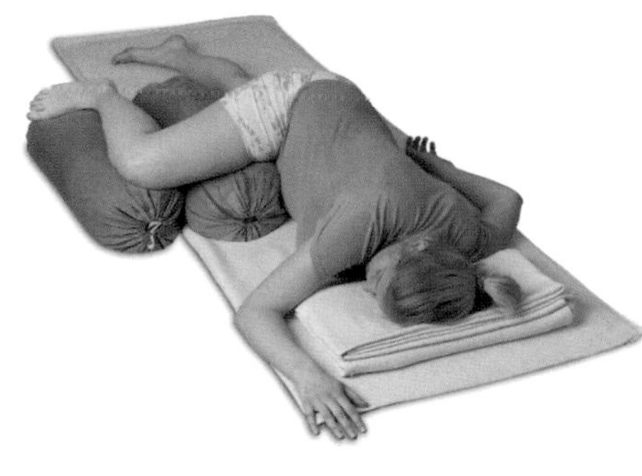

Be very attentive. Concentrate on the rhythm of the contractions and follow them with your breathing using soft, deep inhalations and prolonged exhalations. Use the "so-ham" mantra, which gives undivided concentration for deep and quiet breathing. In your mind, utter "so-o-o-o" while inhaling and "ha-a-a-a-m" while exhaling. Don't remove yourself from the labor, but rather become one with it, so that you don't become short of breath.

Allow your vagina and pelvic floor to expand—literally open the door.

Bear in mind that the birth itself will be the closest moment in your life with your baby. Imagine saying good-bye to a dear friend. You hug him, maybe you cry. But at the same time, you let go, you surrender, and you bless him on his way.

Asana, Pranayama, and Mantra for Birthing and Pushing (Stage 2)

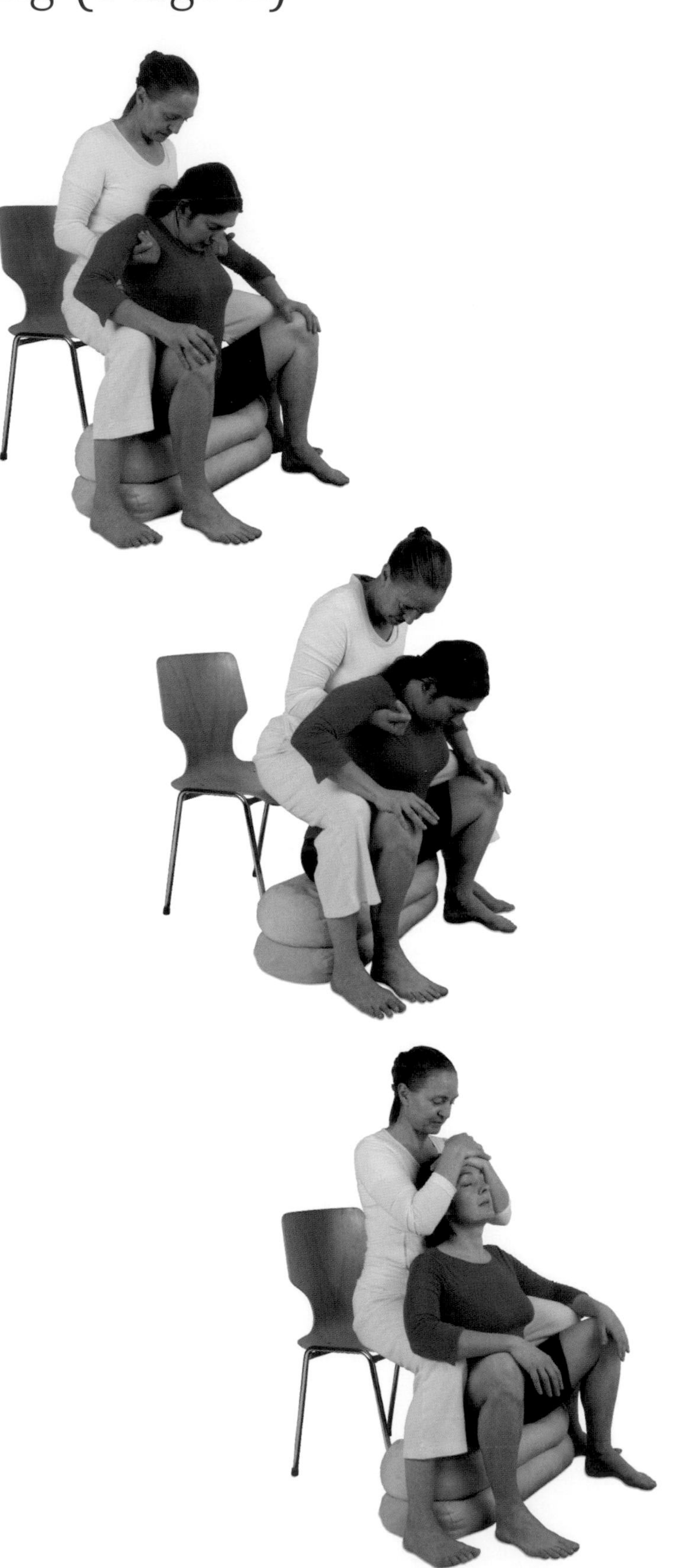

While it must seem that there are many possible asanas you could use, we recommend the half-sitting pose that you practiced in Malasana. Half-sitting keeps the body in an upright position—the position of consciousness, awareness, and presence.

To make sure that the pose is comfortable enough for you to relax, you can sit with your back against the wall or against your partner. Alternatively, your partner can support you as in the photos. Your chest is open, and your diaphragm can expand freely.

After a deep inhalation, put your head down, close your eyes (your throat will close by itself), and slowly but steadily push and guide the baby down the birth canal to the pelvic floor with concentrated exhalations. Here too you can use the "so-ham" mantra. If you have a midwife, follow her instructions regarding the pressure of your exhalations during the pushing stage.

If you find you are unable to deliver in a sitting pose, then lie down on your back with a pillow under your head, your knees bent, and your feet close to your body. Widen your thighs, knees, and feet, hold on to the back of your knees and follow the same pushing instructions as for delivering in a sitting pose.

After the Delivery

The labor will go on to bring out the placenta and umbilical cord, and to stop the bleeding. This takes approximately one hour.

After delivery, it is important that you have mental and physical rest, and that you are in undisturbed union with your newborn baby.

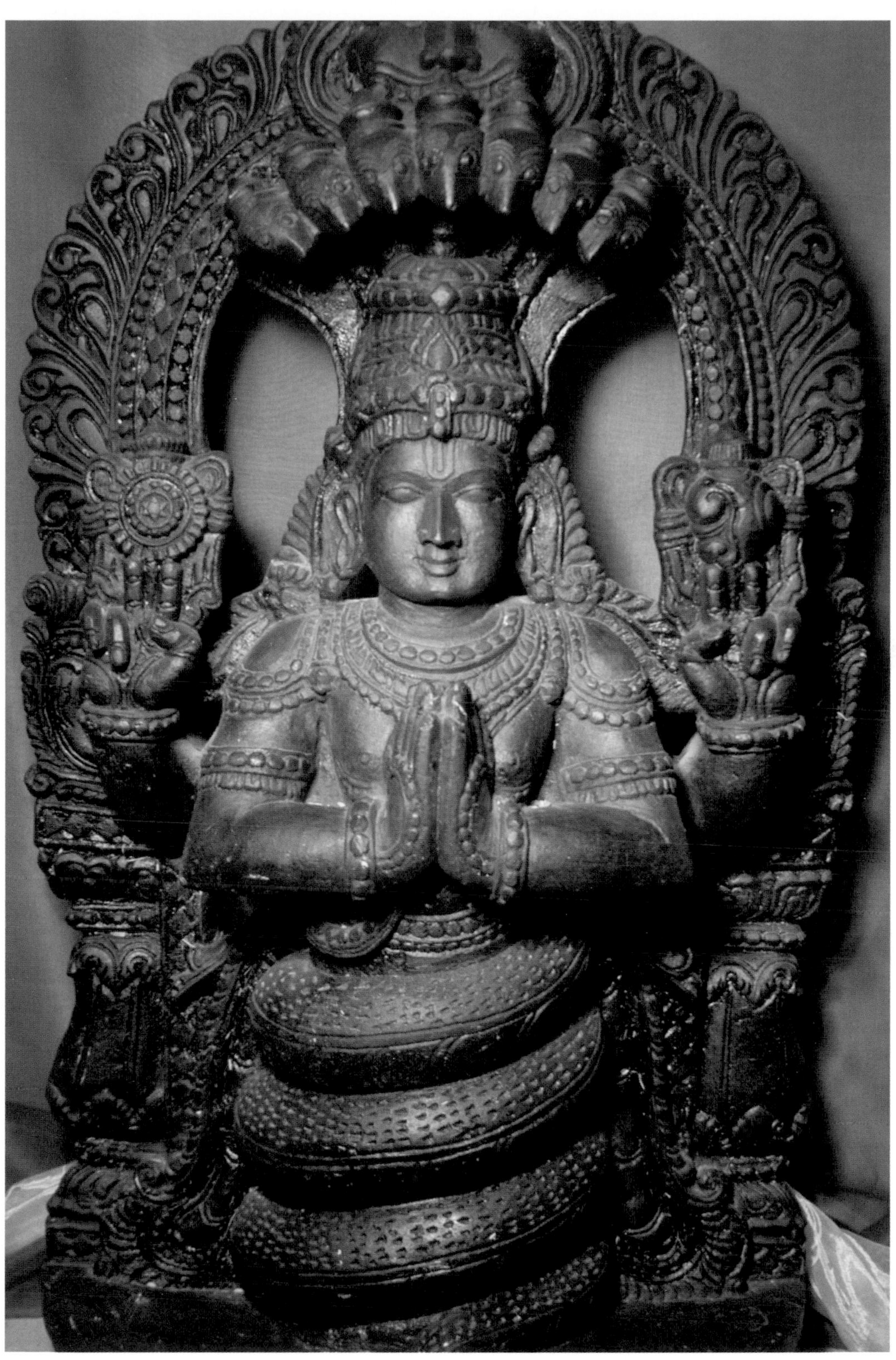

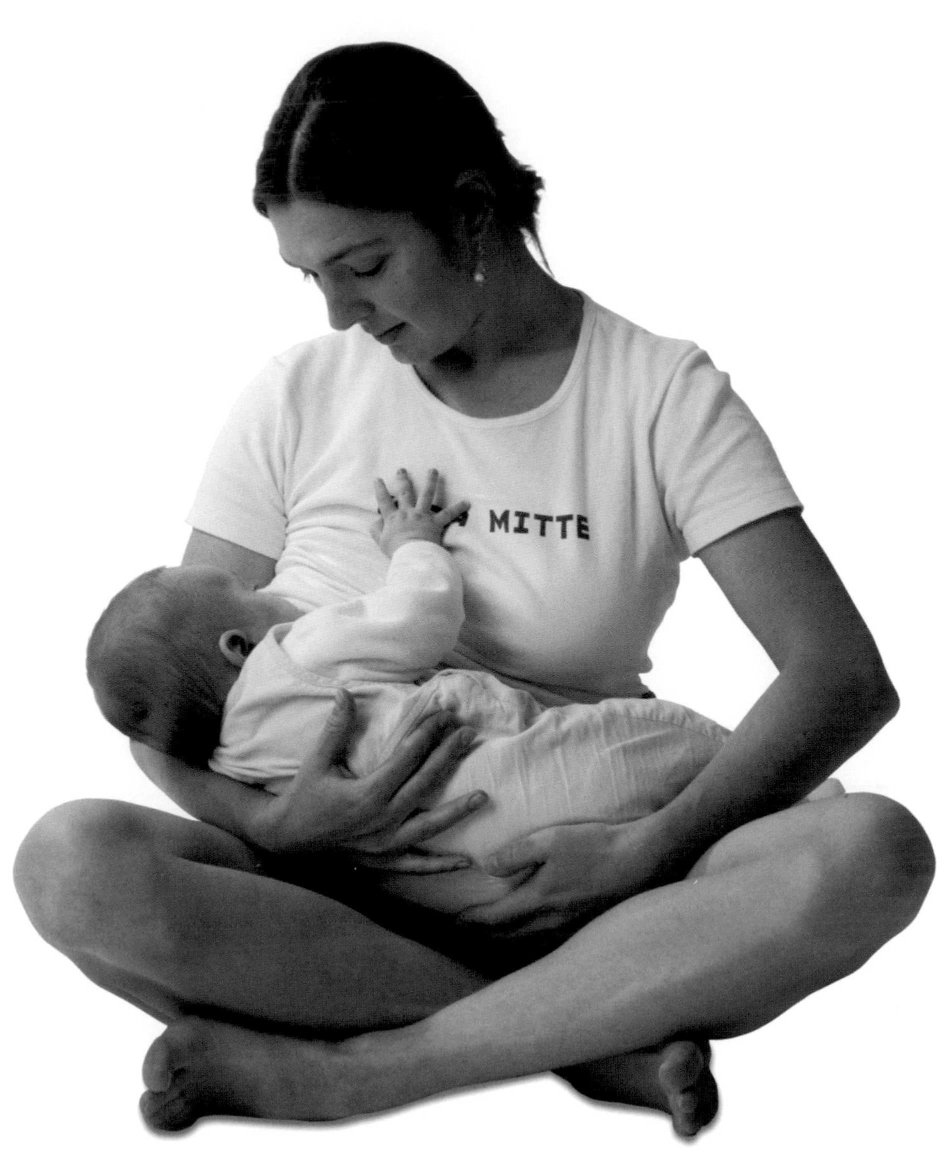
MITTE

PART III

Yoga After Delivery

Chapter 7

Immediately After Delivery

How to Use This Chapter

The terms for after your delivery correspond to the following weeks and months:

1st term	End of vaginal discharge to 12th week	2nd and 3rd month	Sequence: Passive - Active
2nd term	13th week to 25th week	4th to 6th month	Sequence: Active - Passive
3rd term	26th week to 40th week	7th to 10th month	Sequence: Back to normal

Chapter 7 starts with sequences for all three terms after delivery. No distinction has been made between beginners and advanced students as both have to be careful when rebuilding strength and resuming Yoga practice. B. K. S. Iyengar emphasizes that advanced students should especially not overwork themselves. Yoga after delivery is completely different work. Please find detailed descriptions of asanas in Chapter 8.

After delivery, women often forget to take care of themselves. The enthusiasm they felt for protecting themselves and the baby during pregnancy tends to fade in the postnatal stage. It's important, though, that you continue practicing asanas after delivery, which will help you return to normal and maintain your health.

On the other hand, it's not good to be overeager! We often see women who want to do yogasanas immediately after delivery to trim their flab and get back in shape. Both of these attitudes—negligence and overenthusiasm—are bad. After delivery, you must be ensured of mental and physical rest, even with your infant keeping you busy most of the day.

You need rest because in the weeks after childbirth, the reproductive organs return to their approximate prepregnancy condition. In this important change, called "involution," the uterus lowers to its original position in the pelvic cavity. The length of time required for these changes is shorter with mothers who nurse. *Too much activity may not cause an immediate problem, but later on, you could suffer from body pain, bulky uterus, and loose organs.*

It is usually best to refrain from strenuous activity for six weeks after delivery. In order to recover your energy and health, you should practice pranayama.

Resuming Your Yoga Practice

In the first four weeks or so after your delivery, there will be a vaginal discharge, or lochia, which will gradually stop. If you start going about your normal routine too quickly, the discharge is likely to increase.

Until the discharge has stopped and your uterus is dry, you should practice only:

• Shavasana (bolster/s), *page 336*

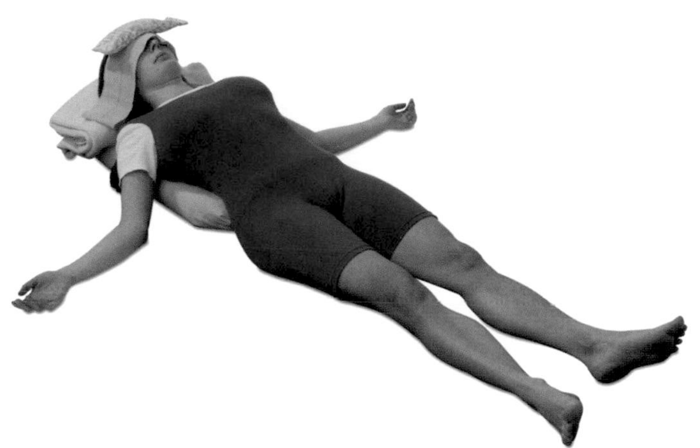

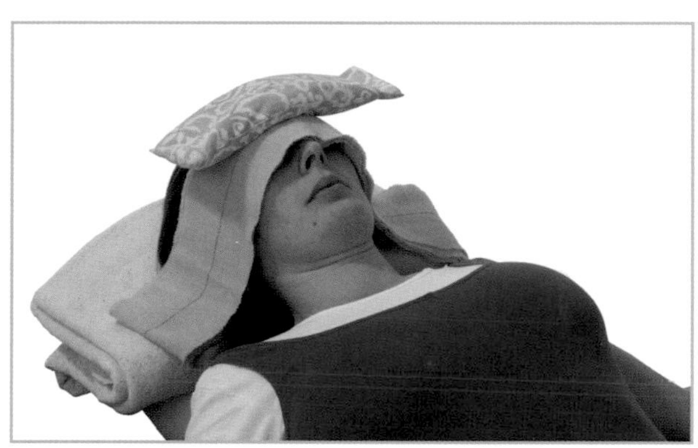

• Ujjayi Pranayama 1 in Shavasana (without retention of breath, on bolster), *page 148*

• Supta Baddha Konasana (bolster crosswise), *page 127*

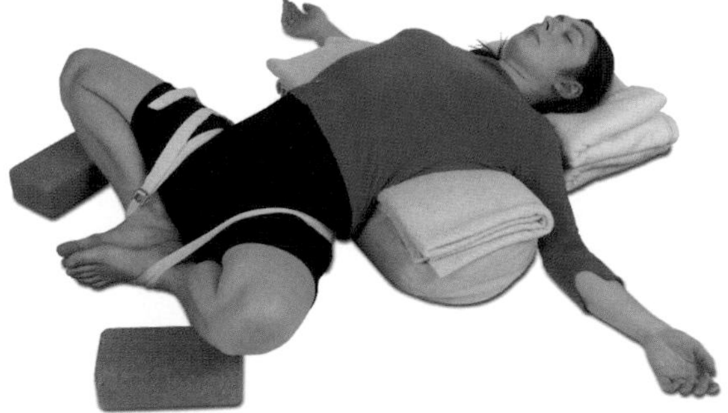

and (pillows/bolsters lengthwise, feet on block)

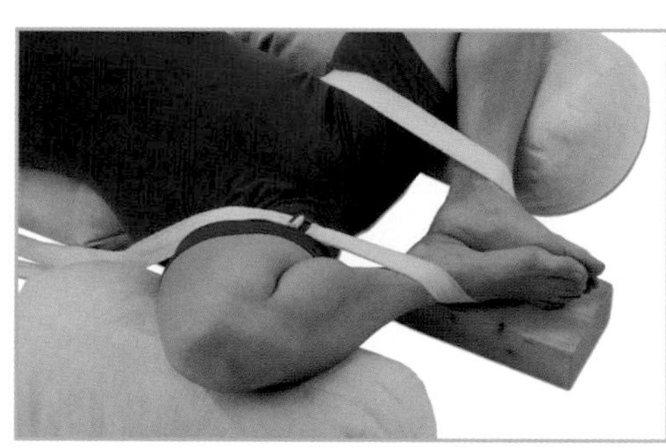

Four weeks after delivery, you can start performing asanas gradually, adding a few in the fifth week and a few more in the sixth week, depending on the limits of your capability and strength.

Mental peace, proper diet and digestion, sufficient rest, and a relaxed body and mind are good not only for you, but also for your baby. If you're agitated and annoyed, you can't provide high quality, nourishing milk. Other factors that can affect your milk include gas-forming food and conditions such as constipation, cold, cough, and fever.

To avoid congestion and hardness of the breasts, practice asanas that open your chest, such as:

- Setu Bandha Sarvangasana (page 334)
- Viparita Karani (page 335)

To increase the oxygen that you need for your milk, practice

- Shavasana (page 366)
- Ujjayi Pranayama 1 (page 369)

In Shavasana, the internal organs are in a restful state. This allows the diaphragm and lungs to expand fully in the deep breathing of Ujjayi Pranayama, increasing your oxygen intake.

Shavasana and Supta Baddha Konasana, and Shavasana plus pranayama, ensure more oxygen and a better quality of milk. These are the only asanas you can practice when your breasts are full.

Use a special pillow for breast-feeding, to avoid straining your body.

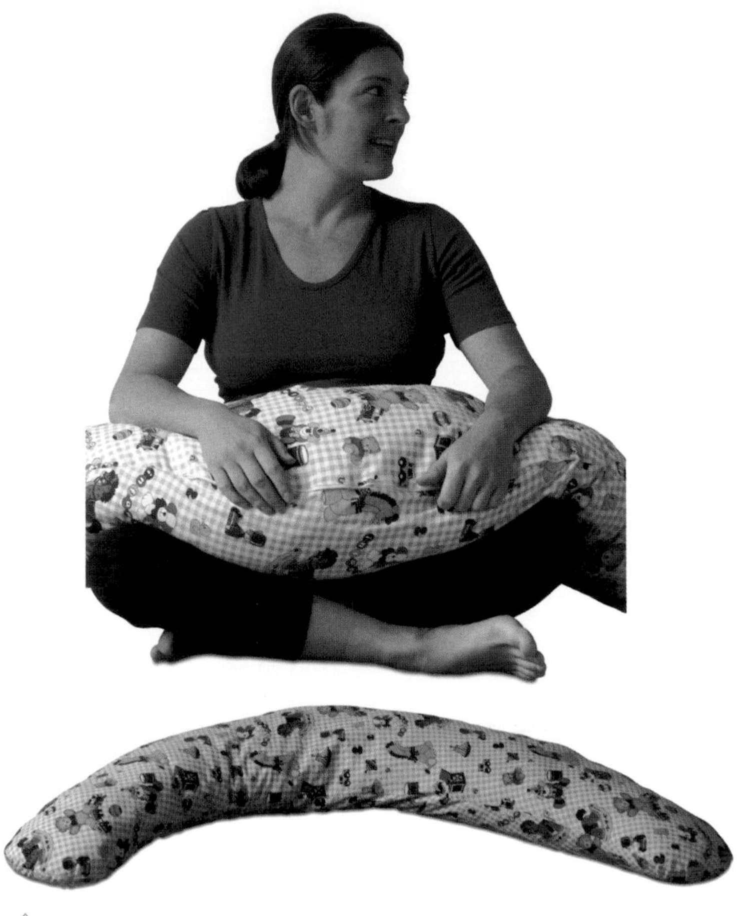

General Guidelines

- Practice Shavasana and Supta Baddha Konasana often to eliminate fatigue and feel rejuvenated.
- Performing Supta Baddha Konasana, Shavasana, and pranayama in Shavasana adds to your energy, and psychologically reduces your urge to overwork. If you tend to return to overactivity too quickly, these will help you stop.
- The asanas and pranayama above also increase lactation and purify your breast milk.
- Don't practice asanas if:
  - It has been less than a month since your delivery.
  - The vaginal discharge (lochia) has not stopped.
  - Your breasts are congested.
- After a Cesarian section or tubectomy, you should do Shavasana, Ujjayi Pranayama 1, and Viloma Pranayama 1 (page 369) for about two months until the incision heals. After that, you can practice Salamba Sarvangasana (page 331), Setu Bandha Sarvangasana (page 334), Parvatasana (page 303), Janu Shirshasana (page 306), and Maha Mudra (page 369).
- Build up your practice gradually and don't overindulge, which may cause pain.

After a Cesarian Section

If you gave birth by cesarian section, you have to be especially cautious.

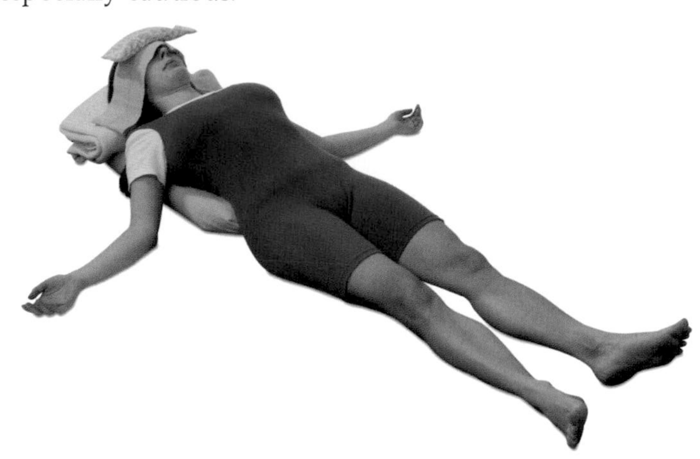

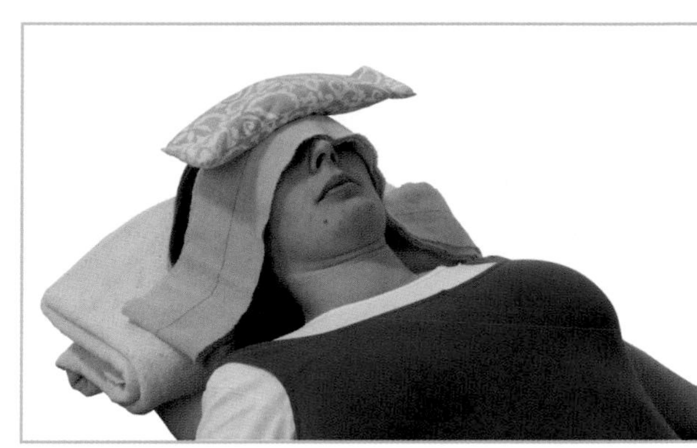

1st Term

You must recover and heal completely before practicing asanas, so you should concentrate on pranayama for the entire first term after your delivery, practicing Shavasana, Ujjayi Pranayama 1, and Viloma Pranayama 1.

Rest as often as possible; you can do Shavasana on a bolster at least twice a day for 15 to 20 minutes. Doing Ujjayi breathing without retention of breath on a bolster is revitalizing on all levels of being. Both the relaxation and the higher intake of oxygen clean your breast milk, increasing its quality.

2nd Term

After 10 to 12 weeks, you can slowly start to practice the sequence bellow:

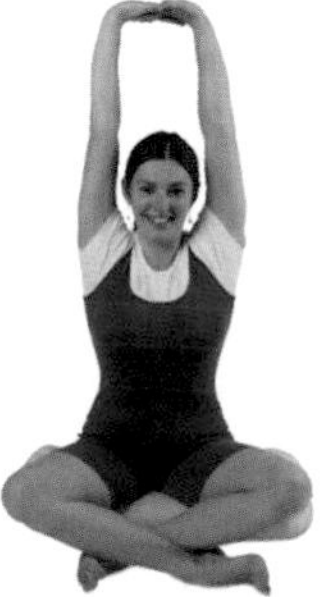

1 Parvatasana from Svastikasana, *page 302*

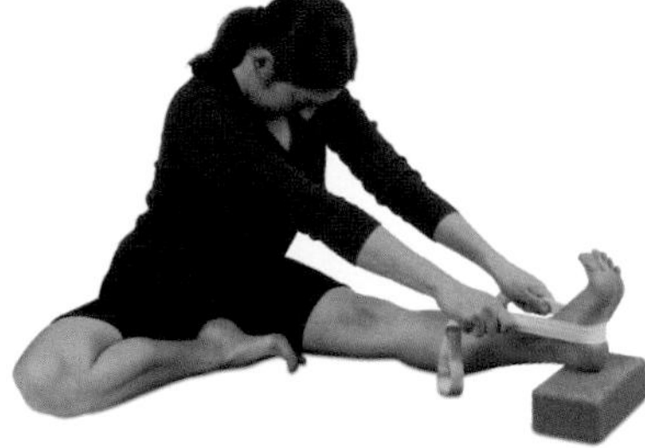

2 Maha Mudra (belt around foot and heel on block), *page 305*

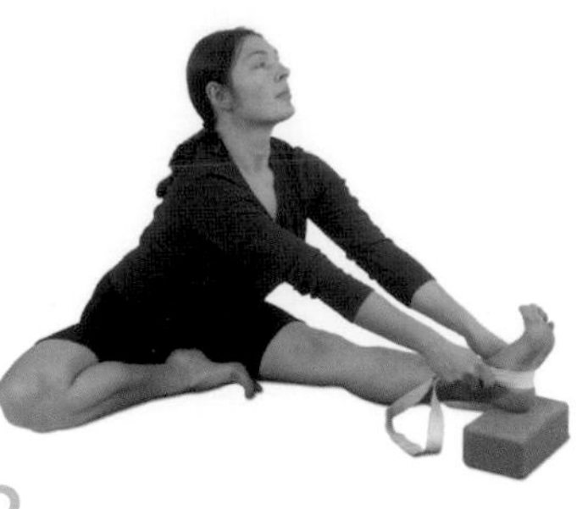
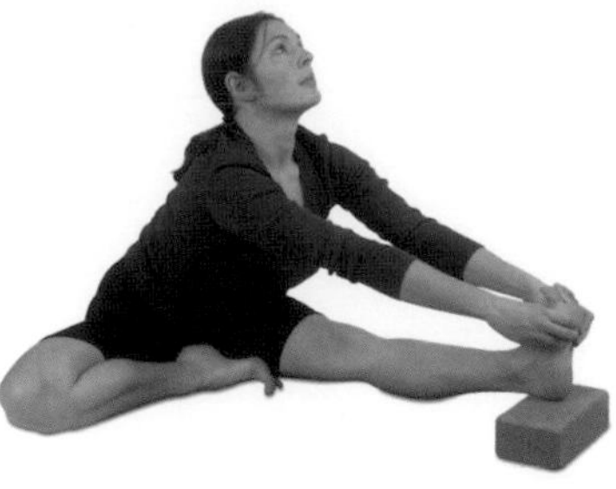
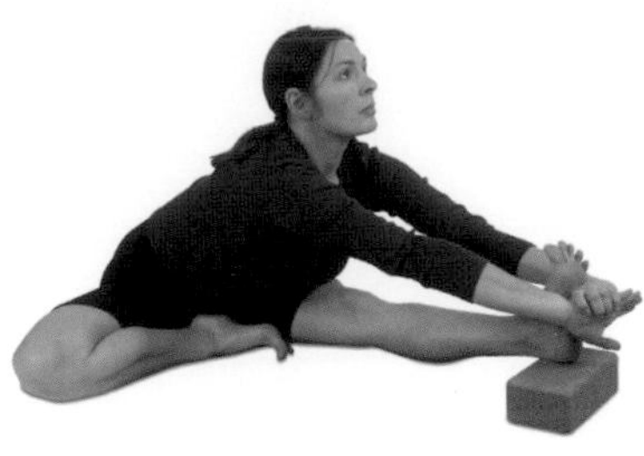

3 Janu Shirshasana (concave back, belt around foot and heel on block), *page 306*

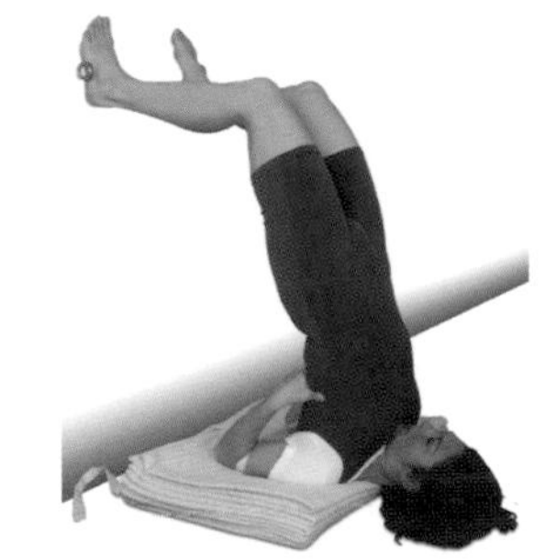

4 Salamba Sarvangasana (from the wall), *page 327*

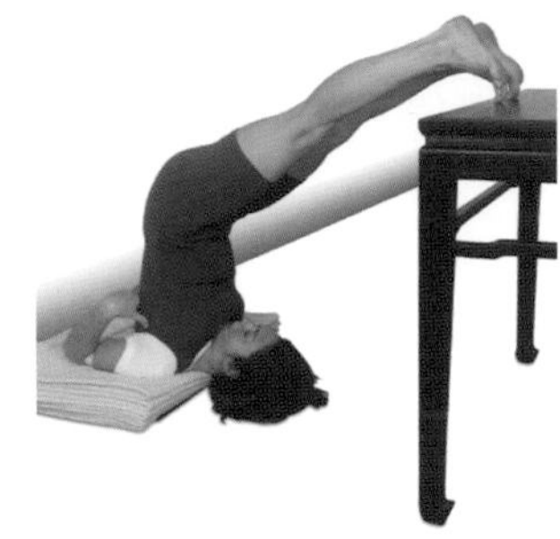

5 Ardha Halasana (toes on table, keep spine lifted), *page 332*

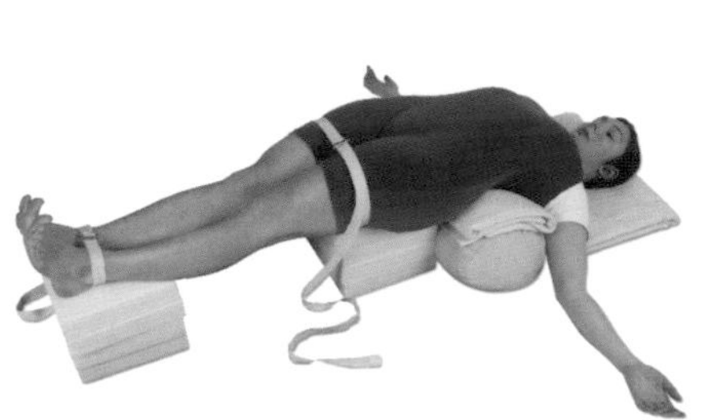

6 Setu Bandha Sarvangasana (bench or similar height), *page 334*

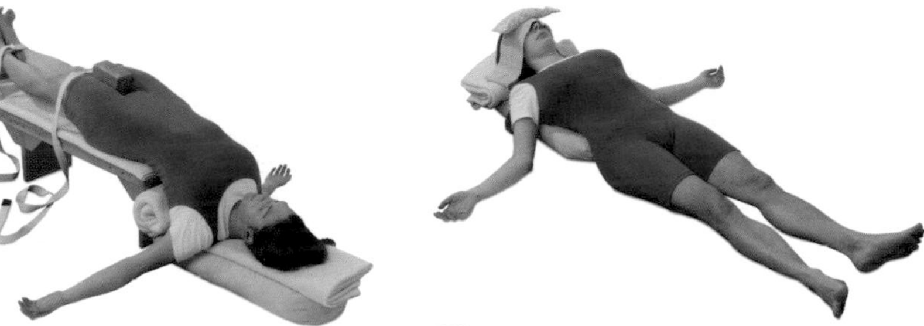

7 Shavasana (bolster/s), *page 366*

8 Ujjayi Pranayama in Shavasana (without retention of breath, on bolster), *page 148*

3rd Term

If you're feeling well, follow the sequence for beginners and advanced students for the second term after delivery. Continue with this program for at least eight weeks before you go on to the sequence for the third term after delivery.

Think of slowly toning and building yourself up.

CHAPTER 8

DETAILED DESCRIPTIONS OF ASANAS FOR BEGINNERS AND ADVANCED STUDENTS

How to Use This Chapter

The terms for after your delivery correspond to the following weeks and months:

1st term	End of vaginal discharge to 12th week	2nd and 3rd month	Sequence: Passive - Active
2nd term	13th week to 25th week	4th to 6th month	Sequence: Active - Passive
3rd term	26th week to 40th week	7th to 10th month	Sequence: Back to normal

Chapter 8 starts with sequences for all three terms after delivery. No distinction has been made between beginners and advanced students as both have to be careful when rebuilding strength and resuming Yoga practice. B. K. S. Iyengar emphasizes that advanced students should especially not overwork themselves. Yoga after delivery is completely different work. Please find detailed descriptions of the respective asanas in this chapter, following the sequences.

◇

When to Begin

After delivery, it is of primary importance that you take care of your health. You have to recover from your post-labor fatigue, tone your abdominal organs, and build up energy again to look after the baby. The opposing effects of physical exhaustion and mental exhilaration may cause adverse reactions on your body and mind.

In the first month after delivery, therefore, you should restrict yourself to pranayama, which brings a balance between body and mind and gives the body a proper rest.

During the second month, you can take up the task of toning your abdominal organs. Normally you might think of toning as exercising the abdomen in order to reduce the pregnancy-induced fat around the waist, thighs, buttocks, and stomach. What we mean here, however, is toning that improves the overall functioning of the organs. The muscles of the organs are strengthened, and the organs are made healthy. This will help you get your strength back and build up energy.

Undernourishment, inadequate rest, and improper exercise at this stage can cause permanent fatigue, as well as looseness of the body, perennial anemia, and chronic low blood pressure. Some women also face depression after delivery, which may occur after the first few days of exhilaration, as a reaction to the burden of responsibility coupled with insufficient energy. For some, the depression remains pent up inside and is not expressed openly.

Consequently, the asanas we recommend for during this month are aimed at strengthening the spine and the spinal column, toning the nervous system, and building up the muscles of the stomach, abdomen, waist, and buttocks, so that later, when you're ready to exercise them to reduce fat, they'll be able to take the strain. The asanas are also designed to overcome depression.

The asanas—a few standing poses, simple forward extensions, and inversions—and their durations, are meant for the average woman. Keep in mind, however, that each individual has different needs and strengths, and you should practice the asanas accordingly. Your Yoga session should not result in fatigue. Practice pranayama along with the recommended sequences.

By the third month, you will have regained the original shape and strength of your organs and postnatal fatigue will be gone. You can then resume the practice of additional asanas.

Sequences for After Delivery

Sequence for the 1st Term: During Your Period

First 48 to 72 Hours

Complete rest is advisable. To remove fatigue and check any excessive flow of lochia, you can practice the following:

1 Ujjayi Pranayama in Shavasana, *page 148*
2 Shavasana, *page 366*
3 Supta Baddha Konasana (bolster lengthwise or crosswise, or even without the bolster), *page 128*

Third, Fourth, or Fifth Day

Practice the following sequence, which is part of the full sequence for the first term after delivery.

1 Parvatasana from Svastikasana, *page 302*
2 Parshvottanasana (hands against wall, front foot on support), *page 285*
3 Setu Bandha Sarvangasana (bench, or similar height), *page 107*
4 Viparita Karani (bent legs on chair), *page 335*
5 Supta Baddha Konasana (bolster lengthwise or crosswise), *page 128*
6 Supta Virasana, *page 367*
7 Matsyasana , *page 131*
and/or
8 Supta Svastikasana (bolster/s), *page 131*
9 Shavasana (bolster/s), *page 366*
10 Ujjayi Pranayama in Shavasana, *page 148*

Sequence for the 1st Term: Passive - Active

Until the lochia, or vaginal discharge, has fully stopped, you should practice only:

- Supta Baddha Konasana (bolster lengthwise or crosswise, or even without the bolster), *page 128*, (Crosswise is preferable, supporting the chest. If you can't, then lengthwise.)

And for a higher intake of oxygen and a better quality of milk:

- Shavasana (bolster/s), *page 366*
- Ujjayi Pranayama in Shavasana (bolster/s), *page 148*

Don't hesitate to practice these asanas when your breasts are full—in fact, they are especially beneficial then. As soon as the lochia has fully stopped, you may start the program below.

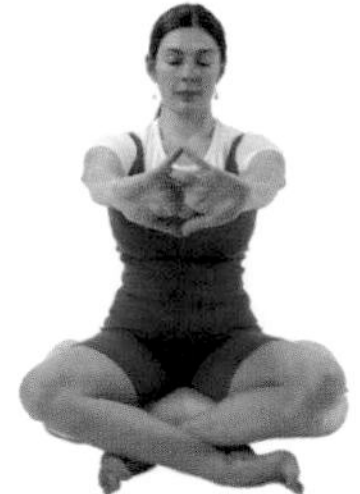

1 Parvatasana from Svastikasana, *page 302*

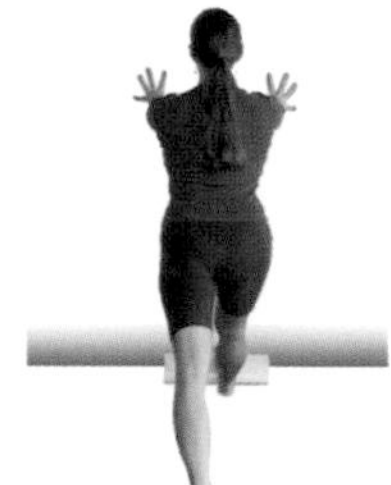

2 Parshvottanasana (hands against wall, front foot on support), *page 285*

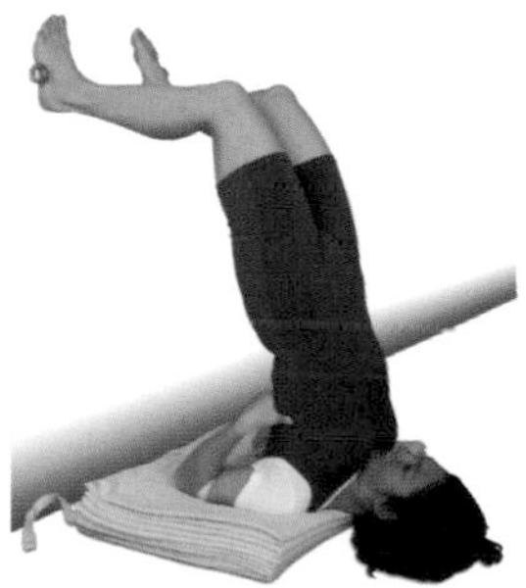

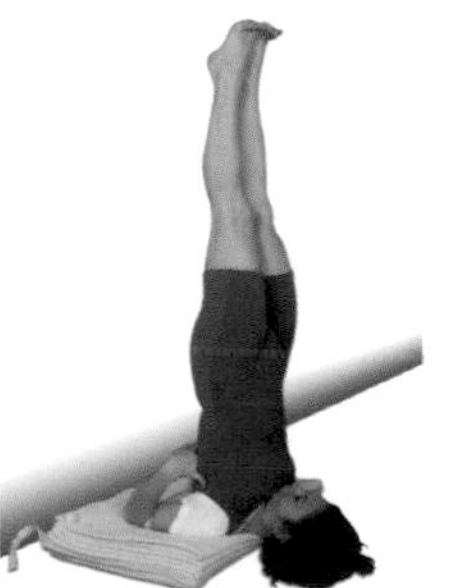

3 Salamba Sarvangasana (from the wall), *pages 327 and 328*

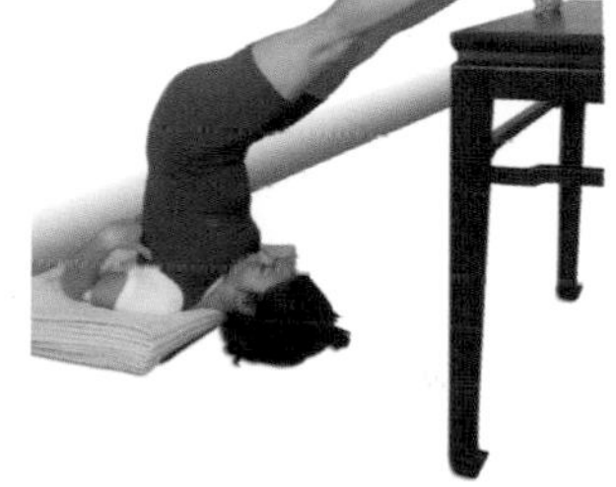

4 Ardha Halasana, (toes on table, keep spine lifted), *page 332*

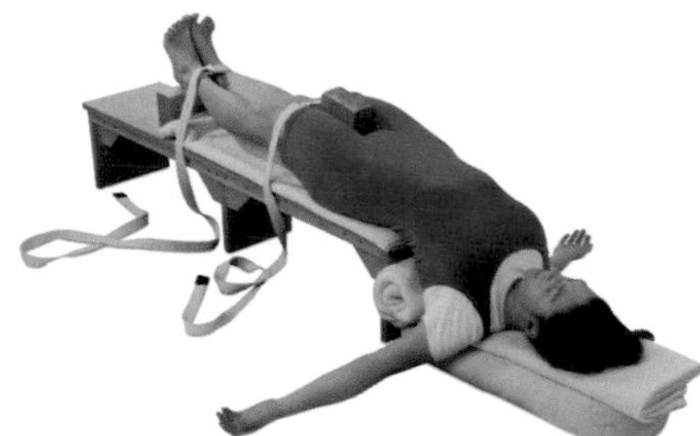

5 Setu Bandha Sarvangasana (bench, or similar height), *page 107*

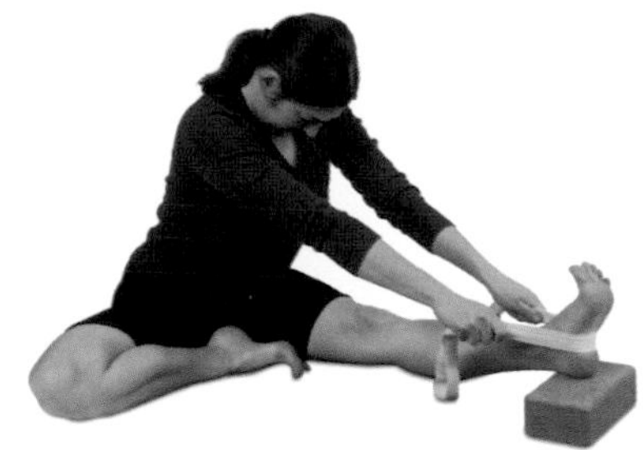

6 Maha Mudra (belt around foot and heel on block), *page 305*

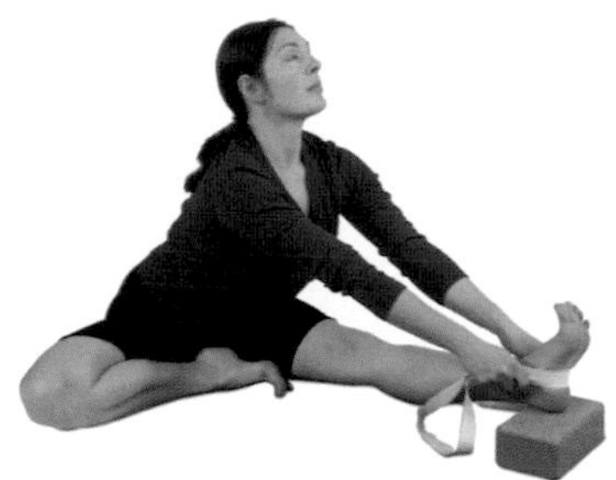

7 Janu Shirshasana (concave back, belt around foot and heel on block, keep abdominal wall lifted), *page 306*

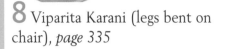

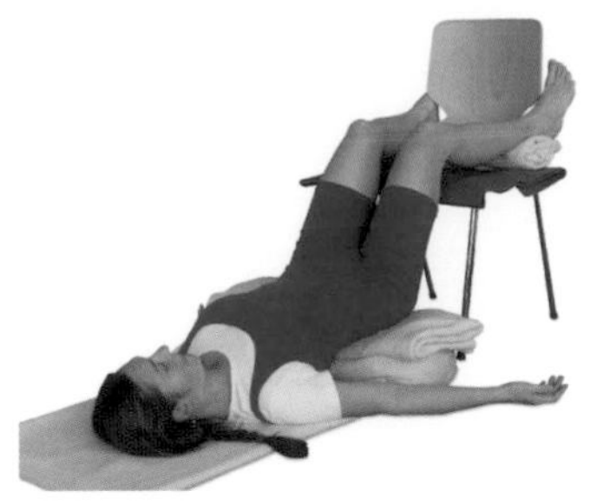
8 Viparita Karani (legs bent on chair), *page 335*

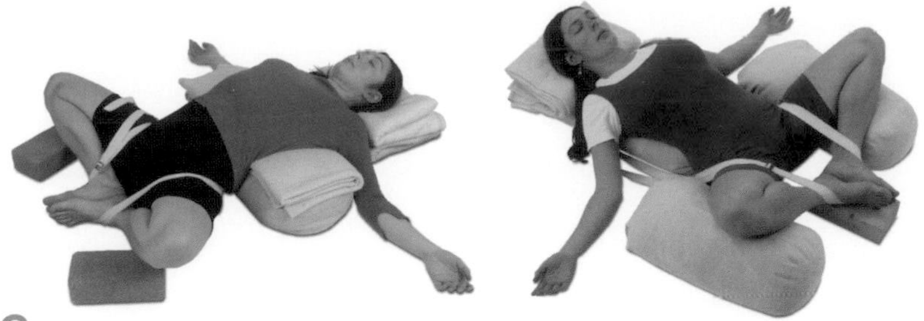
9 Supta Baddha Konasana, *page 128*

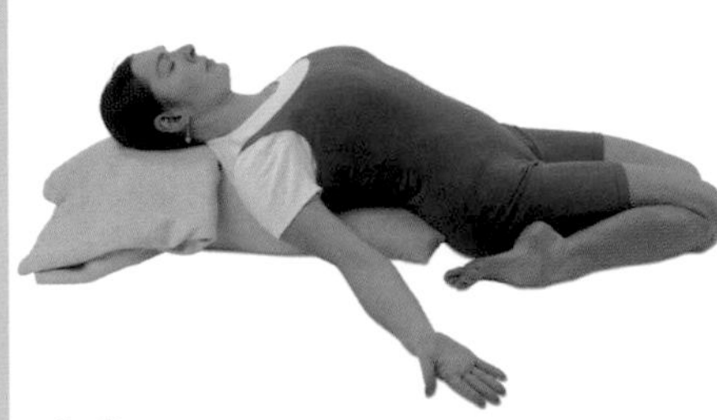
10 Supta Virasana, *page 367*

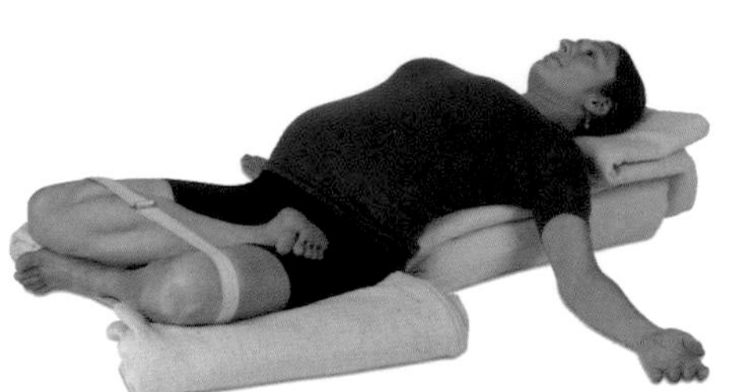
11 Matsyasana, *page 131* and/or

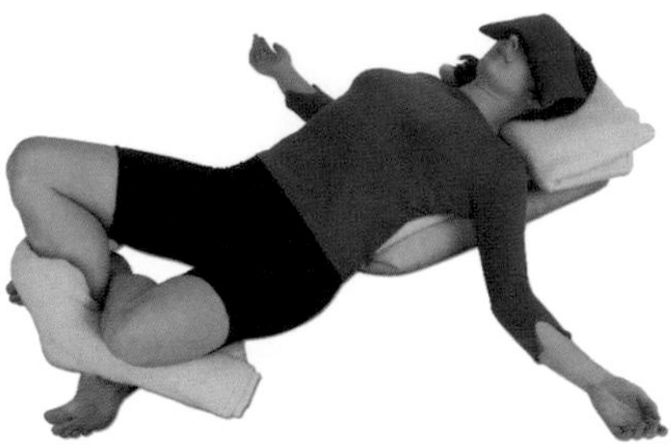
12 Supta Svastikasana (bolster/s), *page 131*

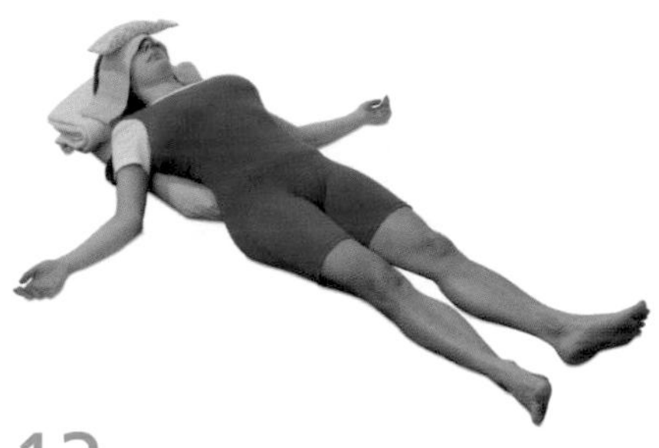
13 Shavasana (bolster/s), *page 366*

14 Ujjayi Pranayama in Shavasana, *page 148*

Durations

Numbers 1, 2, 6, and 7: 30 to 60 seconds on both sides
Numbers 3, 4, 5, 8, 9, 10, 11, and 12, inverted and restorative poses: 5 minutes
Number 13, Shavasana: 15 – 20 minutes

Coming out of the pose

Maintain the lift, width, strength, and calmness that the asana created.

Sequence for the 2nd Term: During Your Period

It's important to adjust your practice of asanas according to your menstrual cycle. Depending on how you feel, you can start this sequence on the third, fourth, or fifth day of your period.

1 Ardha Uttanasana (wall ropes, hands on chair), *page 293*
2 Utthita Trikonasana (back foot against wall), *page 281*
3 Utthita Parshvakonasana (back foot against wall), *page 282*
4 Baddha Konasana (straight back), *page 67*
5 Supta Baddha Konasana (bolster lengthwise or crosswise), *page 128*
6 Virasana, *page 302*
7 Parvatasana in Virasana, *page 303*
8 Supta Virasana (bolster/s), *page 367*
9 Matsyasana (bolster/s), *page 131*
and/or
10 Supta Svastikasana, *page 131*
11 Shavasana (bolster/s), *page 366*
12 Ujjayi Pranayama in Shavasana, *page 148*

◇

Sequence for the 2nd Term: Active-Passive

Reshaping the Body

Use your props as much as possible when you practice this sequence.

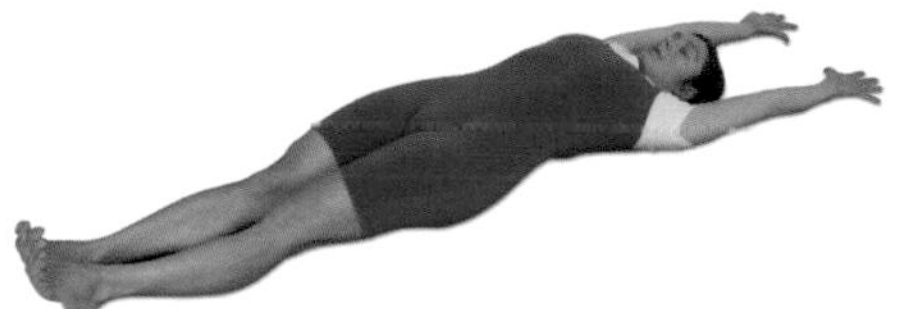

1 Supta Urdhva Hastasana and Supta Tadasana, *page 275*

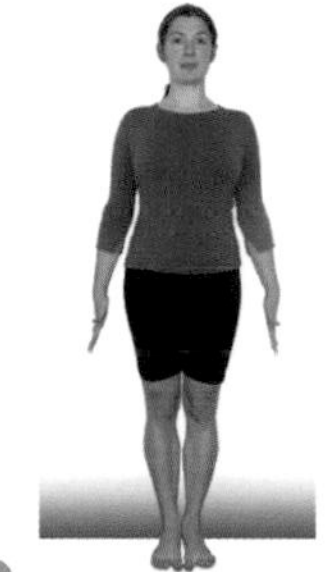

2 Tadasana, *page 275*

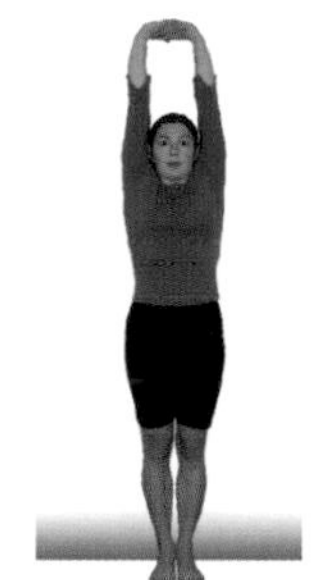

Urdhva Baddhanguliyasana, *page 34*

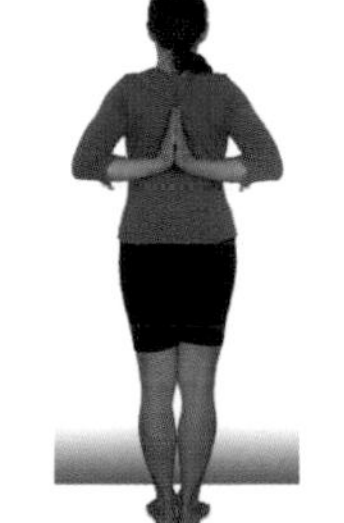

Pashchima Namaskarasana, *page 36*

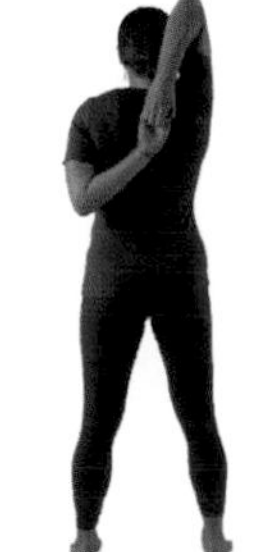

Gomukhasana in Tadasana, *page 37*

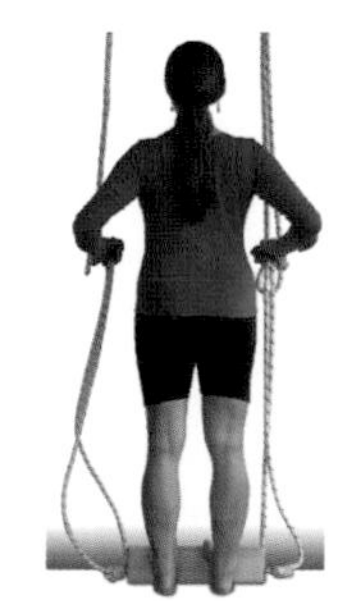

Tadasana (heels down), *pages 33 and 277*

Note

Always start the standing poses from Tadasana. When you finish the pose, come back to Tadasana. If you feel tired, rest in Ardha Uttanasana.

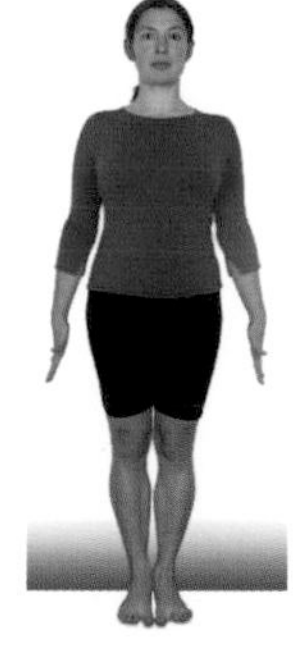

Tadasana

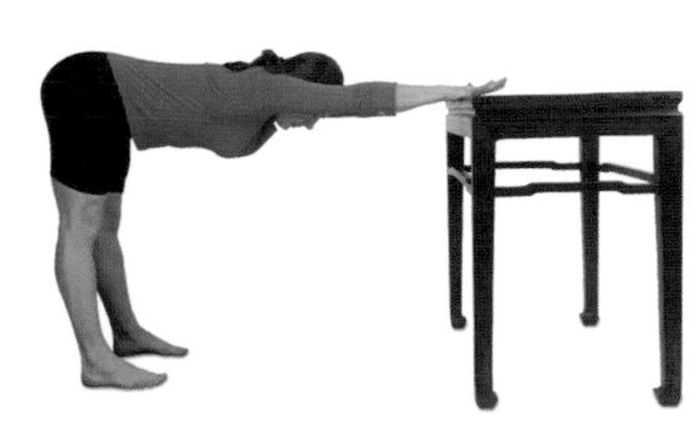

Ardha Uttanasana

See also the variations of Tadasana with a block in between the legs, *page 275*

See also the variations of Tadasana with a block, *pages 275 – 276*

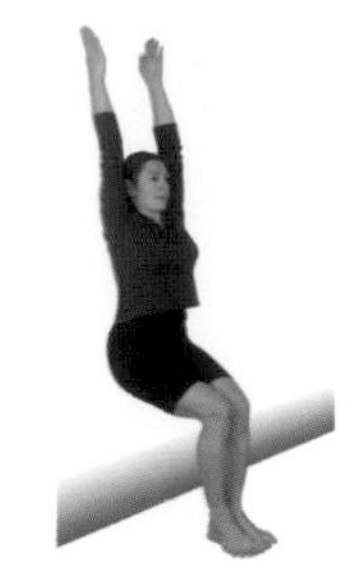

3 Utkatasana (back to the wall), *page 278*

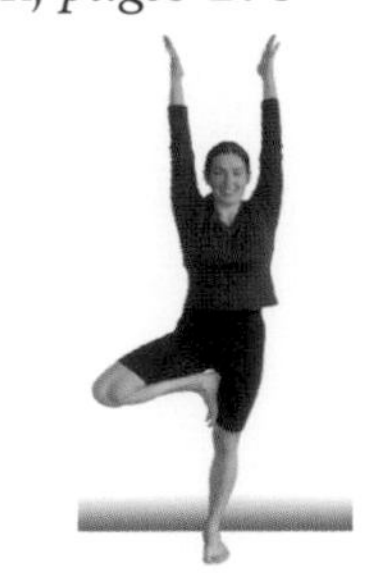

4 Vrikshasana, *page 279*

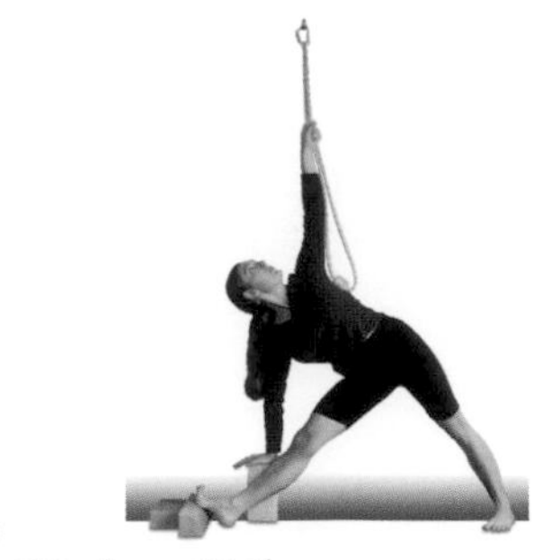

5 Utthita Trikonasana (wall/trestle/block), *page 281*

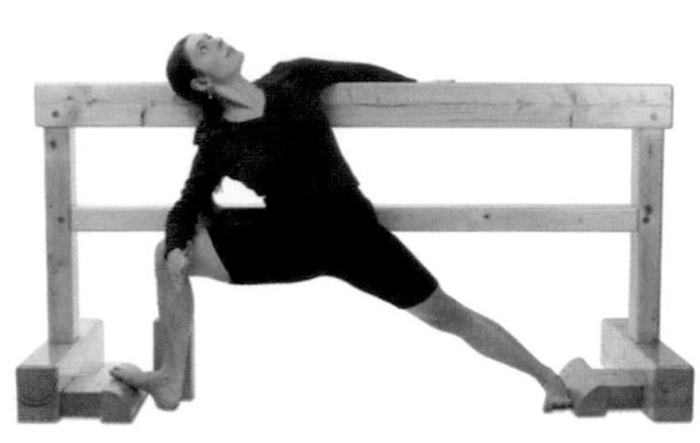

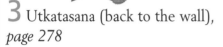

6 Utthita Parshvakonasana (trestle/back foot against wall), *page 282*

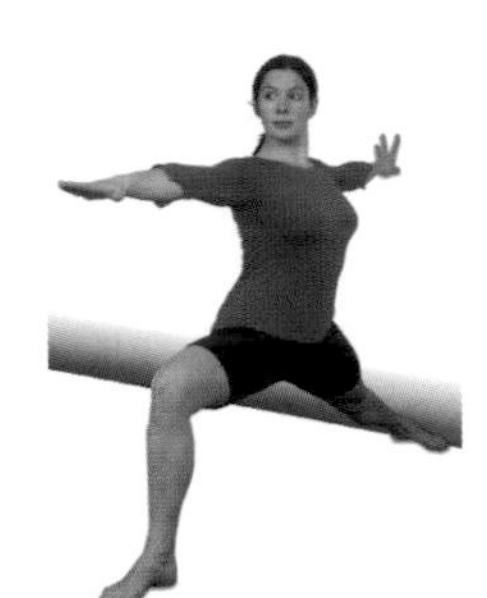

7 Virabhadrasana 2, *page 284*

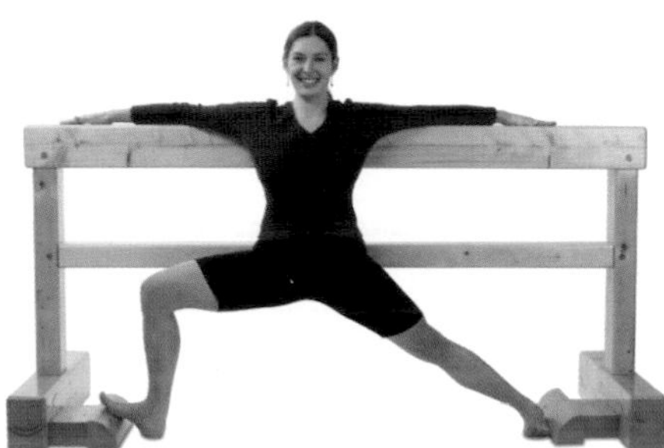

with trestle

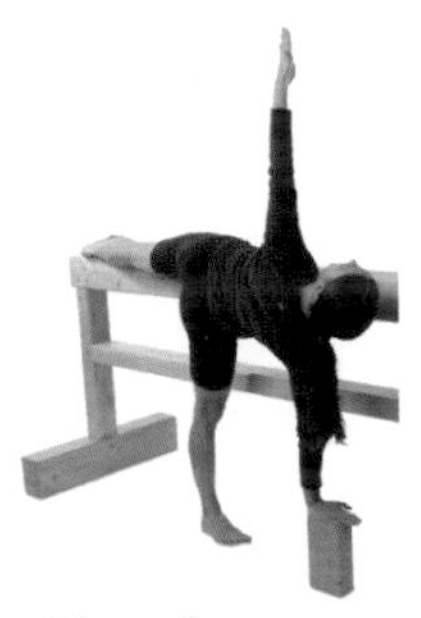

8 Ardha Chandrasana, *page 283*

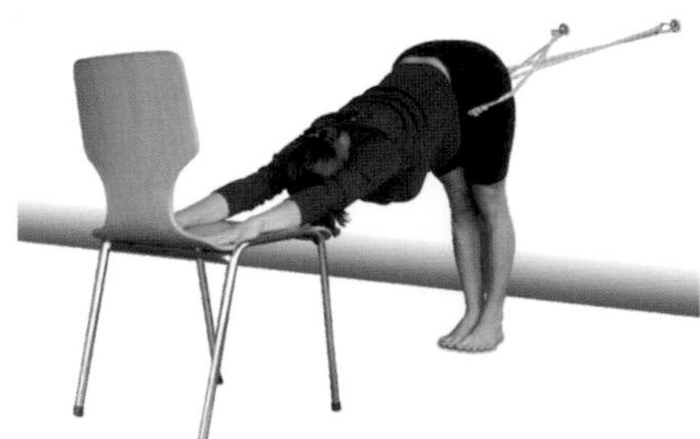

9 Ardha Uttanasana (with ropes and chair), *page 293*

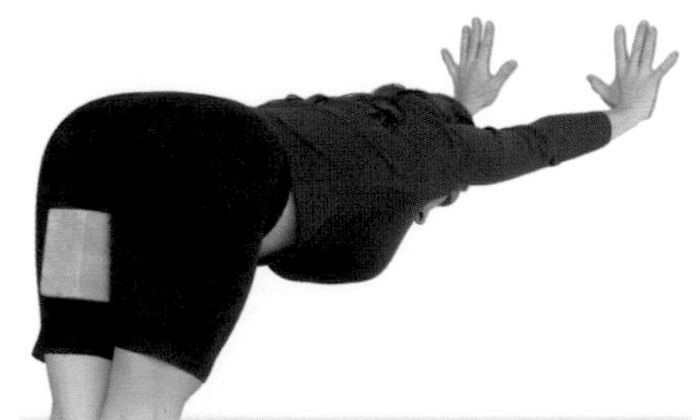

Ardha Uttanasana (hands against wall and block between inner thighs), *page 292*

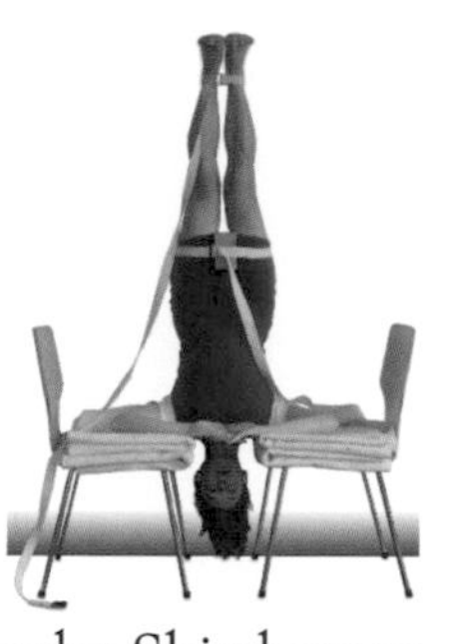

10 Salamba Shirshasana (block between the legs, with 2 chairs or classical pose), *page 340*

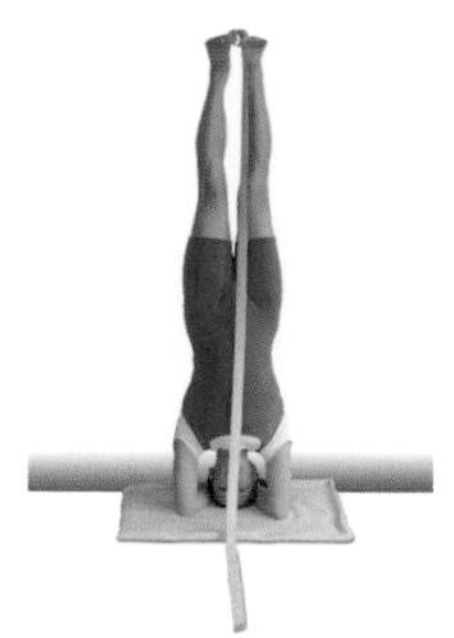

(belt around the big toes), *page 339*

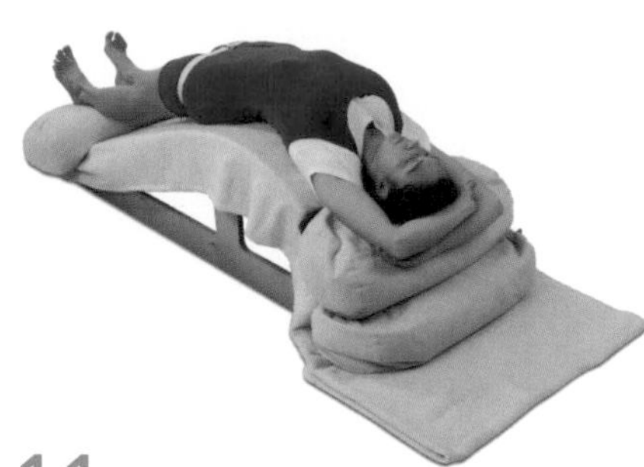

11 Viparita Dandasana (bench/chairs), *page 361*

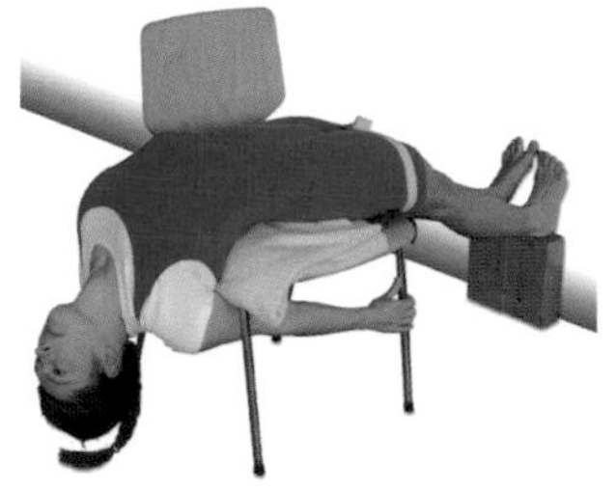

12 Dvi Pada Viparita Dandasana, with a Chair, *page 360*

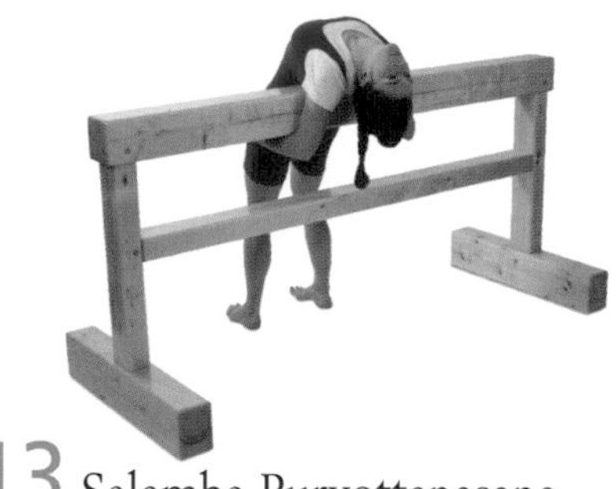

13 Salamba Purvottanasana (trestle), *page 362*

Note

Asanas 12 and 13 are especially good for breast-feeding mothers.

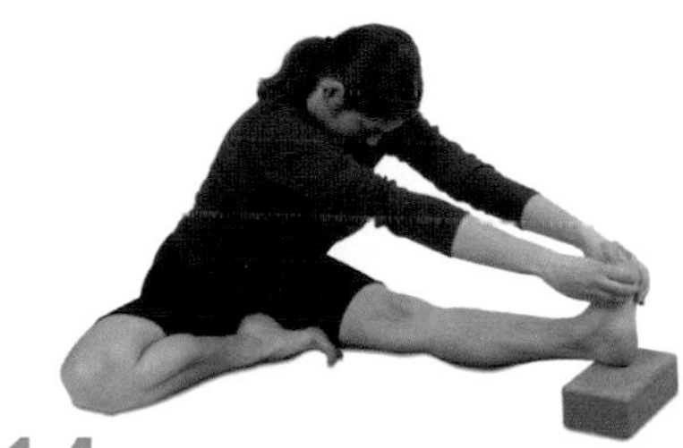

14 Maha Mudra, *page 304*

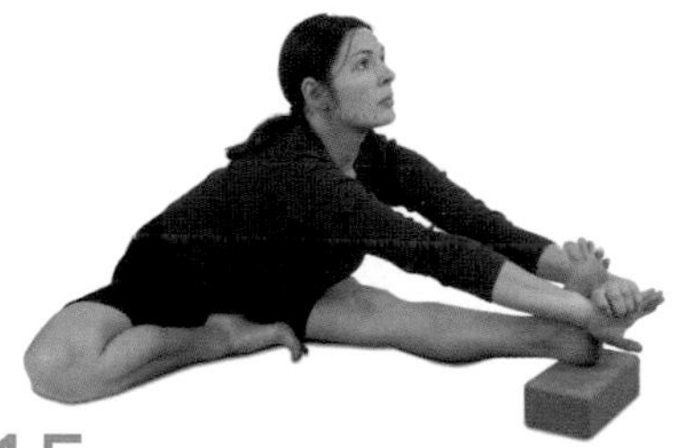

15 Janu Shirshasana, *page 306*

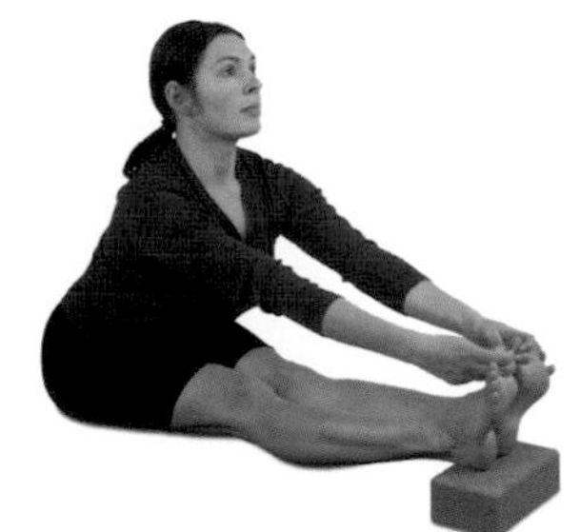

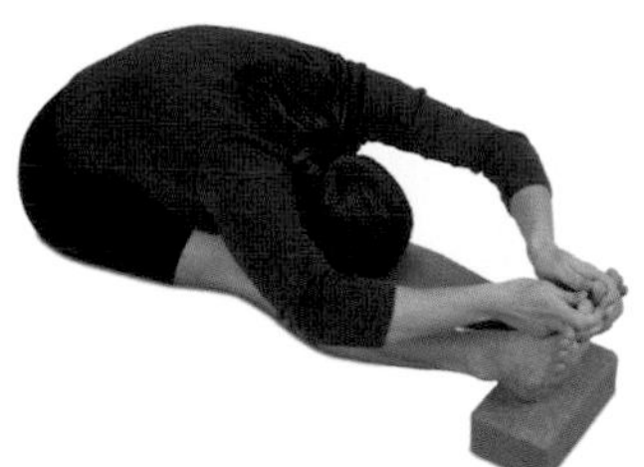

16 Pashchimottanasana, *page 308*

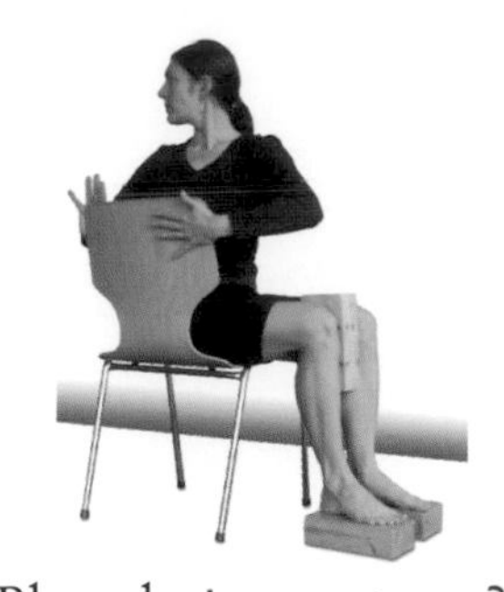

17 Bharadvajasana, *page 319*
(on a chair)

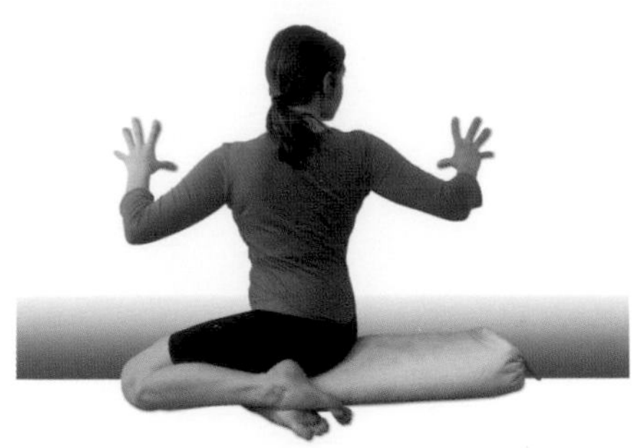

(on a bolster with wall)

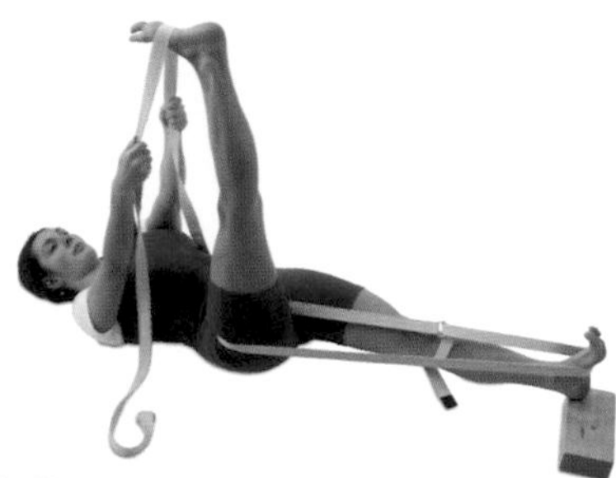

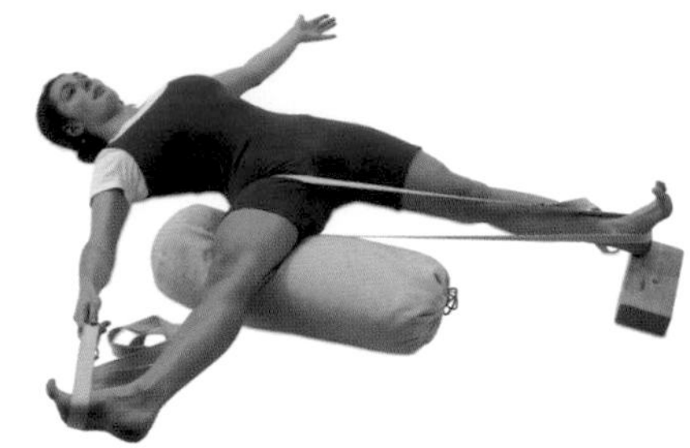

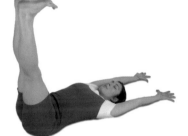

18 Supta Padangushthasana 1 and 2, *pages 342 – 343*

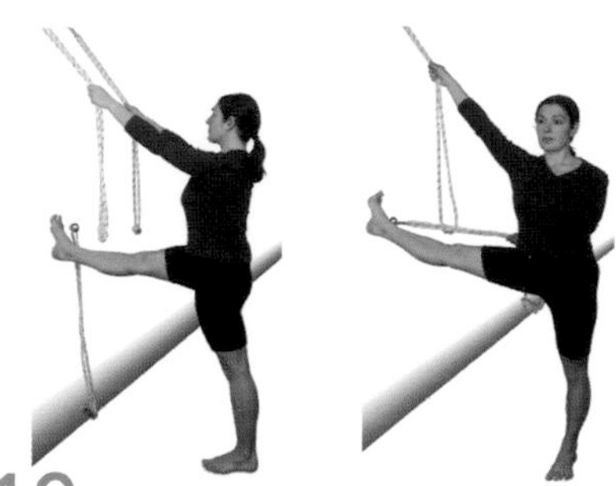

19 Utthita Hasta Padangushthasana 1 and 2, *pages 344 – 345*

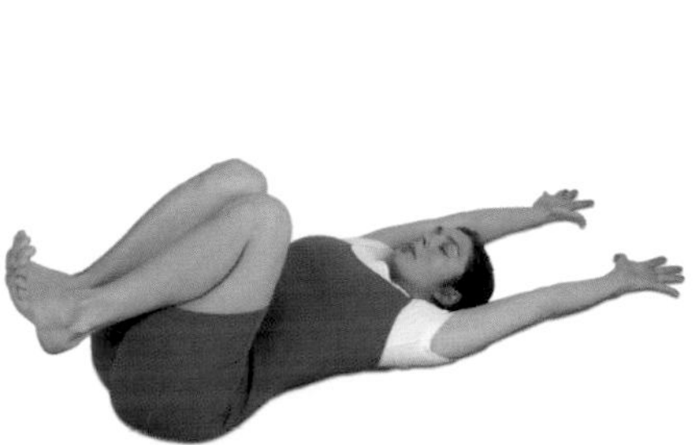

20 Urdhva Prasarita Padasana 90°, *pages 351 – 352*

Note

Begin asana 20 only in the third week of second term, and second version of asana 21, and 22 in the seventh week of second term.

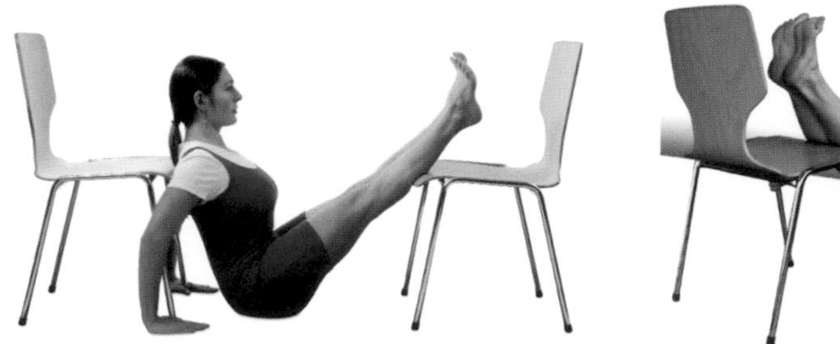

21 Paripurna Navasana (chair/chairs), *pages 348 – 349*

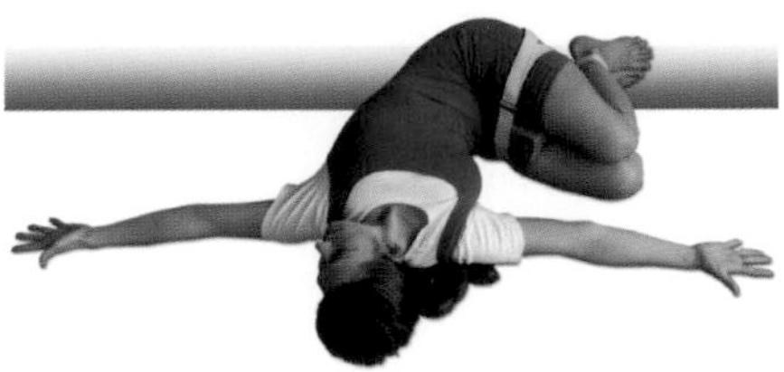

22 Jathara Parivartanasana (bent legs), *page 357*

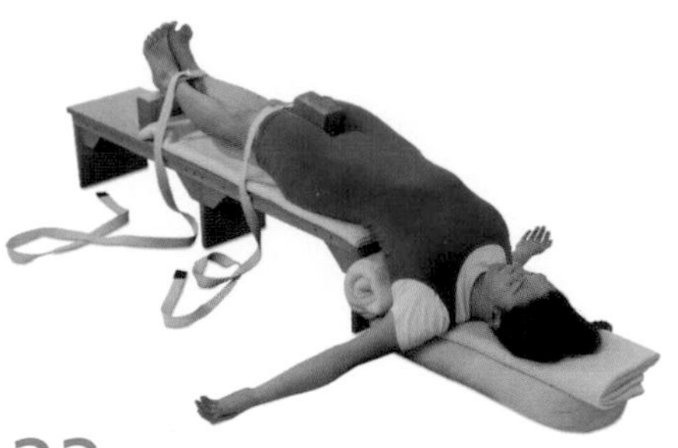

23 Setu Bandha Sarvangasana (bench, or similar height), *page 334*

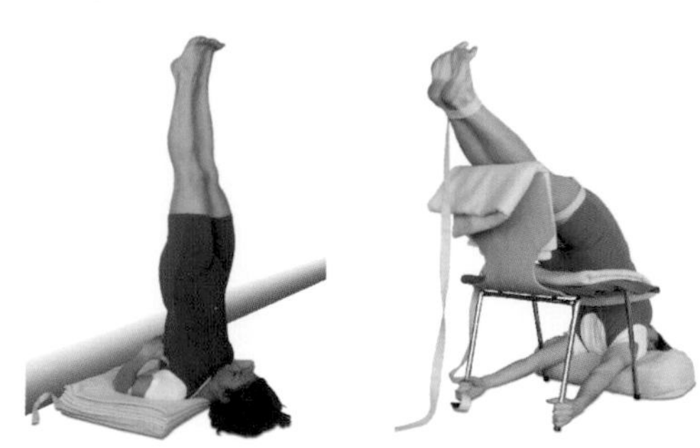

24 Salamba Sarvangasana (from wall), *page 328*, (or with chair), *page 330*

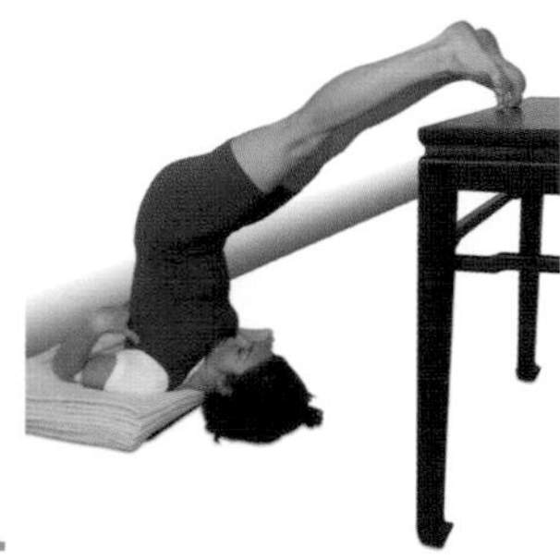

25 Ardha Halasana (toes on table, keep spine lifted), *page 332*

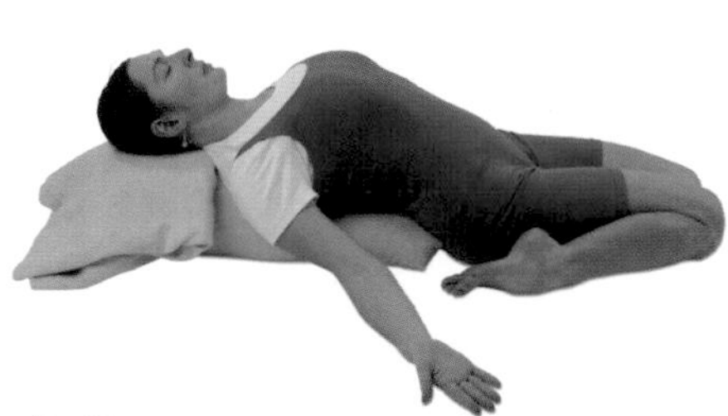

26 Supta Virasana, *page 367*

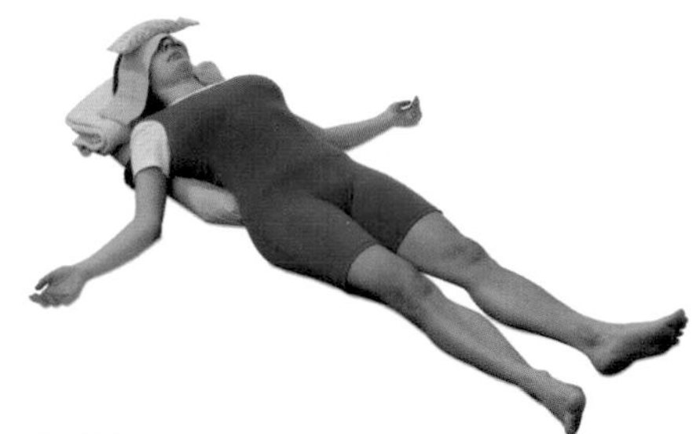

27 Shavasana (bolster/s), *page 366*

28 Ujjayi Pranayama in Shavasana (bolster/s), *page 148*

Notes

- Shavasana and Ujjayi Pranayama in Shavasana increase your oxygen intake and the quality of your breast milk.
- Begin Urdhva Prasarita Padasana, Paripurna Navasana, and Jathara Parivartanasana only after your have practiced Supta and Utthita Hasta Padangushthasana for two weeks with no problem.

Durations

Inversions: 5 to 10 minutes

Note

Salamba Sarvangasana should be practiced two to three minutes longer than Salamba Shirshasana, if you do it without Halasana and Setu Bandha Sarvangasana.

Restorative asanas: 5 minutes
Asanas practiced on both sides: 30 to 60 seconds per side, equally
Forward bends, back bends, twists, or asanas for abdomen and lumbar: 30 to 60 seconds
Shavasana: 15 minutes

Coming out of the pose

Maintain the lift, width, strength, and calmness that the asana created.

Restorative Asanas

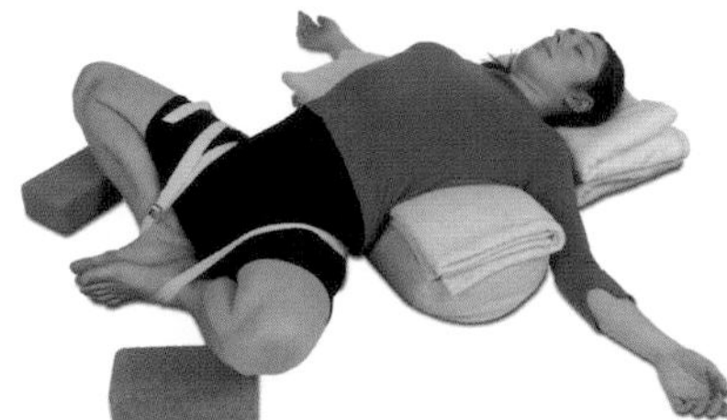

1 Supta Baddha Konasana (bolster crosswise), *page 128*

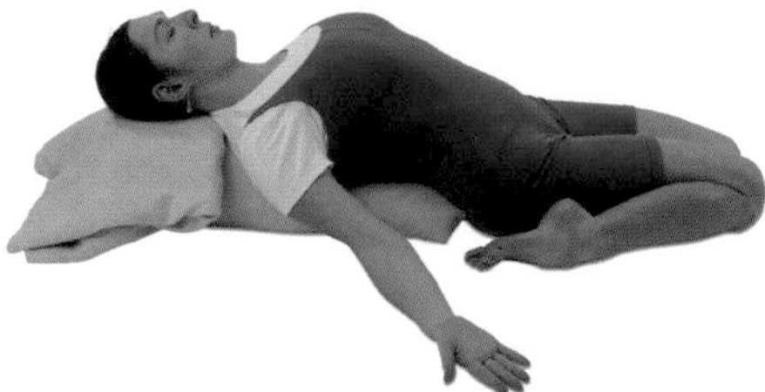

2 Supta Virasana (bolster/s), *page 367*

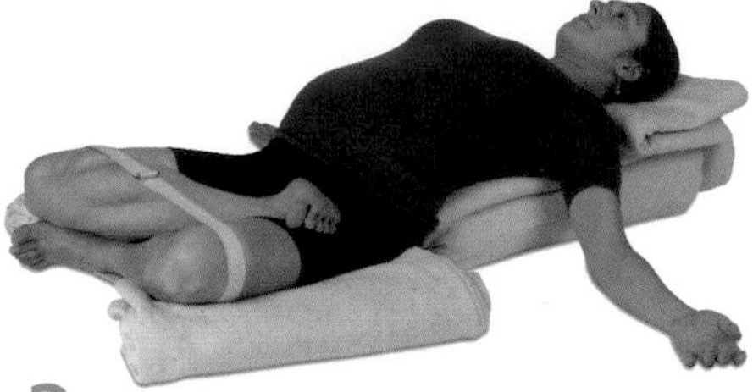

3 Matsyasana (bolster/s), *page 131*

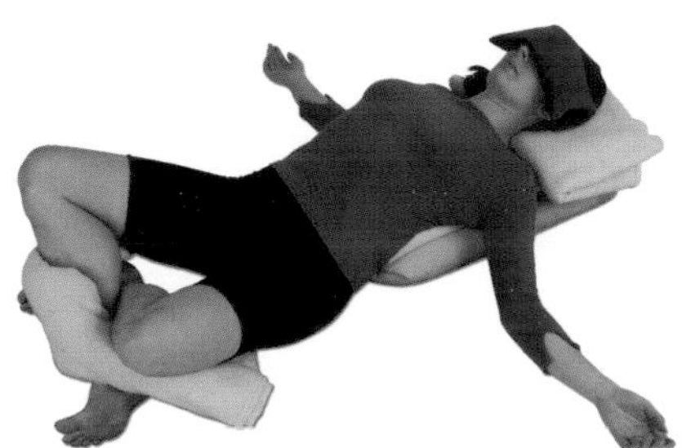

4 Supta Svastikasana (bolster/s), *page 131*

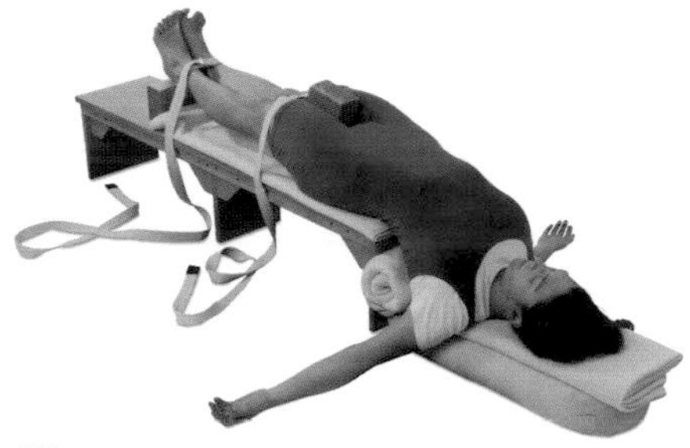

5 Setu Bandha Sarvangasana, *page 334*

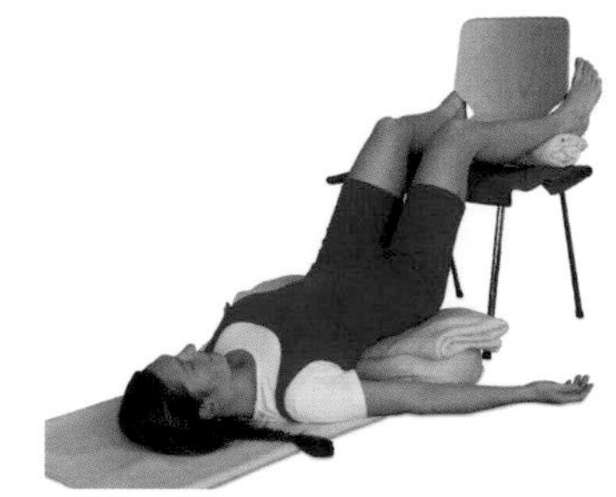

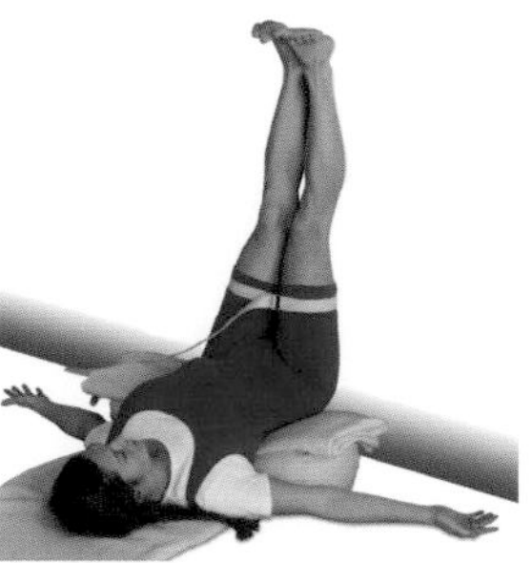

6 Viparita Karani, *pages 335 – 336*

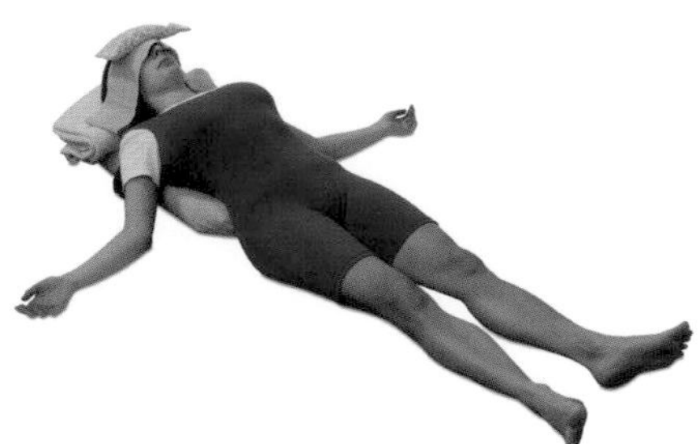

7 Shavasana (bolster/s), *page 366*

Sequence for the 3rd Term: During Your Period

You can start on the third, fourth, or fifth day of your period.

This sequence is also helpful when you suffer from menstrual pain or heavy bleeding.

You should resume practicing inverted poses like Salamba Shirshasana and Salamba Sarvangasana only after your period has fully stopped.

1 Ardha Uttanasana (ropes, with chair), *page 293*

2 Padangushthasana, *page 297*

3 Utthita Trikonasana (back foot against wall), *page 281*

4 Utthita Parshvakonasana (back foot against wall), *page 282*

5 Baddha Konasana (straight back), *page 67*

6 Supta Baddha Konasana (bolster crosswise), *page 128*

7 Upavishtha Konasana (concave back), *page 316*

8 Virasana, *page 302*

9 Parvatasana in Virasana, *page 303*

10 Supta Virasana (bolster/s), *page 367*

11 Matsyasana (bolster/s), *page 131*

and/or

12 Supta Svastikasana (bolster/s), *page 131*

13 Shavasana (bolster/s), *page 366*

14 Ujjayi Pranayama in Shavasana, *page 148*

Sequence for the 3rd Term: Back to Normal

In your third term, you can include all the standing asanas that appear in the classification and detailed descriptions in this chapter.

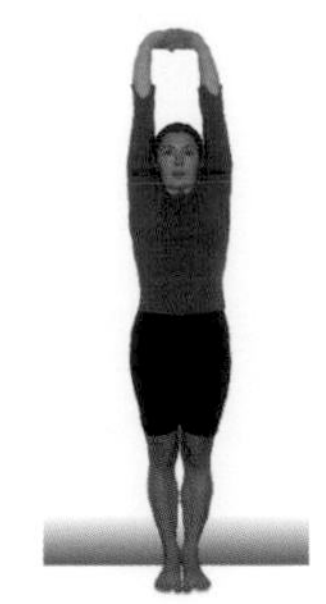

1 Urdhva Baddhanguliyasana, *page 274*

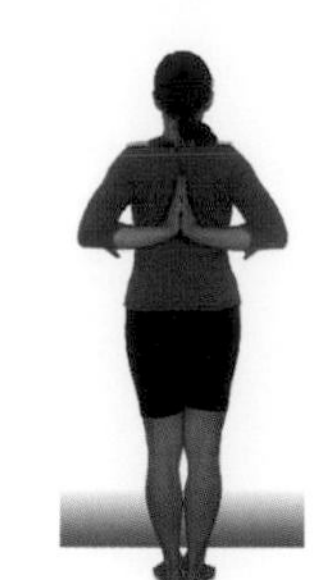

Pashchima Namaskarasana, *page 277*

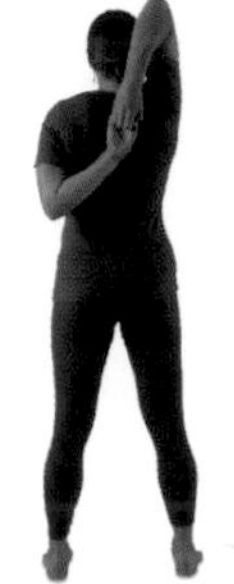

Gomukhasana in Tadasana, *page 37*

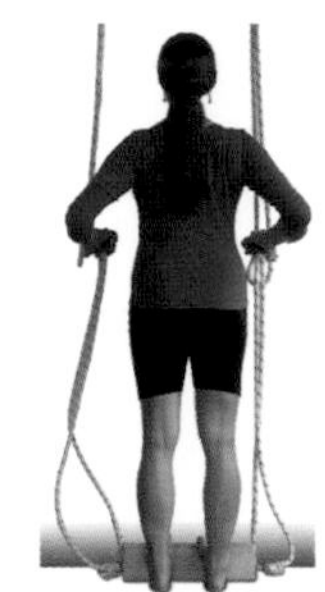

Tadasana (heels down), *page 275*

Note

Always start the standing poses from Tadasana. When you finish the pose, come back to Tadasana. If you feel tired, rest in Ardha Uttanasana.

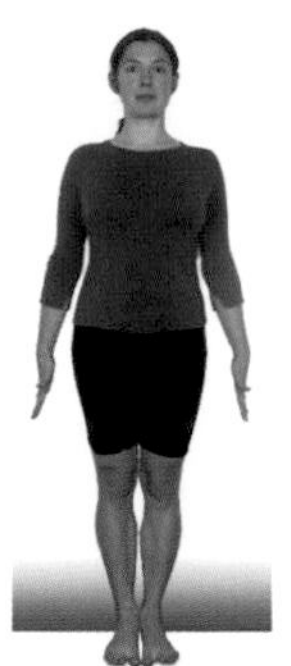

Tadasana

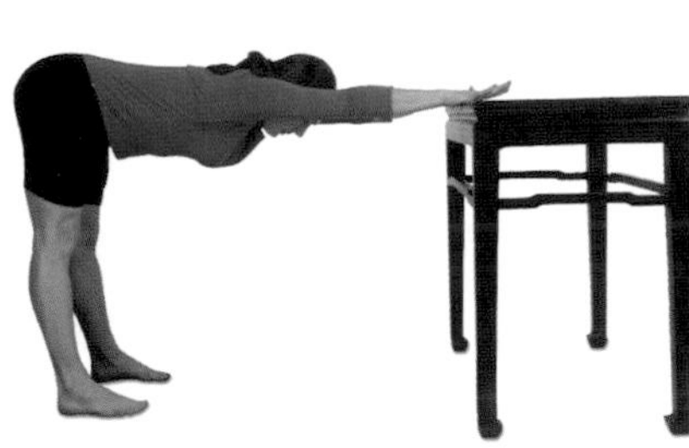

Ardha Uttanasana

See also the variations of Tadasana with a block in between the legs, *page 275*

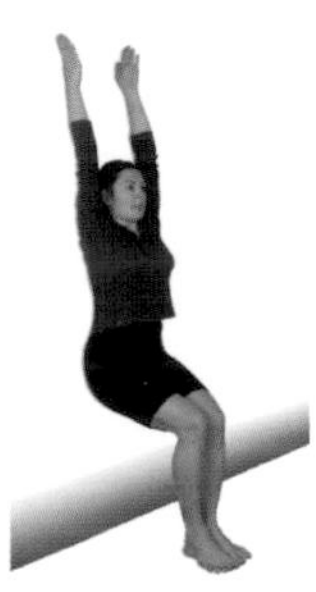

2 Utkatasana (back to the wall), *page 278*

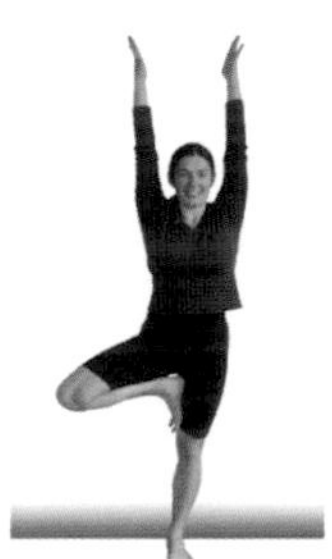

3 Vrikshasana, *page 279*

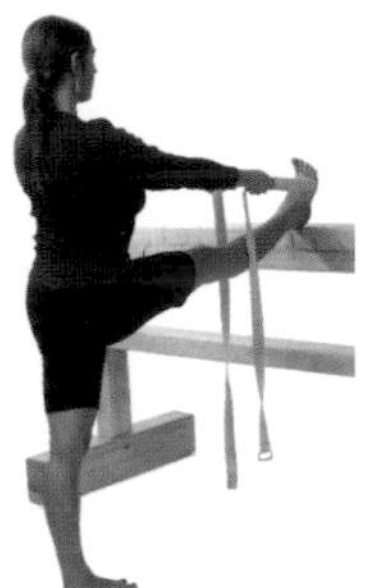

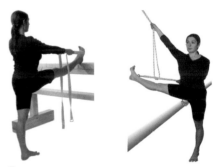

4 Utthita Hasta Padangushthasana 1 and 2, *pages 344 – 345*

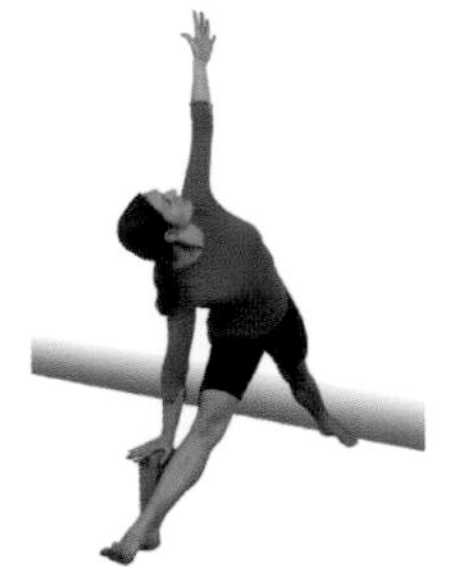

5 Utthita Trikonasana, *page 281*

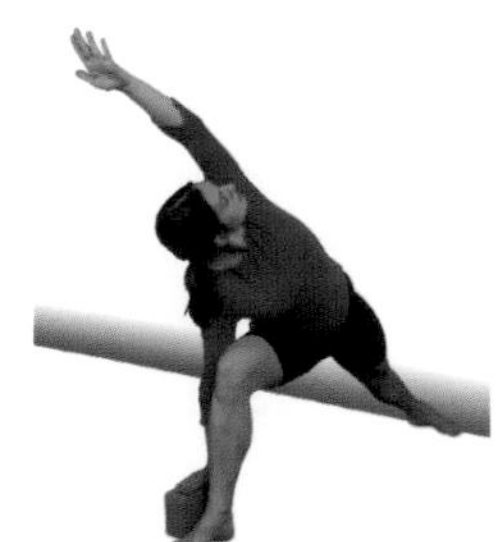

6 Utthita Parshvakonasana, *page 282*

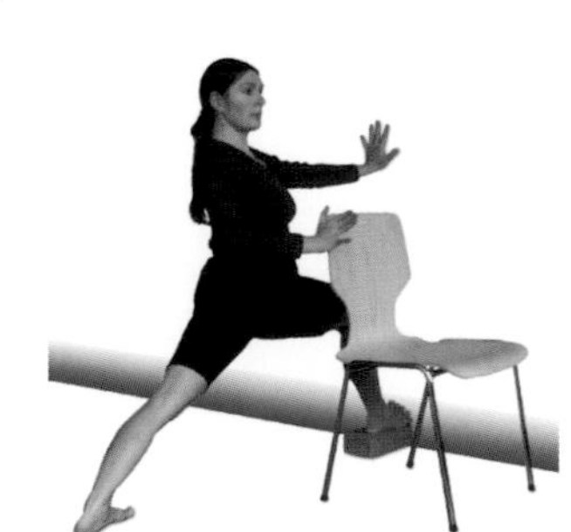

7 Virabhadrasana 1 (twisting in), *page 288*

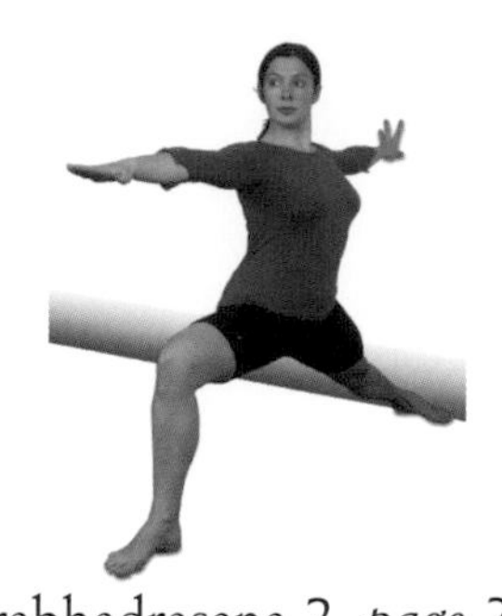

8 Virabhadrasana 2, *page 284*

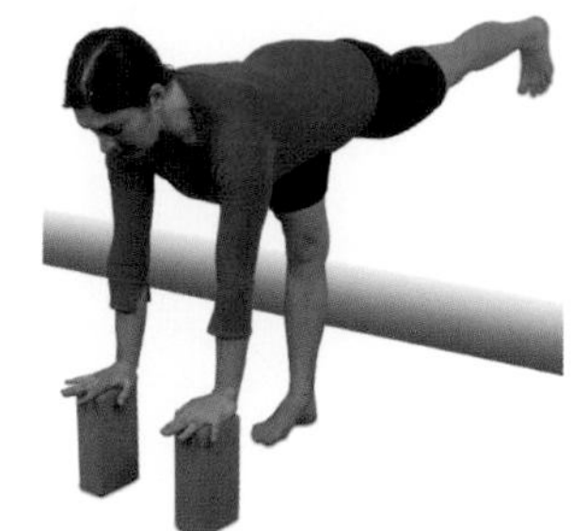

9 Virabhadrasana 3, *page 289*

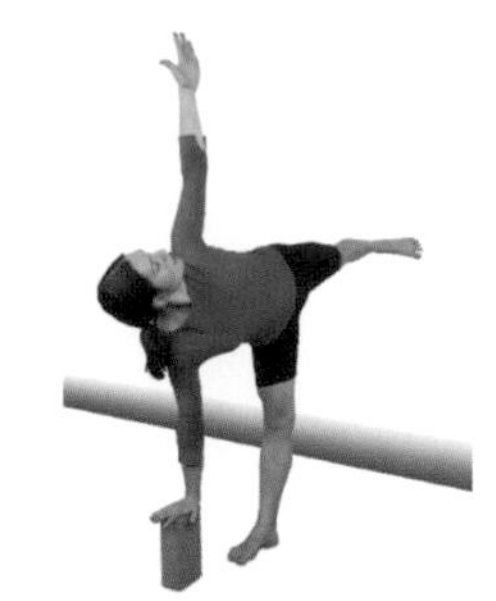

10 Ardha Chandrasana, *page 283*

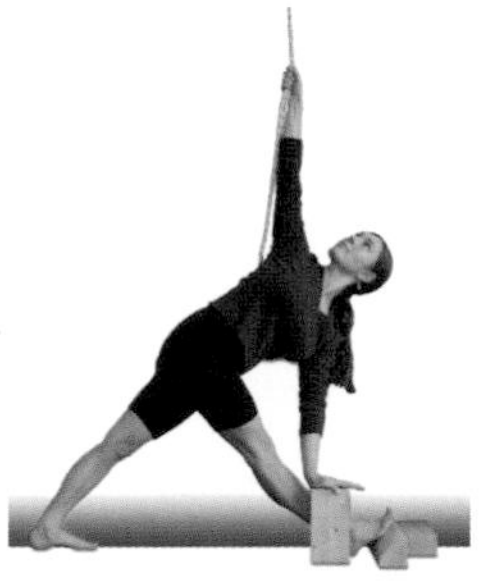

11 Parivritta Trikonasana, *page 290*

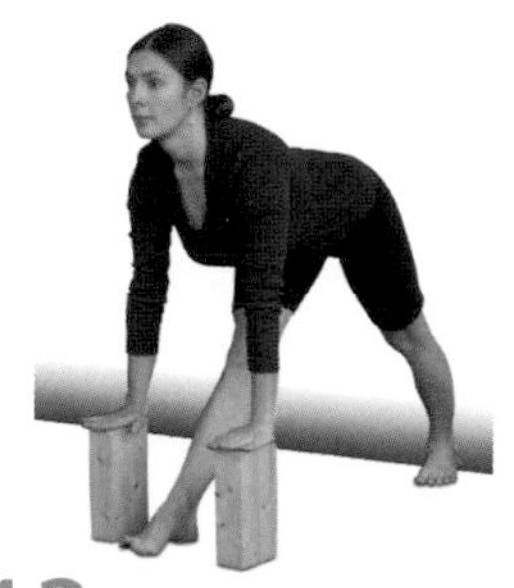

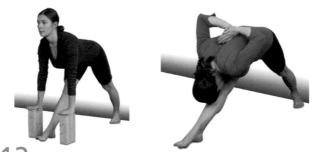

12 Parshvottanasana, *pages 286 – 287*

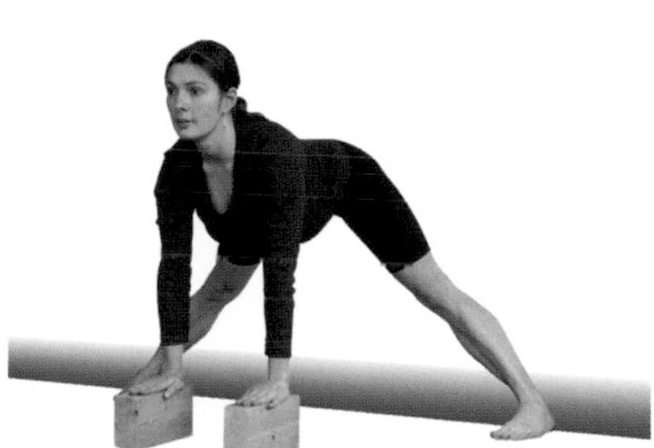

13 Prasarita Padottanasana, *page 296*

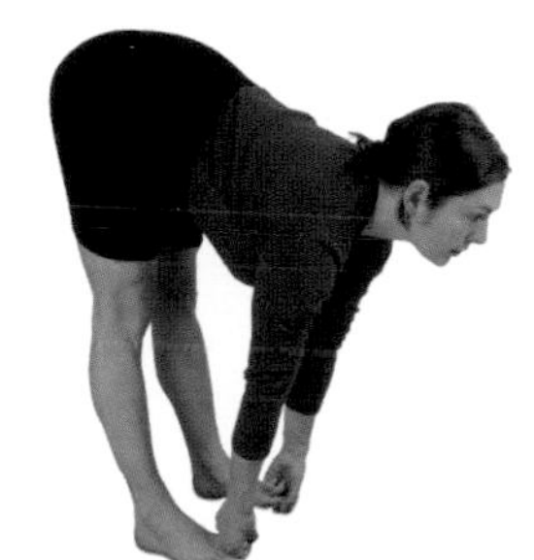

14 Padangushthasana, *page 297*

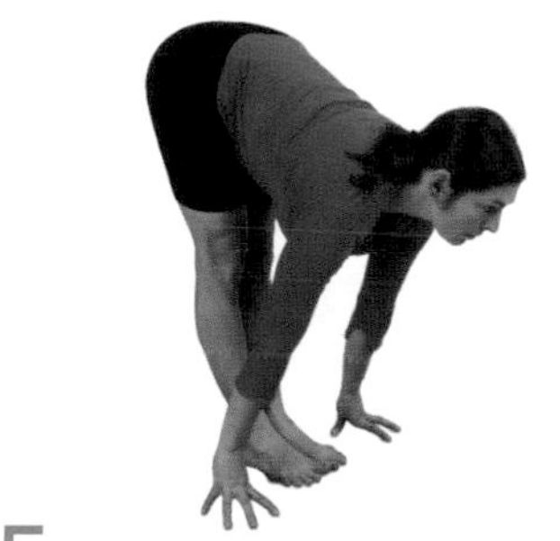

15 Uttanasana, *page 294*

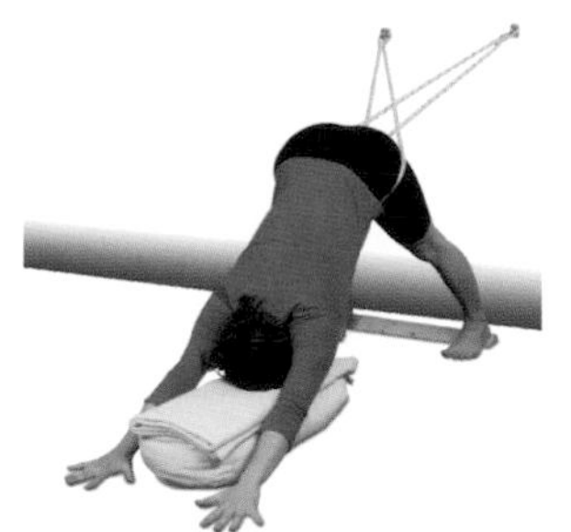

16 Adho Mukha Shvanasana, *page 299*

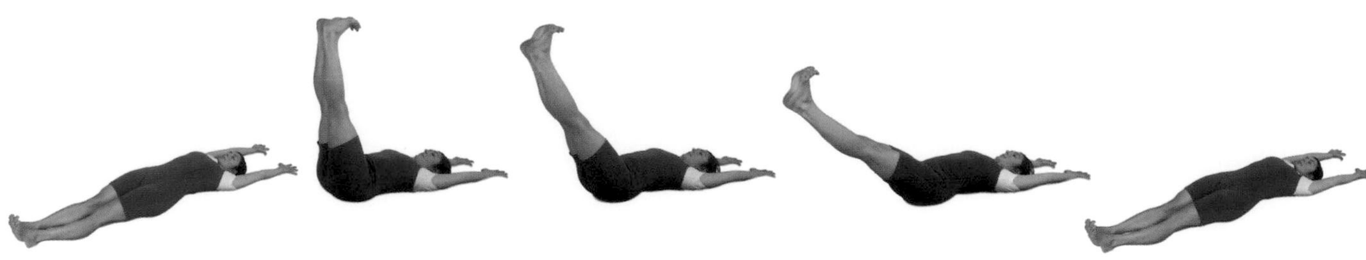

17 Urdhva Prasarita Padasana, 90°, 60°, 30°, *pages 351 – 355*

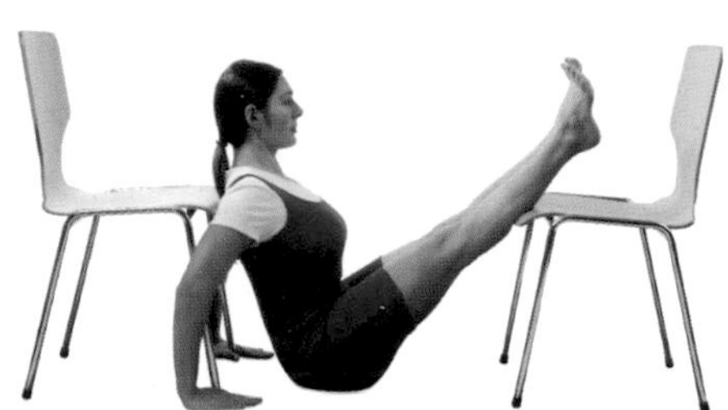

18 Paripurna Navasana (chair/chairs), *page 347*

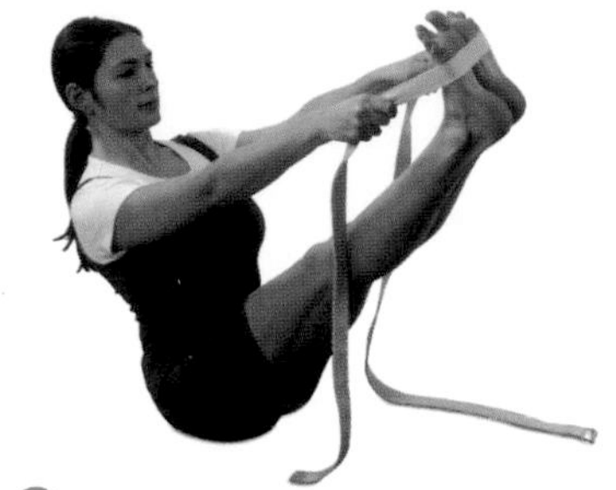

19 Ubhaya Padangushthasana, *page 349*

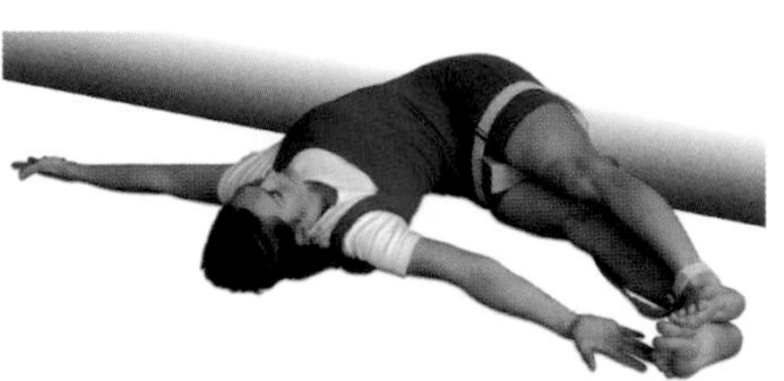

20 Jathara Parivartanasana, *page 358*

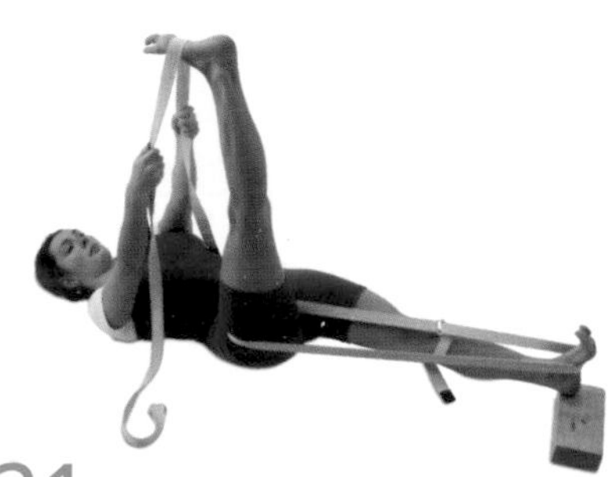

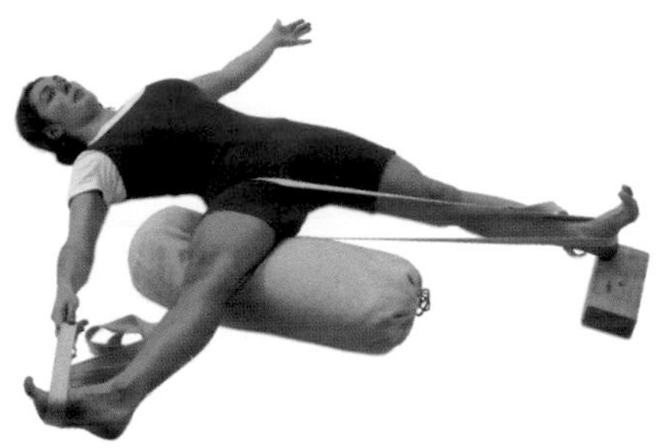

21 Supta Padangushthasana 1 and 2, *pages 342 – 343*

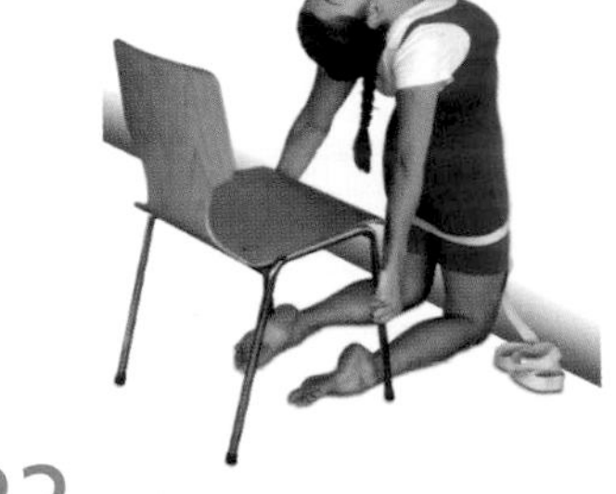

22 Ushtrasana, *page 364*

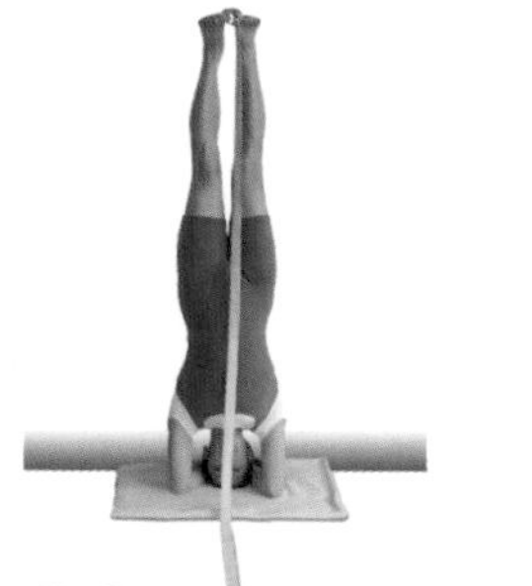

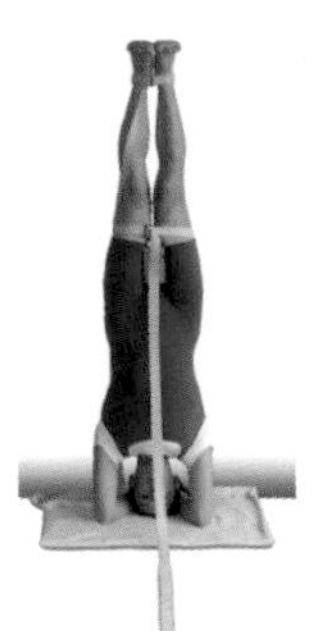

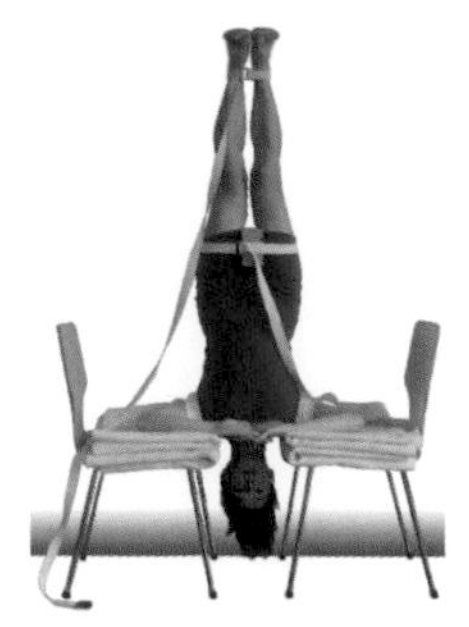

23 Salamba Shirshasana, *pages 339 – 340*

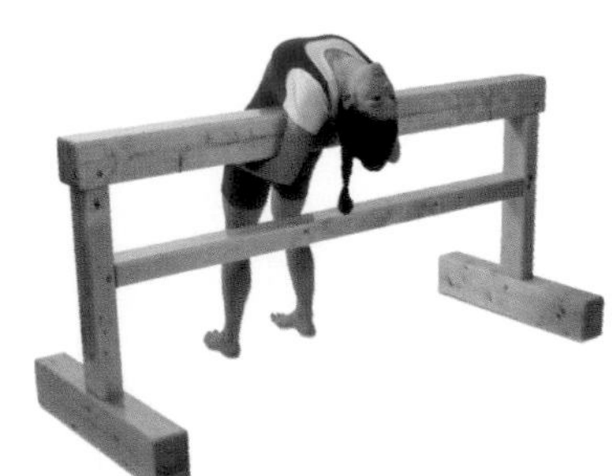

24 Salamba Purvottanasana (trestle), *page 362*

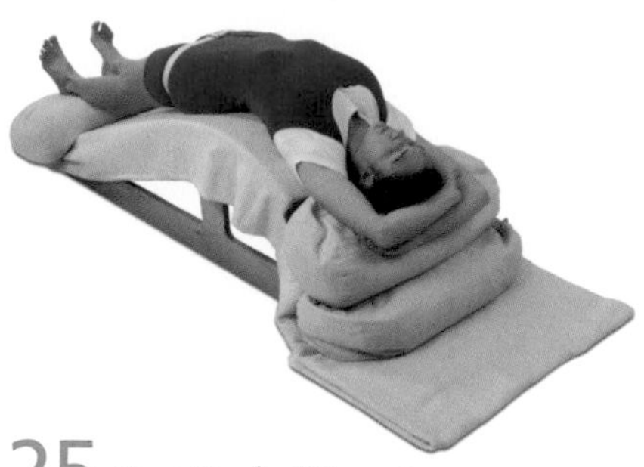
25 Dvi Pada Viparita Dandasana (bench/chairs), *page 361*

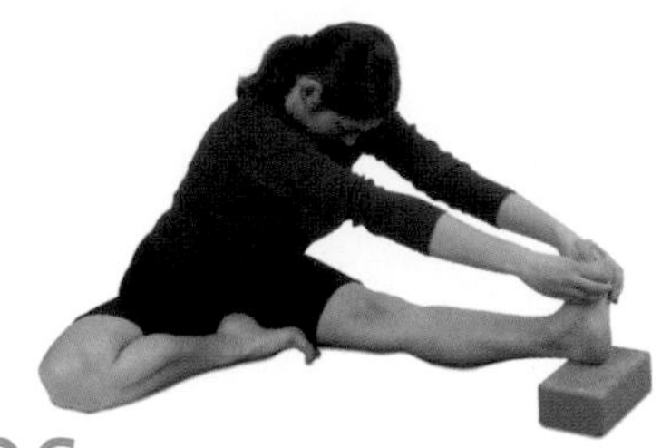
26 Maha Mudra, *page 369*

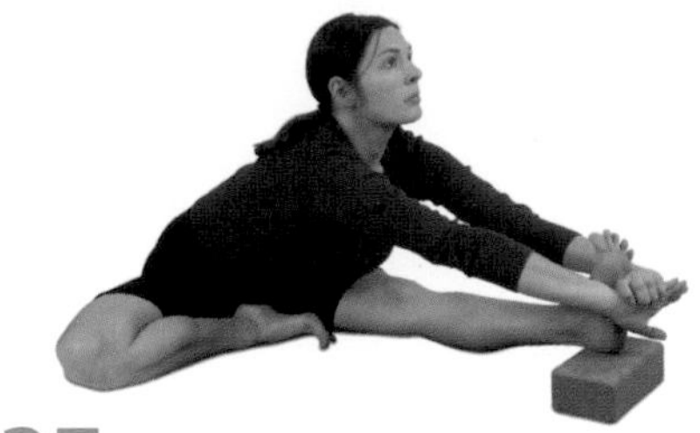
27 Janu Shirshasana, *page 306*

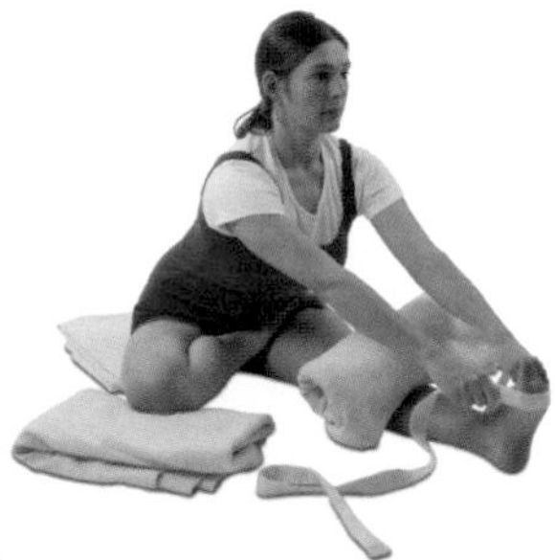
28 Ardha Baddha Padma Pashchimottanasana, *page 311*

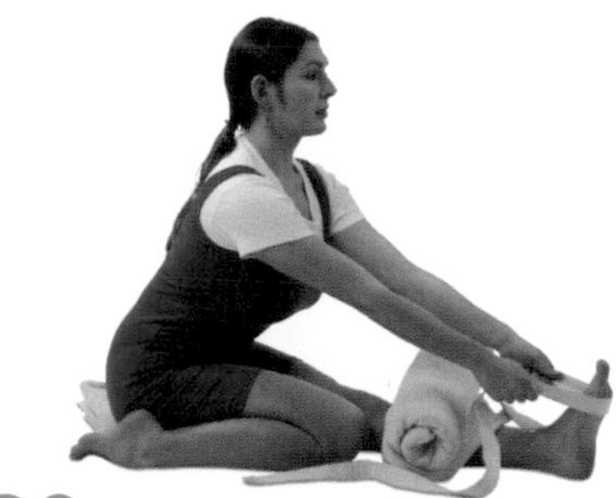
29 Trianga Mukhaikapada Pashchimottanasana, *page 312*

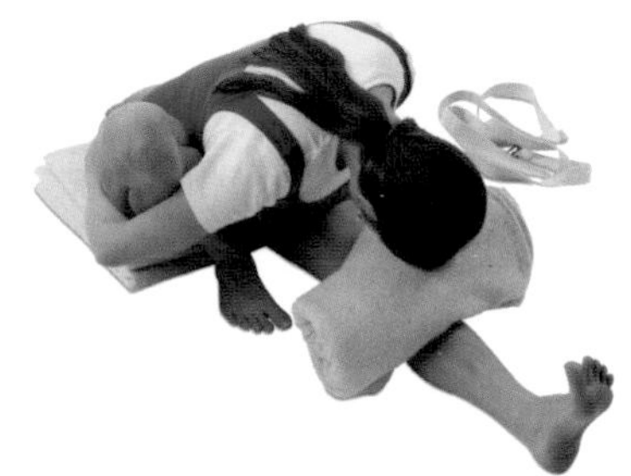
30 Marichyasana 1, *page 315*

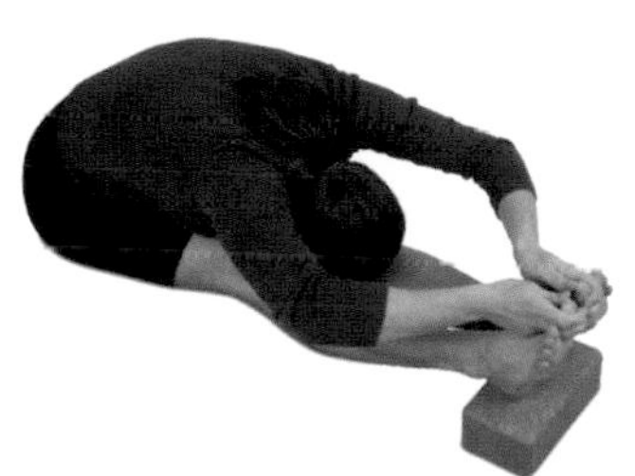
31 Pashchimottanasana, *page 309*

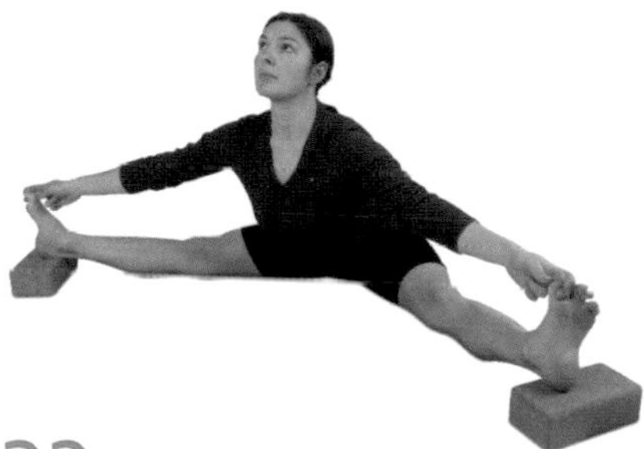
32 Upavishtha Konasana, *page 316*

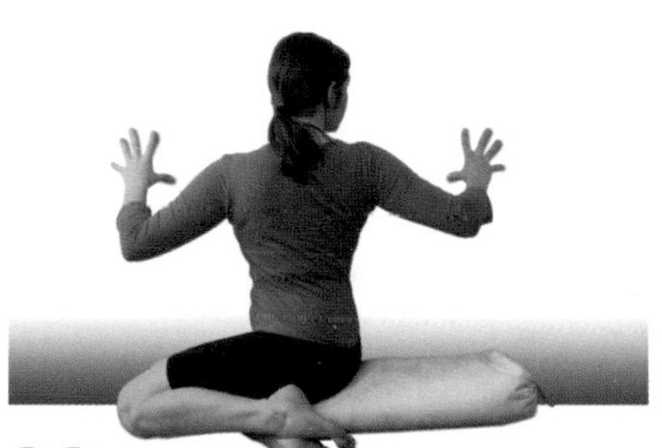
33 Bharadvajasana (chair or bolster), *page 319*

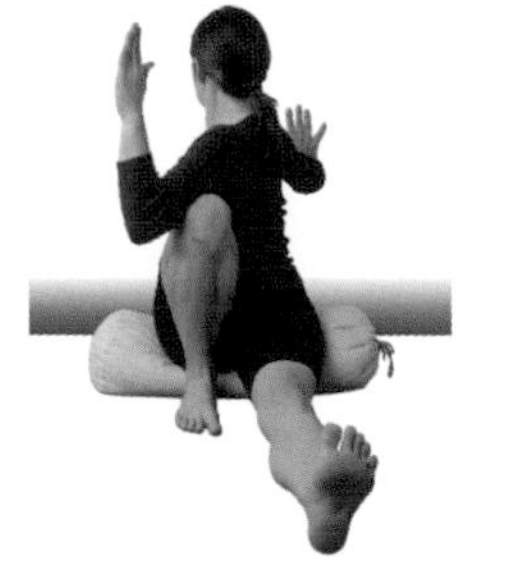
34 Marichyasana 3, *page 323*

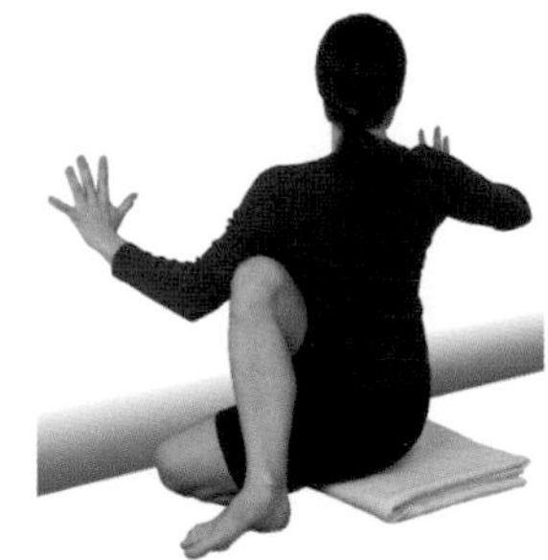
35 Ardha Matsyendrasana, *page 325*

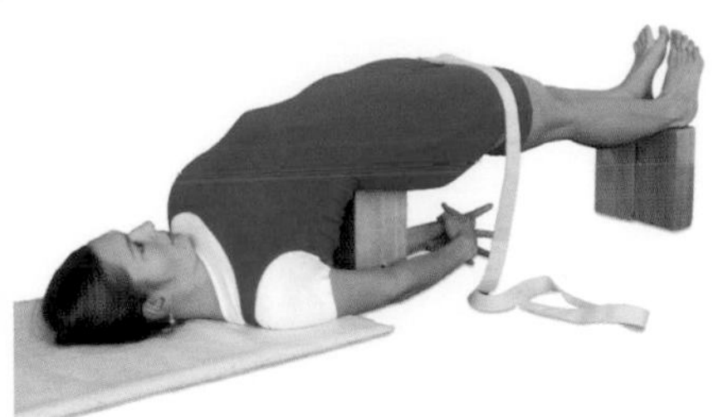

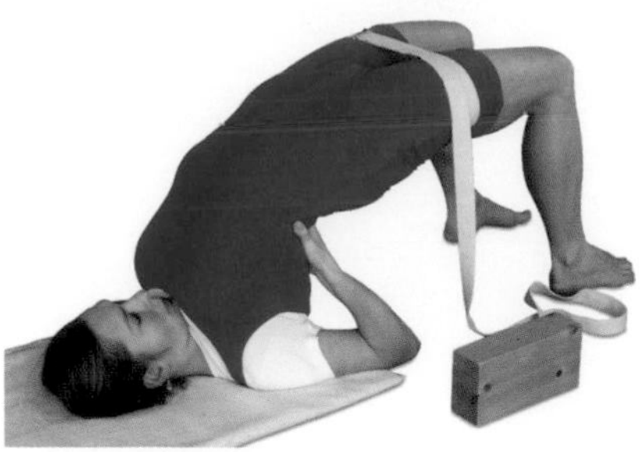

36 Setu Bandha Sarvangasana (blocks), *page 334;* with bent legs

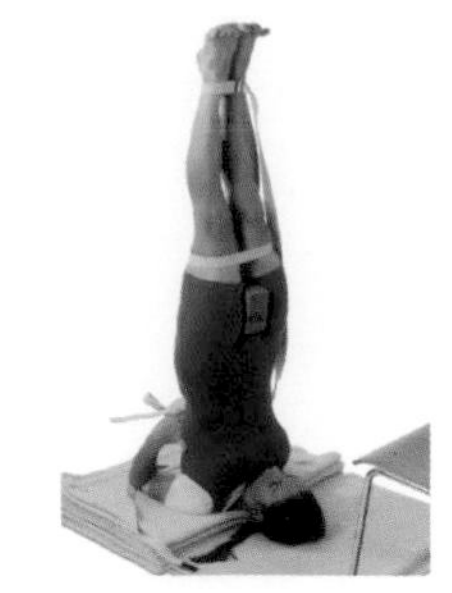

37 Salamba Sarvangasana, *page 331*

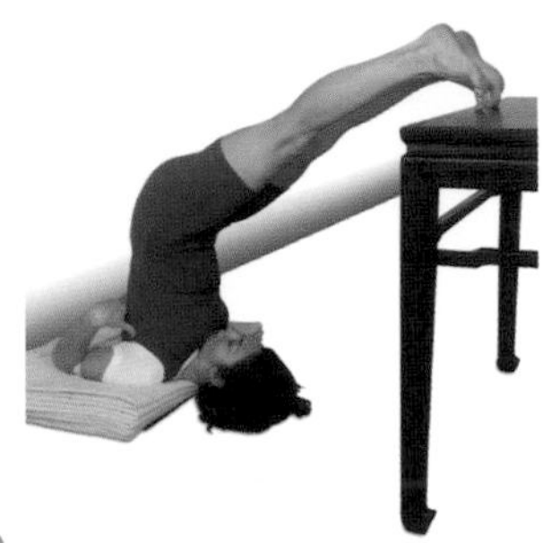

38 Ardha Halasana (with toes on table, keep spine lifted), *page 332*

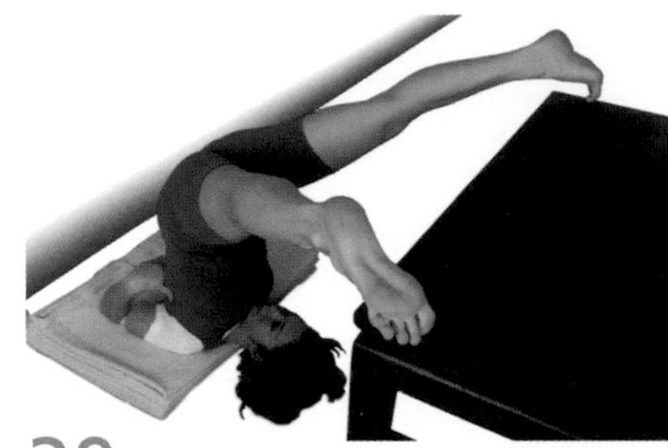

39 Ardha Supta Konasana (toes on table, keep spine lifted), *page 333*

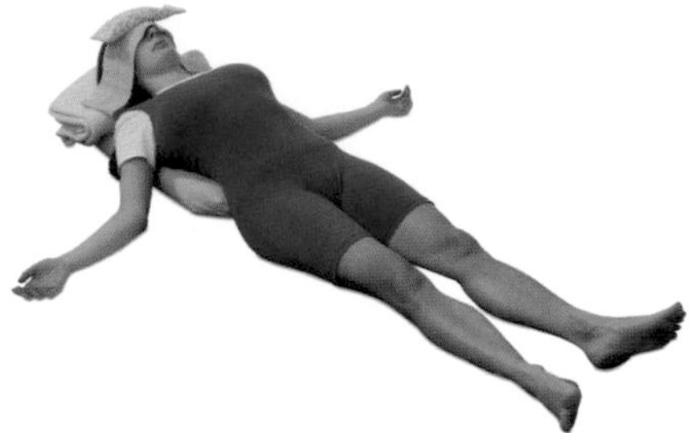

40 Shavasana (bolster/s), *page 366*

41 Ujjayi Pranayama in Shavasana (bolster/s), *page 148*

NOTE

Shavasana and Ujjayi Pranayama in Shavasana increase your oxygen intake and the quality of your breast milk.

Suggestion for Breaking the Sequence into Two

Because the list of asanas is quite long for the third term after delivery, you may practice them in two sequences, as given below, or even break them up into three or four sequences.

1st Sequence

1 Nos. 1 to 18, *pages 264 – 266*
2 Ushtrasana, *page 363*
3 Salamba Shirshasana, *page 338*
4 Urdhva Dhanurasana (trestle), *page 362*
5 Bharadvajasana (wall), *page 319*
6 Setu Bandha Sarvangasana, *page 334*
7 Salamba Sarvangasana, *page 326*
8 Ardha Halasana, *page 332*
9 Ardha Supta Konasana, *page 333*
10 Shavasana, *page 366*

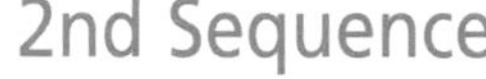

2nd Sequence

Nos. 16 to 40, *pages 265 – 268*

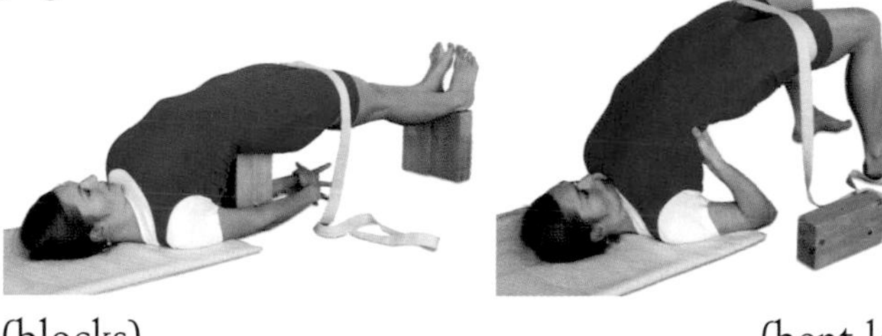

(blocks) (bent legs)

Durations

Inversions: 5 to 10 minutes

Note

Salamba Sarvangasana should be practiced two to three minutes longer than Salamba Shirshasana, if you do it without Halasana and Setu Bandha Sarvangasana.

Ardha Halasana: 2 to 5 minutes
Setu Bandha Sarvangasana: 5 minutes
Restorative asanas: 5 minutes

Asanas practiced on both sides: 30 to 60 seconds per side, equally
Forward bends, back bends, twists, or asanas for abdomen and lumbar: 30 to 60 seconds
Shavasana: 15 minutes

Coming out of the pose

Maintain the lift, width, strength, and calmness that the asana created.

DETAILED DESCRIPTIONS OF ASANAS FOR BEGINNERS AND ADVANCED STUDENTS

Restorative Asanas

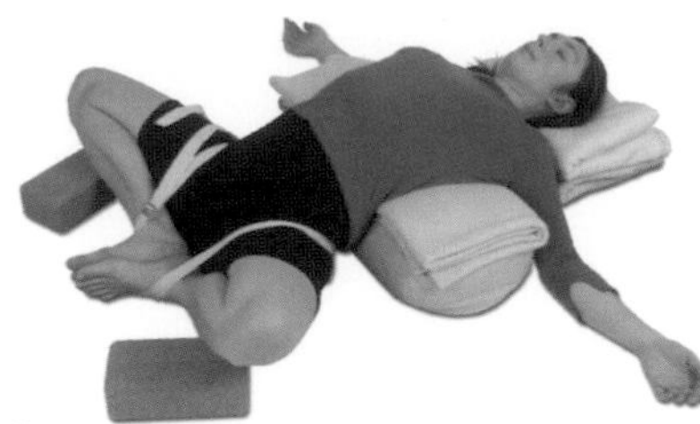

1 Supta Baddha Konasana (bolster crosswise), *page 128*

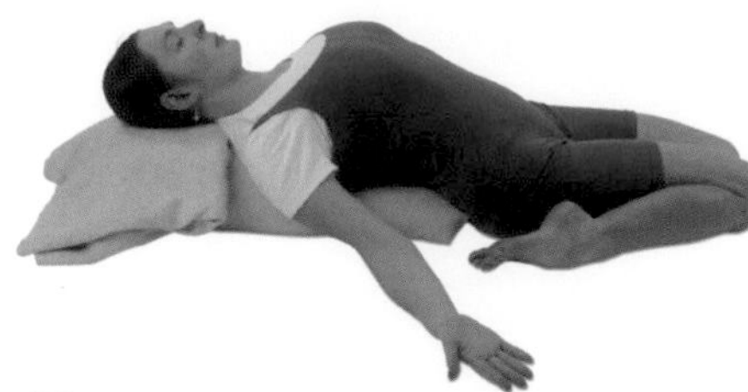

2 Supta Virasana (bolster/s), *page 367*

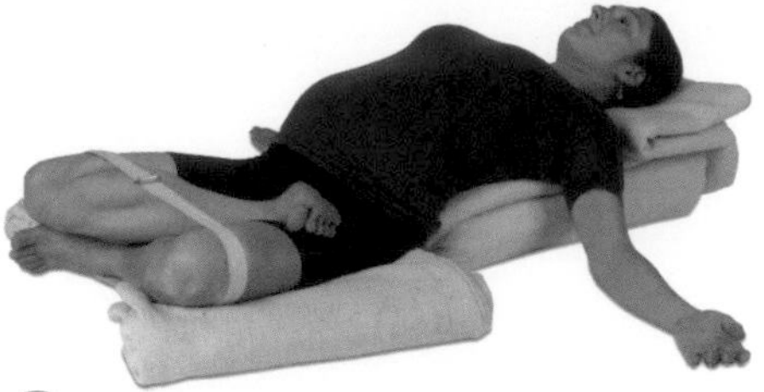

3 Matsyasana (bolster/s), *page 367*

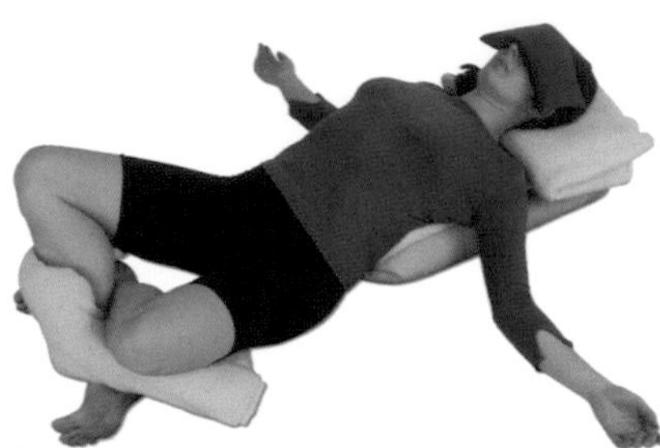

4 Supta Svastikasana (bolster/s), *page 368*

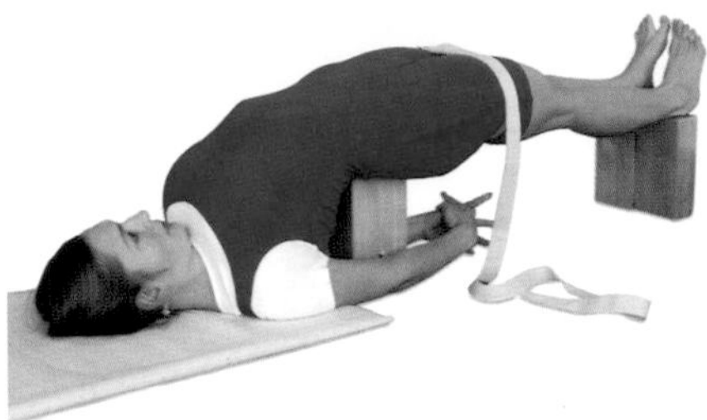

5 Setu Bandha Sarvangasana, *page 334*

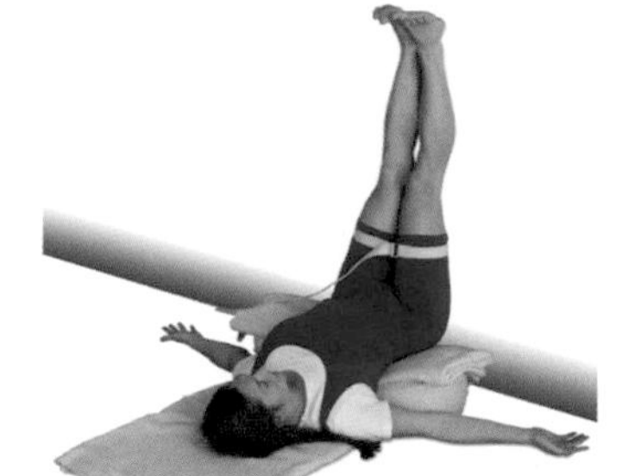

6 Viparita Karani, *page 336*

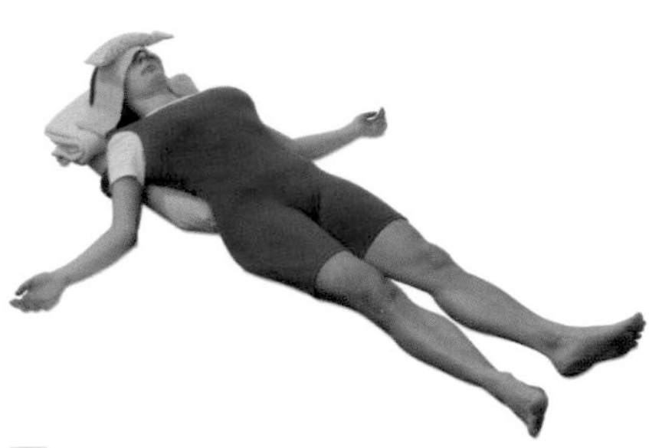

7 Shavasana (bolster/s), *page 366*

Classification of Asanas

Yoga asanas are classified according to the following considerations:

- The anatomic structure of the body
- The radius of movement and action of the body, specifically the spinal column
- How the asanas work on the body, mind, and soul

The asanas here are classified into nine categories, with pranayama appearing as the tenth. The classification gives you a quick and useful reference tool for finding all the asanas and the terms in which they can be safely practiced; it does not, however, show the *order* in which they should be practiced.

The asanas were taken from these categories and brought into practice sequences by the authors.

Although our recommendations are divided into the terms as shown at the beginning of this chapter, feel free to follow your own needs and extend duration of any term if necessary.

Resume your normal Yoga routine only after completing the modified program above for all three terms after your delivery.

Standing Asanas
Uttishtha Sthiti

1st and 2nd terms: practice with wall and props

	1st Term	2nd Term	3rd Term
Parshvottanasana (hands against wall, front foot on support)	√	√	√
Tadasana (lying down)		√	√
Tadasana standing against the wall: Block between wall and sacrum		√	√
Block between thighs		√	√
Block between inner heels and inner ankles		√	√
Tadasana: Urdhva Baddhanguliyasana		√	√
Pashchima Namaskarasana		√	√
Gomukhasana		√	√
On quarter-round block		√	√
Vrikshasana		√	√
Utkatasana (wall)		√	√
Utthita Trikonasana (wall/trestle/block)		√	√
Utthita Parshvakonasana (wall/trestle)		√	√
Virabhadrasana 2 (wall/trestle/block)		√	√
Ardha Chandrasana (wall/trestle/block)		√	√
Ardha Uttanasana (ropes, with chair)		√	√
Virabhadrasana 1 (wall/trestle)			√
Virabhadrasana 3 (wall and chair/blocks)			√
Parivritta Trikonasana (wall/trestle)			√
Parshvottanasana			√
Prasarita Padottanasana			√
Padangushthasana			√
Uttanasana			√
Adho Mukha Shvanasana (ropes/wall)			√

Sitting Asanas
Upavishtha Sthiti

	1st Term	2nd Term	3rd Term
Parvatasana from Svastikasana, Ardha Padmasana, or Padmasana	√	√	√
Virasana		√	√
Parvatasana in Virasana		√	√
Dandasana		√	√

Forward Bends
Pashchima Pratana Sthiti

	1st Term	2nd Term	3rd Term
Maha Mudra (belt around heel, foot on block)	√	√	√
Janu Shirshasana (belt, and foot on block)		√	√
Pashchimottanasana (heels on block)		√	√
Ardha Baddha Padma Pashchimottanasana		√	√
Trianga Mukhaikapada Pashchimottanasana		√	√
Marichyasana 1		√	√
Adho Mukha Virasana Upavishtha Konasana		√	√

Twists
Parivritta Sthiti

	1st Term	2nd Term	3rd Term
Bharadvajasana (chair)	√	√	√
Bharadvajasana (bolster/s)		√	√
Marichyasana 3		√	√
Ardha Matsyendrasana			√

NOTE

Always practice in the above order.

Inversions
Viparita Sthiti

	1st Term	2nd Term	3rd Term
Salamba Sarvangasana (from wall)	√	√	√
Ardha Halasana (toes on table)	√	√	√
Setu Bandha Sarvangasana (bench, or similar)	√	√	√
Viparita Karani (legs bent on chair)	√	√	√
Salamba Shirshasana: Block between legs		√	√
Heels against wall, toes inward		√	√
Belt around big toes		√	√
Salamba Sarvangasana (chair)		√	√
Viparita Karani		√	√
Salamba Sarvangasana (independent)			√
Ardha Supta Konasana (toes on chair, keep spine and groin lifted)			√

Asanas for Abdomen and Lumbar
Supta and Uttishtha Sthiti

	1st Term	2nd Term	3rd Term
Supta Padangushthasana 1 and 2		√	√
Utthita Hasta Padangushthasana 1 and 2		√	√
Urdhva Prasarita Padasana 90°		√	√
Paripurna Navasana: With 2 chairs		√	√
With chair		√	√
Jathara Parivartanasana (bent legs)		√	√
Jathara Parivartanasana			√
Ubhaya Padangushthasana (belt and chair)			√
Ubhaya Padangushthasana (belt)			√
Urdhva Prasarita Padasana 90°, 60°, and 30°			√

Back Bends
Purva Pratana Sthiti

	1st Term	2nd Term	3rd Term
Dvi Pada Viparita Dandasana (chair)		√	√
Dvi Pada Viparita Dandasana (bench)		√	√
Salamba Purvottanasana (chair)		√	√
Salamba Purvottanasana (trestle)		√	√
Note: The asanas above are recommended for breast-feeding mothers.			
Ushtrasana (wall and chair)			√

Rope Asanas
Yoga Kurunta

	1st Term	2nd Term	3rd Term
Ardha Uttanasana		√	√
Adho Mukha Shvanasana			√

Restorative Asanas
Vishranta Karaka Sthiti

	1st Term	2nd Term	3rd Term
Supta Baddha Konasana	√	√	√
Supta Virasana	√	√	√
Matsyasana	√	√	√
Supta Svastikasana	√	√	√
Shavasana (bolster/s)	√	√	√
Setu Bandha Sarvangasana (bench, or similar height)	√	√	√
Viparita Karani (legs bent on chair)	√	√	√
Maha Mudra (belt around heel, foot on block)		√	√
Viparita Karani		√	√
Niralamba Sarvangasana (chair and wall)		√	√
Salamba Sarvangasana (independent)			√

Breathing Techniques
Pranayama

	1st Term	2nd Term	3rd Term
Ujjayi 1 and 2 (lying on bolster)	√	√	√
Maha Mudra	√	√	√

Instructions and Benefits

Standing Asanas

Uttishtha Sthiti

Tadasana

Mountain pose

Follow the instructions given for during pregnancy, page 32.

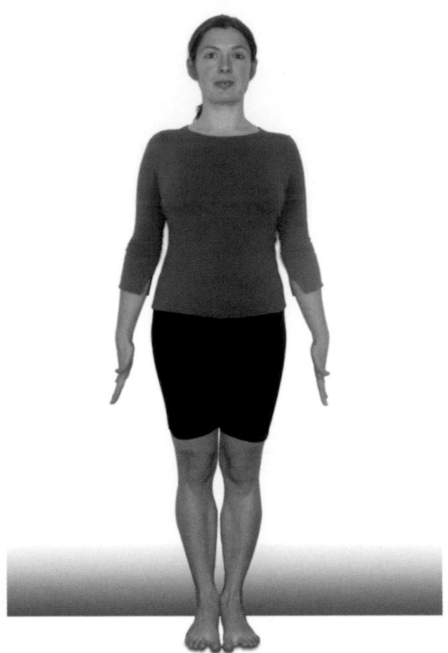

1st term: no
2nd term: yes
3rd term: yes

Benefits

See page 33

Urdhva Baddhanguliyasana, in Tadasana

Upward bound fingers in mountain pose

Follow the instructions given for during pregnancy, page 34.

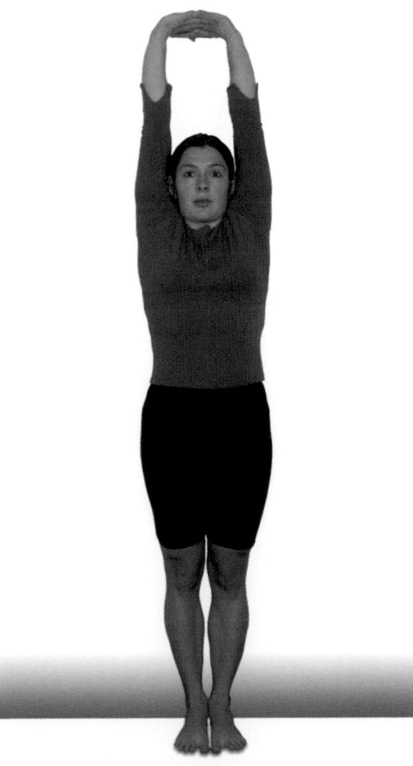

Benefits

Stretching your arms with your fingers interlocked lifts up the abdominal muscles and the breasts. This pose is particularly meant to tone the muscles of the buttocks, abdomen, and breast.

Special Instructions

- Breathe freely while staying in the pose.
- While exhaling, don't loosen the abdominal lift.
- Repeat the pose twice, staying in it for 10 seconds.

Supta Urdhva Hastasana and Supta Tadasana

Mountain or reclined mountain pose

1st term: no
2nd term: yes
3rd term: yes

If you don't feel centered in your body, then start Tadasana lying on the floor, preferably with your feet against the wall.

Tadasana, Block between Wall and Sacrum

Mountain pose

1st term: no
2nd term: yes
3rd term: yes

In this variation, you'll learn to bring in your sacrum (bone plate just above the tailbone).

1 Place a block between the wall and your sacrum to concentrate feeling in the pelvis and the muscles that keep the pelvis erect.

2 Bring your feet back, keeping them about 1 foot apart.

3 Bring your sacrum and tailbone in and lift your spine.

4 Stay for 20 to 30 seconds.

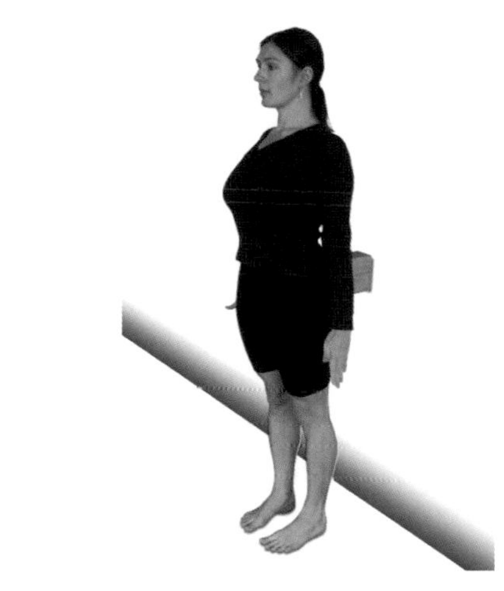

Urdhva Hastasana

Upward hand pose

1st term: no
2nd term: yes
3rd term: yes

Follow the same technique as in Tadasana, Block between Wall and Sacrum (above), and stretch your arms in Urdhva Hastasana.

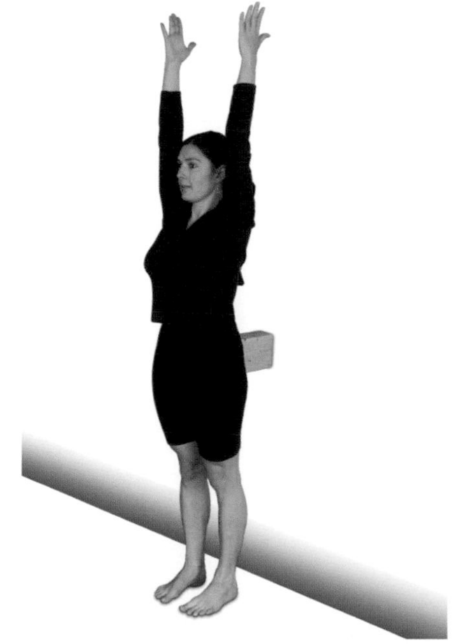

Tadasana, Block between the Feet
Mountain pose

1st term: no
2nd term: yes
3rd term: yes

1 Grip the block with your inner heels and inner ankles. Feel how by doing this, you can grip your whole body. Use this method to lift your inner body and spine.

2 Remain in the pose up to 2 minutes.

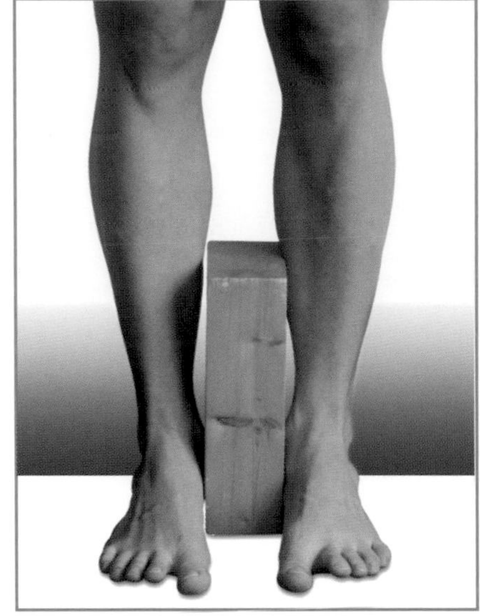

Tadasana, Block between the Inner Thighs
Mountain pose

1st term: no
2nd term: yes
3rd term: yes

1 Put a block between your upper thighs close to the perineum and bring your feet completely together. (If the ball of your big toe keeps you from closing the big toes, move your heels slightly apart.)

2 Grip the block, touching it evenly with the front and back of your upper thighs. Bring your sacrum and the tailbone in and extend your spine upward.

3 Remain in the pose up to 2 minutes.

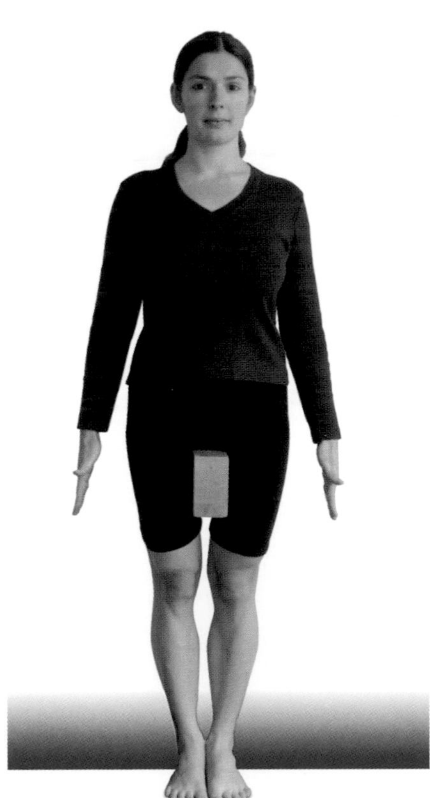

Pashchima Namaskarasana in Tadasana
West-facing prayer in mountain pose

Follow the instructions given for during pregnancy, page 36.

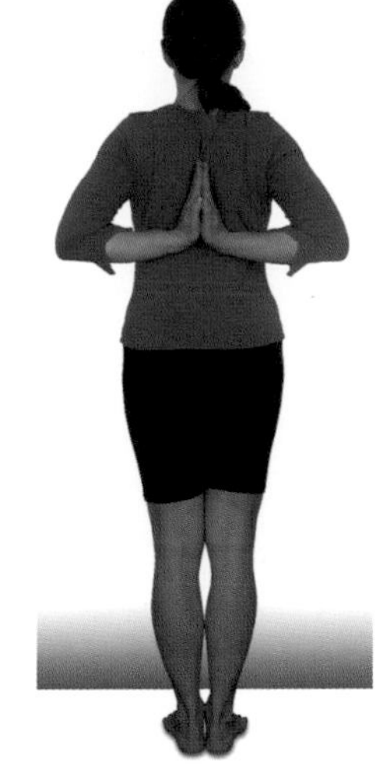

1st term: no
2nd term: yes
3rd term: yes

Benefits

See page 36

Gomukhasana in Tadasana
Cow face in mountain pose

Follow the instructions given for during pregnancy, page 37.

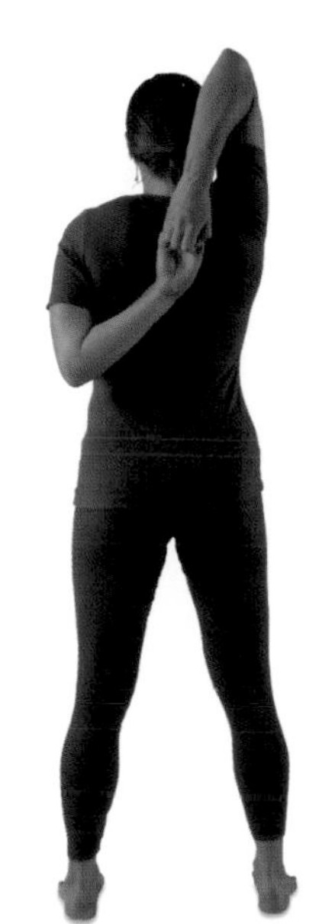

1st term: no
2nd term: yes
3rd term: yes

Benefits

See page 37

Tadasana, with Quarter-round Block
Mountain pose

Follow the instructions given for during pregnancy, page 33.

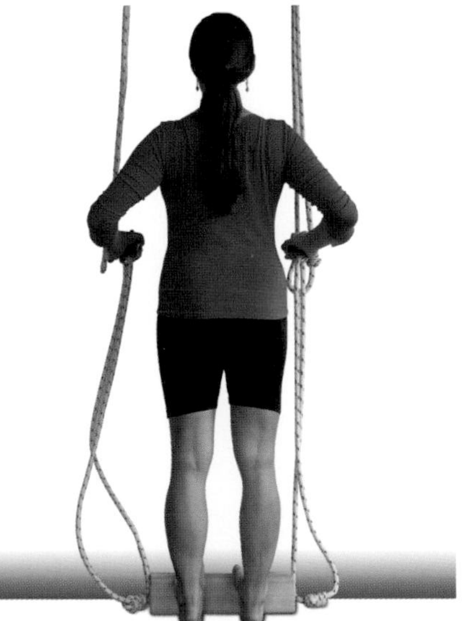

1st term: no
2nd term: yes
3rd term: yes

Benefits

See page 33

Utkatasana, Back to the Wall

Fierce pose

1st term: no
2nd term: yes
3rd term: yes

1 Stand in Tadasana (page 32), 1 to 1½ feet from the wall.

2 Place your fingertips on the wall behind you and rest your back against the wall.

3 Keeping your back against the wall, exhale, bend your knees, and release your buttock bones downward.

4 Inhale and extend your arms upward with the palms facing each other, trying to reach the wall with your thumbs. Keep the back of your waist in touch with the wall, and your chest lifted.

5 Stay for 15 to 30 seconds in the final position.

Coming out of the pose

Inhale, straighten your legs, and come to Tadasana.

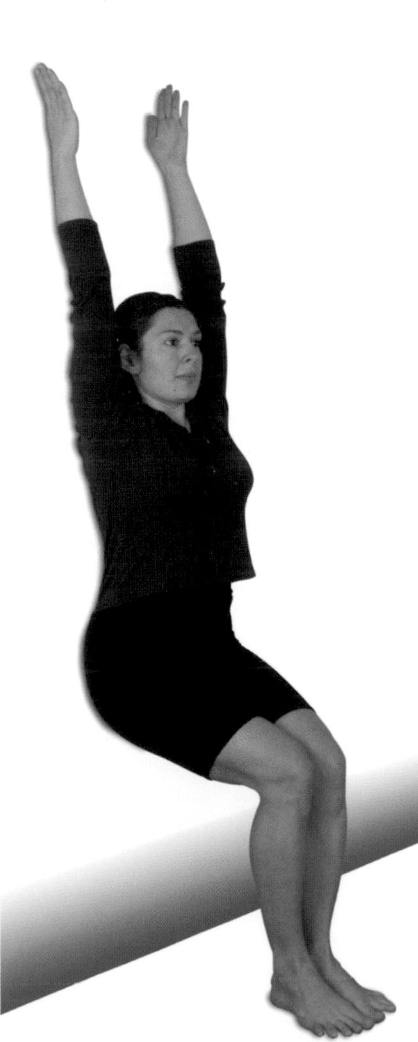

Benefits

- Tones the back muscles and abdominal organs
- Develops the chest muscles
- Extends the gluteal muscles
- Strengthens the exterior spinal muscles
- Lifts the diaphragm, which gives a gentle massage to the heart
- Strengthens the shin, which is the weight-bearing bone in this case
- Develops your ability to flex the thigh, ankle, and knee joints

Special Instructions

- Develop your ability to flex your knees and hip joints without stooping and dropping the spinal muscles, the lower abdomen, and the navel region.
- When bending your knees, bring your buttock bones straight down; don't push them out behind or lean your chest forward. Try to maintain the length of the sides of your torso, as in Tadasana.

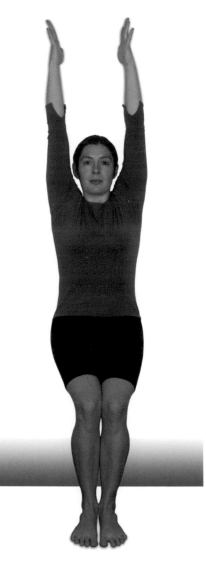

Vrikshasana, Back to the Wall

Tree pose

1st term: no
2nd term: yes
3rd term: yes

Benefits

- Tones the shoulder muscles and gives poise and balance
- Lifts the pelvic organs
- Strengthens the spinal and abdominal muscles

1 Stand in Tadasana (page 32).

2 Bend your right knee, grasp your right foot, and bring your knee out to the right side.

3 Place your right sole high on the inside of your left thigh with the toes pointing downward.

4 Keep your left leg straight and steady.

5 Bring your hands in front of your chest, press the palms evenly against each other, and be in your center.

6 Just as you are pressing your hands evenly together, evenly press your right foot against your left thigh and the thigh back against the foot.

7 Look straight ahead.

8 With an inhalation, extend your arms over your head, keeping your hands as close together as possible.

9 Stay in the pose for 30 seconds.

10 Repeat on the other side.

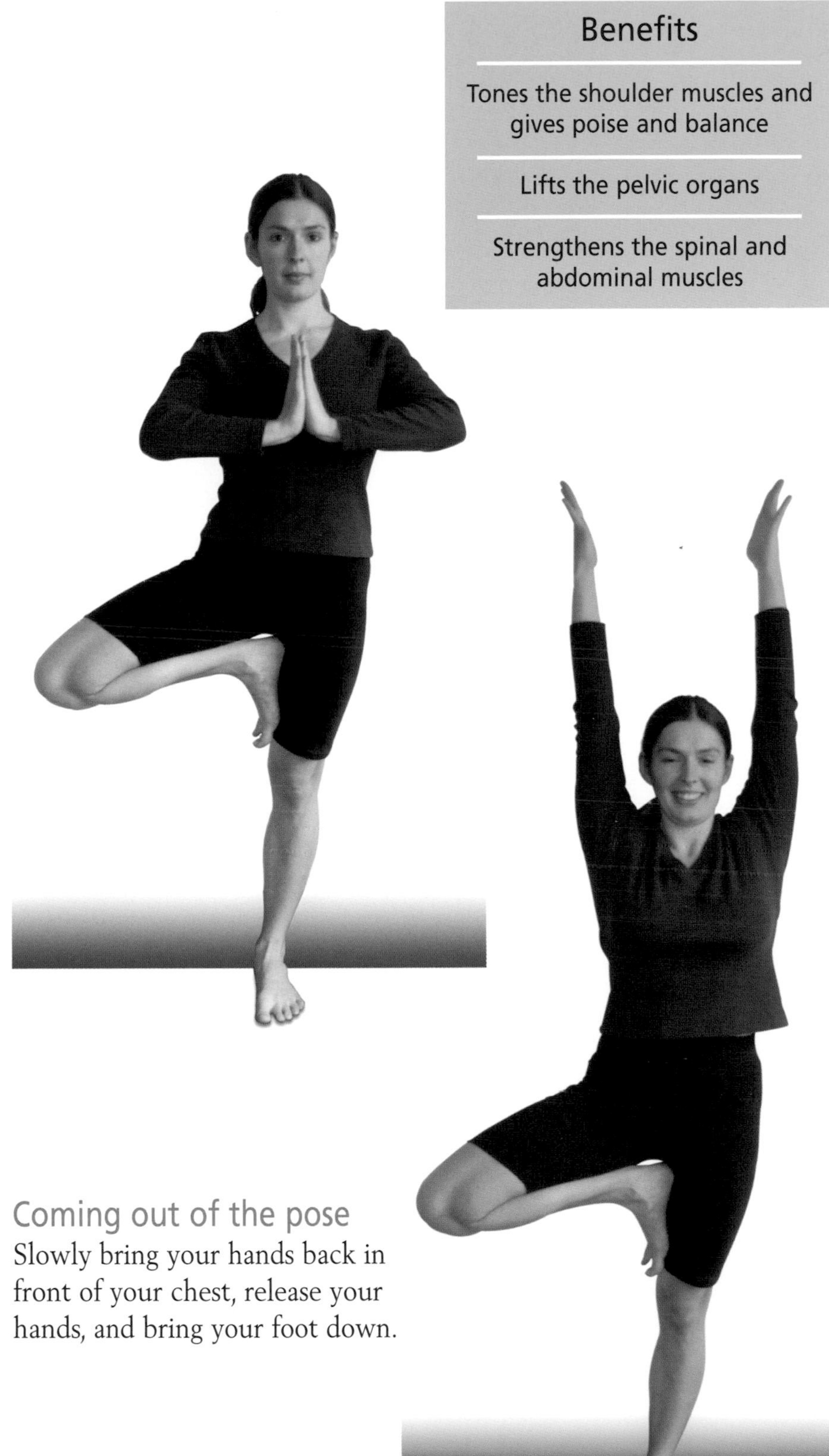

Coming out of the pose

Slowly bring your hands back in front of your chest, release your hands, and bring your foot down.

Utthita Trikonasana
Utthita Parshvakonasana
Ardha Chandrasana
Virabhadrasana 2

Benefits

This group of asanas strengthens the spinal and abdominal muscles. Because the pelvic floor is lifted, the tension on the abdominal organs is lessened. You can feel your body become firmer.

For the general techniques for these asanas, see Chapter 3 (pages 38, 40, 45, and 42). Below we have added additional instructions for each one.

Try them also with a trestle. If you don't have a trestle, you can achieve good alignment with a support for the front foot as shown, a wall in the back, and a wall rope (if possible).

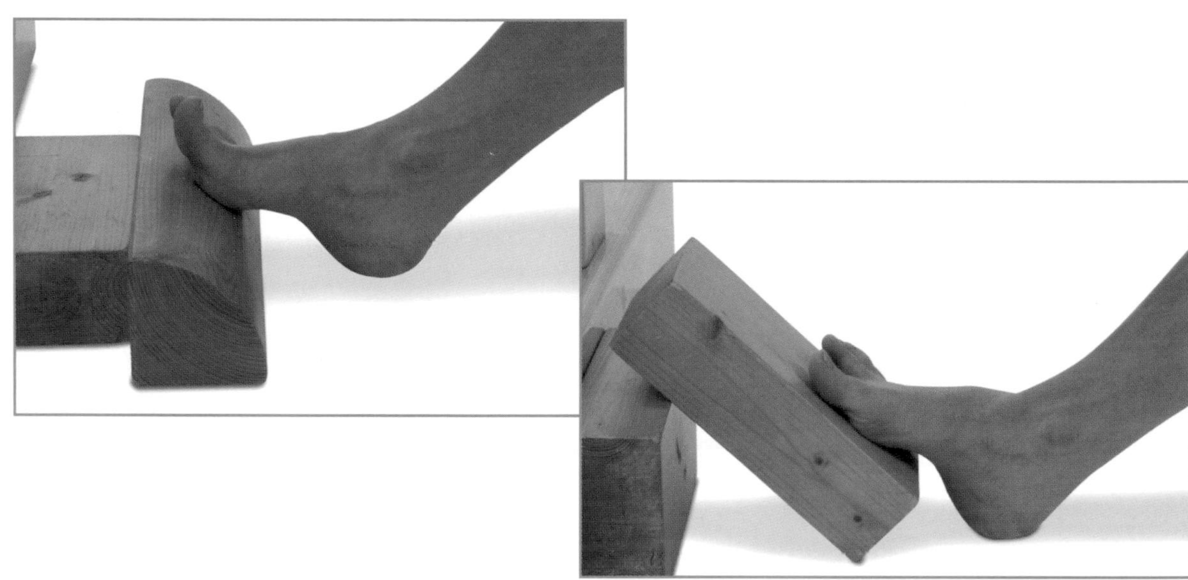

With the back foot against the wall:

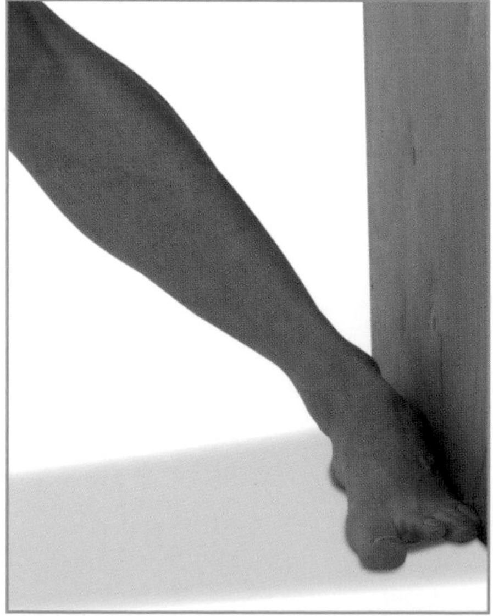

Utthita Trikonasana
Extended triangle pose

1st term: no
2nd term: yes
3rd term: yes

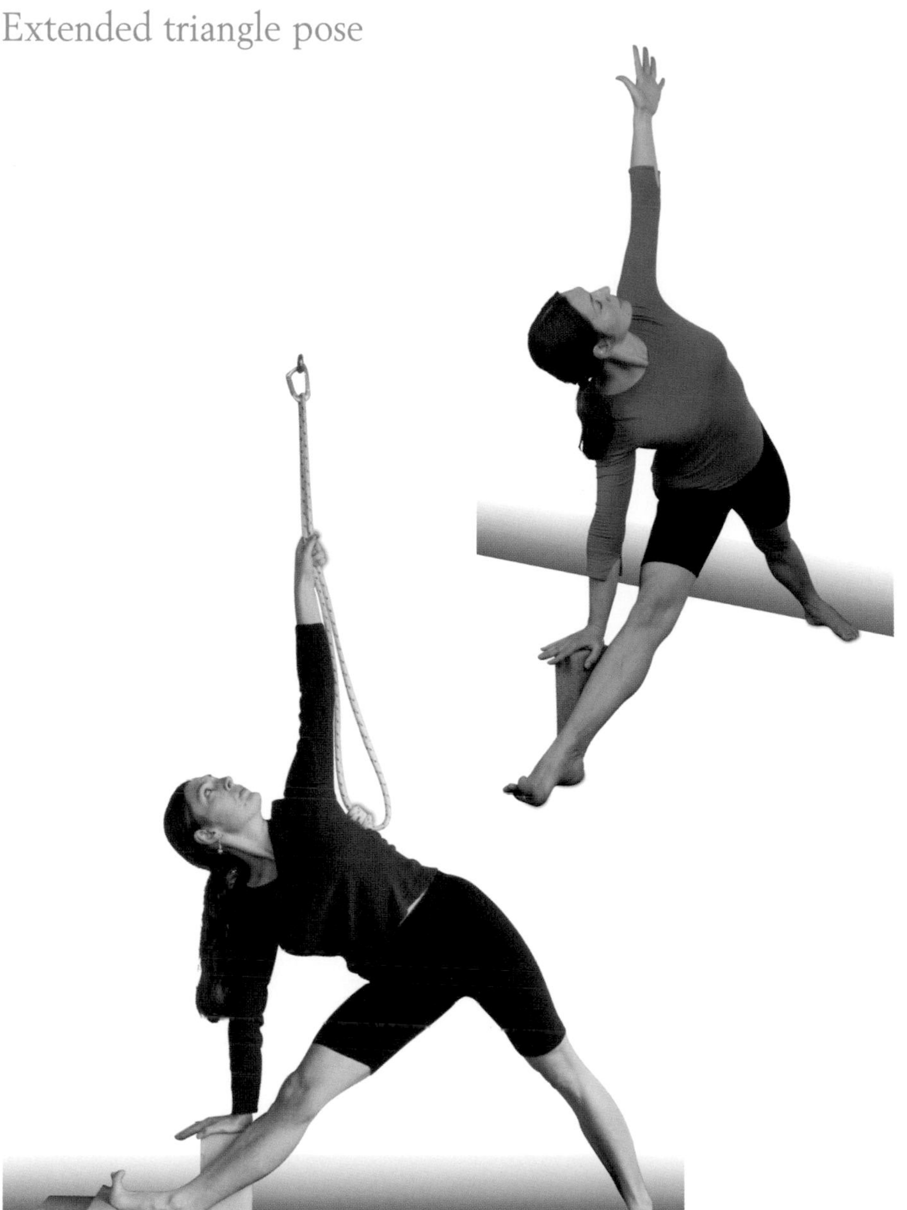

Special Instructions

- While reaching for your ankle, do a long exhalation so that you feel the lightness in your torso and it lowers easily.
- When coming up from the pose, do a long inhalation so that you feel stable.
- While staying in the poses, inhale and exhale slightly more deeply than normal. The sound should not escape from your nostrils; the breathing should occur from your torso. Inhalation should flow from the abdomen to the chest, and exhalation from the chest to the abdomen.

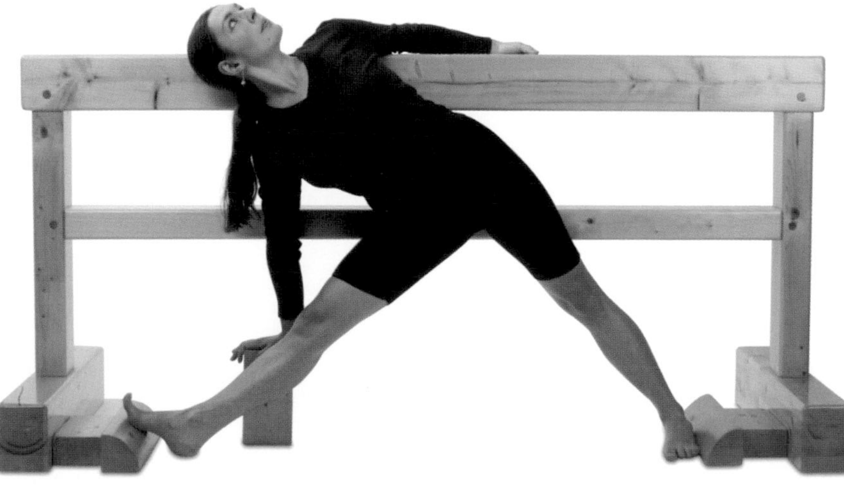

Utthita Parshvakonasana
Extended lateral pose

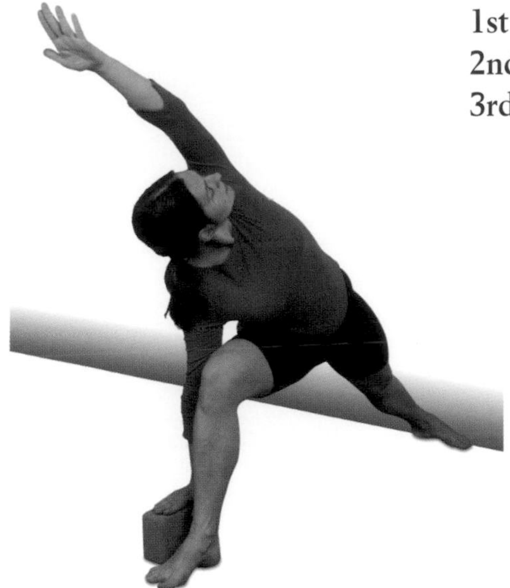

1st term: no
2nd term: yes
3rd term: yes

Special Instructions

- While staying in the pose, although your breathing is slightly deeper than normal, it should be more abdominal than nasal. Your head should not feel heavy.
- When getting up from the pose, inhale and lift your torso.
- While in the pose, the hand that is stretched over your head should be extended from the lower part of the abdomen. The stretch of the arm pulls the abdominal organs up and strengthens them.
- When you're doing the asana on the right, the left side of your pelvis should not drop downward towards the floor. There are two types of stretches on the left side:
  - A full lengthwise extension from the left ankle to the left wrist along the side of the torso
  - A rotational circular stretch of the left thigh and left torso up and outward
- Don't let your left torso drop; be sure to keep it lifted.
- Working with the trestle with both arms wrapped around the upper beam teaches you how to open, lift, extend, and come to proper alignment.

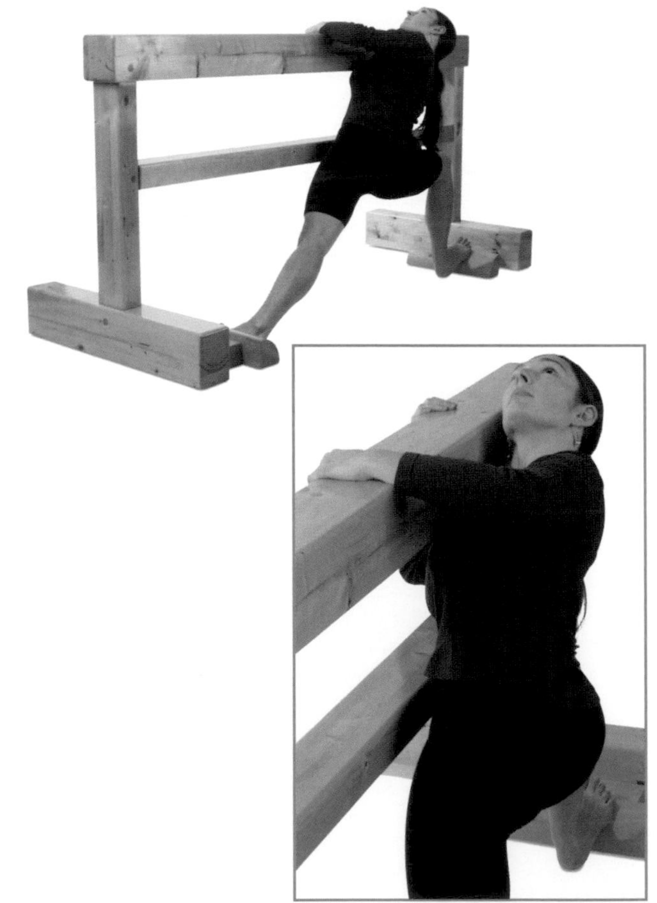

Ardha Chandrasana
Half moon pose

1st term: no
2nd term: yes
3rd term: yes

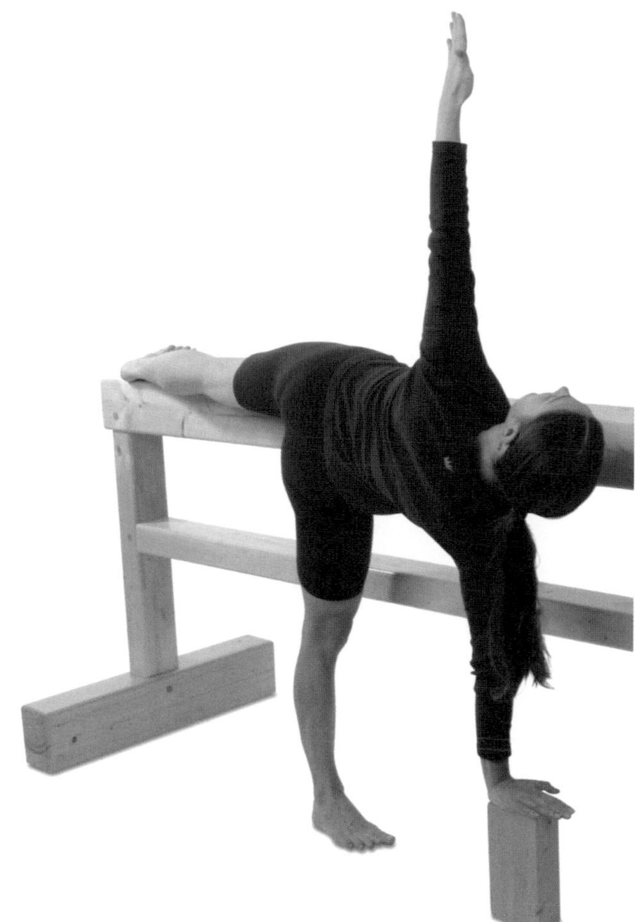

Special Instructions

- Extend the sides of your torso. Press your lower hand onto the block to bring your shoulder blade into your ribs.
- Stretch your upper arm upward to lift your chest. Tighten your buttock muscles, bring your sacrum and tailbone in, lift your chest away from your pelvis, and rotate your torso upward towards the ceiling.

(See also Utthita Parshvakonasana on the previous page and Virabhadrasana 2 on the following page.)

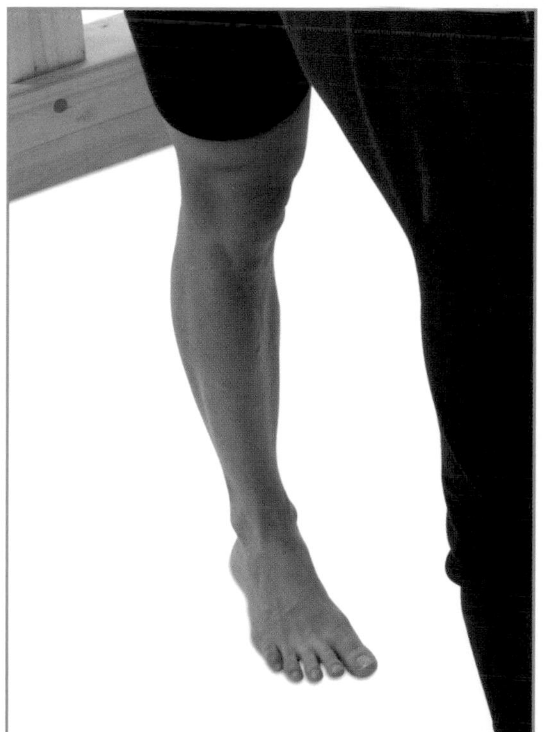

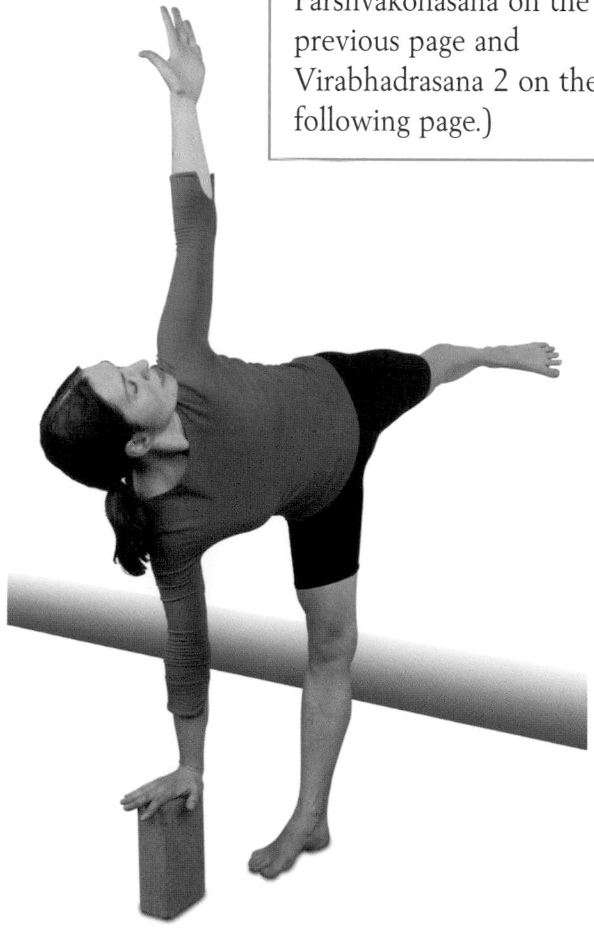

Virabhadrasana 2
Warrior pose 2

1st term: no
2nd term: yes
3rd term: yes

HINT: As you come up from the pose to stand straight, don't let your body loosen; retain the firmness of the muscles while standing erect. If you feel that you failed to achieve a sharp extension or that you let your body sag, give it another try and repeat the pose.

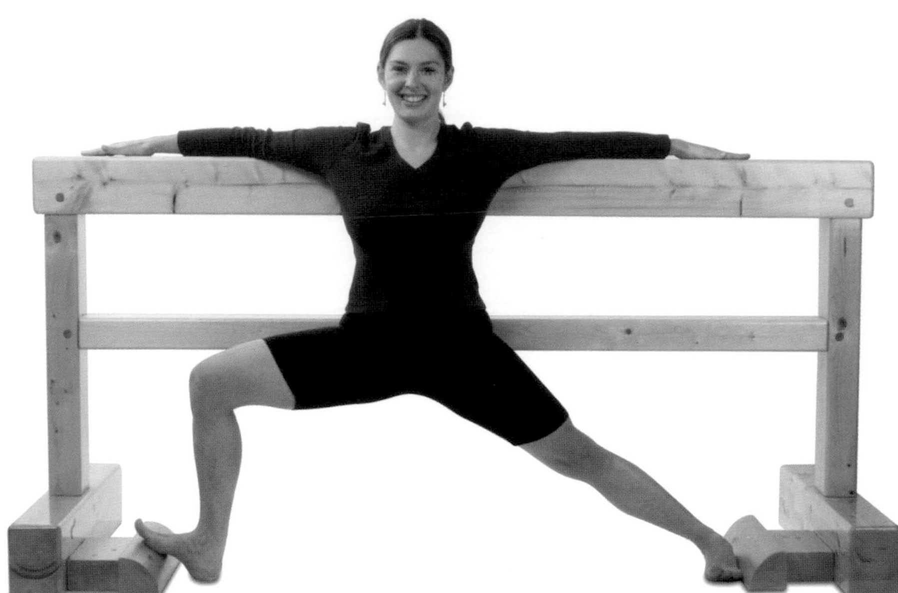

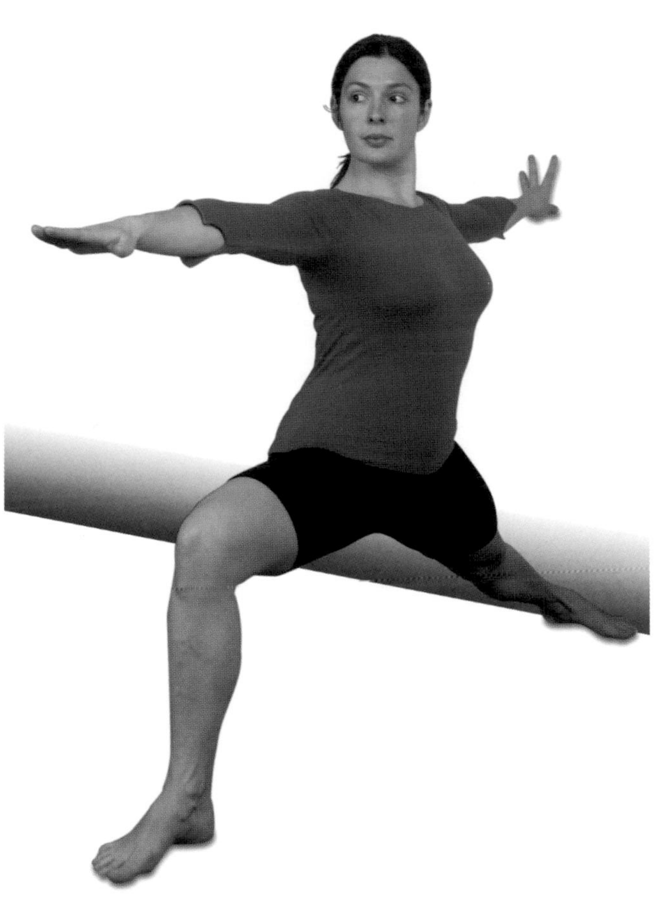

Special Instructions

- Practicing this asana either with your back foot against the wall or with the trestle helps you keep both sides of your torso parallel, turn your torso, stretch your spine, and balance.

- This is particularly useful when you are a new mother who may be weak at this stage. Often pain in the tailbone continues after delivery; the support of the wall relieves your lower back. When you do the asana as presented in this book, your tailbone goes into your body and the outward projection is checked. Although you don't stay in the pose for long, it still takes a concerted effort to tighten your buttock muscles and lift the sides of the pubic bone.

- Don't stay for too long in the pose, letting your body loosen and your abdomen sag. Allow the pose to straighten and lift the spinal column and strengthen your spinal muscles.

Parshvottanasana, Hands against the Wall, Front Foot on Support

Intense chest stretch pose

1st term: yes
2nd term: yes
3rd term: yes

Benefits
Tones the pelvis and spine
Lifts the uterus
Calms the mind
Allows the heart to rest

1 Place your hands against the wall and have a quarter-round block for your front foot, so that you can keep your heel down while the balls of your toes press against the block.

2 Keeping your pelvic bones and hips parallel, extend your right leg from the heel to the buttock and your left leg backward. Putting as much weight as possible on your left outer foot and heel, bring your left buttock down, keeping your left outer hip forward and the right side of your groin backward.

3 Lift your lower abdomen and navel upward.

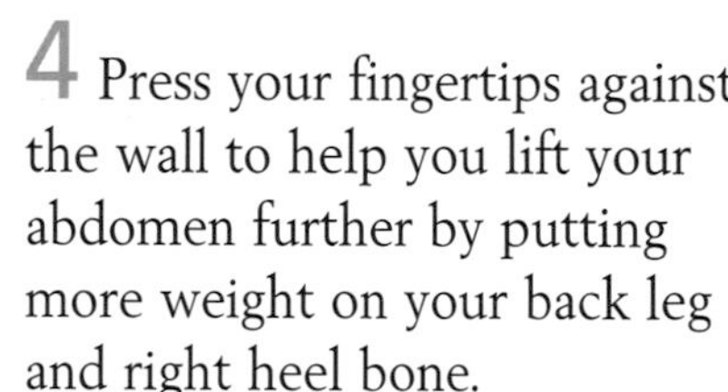

4 Press your fingertips against the wall to help you lift your abdomen further by putting more weight on your back leg and right heel bone.

5 Stay for 20 to 30 seconds per side.

Detailed Descriptions of Asanas for Beginners and Advanced Students

Back Heel against the Wall pose, Hands on Blocks

1st term: no
2nd term: yes
3rd term: yes

Special Instructions

- Practice with your back heel against the wall and your pelvis as described above.
- Follow the technique given for during pregnancy (pages 49 – 50).
- If you can't balance well enough to bring your weight firmly onto your back foot, then use the blocks as shown.
- Practice also Pashchima Namaskarasana standing upright.

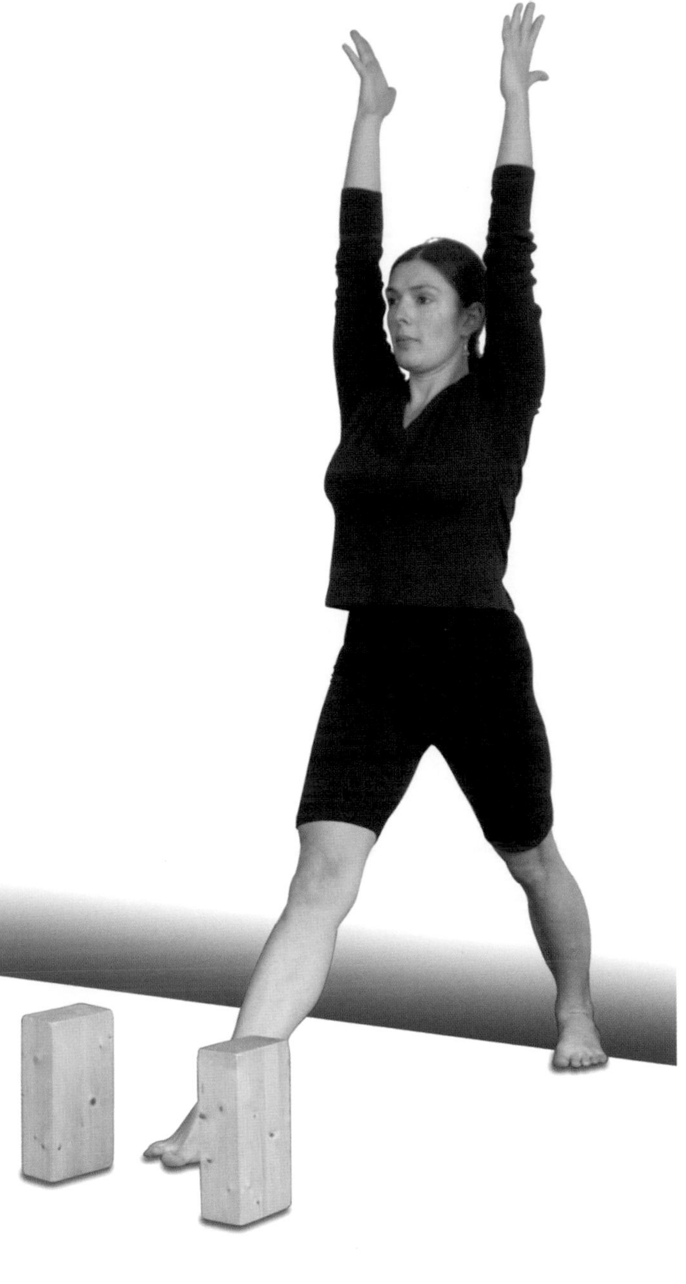

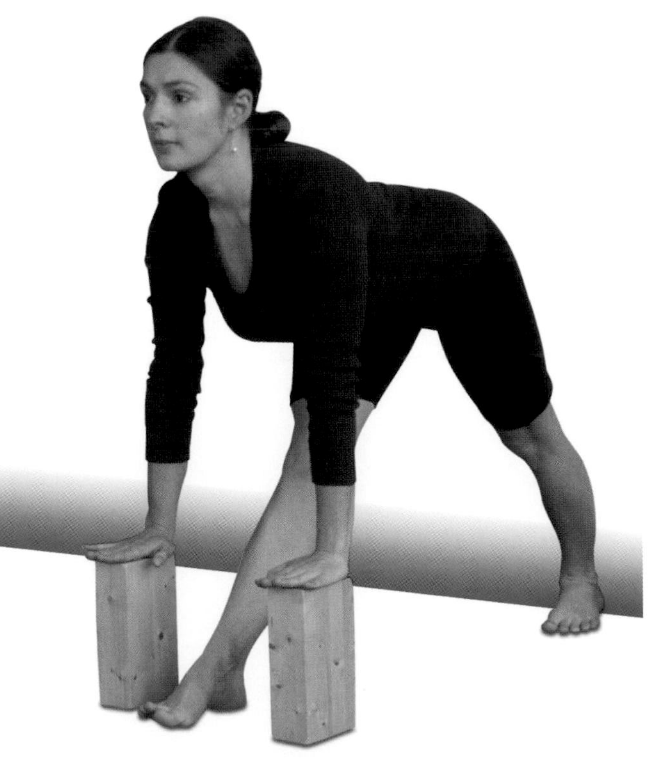

Pashchima Namaskarasana
Hands in cow face pose

1st term: no
2nd term: yes
3rd term: yes

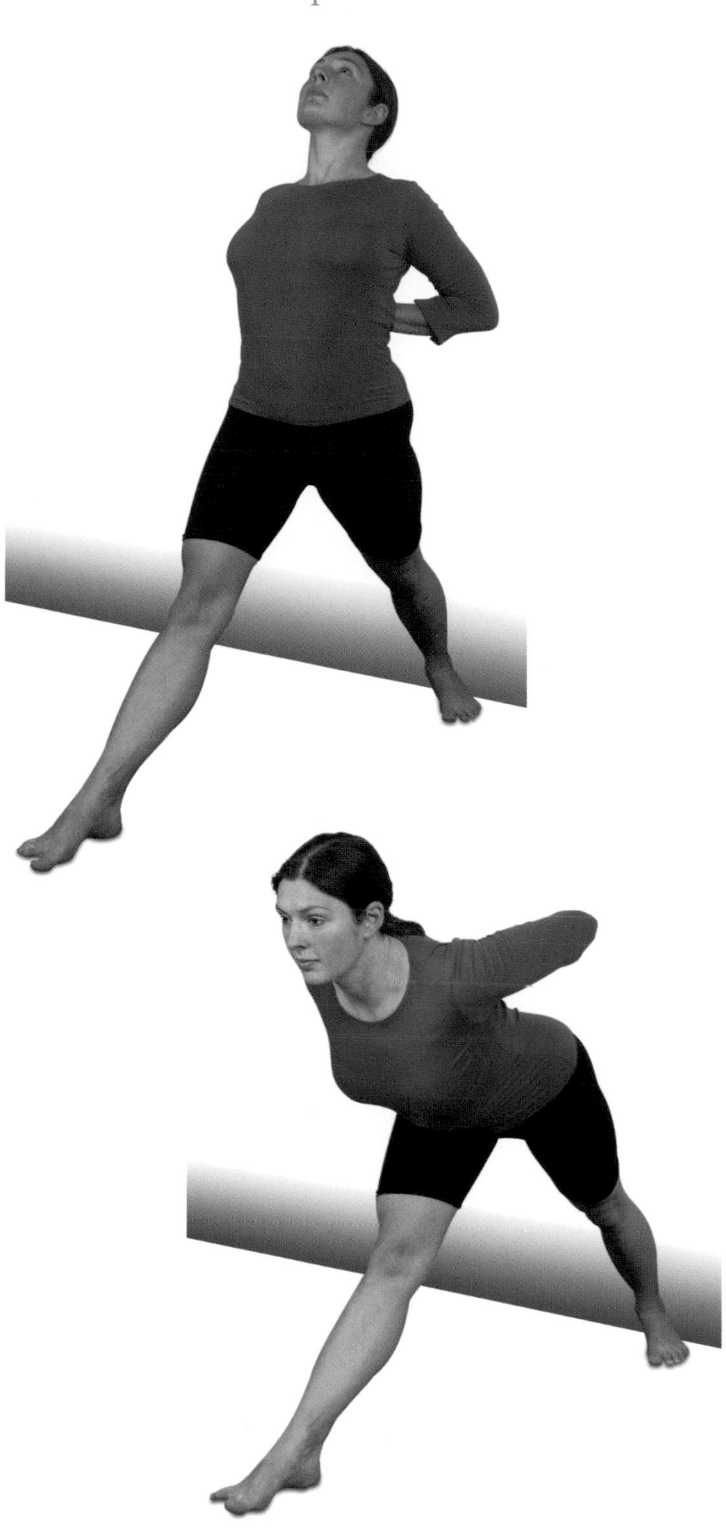

Benefits

Tones the pelvis and spine

Lifts the uterus

Calms the mind

Allows the heart to rest

HINT: Deepen your breath without sharpening it.

Additional Instructions

- Practice with your back heel against the wall and your hands in Pashchima Namaskarasana.
- If you still feel awkward, follow the instructions for the second term.

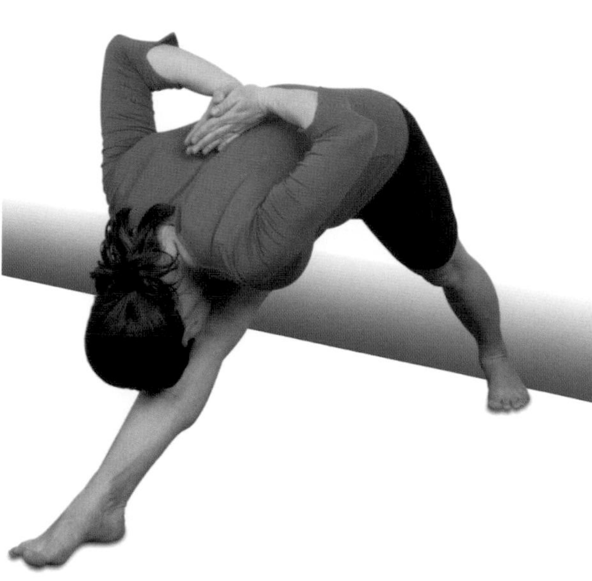

Virabhadrasana 1
Warrior pose 1

1st term: no
2nd term: no
3rd term: yes

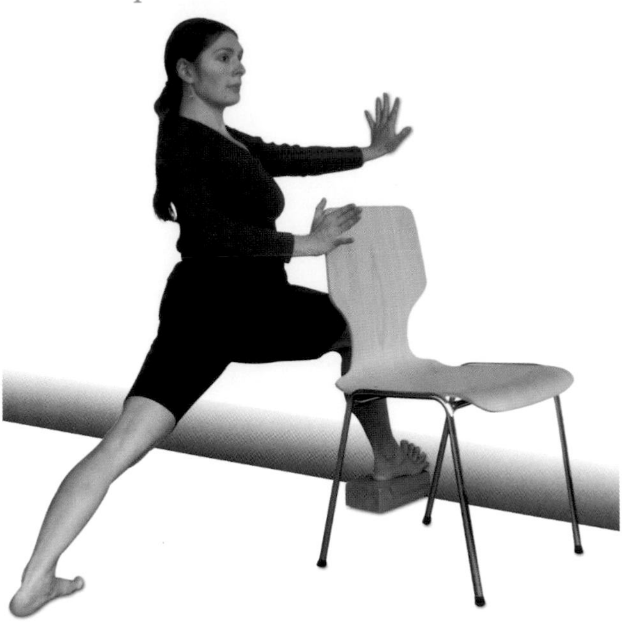

Benefits
Tones the spine
Tones the muscles around the tailbone and sacrum
Calms the brain
Relieves stomach pain
Alleviates depression

Concentrating on your deepened breath, lift your sides, abdomen, and chest.

Additional Instructions

- Begin with the wall and your front foot on a block; or with the wall, a block, and a chair.
- If the left side of your torso (when the right leg is forward) is hanging backward, grip the backrest of the chair with your right hand, move your left hand more towards the right, and press your fingers firmly against the wall.
- Lifting your lower abdomen: Bring your tailbone down and in, bring the sacrum (bone-plate just above the tailbone) in, be firm on the back leg, and press your front heel firmly down on the block.
- With your fingers pressing firmly against the wall, lift your anterior spine upward.
- As in Parshvottanasana, it's important that you keep your pelvic bones and hips parallel to each other, and that the buttock of the back leg moves away from the buttock of the front leg.

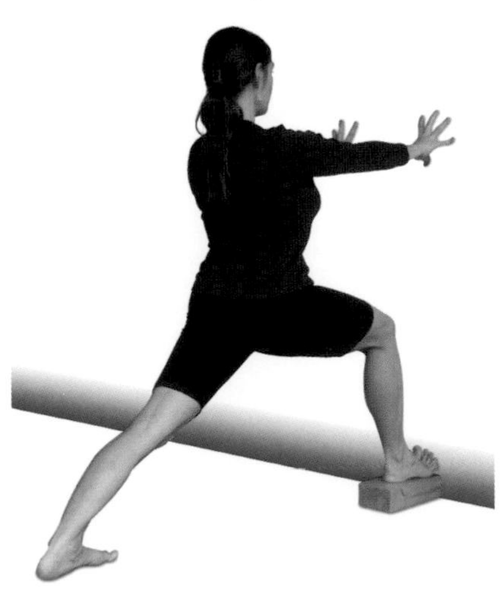

Virabhadrasana 3
Warrior pose 3

1st term: no
2nd term: no
3rd term: yes (Begin with two blocks and a wall behind you.)

Benefits
Tones the spine
Relieves backache and hip problems
Tones the muscles around the tailbone and sacrum
Rests the heart

1 Measure the distance to the wall (1 leg length, see photo below).

2 Stand in Tadasana (page 32). Stretch your arms above your head to Urdhva Hastasana (page 35), with your palms facing forward.

3 Bend forward to Uttanasana and place both hands on the blocks. Feel how your thighbones grip into the hip sockets.

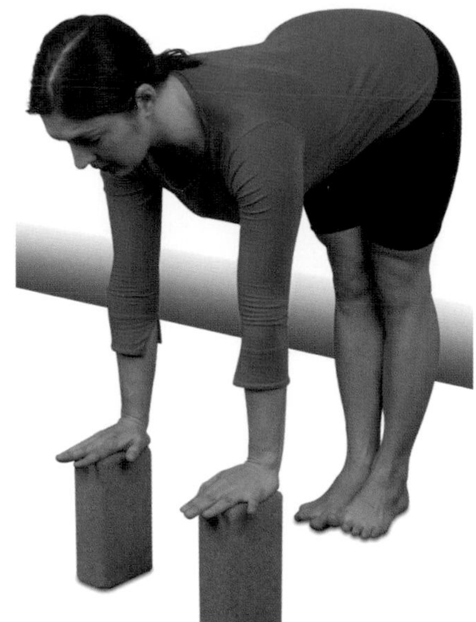

4 Extend the sides of your torso, abdomen, and chest, and your navel, forward.

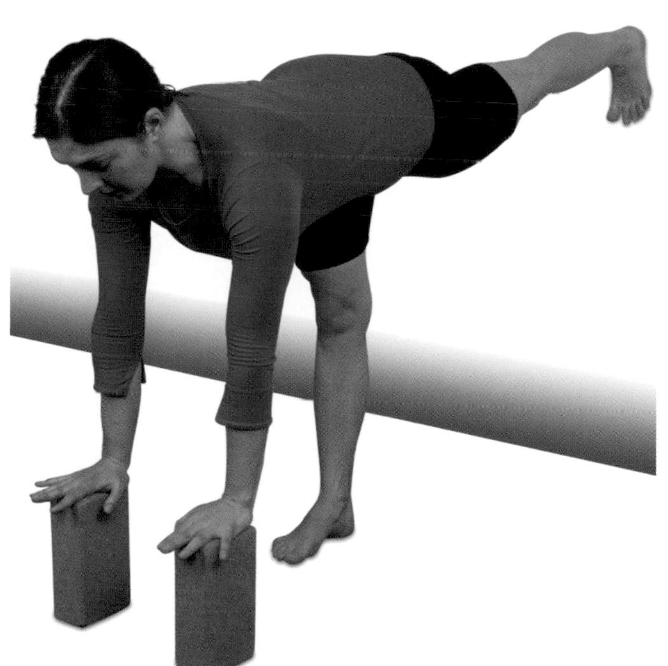

5 Lift your left leg parallel to the floor and place your right foot against the wall with the big toe facing the floor. Let the muscles of your left leg follow the direction of your left big toe.

6 Keep your pelvic bones and hips parallel.

7 Stretch your right leg, bring your right kneecap deep into the knee, and tighten your upper thigh.

8 Looking forward, stay in this position for 20 to 30 seconds. Bring your feet together and repeat on the other side.

Parivritta Trikonasana

Revolved triangle pose

Technique for the 3rd Term

This is a standing twist that offers benefits similar to those of the sitting twists.

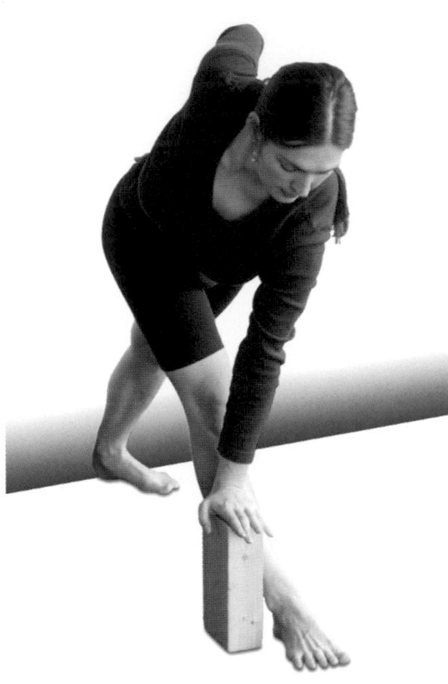

A With wall and block, back heel on the wall

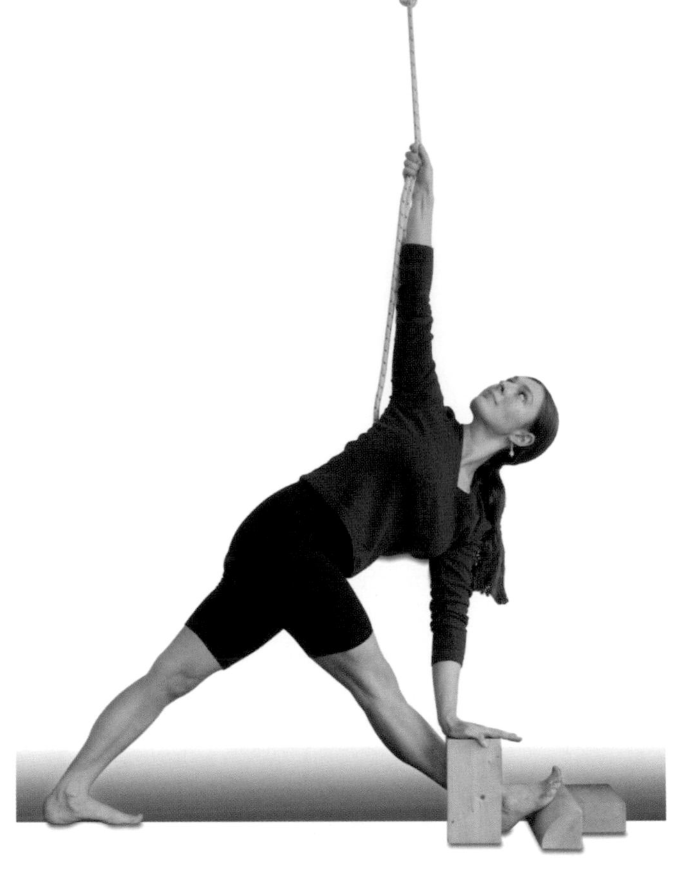

B With wall and block, alongside the wall, front foot up, and wall rope

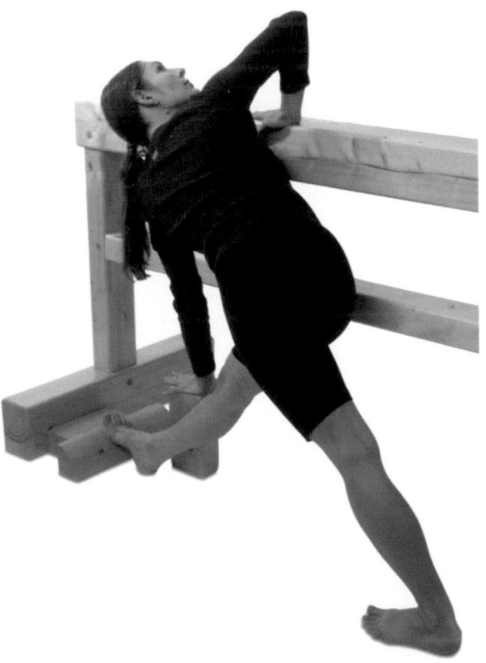

C With front facing trestle and front foot up

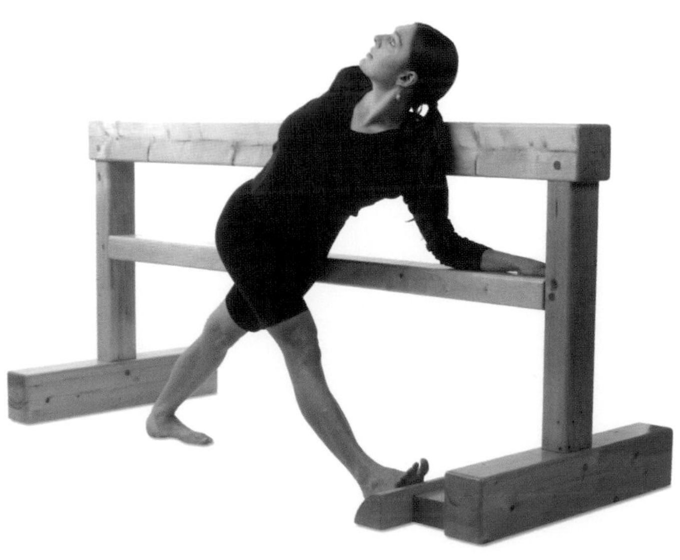

D With back facing trestle and front foot up

1 Stand in Tadasana (page 32) with your heels against the wall.

2 Take a big step forward and turn your left foot inward, with the left outer heel touching the wall. The outer edge of your left foot and the heel should be firmly on the floor.

3 Extend your right foot from the heel bone to the balls of the toes. Extend the toes.

4 Tighten your knees and thighs. Take one or two breaths.

5 Bring your tailbone in, extend your left arm forward, and bring your right arm back.

6 Inhale and lift your lower abdomen and your chest.

7 Exhale, stretch both legs backward, and extend the sides of your torso forward. With the next exhalation, rotate your torso and place the fingers of your left hand on the block (near the outer side of your right foot).

8 Raise your right arm, bringing it in line with your left arm.

9 Extend your chest forward towards your head, move your chin away from your chest, turn your head, and look at your right hand.

10 This is the final position. Breathing normally, stay for 20 to 30 seconds, observing the following points:

- Tighten both legs.
- Tuck in your left shoulder blade and keep your chest expanded.
- Keep both edges of your torso parallel and in line with your right leg.
- Keep your torso in line from your hips to your head.

11 Inhale, take your left hand off the block, and come to Tadasana.

12 Repeat on the left side and come to Tadasana.

Refer also to the techniques given in Chapter 3, "Twists," pages 91 – 95, for during pregnancy. All the variations given there can also be practiced after delivery.

1st term: no
2nd term: no
3rd term: yes

Benefits

Increases the blood supply to the lower part of the torso and invigorates the abdominal organs

Together with the other standing asanas like Virabhadrasana 1 and 3, this asana:

- Has an overall strengthening effect on the body
- Improves the functioning of the organs and reproductive system
- Helps treat stiff shoulders, humpback, rheumatic pain, lumbago, and slipped disk
- Develops stamina, strength, flexibility, lightness, and balance

Special Instructions

- Keep both legs firm when turning the pelvic region.
- Extend your torso towards your head in such a way that your abdominal muscles revolve and also move towards your chest.

Ardha Uttanasana
Half-standing foward bend pose

1st term: no
2nd term: yes
3rd term: yes

Once you've reached the second term after your delivery, you can add Uttanasana and Parshvakonasana to your practice.

Benefits
Aligns the inner and outer body
Lifts and strengthens the pelvic organs
Strengthens the inner legs

Variation 1 with a Block and the Wall

1 Measure the distance so that your feet are one leg length away from the wall (See photo page 289).

2 Stand in Tadasana. Put a block between your upper thighs close to the perineum and grip it evenly with your thighs, bringing your thighbones into the hip sockets.

3 Tighten your knees, stretch both legs, and lift both arms towards the ceiling, palms facing forward. While lifting your arms, stretch your whole body as in Parvatasana in Tadasana. Take one or two breaths.

4 Extend your spine, exhale, bend your torso forward parallel to the ground, and place your hands against the wall (spread them as in Adho Mukha Shvanasana).

5 Breathing normally, stay in this position for 30 to 60 seconds, observing the following points:

- Extend your bottom ribs and back torso forward, and extend the crown of your head towards the wall.
- Bring your abdominal muscles, front torso, diaphragm, and bottom chest forward.
- Maintain your grip on the block throughout the pose and while coming back to Tadasana.

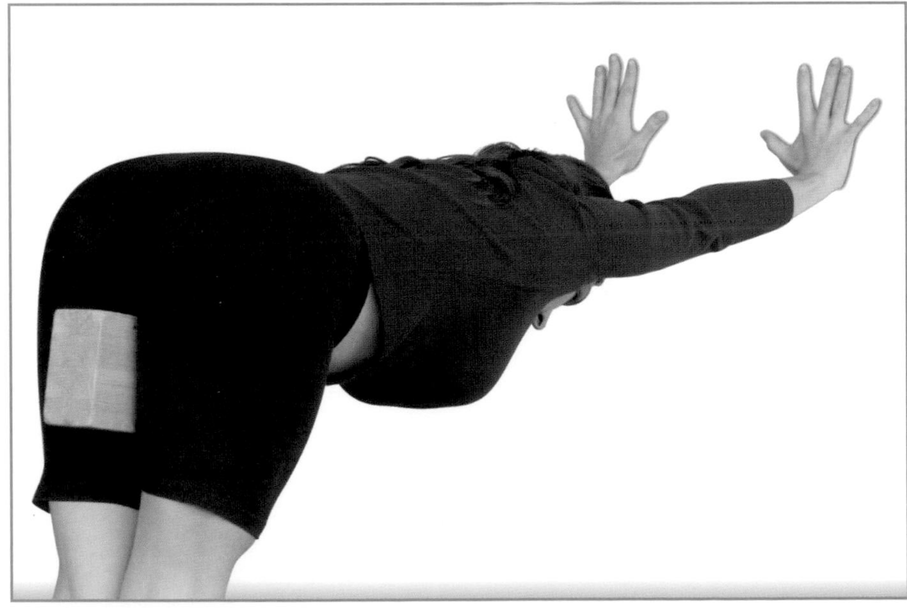

Variation 2 with Wall Ropes and Chair

Follow the instructions for Variation 1. Extend your arms with your palms on the seat of the chair, or over the backrest with your palms facing each other.

Benefits

Realigns and recenters the body after delivery

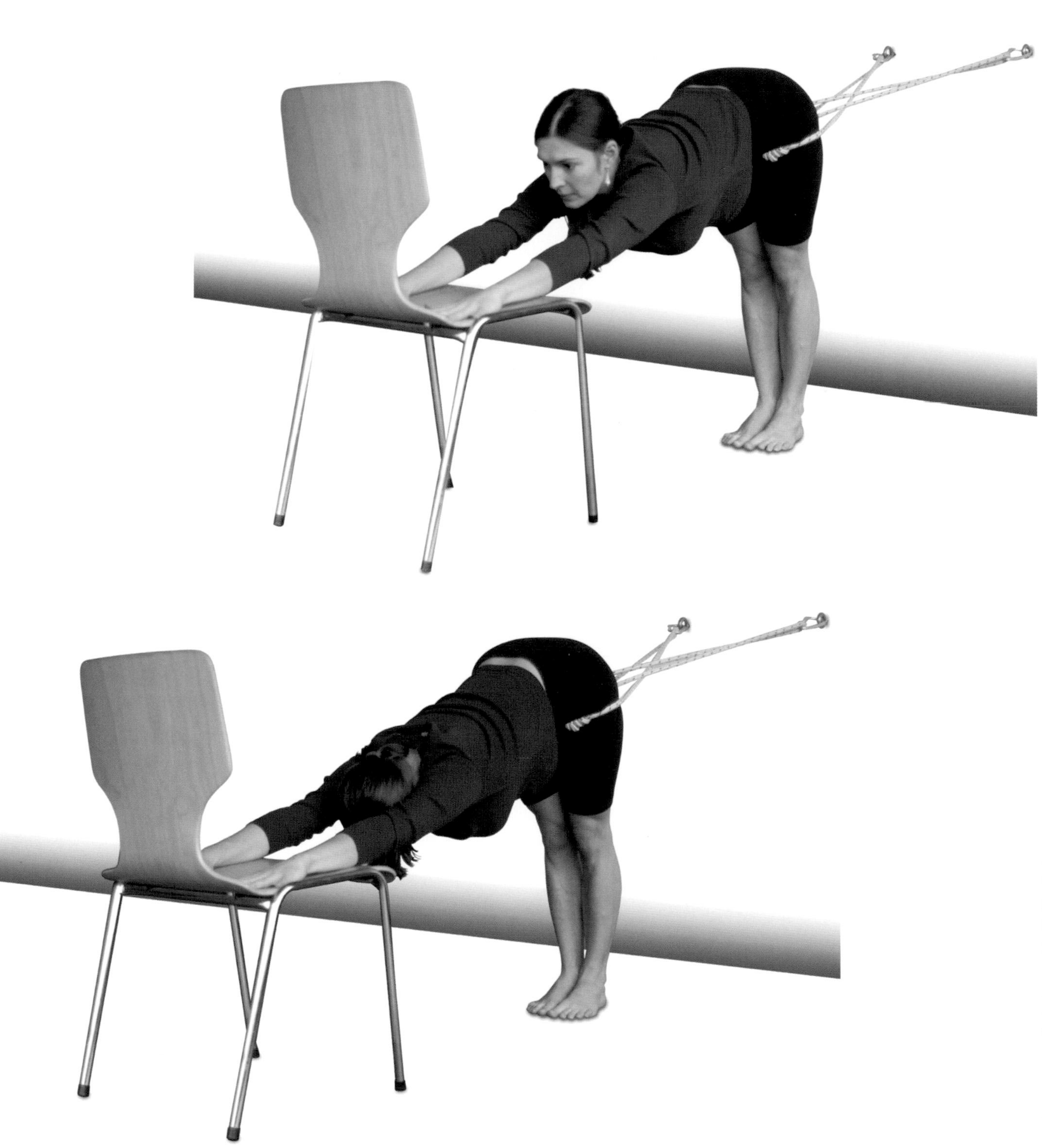

Uttanasana
Intense stretch pose

Technique for the 3rd Term

1 Stand in Tadasana (page 32).

2 Tighten your knees, stretch both legs, and lift both arms towards the ceiling, palms facing upward. While lifting your arms, stretch your whole body as in Vrikshasana. Take one or two breaths.

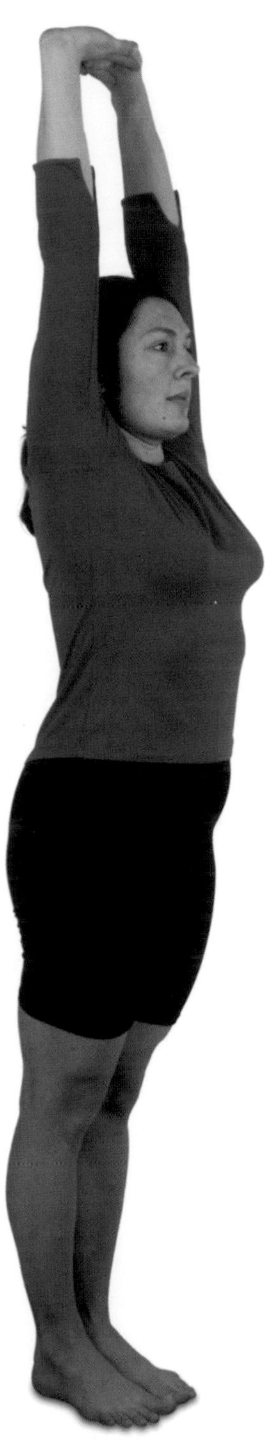

3 Extend your spine, exhale, and bend your torso forward.

4 Rest your palms on the floor by the sides of your feet. Stretch your torso forward by keeping your head up and your spine concave. Take one or two breaths.

5 Exhale and bring your head to your knees.

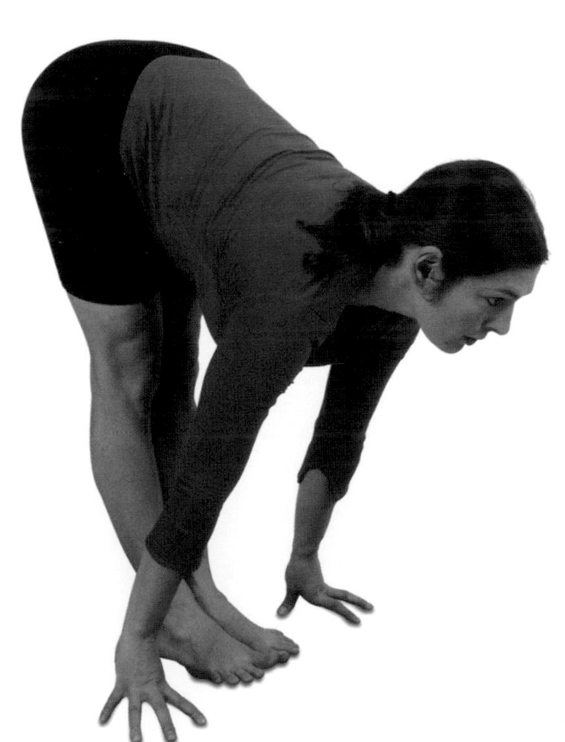

1st term: no
2nd term: no
3rd term: yes

6 Breathing normally, stay in this final position for 30 to 60 seconds, observing the following points:

- Extend your bottom ribs and back torso so that your head rests on your knees.
- Pull your abdominal muscles, front torso, and diaphragm towards the floor.

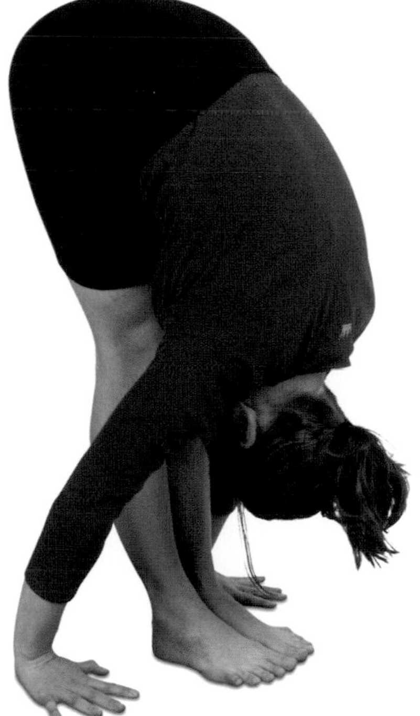

7 Return to the positions in step 4 and then step 3, and finally come to Tadasana.

Special Instructions

- At first, resting your palms on the floor is difficult. Instead, place only your fingertips on the floor, or place your fingers on blocks by the sides of your feet.
- Don't bend your knees to touch your head.
- Don't constrict your neck and chest.

Benefits

Good starter for massaging the abdomen.

Although you may be eager to reduce fat around your abdomen, you can't suddenly start exercising it immediately after delivery. Due to the inverted position of the abdomen in this asana, there is less strain on it and the uterus stays dry. When you bend forward, the abdomen does not contract strenuously; and later, you won't experience adverse effects while doing Navasana, such as sudden bleeding or pain.

The uterus is positioned properly.

Contraindications and Help

If you don't feel dizzy after bending forward, then you're on your way to overcoming the fatigue of delivery. But if you do, then you are still weak, and we recommend the following:

- Continue with this asana, but rest your head on the chair.
- Don't proceed with the sequence of asanas for the third term; instead, follow the asanas for the second term.
- You can perform Pashchimottanasana and Janu Shirshasana.

Use your performance in the second-term asanas to assess whether you're ready for the ones for the third term. If not, postpone them for another week or two.

Prasarita Padottanasana
Extended feet intense stretch pose

1st term: no
2nd term: no
3rd term: yes

Benefits

See page 55

If you still have a loose feeling in the pelvis, place your feet between two blocks to increase both the lift of the inner legs and the sensitivity of the legs and pelvis.

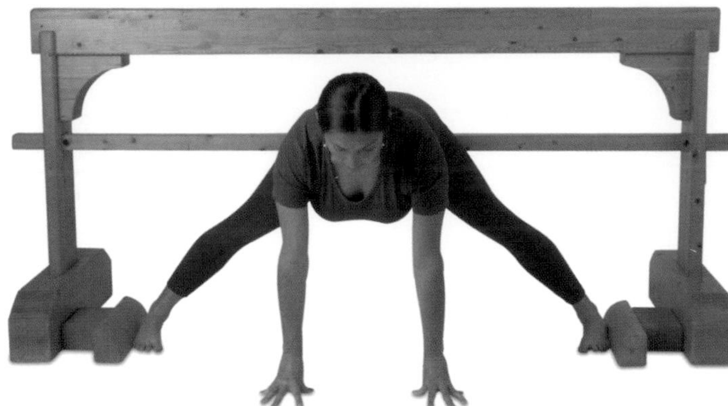

For good alignment, place your heels and buttock bones against the wall.

Practice also with a concave back, with your hands either on blocks or cupped and your head resting in the traditional way with your elbows bent.

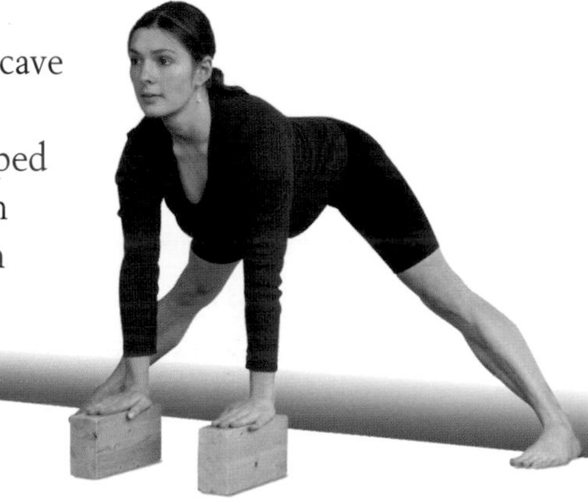

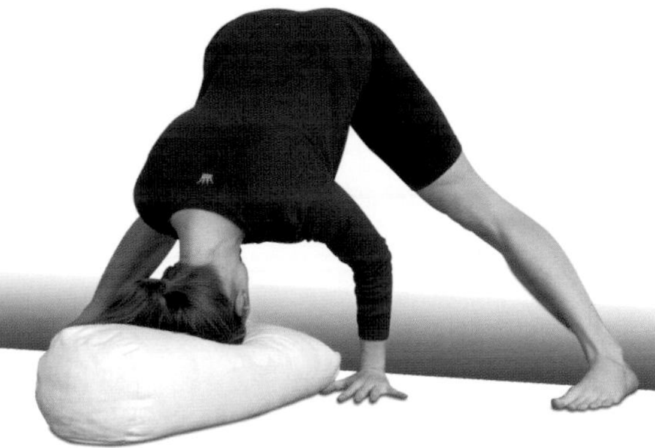

Alternatively, you can extend your hands and arms as in Adho Mukha Prasarita Padottanasana.

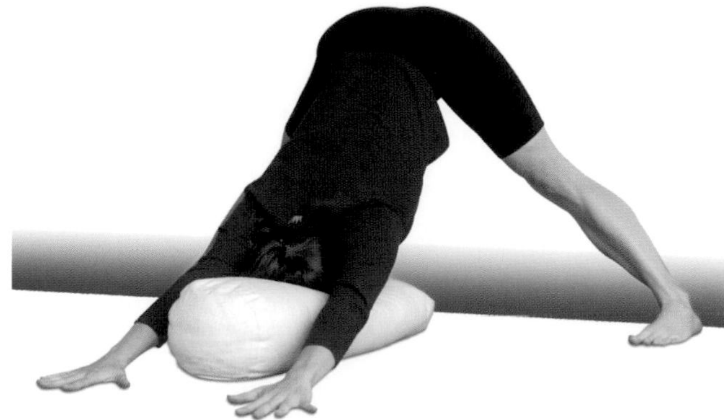

(For further instructions and benefits, see page 55. You can practice all the variations given there from the third term onward.)

Padangushthasana

Big toe pose

Pada means "foot," and *angushtha* means "big toe." In this pose, you grip your big toe with your fingers.

1st term: no
2nd term: no
3rd term: yes

Benefits

Tones the abdominal organs and aids digestion

Adjusts slipped disks (stage 1 only)

1 Stand in Tadasana (page 32) with your feet 1 foot apart. The outer sides of your feet and hips should be in line. Take one or two breaths.

2 Exhale and bend forward without bending your knees.

Stage 1: Concave Back

3 Hook your big toes with your thumbs, index fingers, and middle fingers.

4 Keep your arms straight.

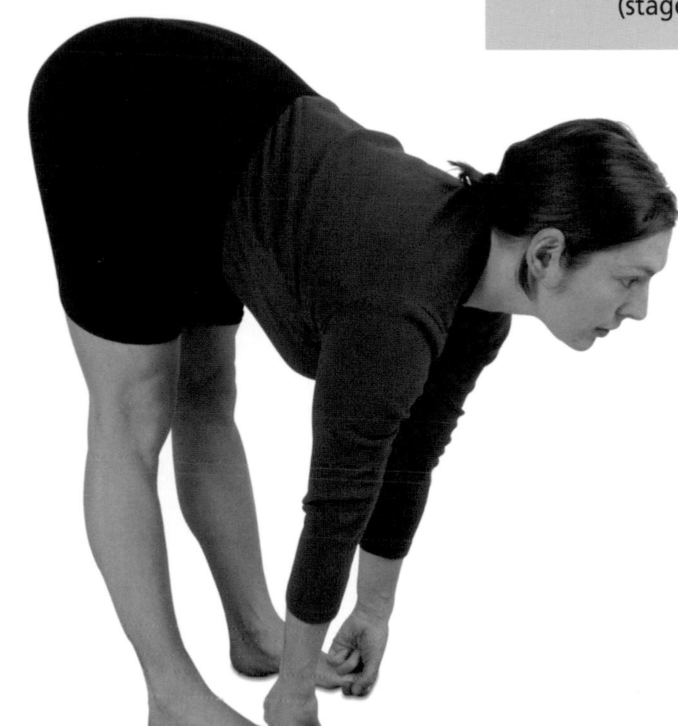

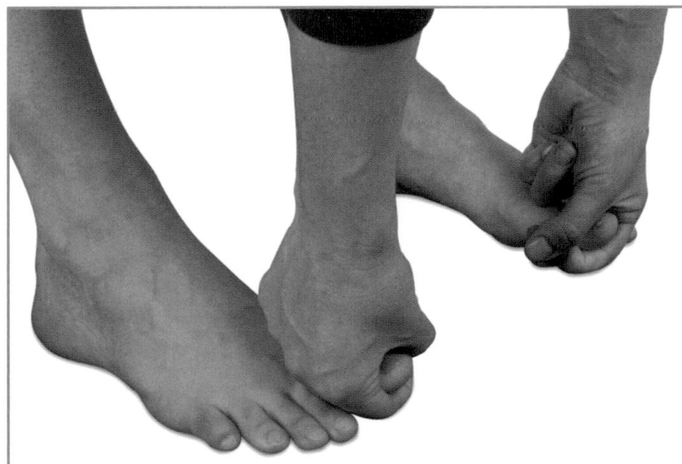

5 Inhale, make your back concave by lengthening your spine from your hips towards your neck, raise your chest, lengthen your neck, and look up.

6 Breathing normally, stay in this position for 5 seconds. If you're going to do only stage 1, then stay for 15 to 20 seconds.

7 Develop your ability to create space between your armpits and leg sockets at the groin, so that the sagging organs of the abdomen are lifted and are supported by the spine.

Stage 2: Head Down

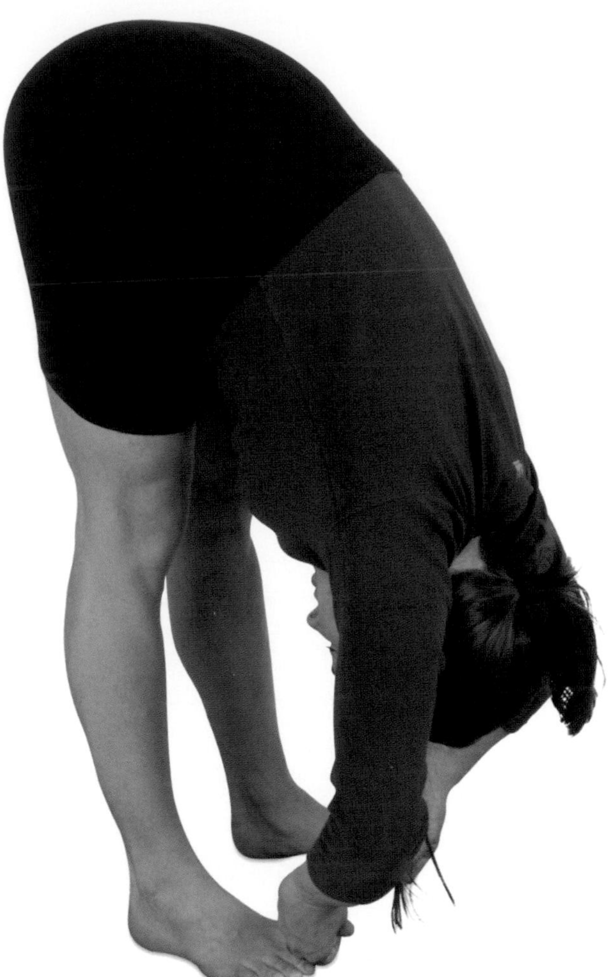

8 While exhaling, bend your elbows out to the sides and lower your head and torso down, head towards your shinbones.

9 This is the final pose. Breathing normally, stay for 15 to 20 seconds, observing the following points:

CHECK YOURSELF

> Pull your spine towards the floor by bending and widening your elbows.
> Tuck in your shoulder blades towards your chest.
> Develop your ability to bend farther forward while gripping your toes.
> Stretch your back and press your abdominal organs towards your thighs; your abdomen and thighs should seem fused together.

10 Inhale, make your back concave, raise your head, release your grip on your big toes, and come up to Tadasana.

Special Instructions

- If you can't grasp your toes with your fingers, you can start by holding your ankles, and later, with practice, work up to gripping your toes.
- Don't try to touch your head to your knee by caving in your chest. This not only causes cramps in the chest and abdomen, but also makes your neck stiff and causes headaches.

Adho Mukha Shvanasana
Downward-facing dog pose

1st term: no
2nd term: no
3rd term: yes

1 With wall ropes, slanted plank or block under the heels, and head supported

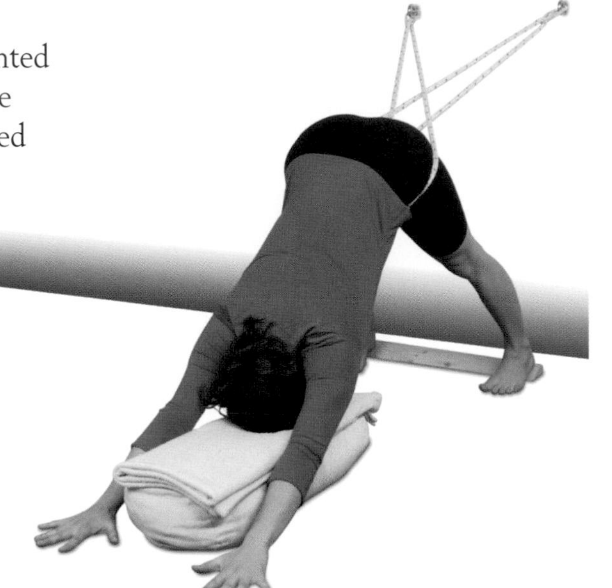

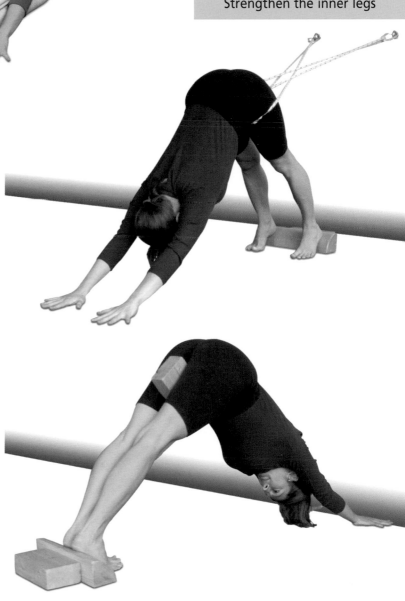

Benefits

In addition to the benefits of Adho Mukha Shvanasana, before delivery (page 62), the three ways of practicing the asana shown here:
Realign the inner and outer body

Lift and stengthen the pelvic organs

Strengthen the inner legs

2 With wall ropes and a block under the heels

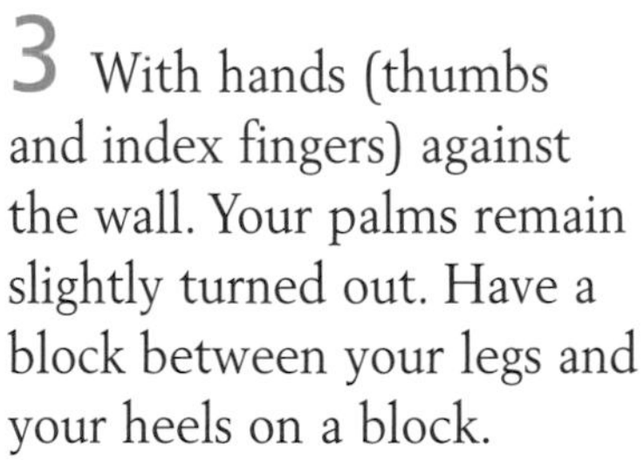

3 With hands (thumbs and index fingers) against the wall. Your palms remain slightly turned out. Have a block between your legs and your heels on a block.

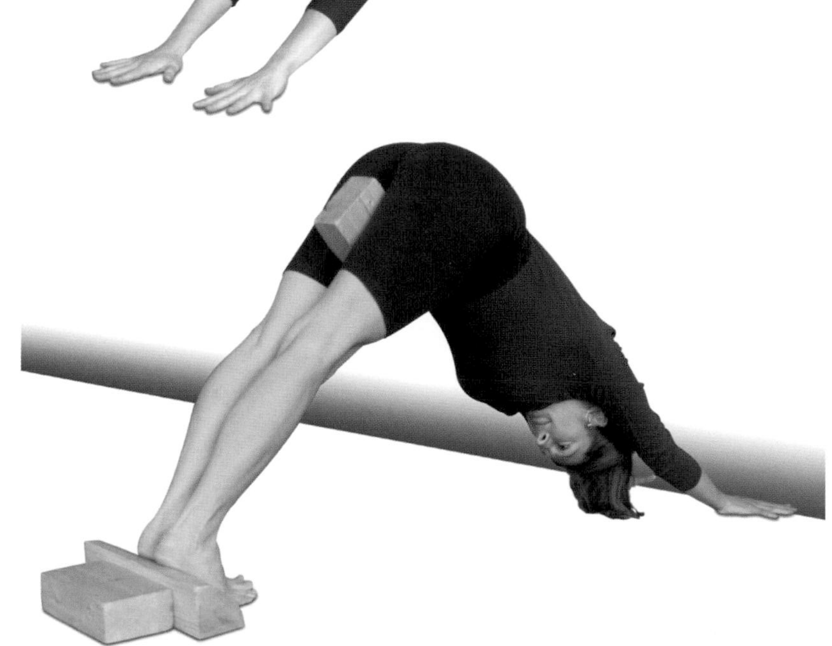

(For further information, see the detailed description of Adho Mukha Shvanasana, page 62, and page 214.)

DETAILED DESCRIPTIONS OF ASANAS FOR BEGINNERS AND ADVANCED STUDENTS

Special Technique for the 3rd Term

HINT: Develop your ability to stretch from your hands to your buttocks, and from your heels to your buttocks.

With hands flat on the ground or on blocks against the wall, and head supported

1 From Uttanasana, place your hands on the floor.

2 Step back one leg at a time so that there is a distance of 3 to 4 feet between your hands and feet.

3 Your hands are shoulder-width apart.

4 If you practice without a block, your feet are in line with your palms.

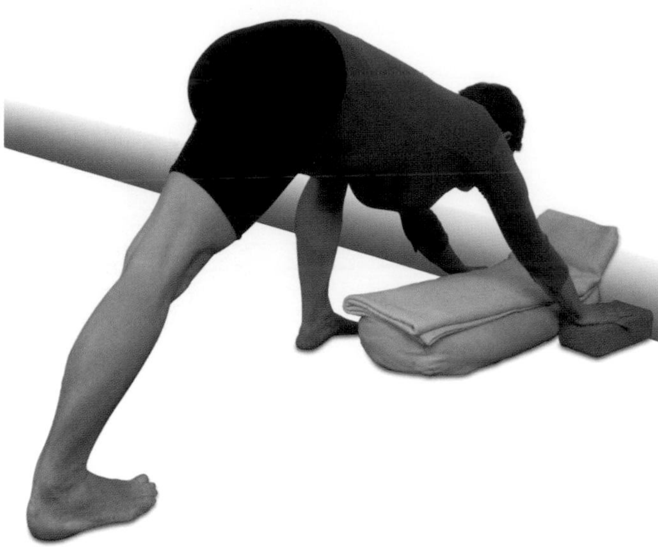

5 Open your palms, spread your fingers, and press them evenly on the floor.

6 Exhale, stretch your arms keeping your elbows straight, and lengthen your spine up towards your hips.

7 Keeping your legs straight and the back of your knees open, lift your thighs up and push them back. Lift your hips so there is space to bring your torso in towards your thighs.

8 Stretching your calf muscles, bring your heels towards the floor.

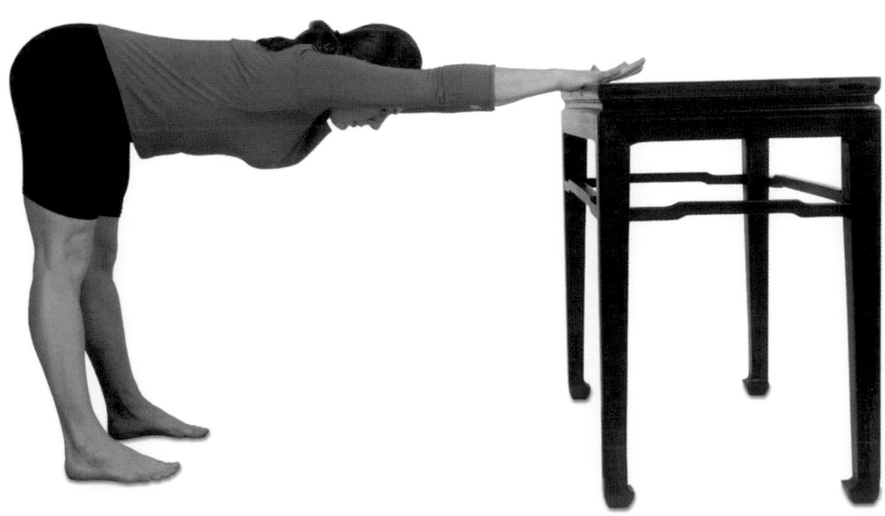

Sitting Asanas
Upavishtha Sthiti

For the general techniques for these asanas, see Chapter 3, pages 64 – 75. Below we have added special recommendations for after your delivery.

The joints of new mothers are especially susceptible to arthritic or rheumatic attacks. The movements of the knees, shoulders, elbows, wrists, and knuckles in the poses that follow help you protect yourself against these conditions.

◇

Parvatasana
Mountain pose

When practicing the poses on the following pages, we recommend that you take note of the instructions below:

Special Instructions

This asana, when done sitting in Svastikasana, Padmasana, or Virasana, is basically a different movement of the feet, knees, hips, and back for each and the same action of the arms and hands.

- In Virasana, because your legs are folded backward, your lower back moves upward freely without resistance; you experience longitudinal extension.
- In Ardha Padmasana or Svastikasana, however, because your legs are crossed, your legs act as a fulcrum and the extension takes place against the resistance of the legs. This position is more effective for the abdominal organs than in Virasana.
- Parvatasana in Virasana, however, is more effective for the back muscles. After delivery, weak back muscles can cause you pain. The lumbar (lower) spine and the sacrum in particular require toning.

Parvatasana from Svastikasana or Padmasana
Mountain pose from cross-legged pose or lotus pose

1st term: yes
2nd term: yes
3rd term: yes

Follow the instructions given for during pregnancy, page 74.

Benefits

See page 75

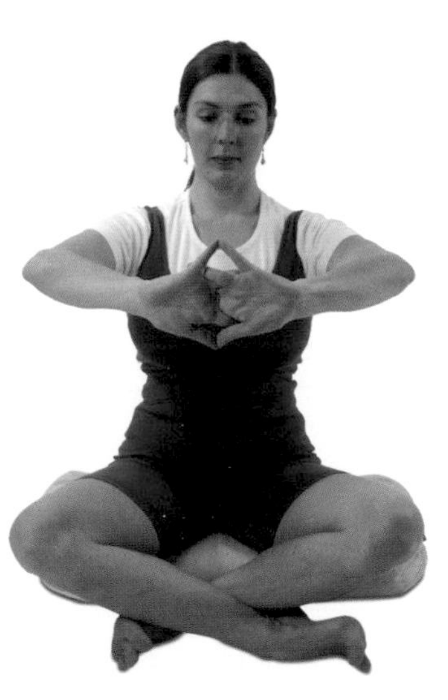

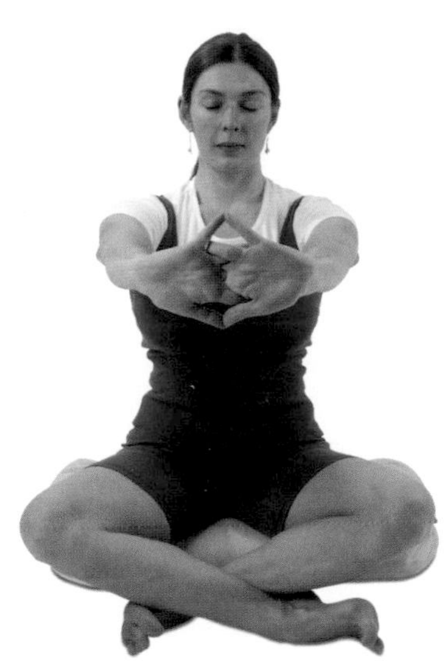

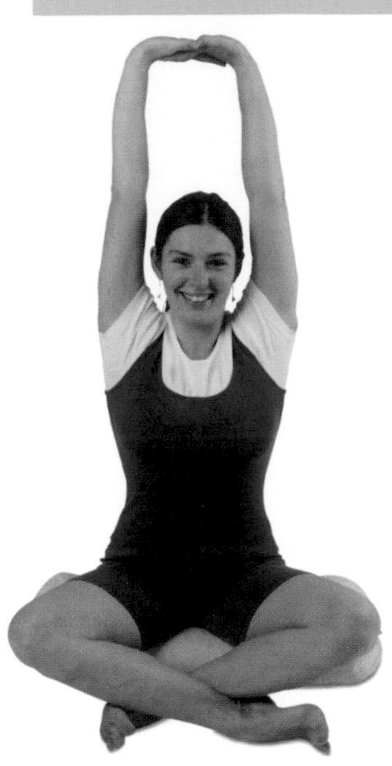

Virasana

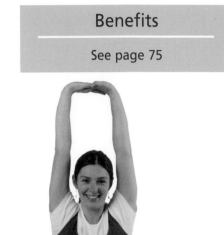

1st term: no
2nd term: yes
3rd term: yes

Follow the instructions given for during pregnancy, page 72.

Benefits

See page 73

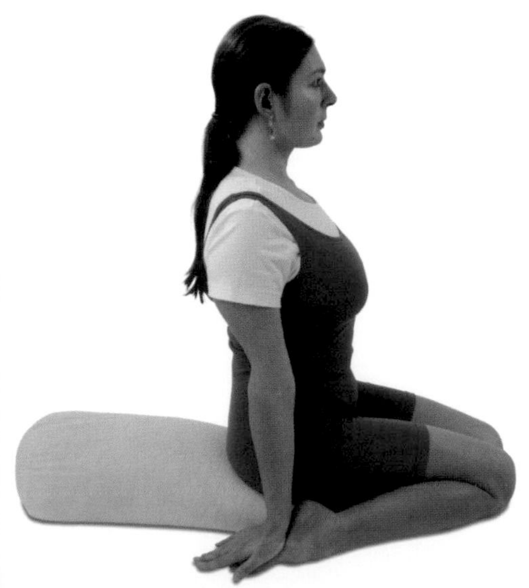

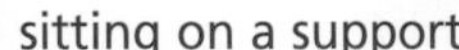
sitting on a support

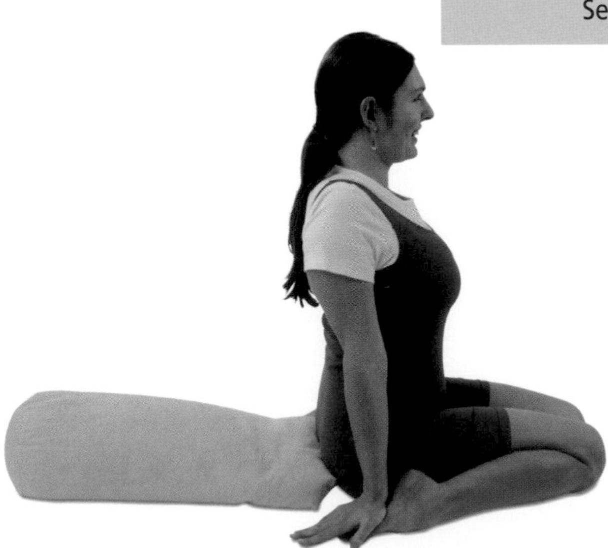
sitting on the ground

Parvatasana from Virasana
Mountain pose from hero pose

Follow the instructions given for during pregnancy, page 74.

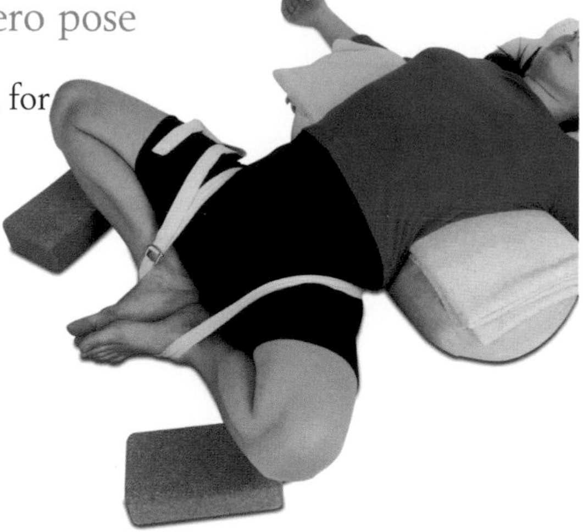

1st term: no
2nd term: yes
3rd term: yes

Benefits

See page 75

Dandasana

Follow the instructions given for during pregnancy, page 64.

1st term: no
2nd term: yes
3rd term: yes

Benefits

See page 65

Special Instructions

- Close your feet completely as shown.
- Make use of the wall and supports to give a proper extension to your legs, pulling the outer side of your feet towards you and extending the inner arches away from you. Spread the balls of your feet and your toes, bringing your legs from the outside in and down.
- Using the resistance in your buttock bones, legs, and fingers, lift the abdominal wall and the sides of your torso and broaden your chest.

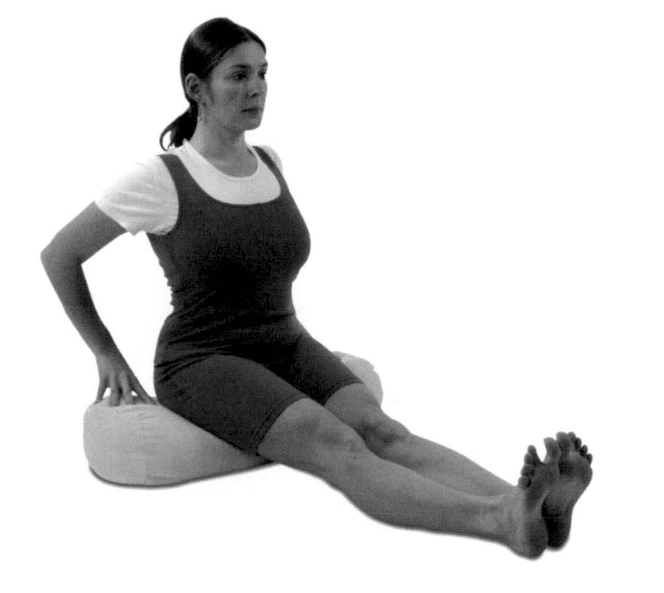

Forward Bends
Pashchima Pratana Sthiti

Maha Mudra, Belt around Foot and Heel on Block
The great seal pose

Drying, replacing, and strengthening

Now that your childbirth is behind you, you'll practice Maha Mudra differently than you did during pregnancy, as you can see in the technique below.

When you practiced Maha Mudra during pregnancy, the emphasis was on expanding the chest. You didn't tighten your abdominal muscles. After delivery, however, you do want to strengthen these muscles. Now, while performing Maha Mudra, you'll concentrate on your spine, abdomen, and chest. The action of lifting the spinal muscles is equally important both before and after delivery.

Maha Mudra reduces flatulence and organically tones the stomach, liver, spleen, and intestines, which in turn improves metabolism. The body shows rapid recovery from fatigue.

◇

1 Have a block and a belt, and spread a blanket on the floor.

2 Sit in Dandasana and put a block in front of you.

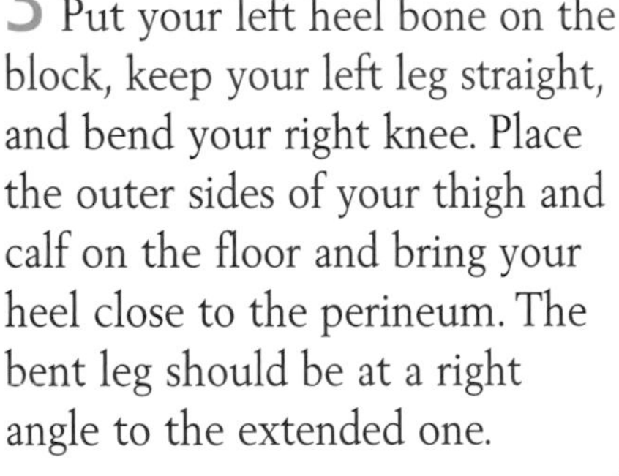

3 Put your left heel bone on the block, keep your left leg straight, and bend your right knee. Place the outer sides of your thigh and calf on the floor and bring your heel close to the perineum. The bent leg should be at a right angle to the extended one.

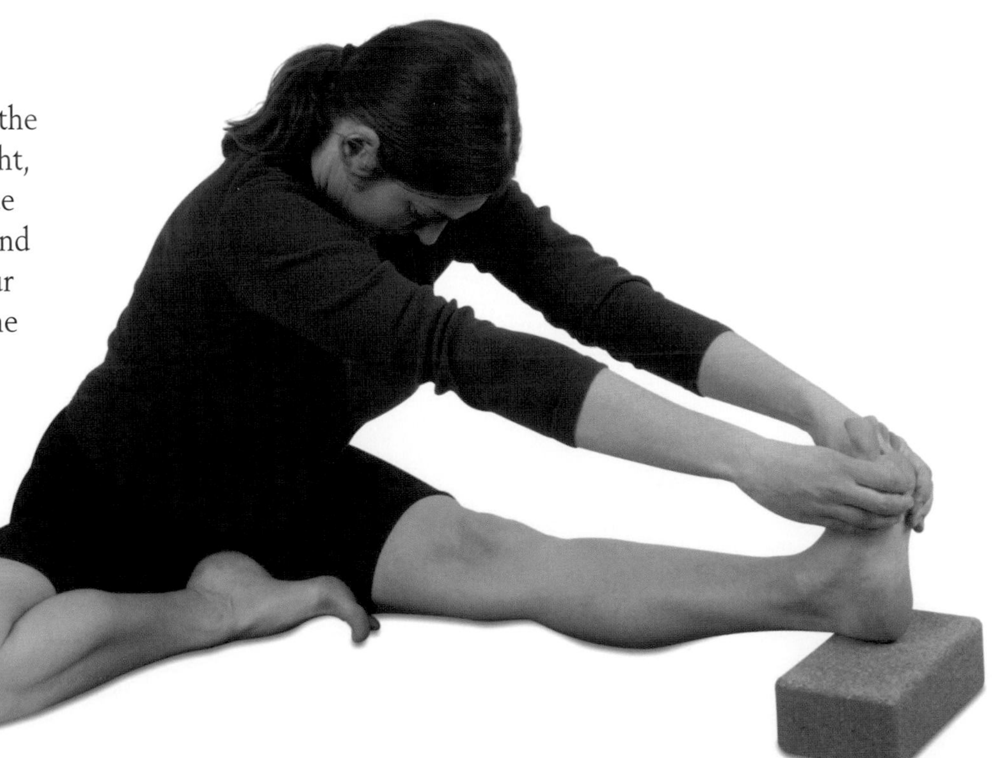

4 Extend your arms and hook your big toe with both thumbs, index fingers, and middle fingers.

5 Straighten both arms at the elbows.

6 Grip your toes well to lift up your torso and extend your spine. Raise your torso more by maintaining your grip and pressing your thighs to the floor.

7 Inhale softly and raise your frontal chest upward by expanding your intercostal (rib) muscles. Lower your head from the nape of the neck until your chin rests in the hollow between your collarbones.

8 From here, continue with the practice you became used to during pregnancy (pages 79 – 81).

Help

If you can't reach your big toe, use a belt for your foot and grip it as tightly as possible.

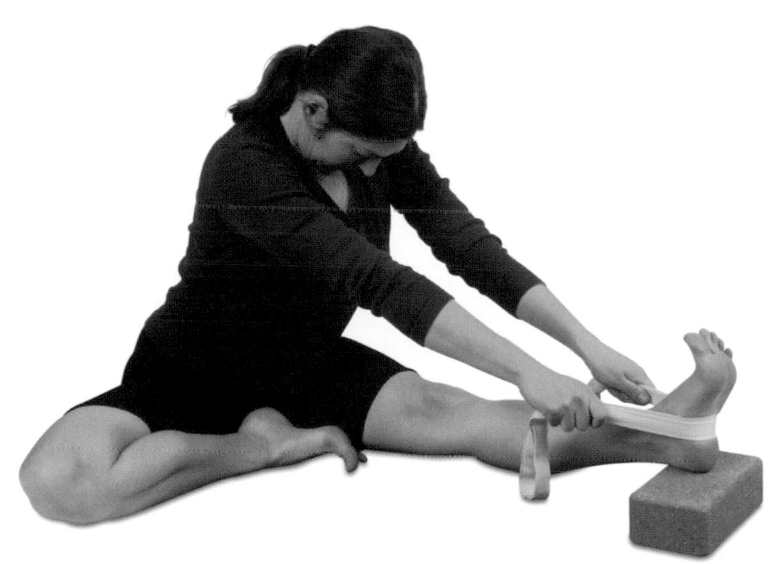

1st term: yes
2nd term: yes
3rd term: yes

Benefits

Maha Mudra as a Preparatory Asana

Maha Mudra offers good preparation for the asanas that come under the category of abdominal contractions, such as Navasana, for the second and third terms onward. It strengthens the abdominal muscles and the uterus. Along with Shirshasana and Sarvangasana, Maha Mudra dries the uterus, so that hemorrhaging does not occur. If a new mother with a weak uterus were to take up abdominal exercises too suddenly, her uterus could easily become displaced, resulting in heavy bleeding. Maha Mudra protects from this danger.

After delivery, the uterus tends to sag downward and the internal organs and muscles of the pelvis and the abdomen are in a weakened state. Maha Mudra and Janu Shirshasana strengthen those areas and bring them back to normal.

Other positive effects shared by these positions include reducing excessive menstrual flow, strengthening the entire back and neck, helping treat high blood pressure, soothing the nerves, and calming the mind.

HINT: While retaining your breath, be careful not to tilt your head or contract your chest, which may cause fatigue and depression.

Janu Shirshasana
Head on knee pose

Janu Shirshasana is also practiced differently after delivery. You'll sit on the floor with the heel bone of your straight leg on a block.

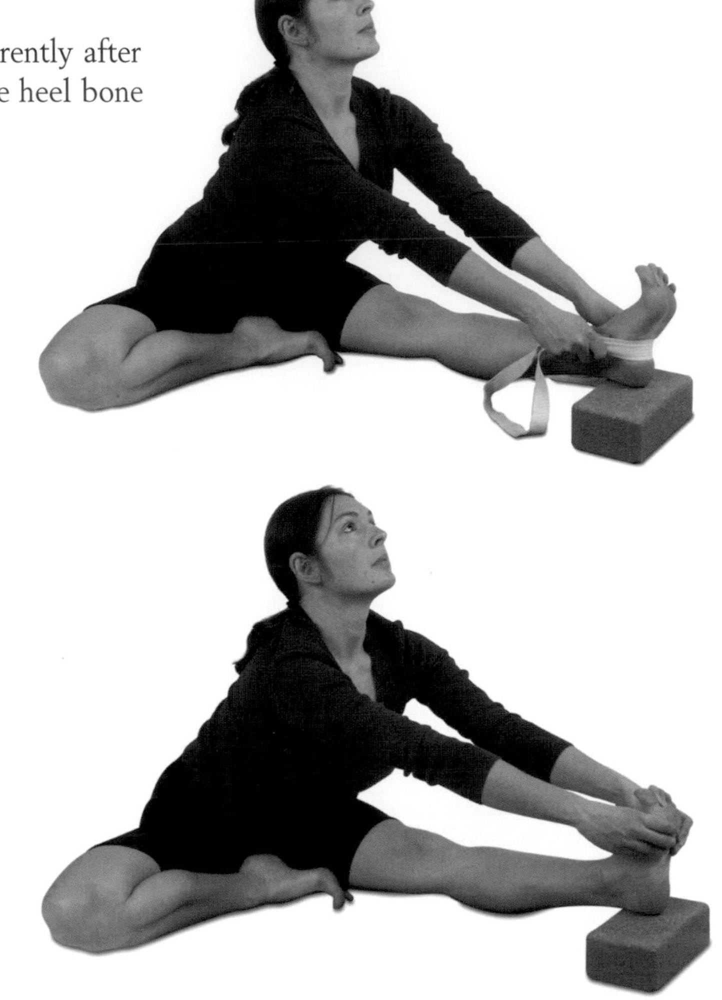

1 Have a block and a belt, and spread a blanket on the floor.

2 Sit in Dandasana and put a block in front of you.

3 Place your left heel bone on the block and keep the leg straight. Bend your right knee, place the outer sides of your thigh and calf on the floor, and bring your heel close to the right side of your groin. Pull your right knee back.

4 Inhale and stretch your arms toward the ceiling in Urdhva Hasta.

5 Exhale, extend both arms forward beyond your left foot, and grasp the sides of the foot with both hands in Urdhva Mukha. Breathe normally.

6 After holding the foot with straight arms, inhale, and extend and lift your spine. Press your right knee down and raise your hips. There should be an angle of 45° between your left leg and your torso. Bring your head back. Breathe normally and stay for 15 seconds.

7 If you can reach far enough, grip your right wrist with your left hand.

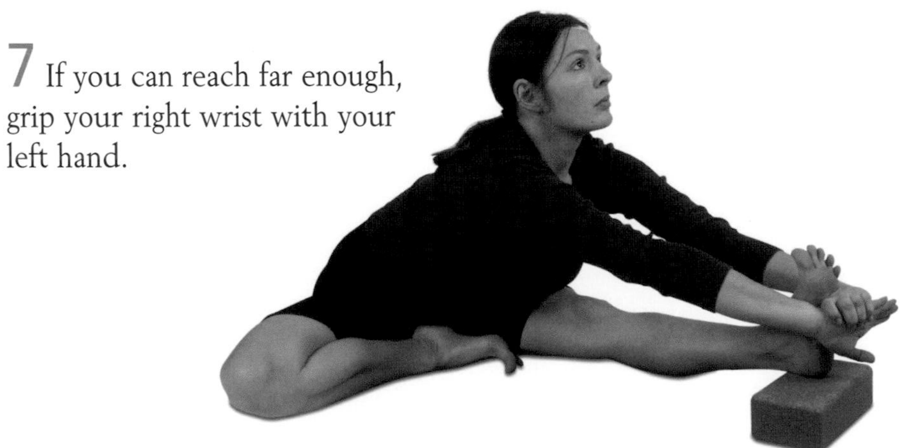

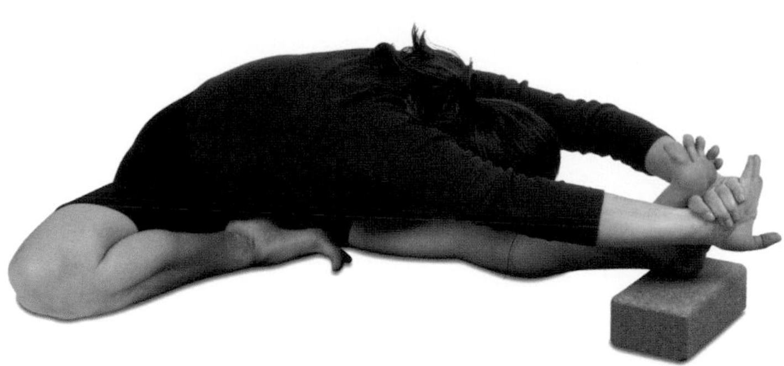

1st term: yes
2nd term: yes
3rd term: yes

Benefits

See page 83

8 Exhale, bend your torso forward by bending your elbows to the sides, and place your forehead on your shin-bone. Stay in this final position for 30 to 60 seconds or longer, while breathing normally and observing the following points:

- Keep your elbows out, widening them to increase the expansion of your chest, and stretch forward.
- Move your floating ribs (two lower ribs on each side) forward and extend them to your chest.
- Your breastbone and the middle of your abdomen must rest on your left thigh as though your torso were merged with the leg.
- While bending forward, keep your stretched left leg and bent right leg firmly on the floor and pull your right knee back as far as possible.

9 Inhale, lift your head and torso, release your palms, and come to Dandasana. Perform the asana on the other side. Remain for the same length of time and return to Dandasana.

Help

If you're a beginner, you may find it difficult to hold your foot with your hands and place your forehead on your knee. Develop your ability to stretch every part of your body gradually—buttocks, back of the torso, ribs, spine, armpits, elbows, and arms. Start with the instructions as given below and gradually move to the technique for the full, classic pose as your spine becomes more supple.

1 Stretch your spine fully so that holding your legs becomes easier.
2 First, let your hands reach your shin.
3 Second, hook your big toe with your index and middle fingers.
4 Third, grasp your sole with your fingers.
5 If you still can't reach, put a belt around your foot, pull it firmly with both hands, and then proceed as instructed above, trying steps 1 to 4 again.
6 It is very important that your spinal column be fully extended.

CHECK YOURSELF

> *The outer edge of your heel should be in line with the outer edge of your thigh.*
> *Your heel bone should firmly press down onto the block.*
> *There should be an extension of the spine from your tailbone to your armpits.*
> *Elongate your spine while exhaling.*
> *Most important:*
- *Don't contract your chest, abdomen, or stomach.*
- *Develop your ability to release your abdomen, stomach, and chest and to extend them forward.*

Pashchimottanasana, Heels on Block

Intense west chest pose

Pashchima means "west," which when applied to the body means "back." This asana has a backward extension.

For this asana, you'll use a block.

1 Sit in Dandasana with your heel bones on the block.

2 Inhale and stretch your arms toward the ceiling in Urdhva Hasta.

3 Exhale, extend your arms, and hold the outer edges of your feet with both hands or grip one of your wrists beyond your feet in Urdhva Mukha. Keep your elbows straight.

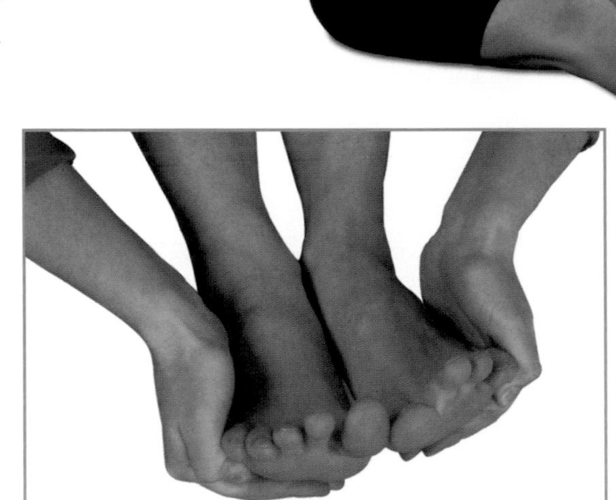

4 Inhale and stretch your spine upward, making it concave. Raise your back, waist, and breastbone and lift your head. Stay for 5 seconds and take a few breaths.

5 Exhale, bend your elbows slightly, and extend your upper arms outward. Extend the sides of your torso and bend forward, touching your thighs. Your head should rest beyond your knees.

Help

If you're a beginner and can't reach your feet without bending your legs, try this:

- Using the block as in the technique above, grasp your big toes: the right one with your right thumb, middle finger, and index finger, and the left one with the same digits of your left hand.
- If this is also too difficult, pull a belt around your feet as shown in Janu Shirshasana above.
- Gradually work up to encircling the soles of your feet with your fingers.
- In the beginning, your back may be hunched. To correct this, raise your torso from the small of your back and raise your head.

6 In this final stage, your head and torso rest on your legs. Stay in this position for 1 minute, breathing normally. Gradually increase the time to 5 minutes, observing the following points:

- Widen your elbows so that your chest expands.
- Rest your abdomen and chest on your thighs.
- Bend your elbows and lift them upward; use the grip of your hands as a lever to extend your torso.
- Don't cave in your chest or pull into your breastbone.
- Keep your neck muscles soft and your head passive.

7 Inhale, raise your head, and come to Dandasana.

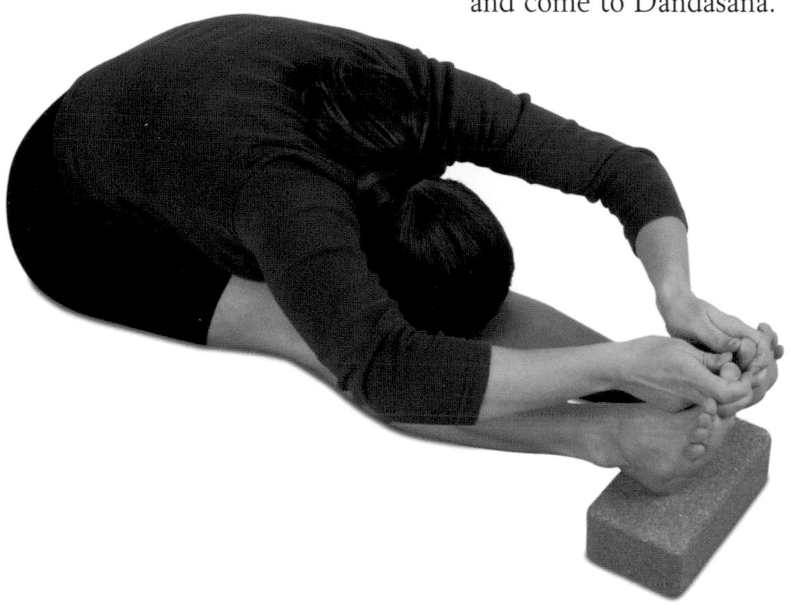

1st term: no
2nd term: yes
3rd term: yes

Benefits

Massages and strengthens the abdominal muscles and organs

Helps treat kidney disease and sluggish liver

Stretches the pelvic region and stimulates its blood circulation

Revitalizes and enhances the efficiency of the entire reproductive system

Rests the heart (heart and spine are horizontal and parallel to the floor)

Soothes an upset, irritated, and restless mind

Calms angry and overemotional moods

Sharpens the memory and brings clarity of thought

Special Instructions

Using a stool or chair against the wall will help you stretch your torso. Try the following:

- Rest your feet on the lower plank of the stool or as shown in the photo below and hold the stool with your hands.
- Don't cave in your chest to touch your knees.
- Don't rest your elbows on the chair; this hinders the extension of the body.
- Make sure that your outer thighs roll inward, and that there is extension of the abdomen.
- If you can't keep your feet together, you can keep them 1 foot apart, which softens the groin and frees the sacrum.

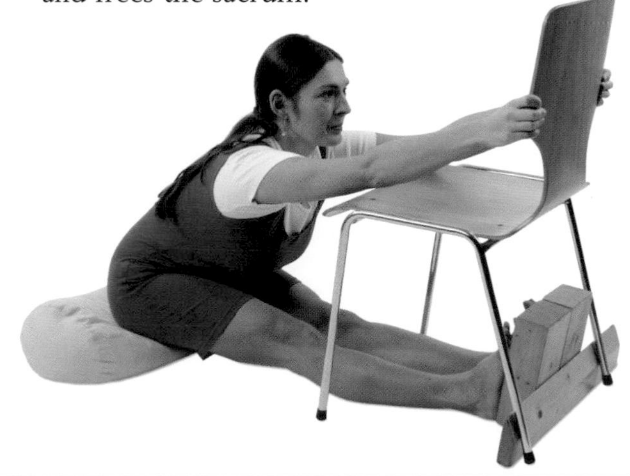

Ardha Baddha Padma Pashchimottanasana

Half lotus forward fold pose

Ardha means "half," *baddha* means "caught," and *padma* means "lotus." In this pose, one leg is in Padmasana, see page 94, the other is stretched, and the back of the torso is extended. This pose works the abdomen.

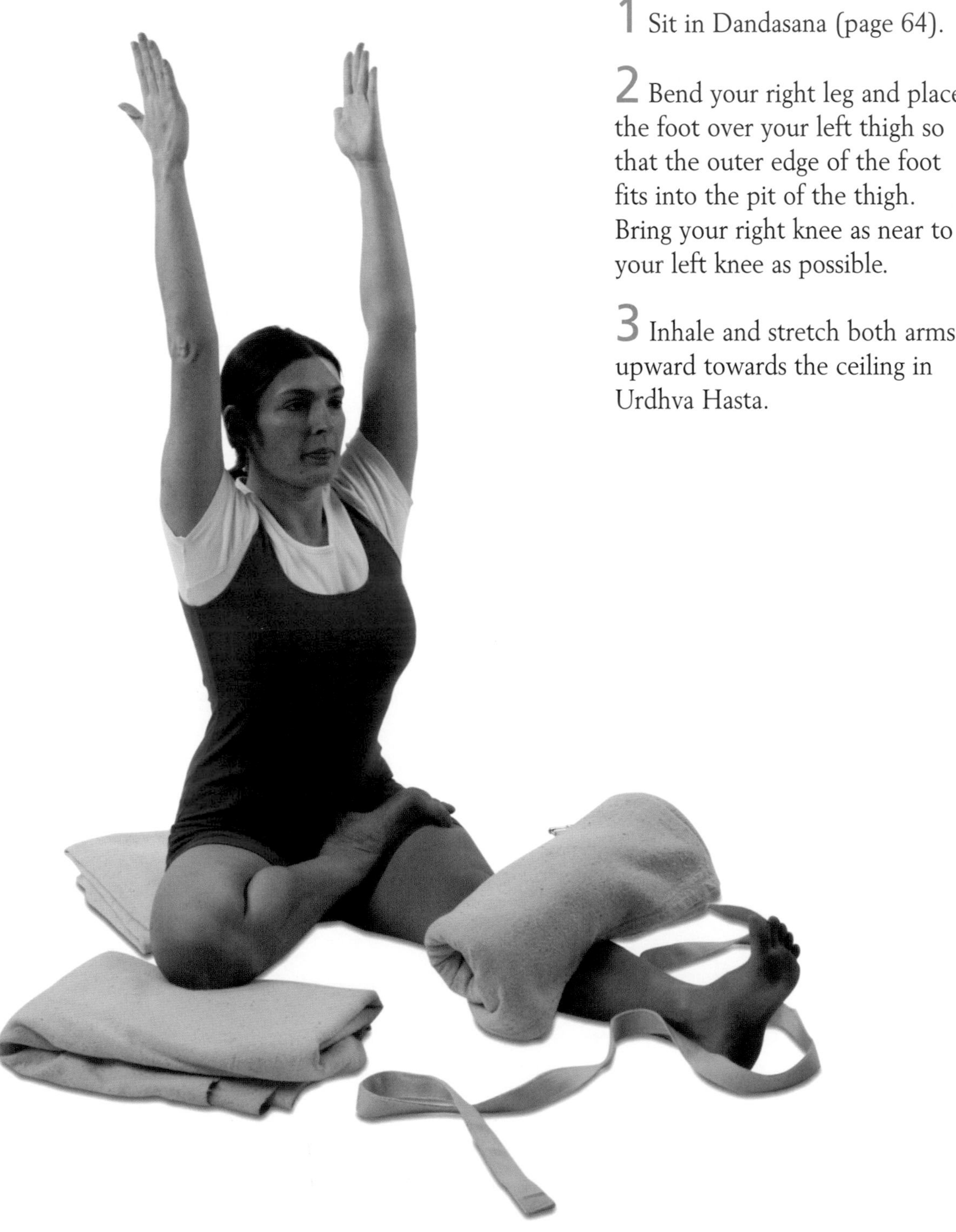

1 Sit in Dandasana (page 64).

2 Bend your right leg and place the foot over your left thigh so that the outer edge of the foot fits into the pit of the thigh. Bring your right knee as near to your left knee as possible.

3 Inhale and stretch both arms upward towards the ceiling in Urdhva Hasta.

4 Exhale and stretch both arms forward towards your left foot. Grasp the foot with both hands; if you can reach farther, entwine your hands behind the foot in Urdhva Mukha. Straighten your arms.

5 Inhale, raise your head, and look up. Extend your spine, expand your chest, and lift your breastbone. Stay for 5 seconds, breathing normally.

6 Exhale, extend your spine forward by bending your elbows to the outside, and place your chin on or beyond your left knee.

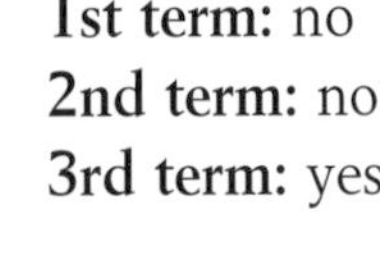

1st term: no
2nd term: no
3rd term: yes

Benefits

Alleviates unsettled stomach and flatulence

Strengthens the abdominal muscles

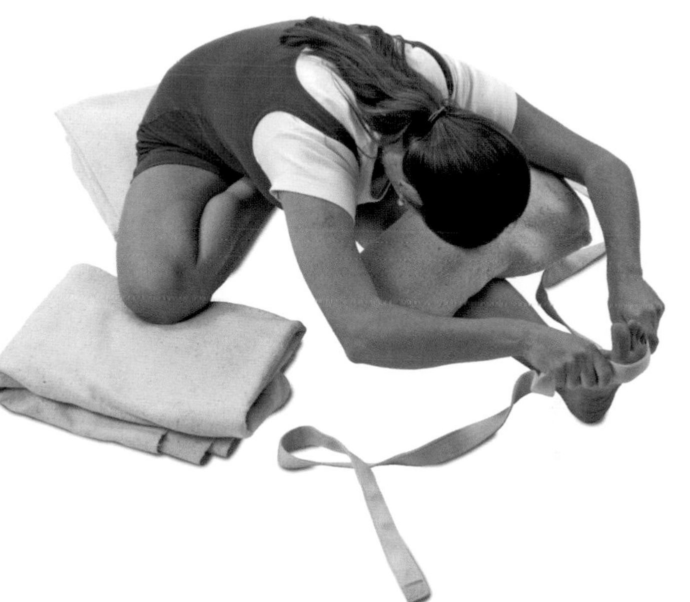

7 Stay in this final position for 30 to 60 seconds, breathing normally and observing the following points:

- Bring your pelvis forward, beyond your right foot and ankle.
- Rest your stomach and chest on your thigh, with your chin beyond the knee.
- Your torso should merge more and more into your thigh.

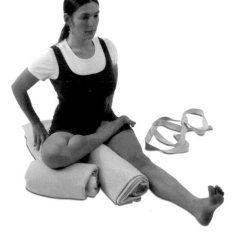

Help

- If the bent knee is not reaching the floor, put a rolled blanket under it and another one under the lower shin and ankle.
- Try putting the block under the heel of your stretched leg, as in Pashchimottanasana above.

Coming out of the pose

1 Inhale, raise your head, and come to Dandasana.

2 Practice the asana on the other side and come back to Dandasana.

DETAILED DESCRIPTIONS OF ASANAS FOR BEGINNERS AND ADVANCED STUDENTS

Trianga Mukhaikapada Pashchimottanasana

Three limbs intense west stretch pose

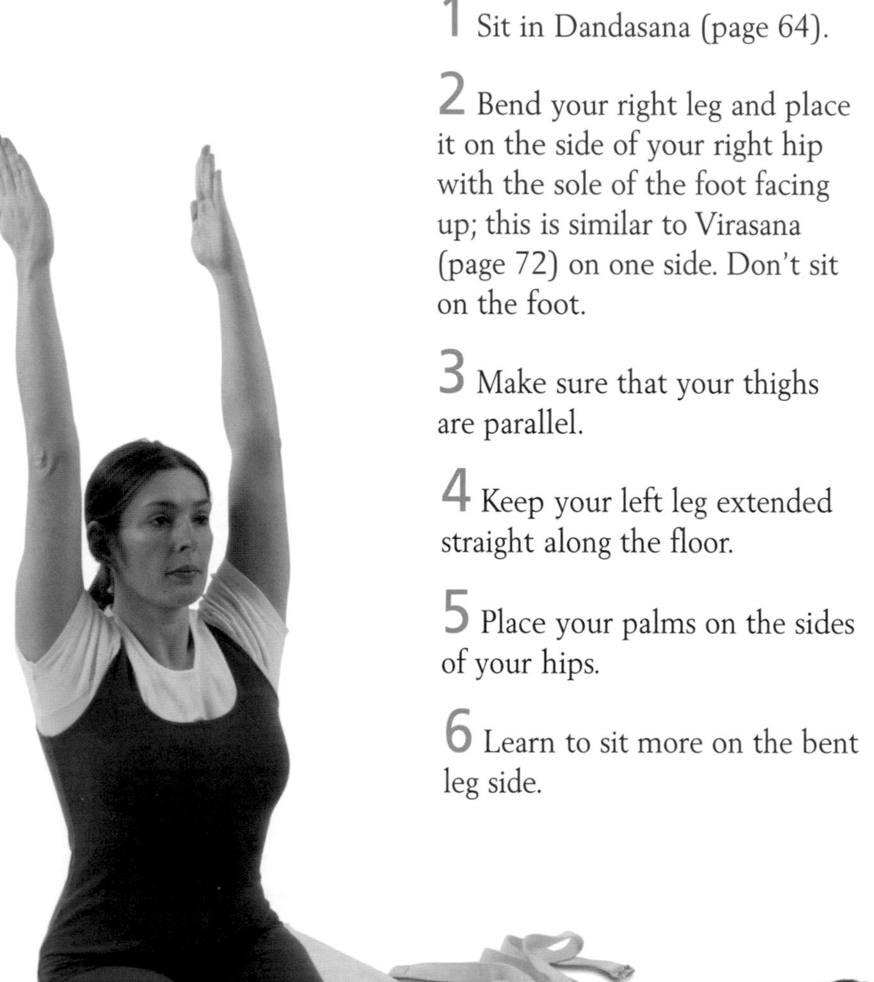

1 Sit in Dandasana (page 64).

2 Bend your right leg and place it on the side of your right hip with the sole of the foot facing up; this is similar to Virasana (page 72) on one side. Don't sit on the foot.

3 Make sure that your thighs are parallel.

4 Keep your left leg extended straight along the floor.

5 Place your palms on the sides of your hips.

6 Learn to sit more on the bent leg side.

7 Inhale and extend your arms up towards the ceiling in Urdhva Hasta (page 66).

8 Exhale, extend your torso forward, and grasp your left foot with both hands or hold your wrists beyond the foot in Urdhva Mukha (page 90, step 6).

9 Inhale, raise the sides of your chest (lengthening the waist), and look up.

10 When you're bending forward, your weight tends to drop more to the stretched leg. Learn to level the sides of your pelvis and torso evenly.

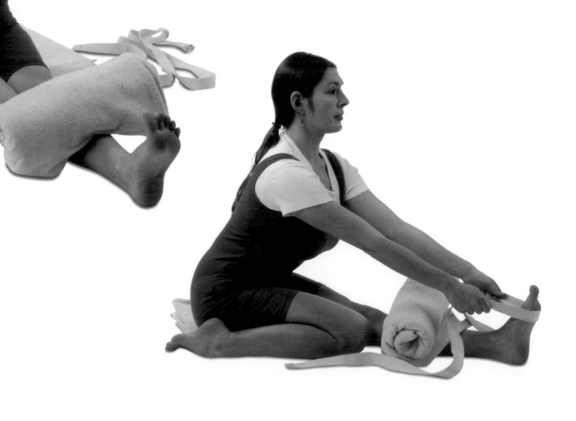

11 Exhale and bend your elbows, lifting the sides of your torso up and forward to rest your abdomen and chin along your left leg.

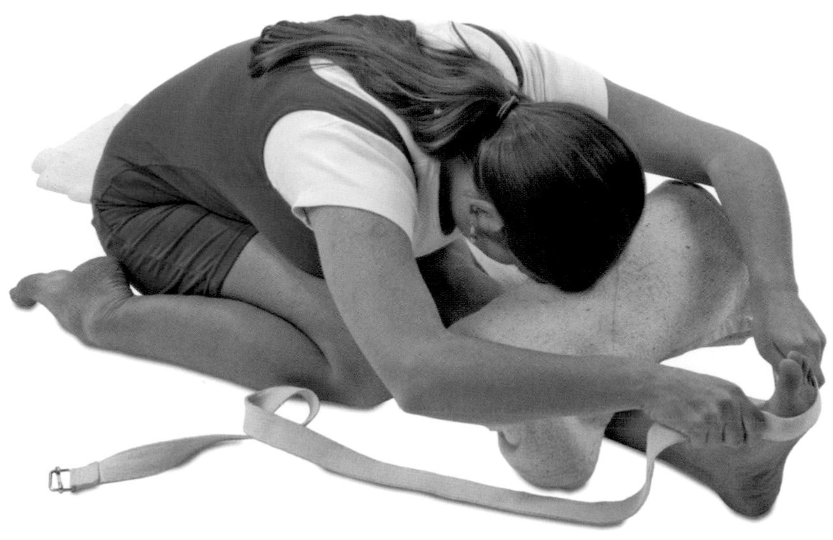

1st term: no
2nd term: no
3rd term: yes

Benefits

See page 89

Coming out of the pose

1 Inhale and raise your head and chest to come up.

2 Release your right leg and sit in Dandasana.

3 Repeat on the other side.

CHECK YOURSELF
Develop your ability to:
> *Balance the sides of your torso evenly.*
> *Keep your torso in the center without tilting.*

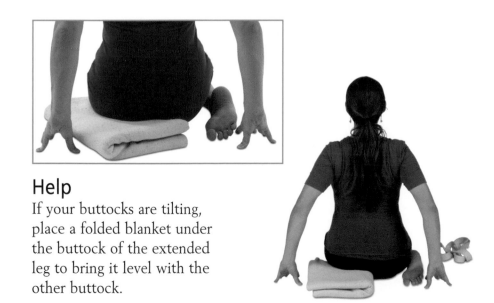

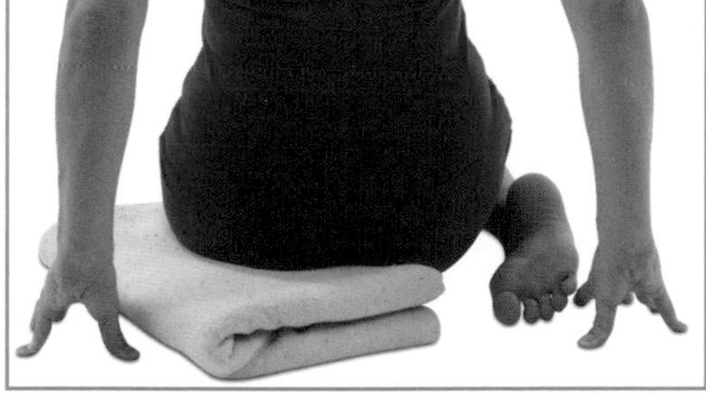

Help

If your buttocks are tilting, place a folded blanket under the buttock of the extended leg to bring it level with the other buttock.

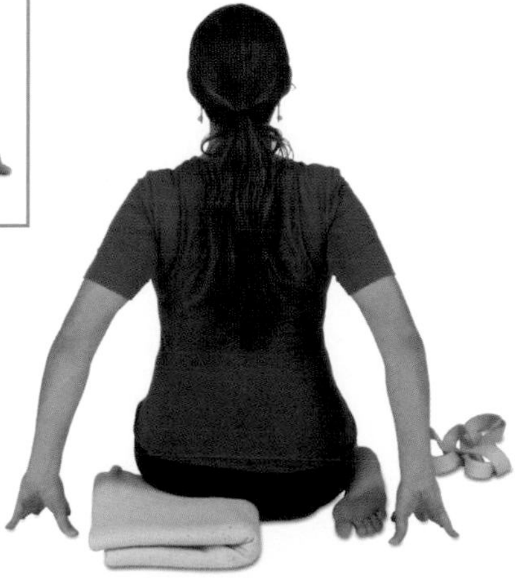

Marichyasana 1
Spinal twist 1 pose

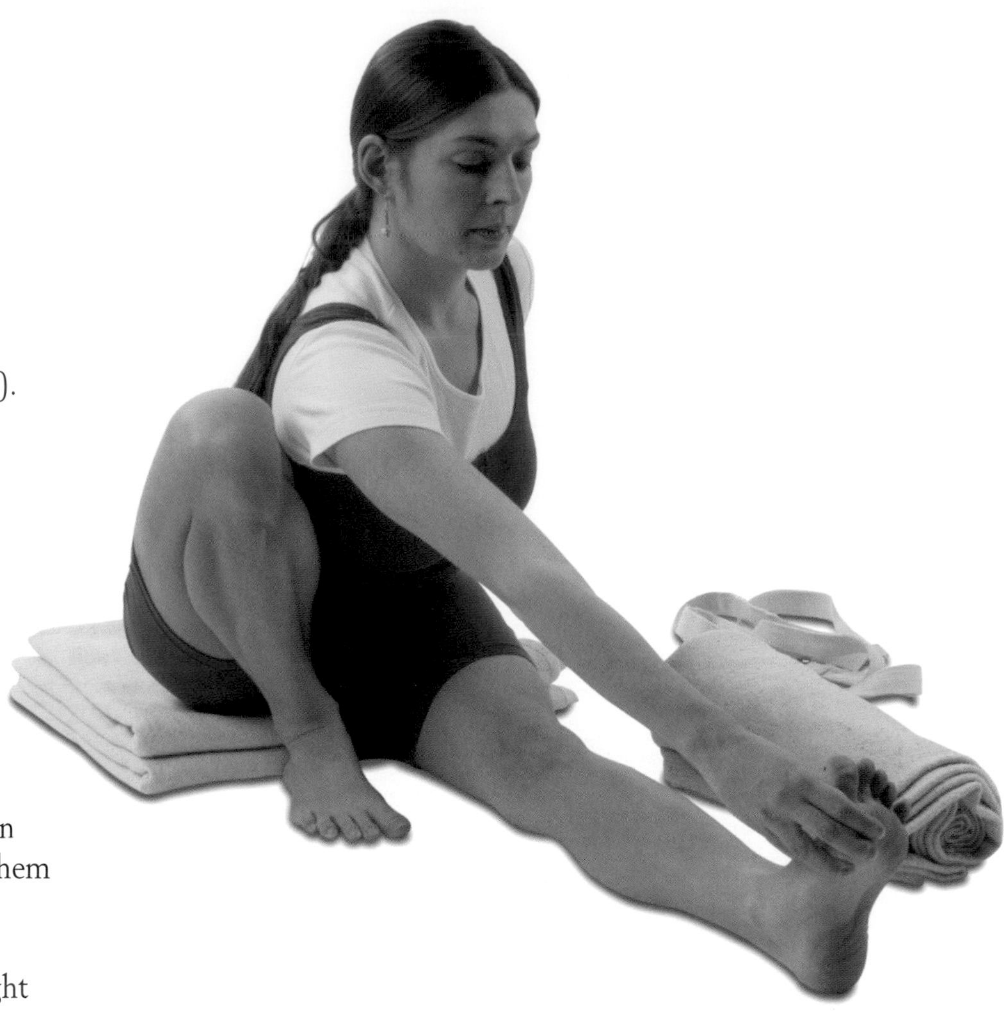

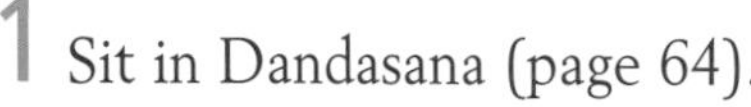

1 Sit in Dandasana (page 64).

2 Bend your right knee so that it faces up towards the ceiling. Your right heel is in line with the right buttock, toes pointing forward.

3 Keep your arms in Dandasana.

4 Level the spinal muscles on both sides evenly, spreading them horizontally.

5 Inhale and extend your right arm straight towards the ceiling.

6 Exhale and extend the arm and the right side of your torso forward along the inside of your right thigh.

7 The inside of your right thigh and your right torso should touch.

8 Hold the ball of your left big toe with your right hand.

9 Extend your right side forward.

10 Make sure that your right knee does not drop out.

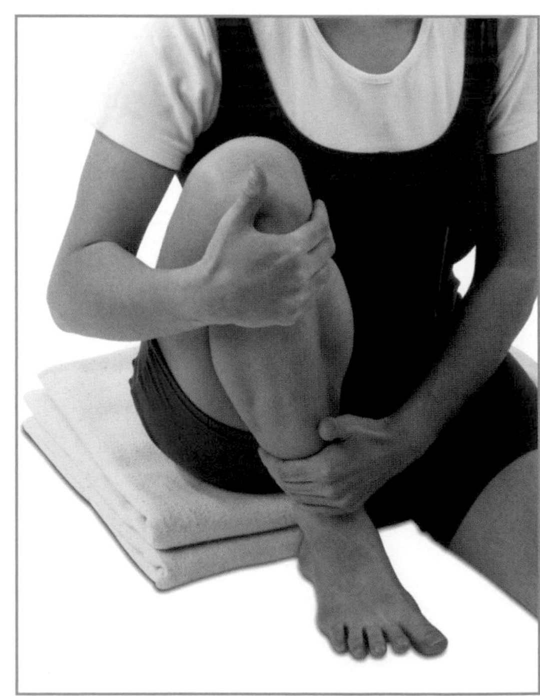

1st term: no
2nd term: no
3rd term: yes

Benefits

See page 321

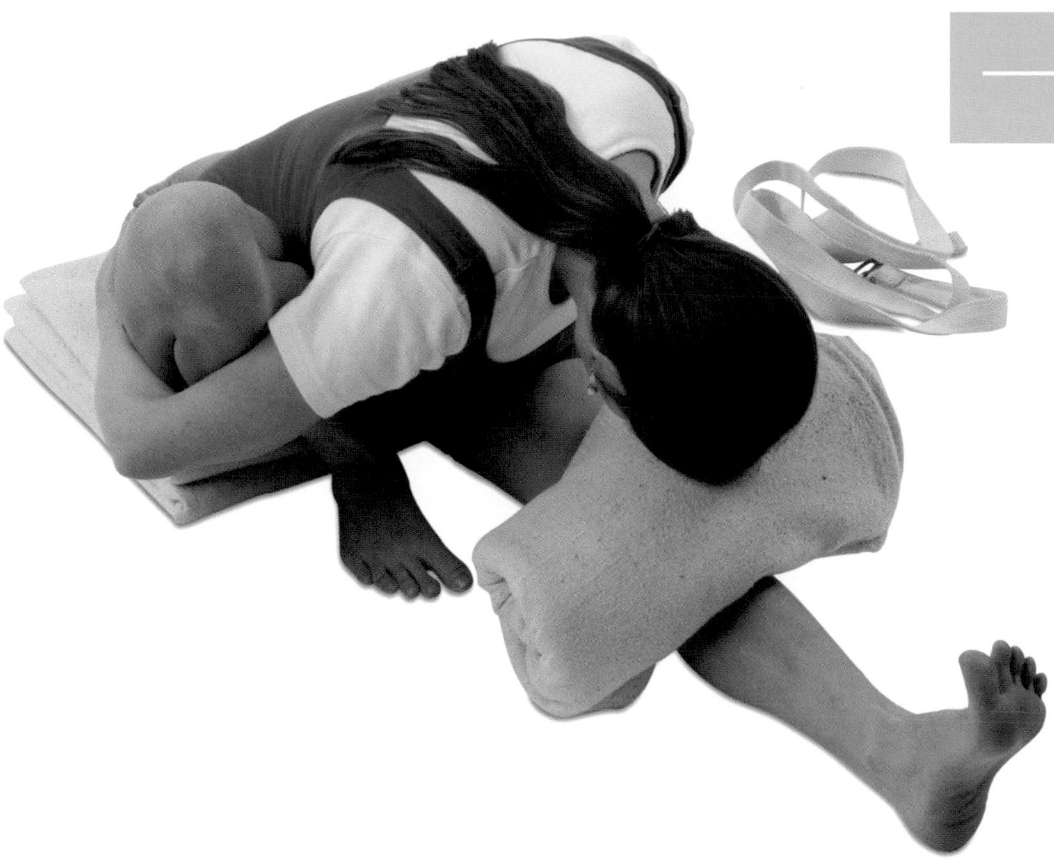

11 Bring your right arm behind by moving it around your right shinbone and thigh.

12 Turning your left shoulder to the left, swing your left arm behind your back to catch hold of your right hand. Lift your chest.

13 Turn your entire torso to face forward.

14 Exhale, and maintaining the lift of your outer shoulders into your back, bring your shoulders in line with each other. Bring your abdomen, sternum, and chin forward towards your left shin, and rest your forehead.

15 Repeat on the other side.

CHECK YOURSELF

> *Keep the pit of your groin on the side with the bent leg down.*

> *Extend the sides of your torso evenly.*

> *Grip your interlocked hands firmly while bending forward. Don't loosen your grip or allow the bent leg to tilt to the outside.*

Upavishtha Konasana
Seated wide-angle pose

1st term: no
2nd term: no
3rd term: yes

1 Sit in Dandasana (page 64).

2 Spread your legs and widen the distance between them. This is shown with blocks under the heels.

3 Make sure that the centers of your thigh, knee, and foot exactly face the ceiling.

4 Keep the back of your thighs, knees, and calf muscles pressing down.

5 Place your hands on either side of your hips.

6 Lift your spine and chest and pull your shoulder blades into your back.

7 Widen your legs and keep the center of the back of your thighs, calves, and heels on the floor.

8 Sit exactly on your buttock bones to avoid a cramp in the hip joint.

9 Keeping your legs extended, lift your spine and raise your arms above your head, upper arms in line with your ears, in Urdhva Hasta.

10 Exhale, bend forward, and grasp your big toes with your index fingers, middle fingers, and thumbs in Padangushthasana. Keep your thumbs on the outside of the big toes and the index and middle fingers on the inside, in Urdhva Mukha. (This is shown with blocks under the heels.)

11 Press your thighs down to the floor and extend your inner heels.

12 Raise the sides of your torso.

13 Move the dorsal (mid) spine into your body between your shoulder blades and further lift your chest, inhale, raise your breastbone, and look up.

14 Exhale, lengthen your torso, and bring your head down.

Coming out of the pose
Inhale, raise your head, chest, and torso, come up, bring your legs together, and return to Dandasana.

Benefits

In addition to the benefits of Upavishtha Konasana before delivery (page 85), working with your heels on a block:

- Gives extra stability to the pelvis
- Strengthens the inner legs and the pelvic muscles
- Realigns the inner and outer body
- Safely lifts the pelvis

Help
- If you can't grip your toes, use a belt for your feet.

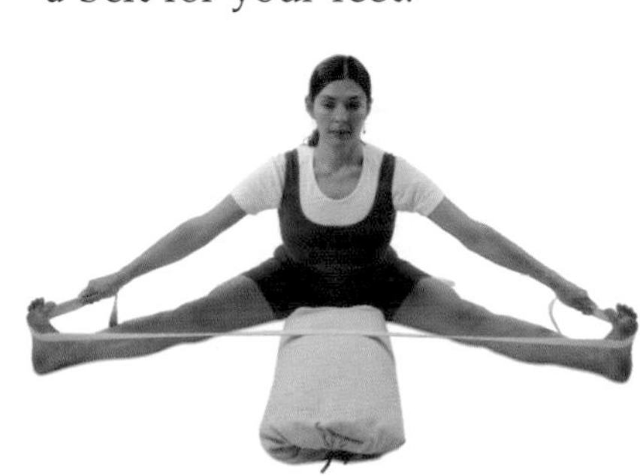

- If your head doesn't reach the floor, use a support such as folded blankets for your head.

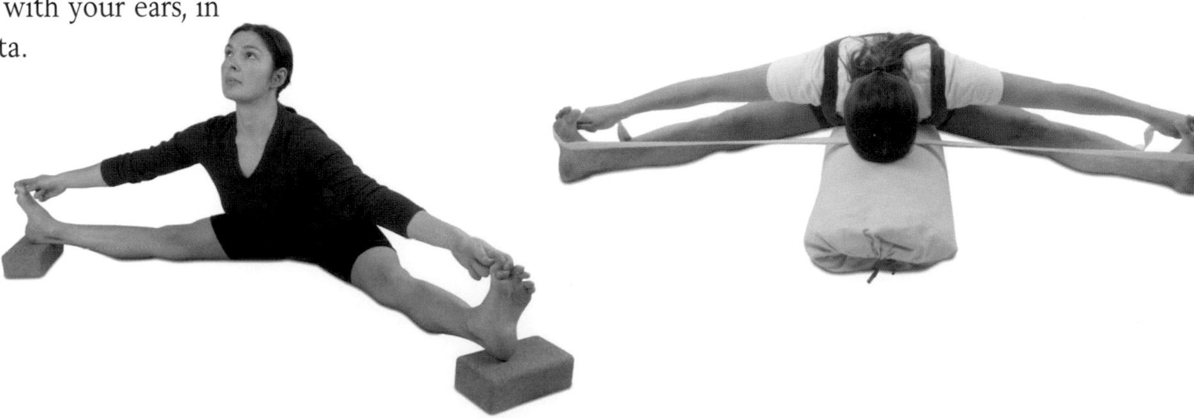

Adho Mukha Virasana
Downward-facing hero pose

1st term: no
2nd term: no
3rd term: yes

Benefits

See page 76

1 With your big toes touching and your knees apart, roll your calf muscles to the outside.

2 Sit between your inner heels.

3 Bring your arms forward, stretch your spine and the sides of your torso forward, and rest your forehead on the floor.

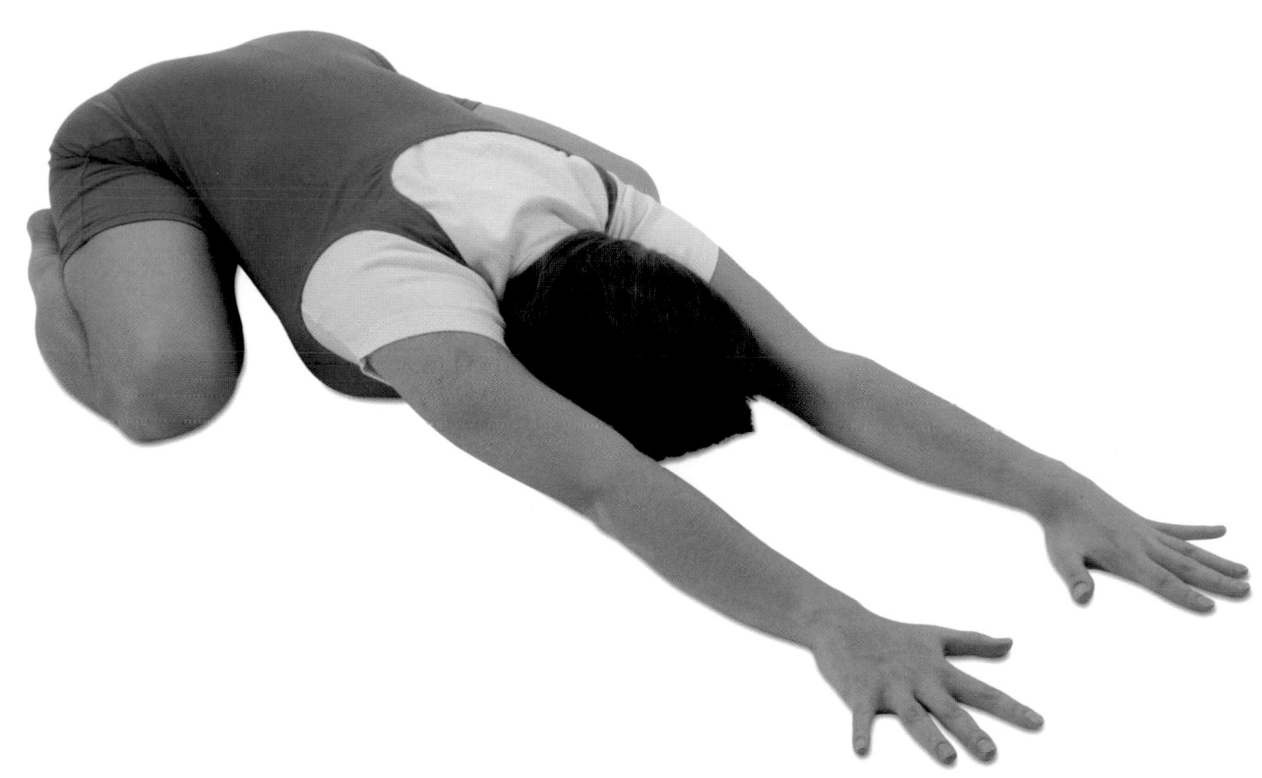

Twists
Parivritta Sthiti

The twisting asanas bring a wide array of benefits, especially for the time after your delivery. They come with cautions, however, and it is very important to perform them correctly.

Dos and Don'ts

Do
- Enjoy the lightness of body that the asanas bestow by creating freedom in your abdomen and chest
- With practice, obtain flexibility of the spinal muscles

Don't
- Allow your lower spine to sag or collapse
- Compress your abdomen downward
- Contract your chest muscles

If you don't heed these "don'ts," and you achieve a pose by force rather than by doing it properly, the result may be bleeding or hernia.

1 Bharadvajasana (chair)
2 Bharadvajasana (bolster/s)
3 Marichyasana 3
4 Ardha Matsyendrasana

Always practice in the above order.

Benefits
(for all twists)

Relieve rheumatism, backache, pain in the spinal column, and humpback. For back sprain or slipped disk, practice against a wall.

Increase the mobility of the shoulders and shoulder blades and expand the chest

Create shapely ankles and calves

Massage and rejuvenate the abdominal organs

Alleviate indigestion, acidity, irritable bowels, diabetes, and flatulence

Help treat kidney, liver, spleen, gallbladder, and bladder disorders

Regulate peristaltic movement

Strengthen the uterus and the waist

Remedy menstrual disorders and malfunctioning of the endocrine glands, and counteract obesity

Reduce exhaustion due to over-work or menstruation

Protect against hernia and displacement of the uterus

Bharadvajasana
Torso stretch pose

1st term: no
2nd term: yes
3rd term: yes

Backache and shoulder pain are common complaints, especially after delivery.

At this stage, your spinal muscles need toning. We'll begin with simple lateral movements of the spine, which will become the foundation for the rest of the twisting asanas. Bharadvajasana is a stepping-stone to correct lateral spinal movement.

After several deliveries, you may face problems related to middle age such as accumulation of fat, loosening of the muscles, and digestive disorders. Especially at this time, poses with lateral spine rotation are very important for maintaining the body's metabolism.

For detailed instructions, see Bharadvajasana for during pregnancy, pages 91 – 93.

Special Instructions

Try the following variations of Bharadvajasana with support:

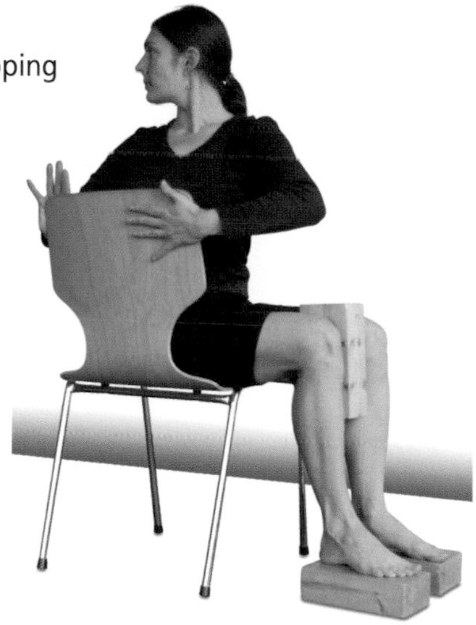

sitting on a chair, gripping block with knees

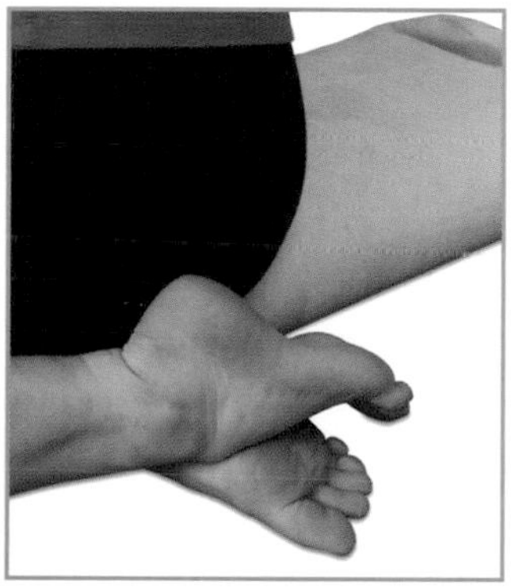

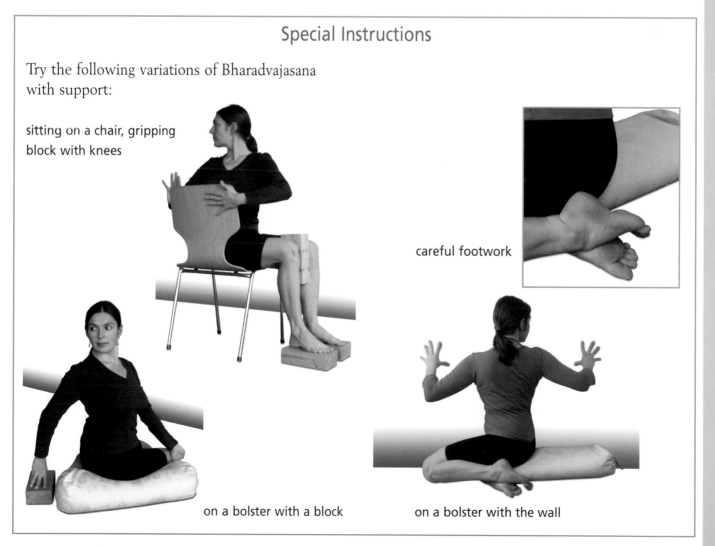

careful footwork

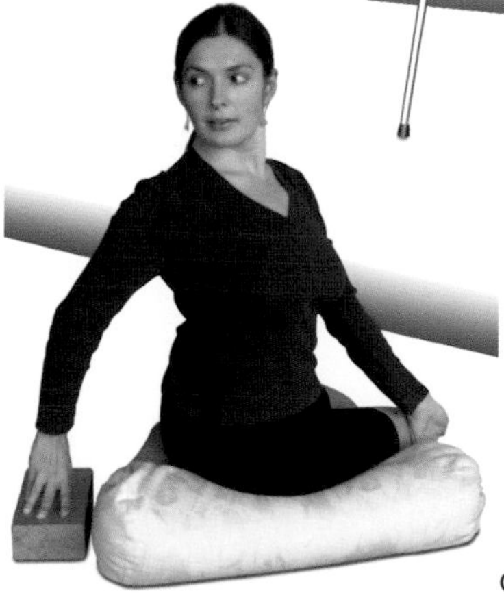

on a bolster with a block

on a bolster with the wall

Marichyasana 3
Spinal twist 3 pose

As a safety measure, you can switch over to Marichyasana after having extended your torso and the internal organs in Supta Baddha Konasana, Supta Virasana, or Setu Bandha Sarvangasana.

1 Sit in Dandasana (page 64).

2 Bend your right leg with the shin perpendicular to the floor and pull the foot to the thigh. Your right calf and thigh should be in close contact. Keep the toes pointing forward and the sole and heel on the floor. Keep your left leg outstretched. Take one or two breaths.

3 Exhale fully, raise your spine, and rotate your torso to the right so that its left side is close to your right thigh. Rest your right arm 8 to 10 inches away from your buttocks behind your back.

4 Raise your left arm and extend it beyond your right thigh in one of the following ways:
- Move your right thigh slightly towards your left leg.
- Push your right thigh with your left arm and entwine your arms round the knee. The left side of your torso and the armpit will now be locked between your right knee and the top of your right thigh.

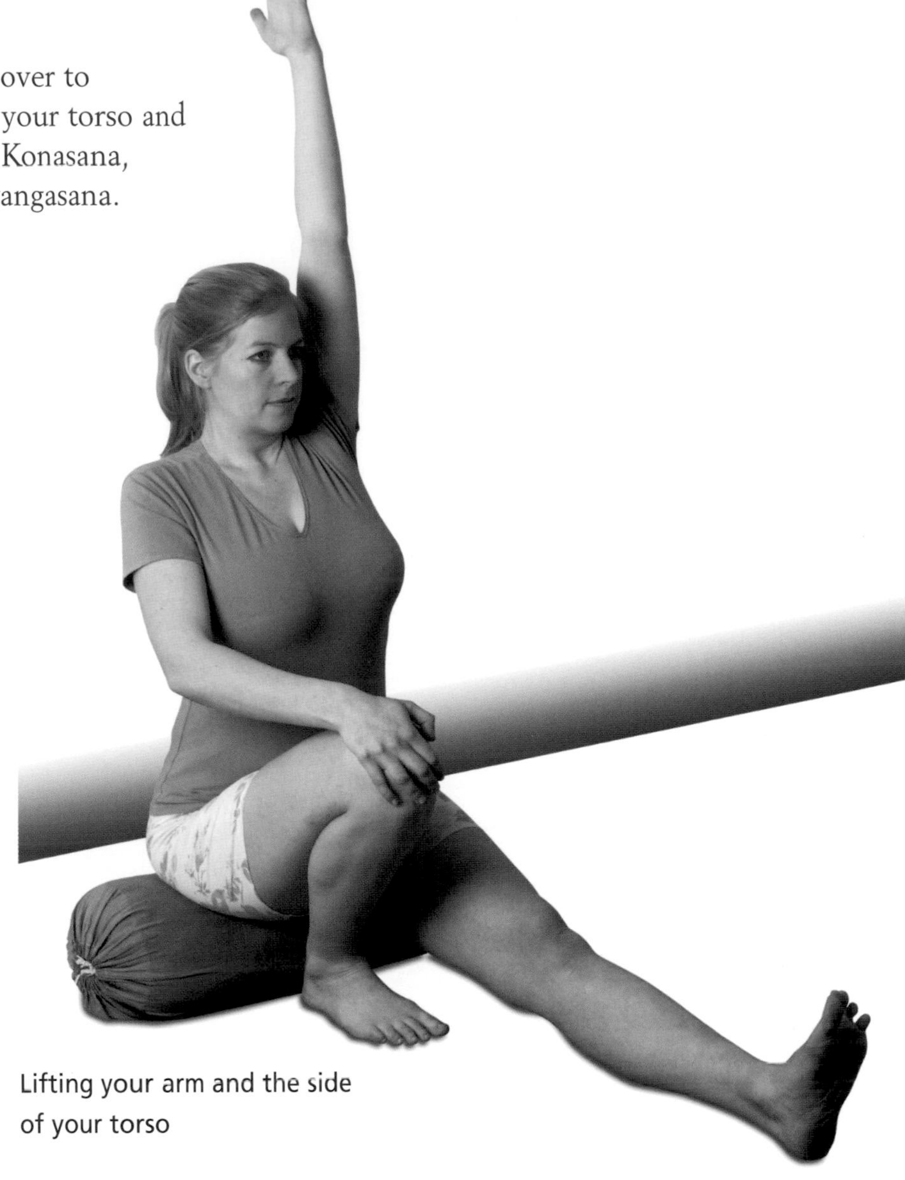

Lifting your arm and the side of your torso

5 Extend your left arm further towards the left leg so that your left forearm, armpit, and left side of your torso come still closer to your right thigh.

6 Bend your left arm, turn it at the wrist, and encircle your right leg, placing your palm on your back. Take a breath or two.

7 Exhale, raise your right arm from the floor, extend it backward from the shoulder, bend it at the elbow, and bring it near your left palm behind your back. With your right hand, firmly clasp in the following order: the fingers, palm, and wrist of your left hand.

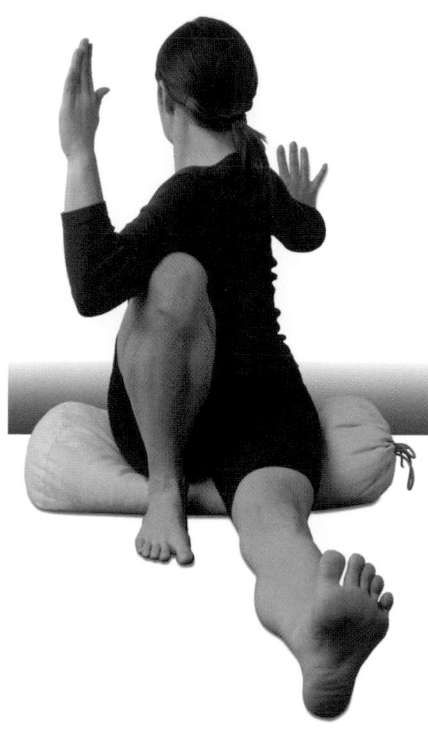

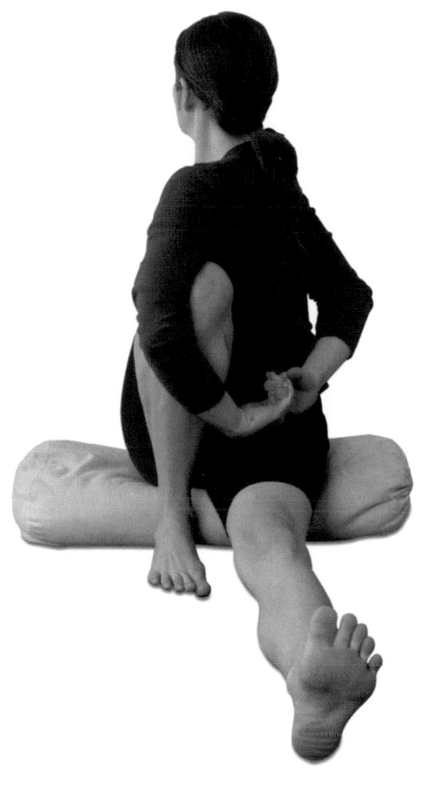

8 Raise your torso and turn it to the right. Turn your neck and gaze to the left.

9 Stay in this position for 20 to 30 seconds. For the first few moments only, your breathing will quicken because your diaphragm is compressed. Observe the following points:

- Stretch the extended leg further.
- Tuck in your shoulder blades.
- Don't leave any space between the armpit of the intertwining arm and the thigh of the bent leg.
- Don't loosen the grip of your fingers in the back.

10 Turn your head to the front, release your hands, and return to Dandasana.

11 Repeat the pose with your right leg straight and your left leg bent. The duration should be the same on both the sides.

1st term: no
2nd term: no
3rd term: yes

Benefits

(for Marichyasana 1, 3 and Utthita Marichyasana)

Reduces fat around the abdomen

Relieves backache, lumbago, and neck and shoulder sprain

Tones the abdominal organs

For beginners, Marichyasana relieves the backache that can result from performing Urdhva Prasarita Padasana with weak muscles. This is a good example of the reason for practicing asanas in their recommended sequences. If an asana causes a problem or pain, you don't have to give it up, because other poses can correct the difficulty. After Urdhva Prasarita Padasana, the supine poses are prescribed to extend the abdominal muscles and then Marichyasana is introduced to remove backache.

Technique Using the Wall

If you can't do this asana independently, use the wall for support as follows:

1 Sit in Dandasana sideways to the wall, so that your right leg is extended along the wall. Sit on a folded blanket or bolster.

2 Bend your right leg and keep the shin perpendicular. Your right heel should remain on the floor and not on the blanket. Take one or two breaths.

3 Inhale, lift your left arm, exhale, and turn your torso to the right so that its left side comes closer to your right thigh.

4 Extend your left shoulder and armpit towards your right leg.

5 Keep your left palm on the wall and push your right thigh with your left arm. Keep your right palm on the floor and maintain the rotation of your abdomen.

6 After achieving a good balance, raise your right arm and place the palm on the wall.

7 Press the wall with both palms, lift your torso up, and turn it as in Ardha Matsyendrasana (page 324).

8 Repeat the asana with your left leg along the wall, reversing all the processes.

Help

If your abdomen is still heavy, bring your leg out to the side at a 45° angle and either practice as instructed above or hold only with your hand and use a wall behind you for support.

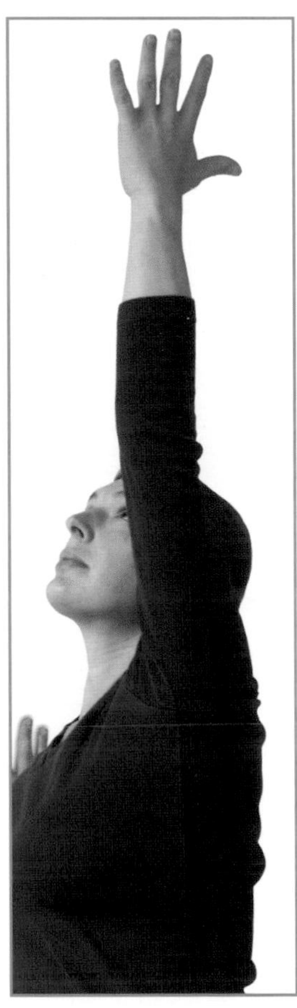

Lifting your arm and the side of your torso

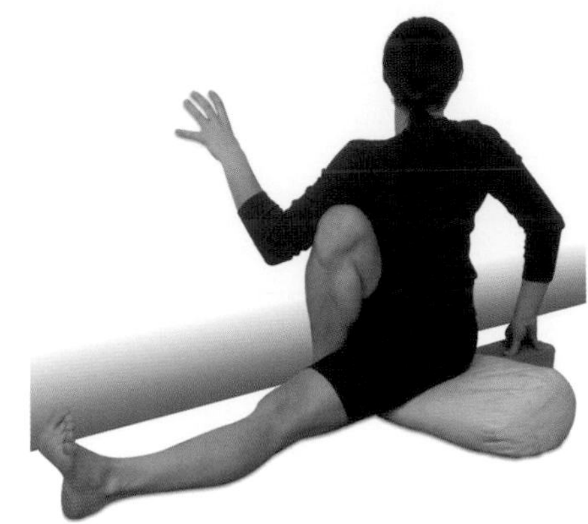

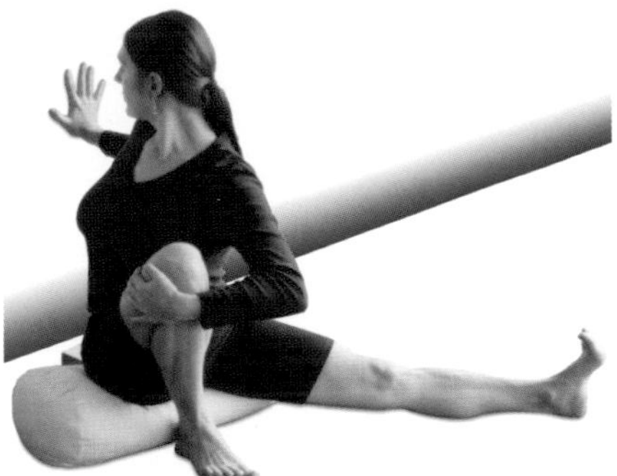

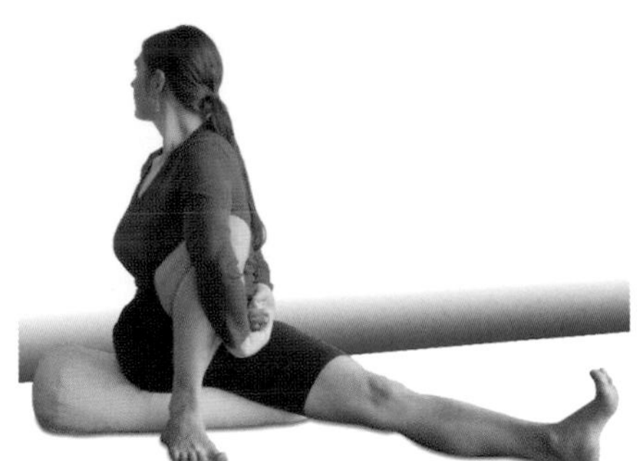

Utthita Marichyasana
Standing spine twist pose

1st term: no
2nd term: yes
3rd term: yes

Follow all the previous instructions, standing instead of sitting.

1 Stand with your left heel on a block and your right leg bent.

2 Keep your left leg straight and your right hip against the wall. Lift your left arm, the side of your torso, and your abdomen.

3 Either work with your hands against the wall as in Ardha Matsyendrasana, or grip your right knee with your left hand, pulling with the hand and resisting with the leg.

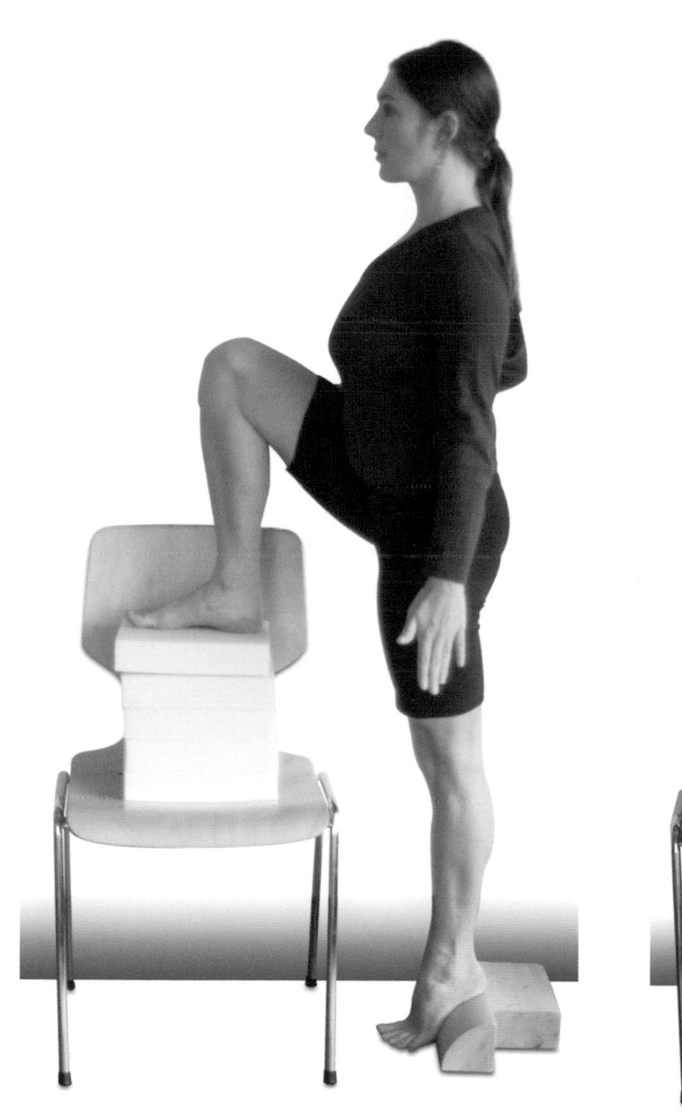

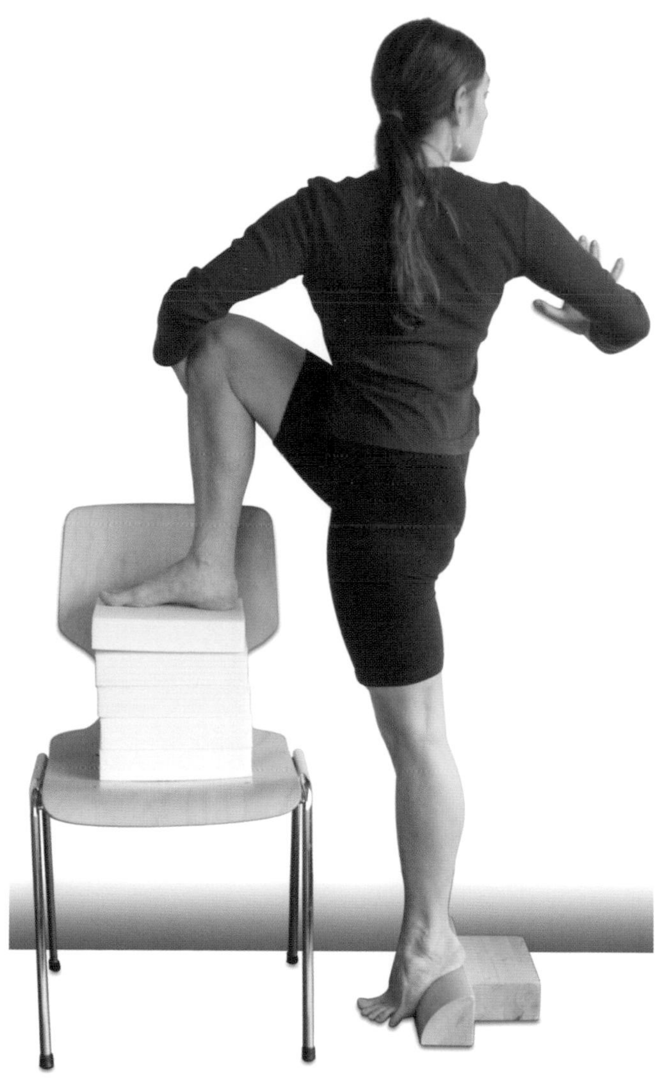

Ardha Matsyendrasana
Half Lord of the Fishes pose

Ardha Matsyendrasana helps massage the lower abdominal organs and strengthens the lower back. The technique below is for the classic pose.

1 Sit in Dandasana (page 64).

2 Bend your left leg and bring your shin backward to the left, so that your left foot is adjacent to your left hip.

3 Lift your buttocks off the floor and place your left foot under them. The foot should be horizontal so that it forms a seat and acts as a cushion. Place the left outer buttock on your heel and the inner part on the sole.

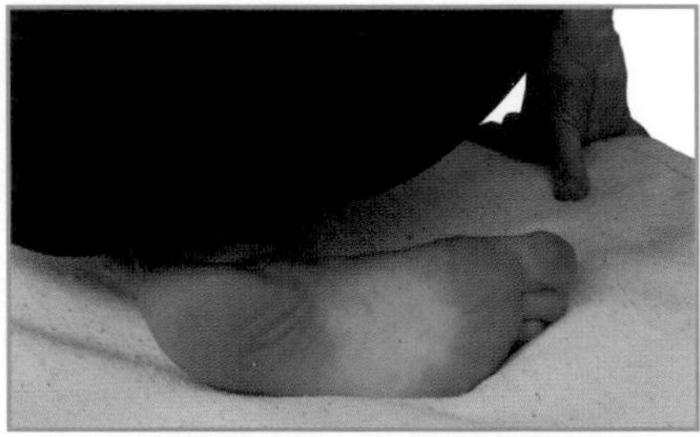

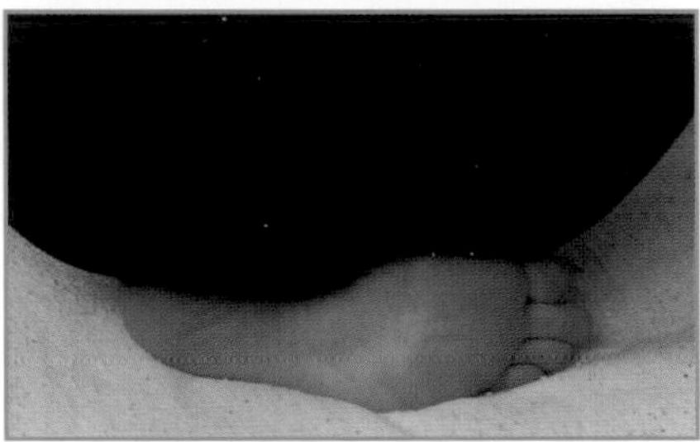

4 Bend your right leg and place your shin by the outer side of your left leg, so that your right outer ankle is close to your left outer thigh. Your right foot and left knee should point forward. Keep your hands by your sides as in Dandasana, maintaining your balance. Take a few breaths.

- If your buttocks are not properly placed on your left foot, or if the foot has not formed a good seat, then your body will tilt.
- If your pelvis is heavy, the leg that is perpendicular will tilt at the wrong angle.

5 Exhale and revolve your torso 90° to the right. Place your right hand 4 to 6 inches behind your right buttock. Turn your spine so that your chest, stomach, and pelvis turn to the right, beyond the perpendicular right thigh.

6 Inhale, lift your left arm, exhale, bend the arm, and bring it beyond the outer edge of your right thigh so that your left armpit and left side of your torso come close to your right knee and thigh.

7 Encircle your right leg with your left arm. Take a breath.

8 Exhale, lift your right hand off the floor, extend it from the shoulder without losing your balance, swing the arm back, and place your hand on your left hip.

9 Grasp the fingers of your left hand with the fingers of your right hand; as your body revolves, gradually extend your grasp and catch your palm and wrist.

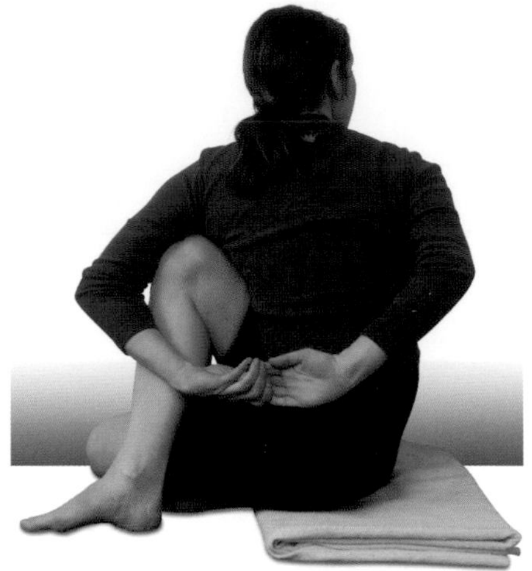

10 Turn your head towards your right shoulder and look to the right. Stay in this final position for 20 to 30 seconds.
At first, your rate of respiration will rise, but it will gradually return to normal. Observe the following points:

CHECK YOURSELF

- *To maintain your balance, make sure that your grip is strong, your chest is lifted and broadened when you turn your arms backward, and your waist and hip muscles are stretched upward.*
- *Your left bottom ribs (floating ribs) should not get caught behind your right thigh; this could hinder your breathing.*
- *Exhale and continue to rotate further until the floating ribs are released.*
- *At the same time, make sure there is no gap between your right leg and left arm. The closer they are, the better the rotation.*

Coming out of the pose

1 Release your hands, and in the following order: bring your torso forward, straighten your right leg, and straighten your left leg.

2 Repeat the asana on the other side, sitting on your right foot and reversing all the processes. Remain for the same length of time.

3 Come back to Dandasana.

1st term: no
2nd term: no
3rd term: yes

Special Instructions

- If you're overweight, you may find it difficult to sit on your foot. Put your heel next to your buttock and place a blanket that is 2 or 3 inches thick under the buttock, so that the buttock is raised and the heel is on the floor.

- You can also use a block as shown.

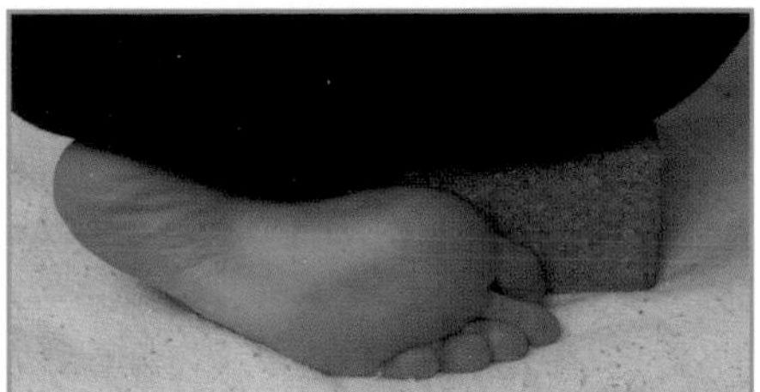

- If you can't hold your hands behind your back, place the perpendicular leg near your left knee so that your abdomen is not compressed. Instead of turning your left arm backward, stretch it and hold the big toe of your right foot. With practice, you'll be able to place your palm under the foot. Bring your right arm back around your waist.

- If the instructions above don't help enough, then practice the asana near the wall as follows:
  1. Sit in Dandasana with your right leg along the wall.
  2. Bend your left leg and sit on your left foot. Your right buttock will remain adjacent to the wall.
  3. Bend your right knee and place your right shin at the outer edge of your left thigh; it will now be away from the wall. Take one or two breaths.
  4. Exhale, turn your torso to the right, and bring its left side towards your right thigh.
  5. Press your left upper arm to the outer edge of your right leg, bend your elbow, and place your palm on the wall. Don't let your right arm slip.
  6. Raise your right arm and place the palm on the wall. Press both palms against the wall, raise your torso, and twist it.

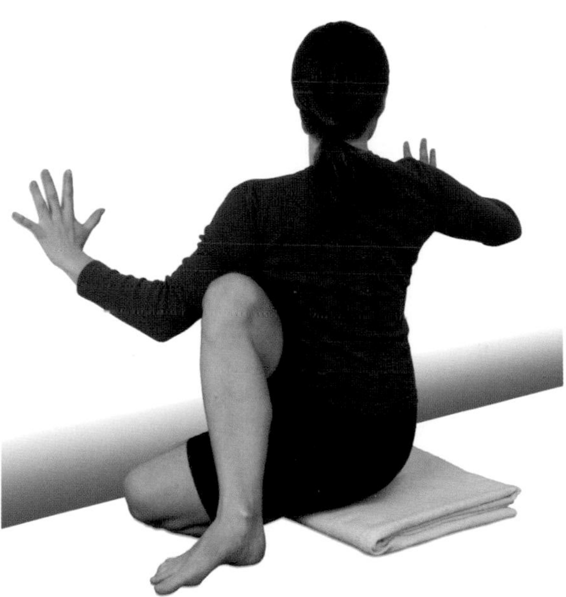

- Even if you can do the asana without the wall, try it against the wall for an intense massage of the abdominal organs and spinal column and for a better lateral twist of the spine.

- For better abdominal rotation and lift of the lower back, try placing a folded blanket under your buttocks. This prevents you from pressing your abdomen down, which can cause hernia or displacement of the uterus.

Inversions
Viparita Sthiti

Salamba Sarvangasana, from the Wall
Shoulderstand pose

Some women attain balance quickly, while others find it very difficult. Besides a good sense of balance, it requires firmness of the muscles. Feeling weak and shaky may cause you to balance incorrectly in Sarvangasana with your body not straight, your legs remaining forward, your buttocks projecting backward, and your chest caving in. This type of balance is harmful to your chest, heart, back, and neck.

"Balance" in any Yogic asana has a special meaning. You are not expected merely to balance, but also to achieve a proper distribution of weight. The lift in Sarvangasana should be such that you feel light and your body does not sink. Your body weight should not be on your neck alone, but should be shared by your shoulders and elbows. It's very important to keep your torso and legs in line with your shoulders.

To make sure that you achieve the right lift, practice in the first term with your feet on the wall, learning to bring your weight onto your shoulders and to lift your spine upward. Later, in the second term, you can use a chair.

Pay special attention to the points in "Check Yourself," which will guide you.

1 Place 3 or 4 folded blankets $1^{1}/_{2}$ feet away from the wall.

2 Bend your legs and place your shoulders on the blankets and your head on the floor.

3 Hold the belt in your right hand.

4 Press your shoulders and upper arms down.

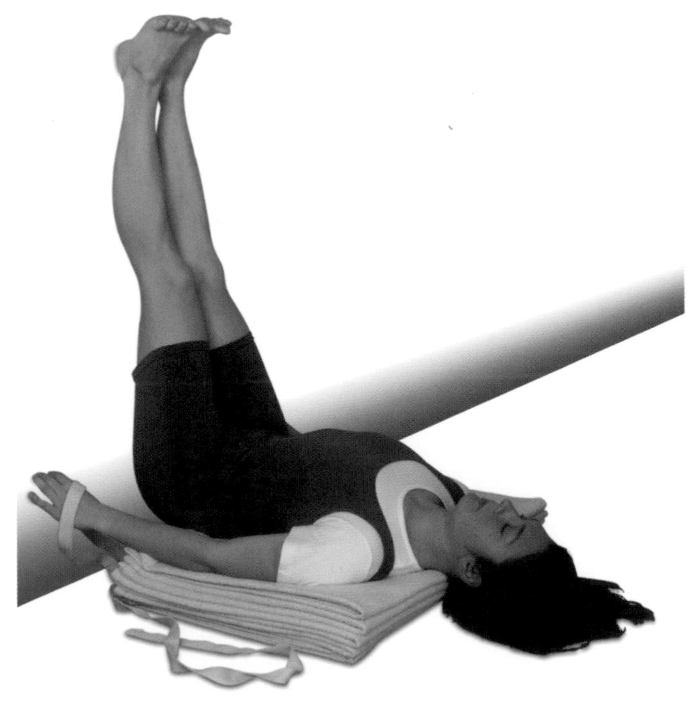

5 Keeping your legs bent, walk up the wall and put your feet firmly against it, with the outer edges of your feet facing up, so that your upper thighs roll inward.

6 Extend your soles from the heel bone towards the balls of your toes.

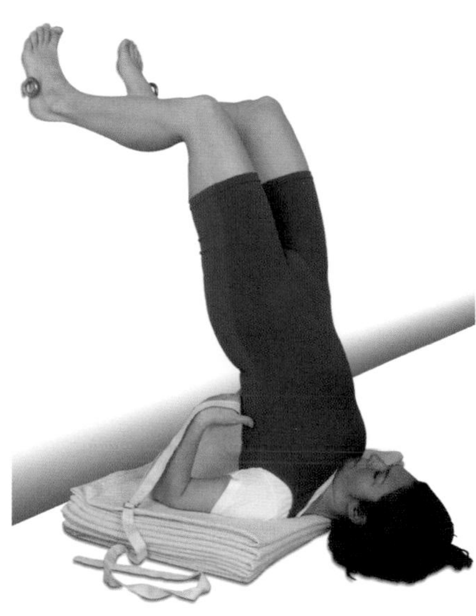

7 Tie the belt around your elbows. Putting weight onto your shoulders, extend your arms towards the wall with the palms facing up and the thumbs turning out.

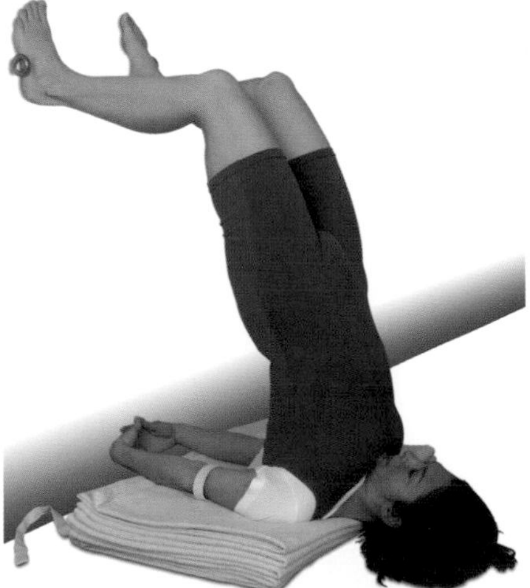

8 Bend your elbows and place your hands on your back, with the thumbs pointing front and the fingers pointing towards your spine.

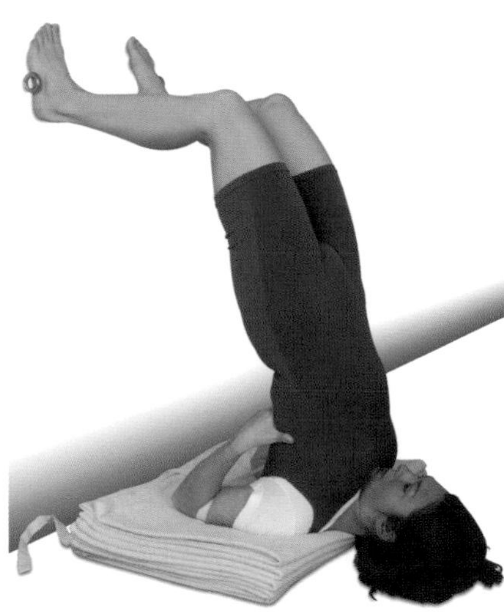

9 Putting weight onto your shoulders, upper arms, and elbows, press your feet against the wall and lift your buttocks, spine, sides of the chest, and chest and extend your knees towards the wall. The top of your breastbone should touch your chin.

1st term: yes
2nd term: yes
3rd term: yes

Benefits

(Refer to all variations on the following pages)

- Expands the chest, frees it of tension, and aerates the lungs
- Purifies breast milk
- Brings firmness to the body
- Stabilizes the nerves and brings back energy after delivery
- Helps treat anemia
- Improves circulation, which helps with cramps and numbness, especially after delivery
- With regular practice, alleviates urinary disorders or infection and uterine displacement

Contraindications

- During menstruation (Don't practice any inverted poses)
- High blood pressure
- If you can't balance your body perpendicular to the floor, stay in the first position with your feet against the wall

10 Maintaining the lift, take one leg after the other away from the wall and stretch up.

11 Contract your buttocks so that your tailbone remains tucked in and straighten your whole body from the armpit to the toes, bringing your toes in and your heels out.

12 Stay in this final position for 5 minutes, breathing normally.

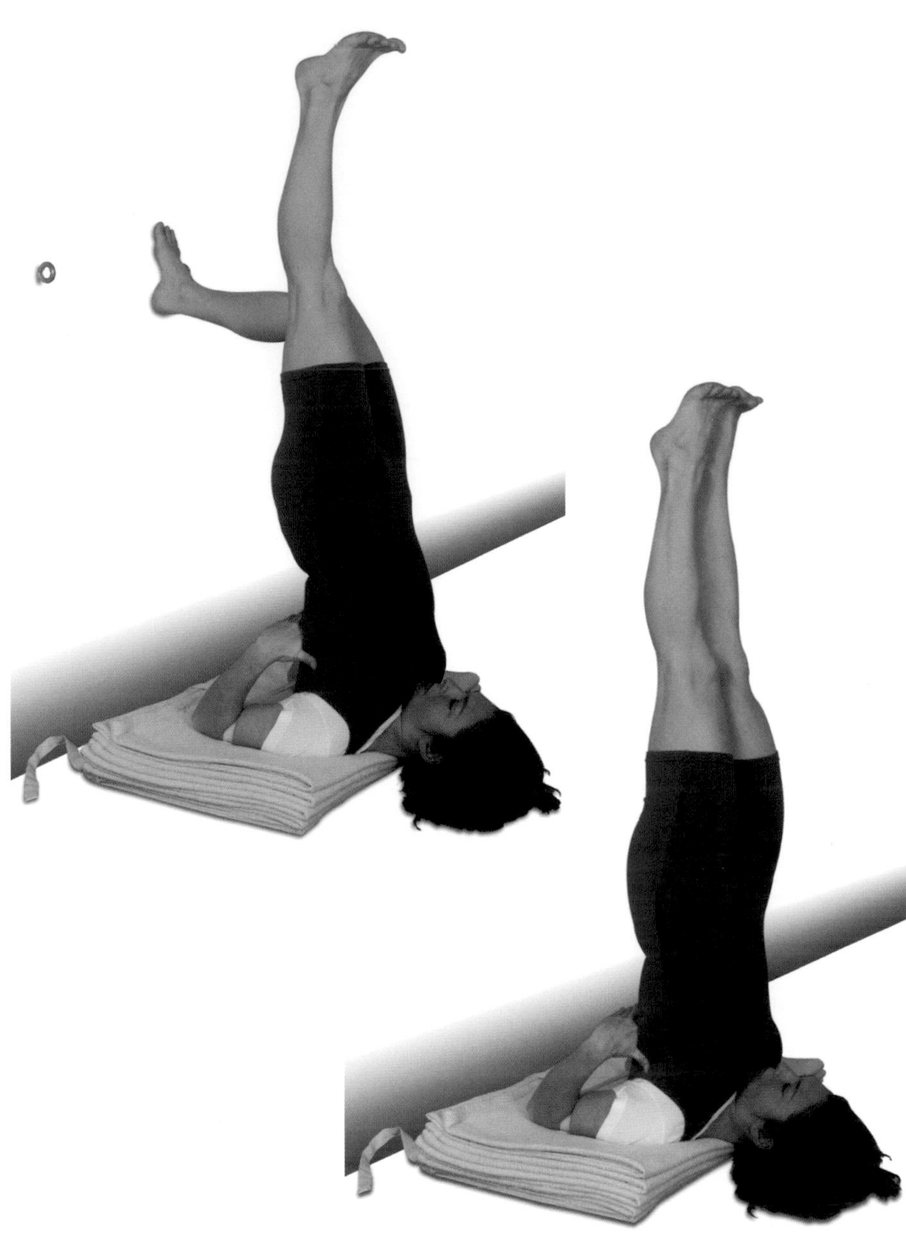

Coming out of the pose

1 Bend your knees, put one foot after the other against the wall, maintain the expansion and lift of your chest, remove the belt, and slowly lower your spine down to the floor. Move your shoulders away from the blanket and bring them to the same height as your head.

2 Rest with your legs in Svastikasana.

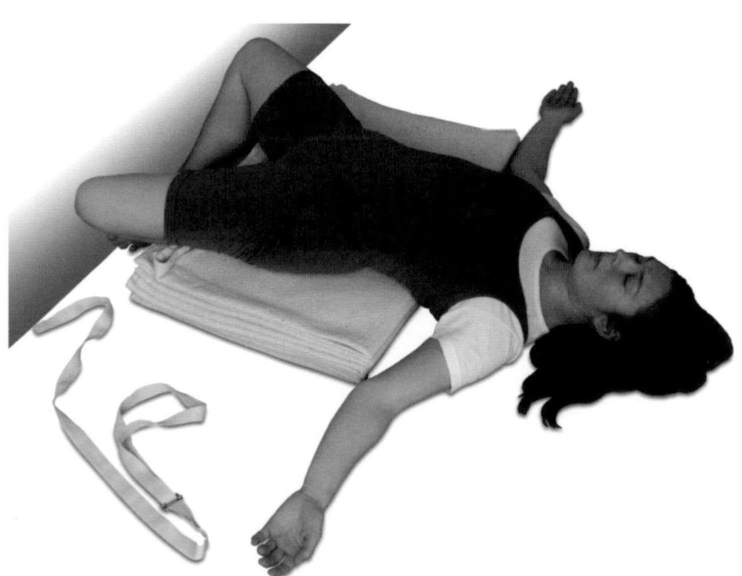

CHECK YOURSELF

- *Keep your hips perpendicular to the floor.*
- *Tighten your buttock muscles.*
- *Elongate your neck.*
- *Press your upper arms into the floor.*
- *Raise your lower ribs and your chest near the armpit.*
- *Your trapezius (upper back) should be raised off the floor by the lift of your back.*

Salamba Sarvangasana, with a Chair

Shoulderstand pose

1st term: no
2nd term: yes
3rd term: yes

You're already familiar with this modification of Sarvangasana. Working with the chair ensures that your spine and neck are lifted, that the weight of your body does not fall on your neck, and that you achieve an upward lift. It is also easier for those who are heavy or just feel heavy.

1 Put a blanket on the seat of a chair and a blanket on the backrest. Place a bolster in front of the chair.

2 Sit on the chair facing its back and put your legs over the backrest.

3 Exhale, hold onto the chair, and recline slightly backward.

4 As you exhale, lower your back until your shoulders reach the bolster.

5 Pause and take a few normal breaths.

6 Put your arms underneath the chair, hold its back legs, and straighten your legs.

7 Stay in this position for 5 minutes breathing normally.

8 If your diaphragm gets compressed, then keep your legs apart.

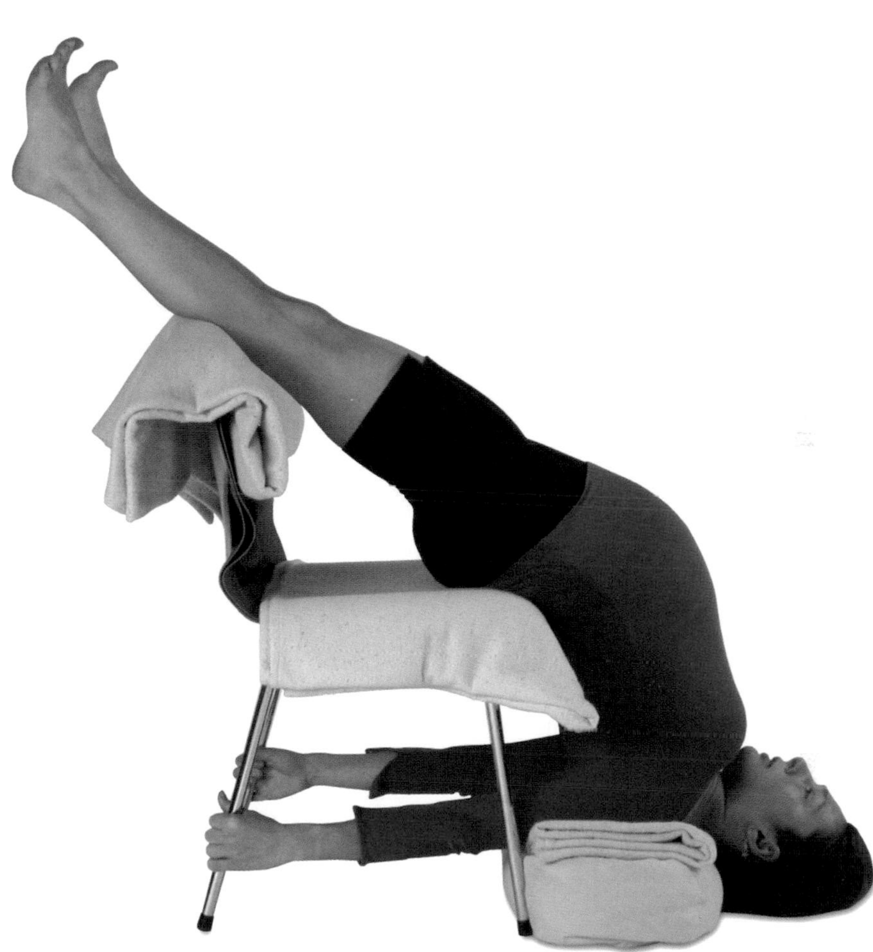

Coming out of the pose

1 Bend your knees, loosen your grip on the chair legs, and let go of them gradually, sliding down towards your head without any sudden movements.

2 When you get up from the floor, first turn onto your right side and then get up. Don't sit straight up suddenly.

CHECK YOURSELF

> *Keep your back, from the waist to the buttocks, on the seat of the chair.*
> *Don't let your throat get compressed.*
> *Don't cave in the chest.*
> *Relax your face, eyes, mouth, and jaw.*

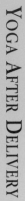

Special Instructions

- A teacher or friend can help you use a block and 2 belts. Grip the block and extend your inner arches as in Pashchimottanasana. This has a rejuvenating effect on the pelvis. You'll be safe in this form of Sarvangasana, because your back is held up by the chair.
- As you can see in the photo with the block and belts, the chair is close to the wall. From that position, you or a helper can place your toes on the wall, extending your heels, in Niralamba Sarvangasana. This gives you a very good grip and lift of the outer and inner muscles—in fact, helps you feel the meaning of inner and outer alignment.

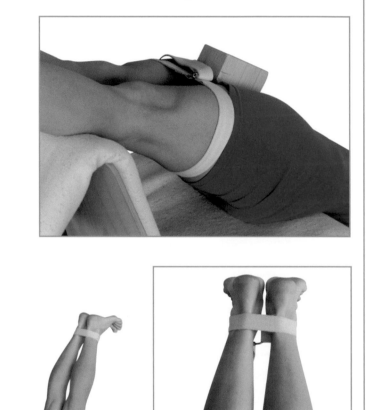

Coming out of the pose

To come down, grip the front legs of the chair, push it away, and slowly slide down.

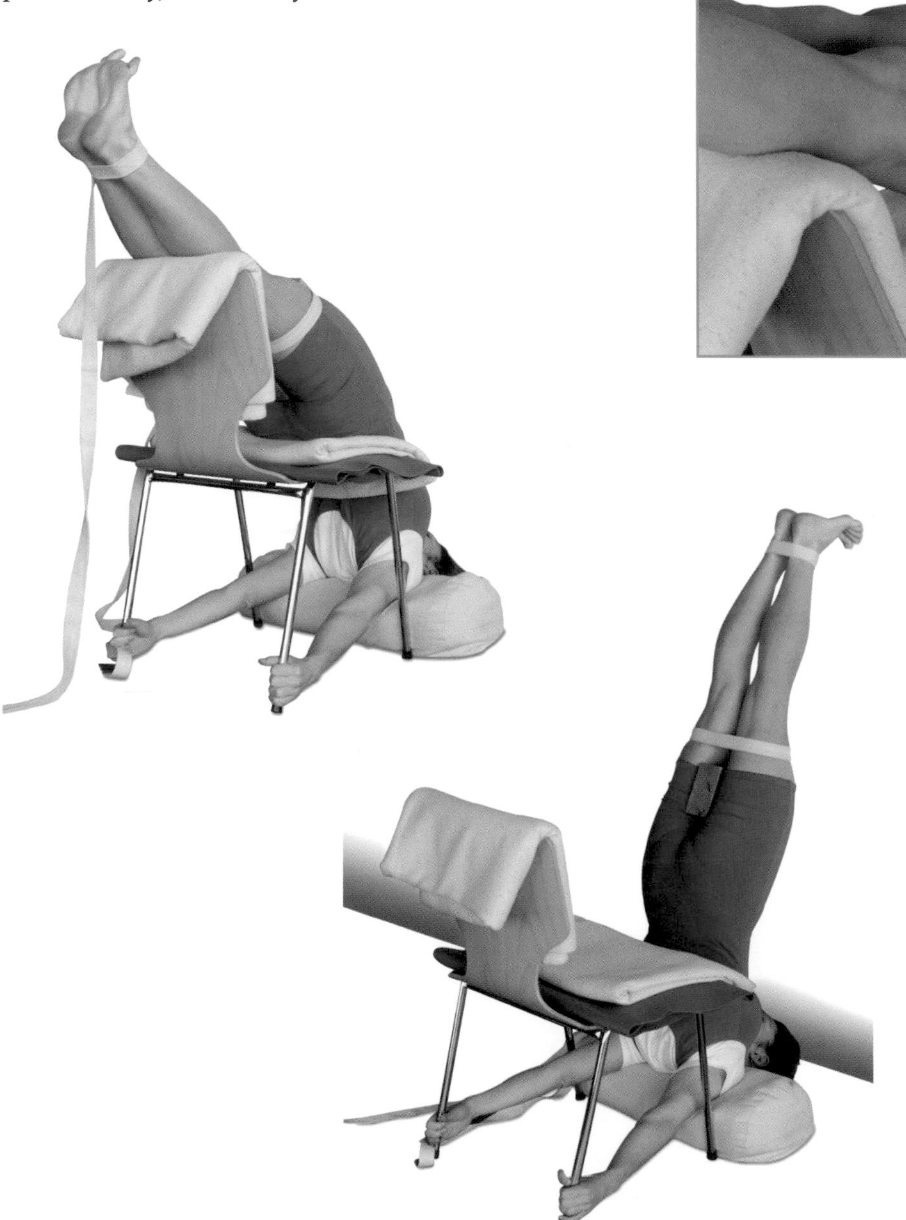

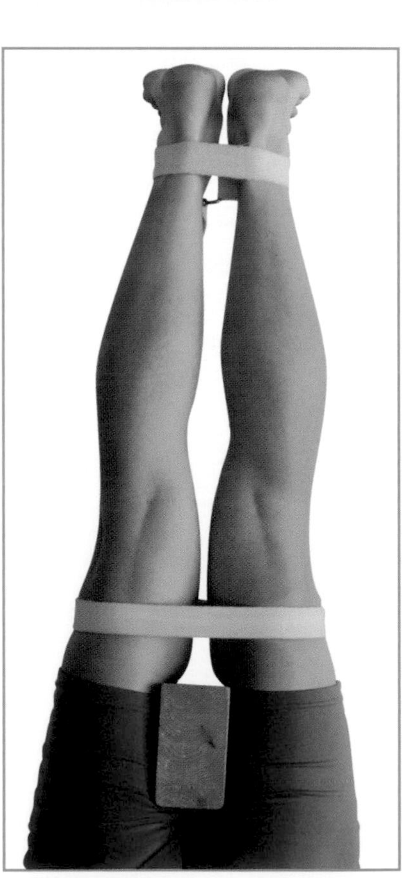

Salamba Sarvangasana, Independent
Shoulderstand pose

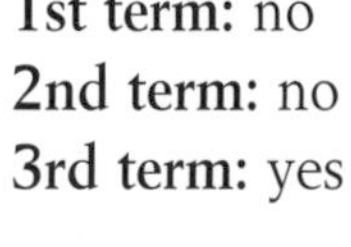

1st term: no
2nd term: no
3rd term: yes

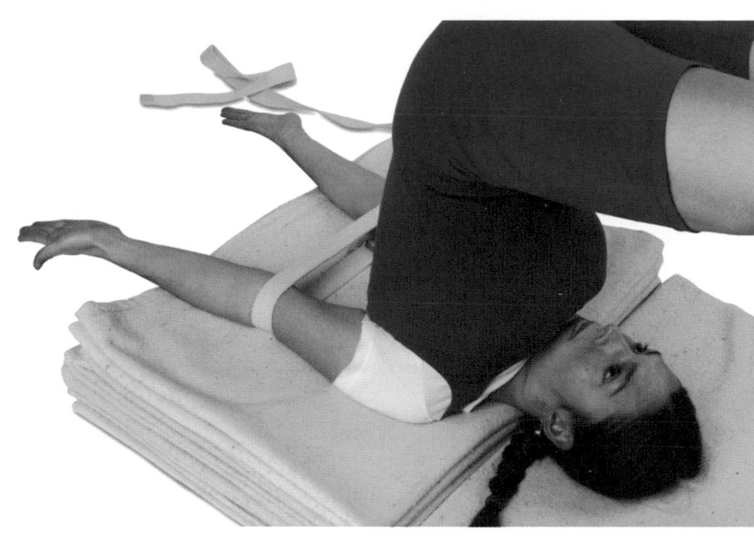

1 Have 3 or 4 folded blankets ready and a belt for your elbows.

2 Lie flat on the floor with your shoulders on the blankets, your head on the floor, and your legs and feet together.

3 Tighten your knees and stretch your arms alongside your body with your palms facing up. Keep your shoulders down and move them away from your head. Your head and neck should be in line with your spine.

4 Exhale and bend your knees over your chest.

5 Press your hands down and with a slight swing, raise your waist and hips, keeping your knees bent and letting them reach beyond your head.

6 Support your hips with your hands and raise your torso.

7 Raise your hips and thighs farther and support your back with your hands. Your body from shoulders to knees is now perpendicular to the ground. The top of your breastbone touches your chin. Keep your palms on your back, with your thumbs pointing front and your fingers pointing towards your spine.

8 Contract your buttocks so that your lumbar (lower) spine and tailbone remain tucked in, and straighten your legs towards the ceiling.

9 Press your palms and fingers into your back to straighten your whole body from the armpits to the toes.

10 Don't let your elbows spread outward; use a belt to keep your shoulders and elbows in line.

11 Keep your shoulders back and away from the direction of your head. Move your upper arms towards each other.

Coming out of the pose
Exhale, bend your knees, and gradually slide your buttocks and back downward without jolting your spine.

Help
To improve the lift of the inner body:

- Put a block between your upper thighs close to the perineum.
- Use a belt for your upper thighs and one for your ankles.
- Develop your ability to grip the block firmly, extend your inner legs upward into the inner arches of your feet, and narrow the space between your inner calves.

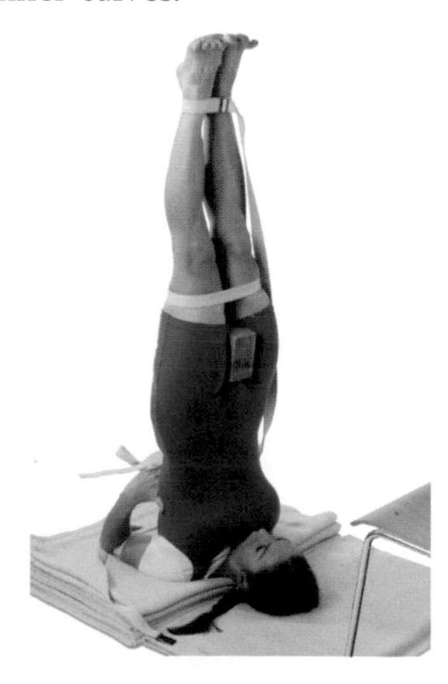

DETAILED DESCRIPTIONS OF ASANAS FOR BEGINNERS AND ADVANCED STUDENTS

Ardha Halasana, Toes on Table
Half plough pose

1st term: yes
2nd term: yes
3rd term: yes

Performing this asana with your toes resting halfway or more on a table lifts your thighs and spine, strengthens them, and corrects the natural collapse that occurs after delivery.

- Although this asana begins in Sarvangasana from the wall, in the third term you can also start from Salamba Sarvangasana without support (*see Sarvangasana, from the Wall and Salamba Sarvangasana, Independent earlier in this chapter*).

Coming from Sarvangasana (page 326):

1 Have a table or similar support $1^1/_2$ to 2 feet behind you.

2 Bring down first one leg, then the other. Stay on the tips of your toes and extend your heels.

3 Support your back with your hands and lift your hips and the sides of your torso away from your armpits and upper arms.

4 Keep your arms in the back or extend them backward, or hold the edge of the blanket you're lying on, and press your arms and elbows down to raise your torso.

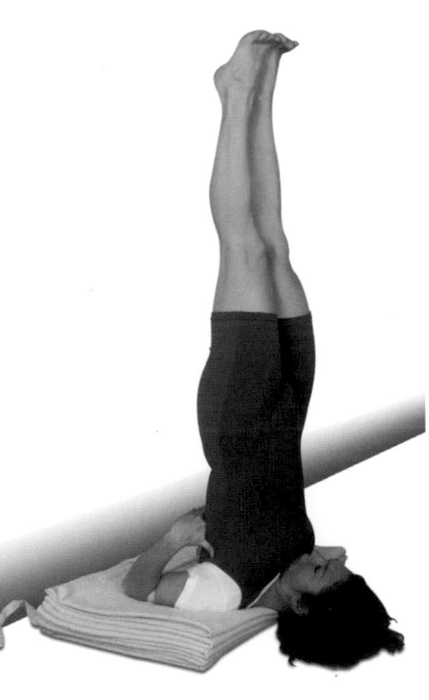

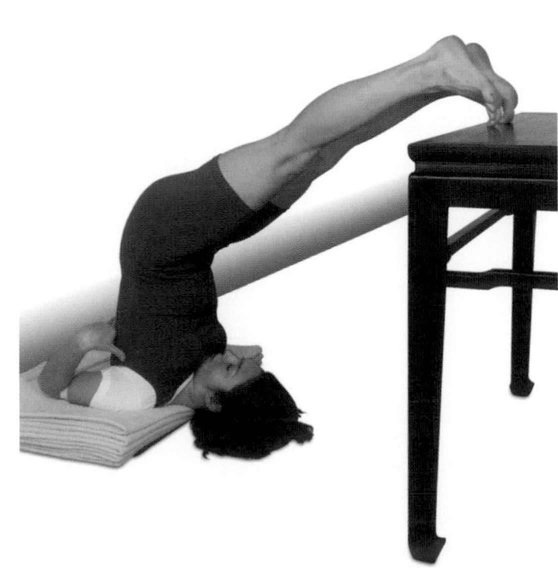

Benefits
Improves digestion
Checks bleeding
Improves circulation in the abdomen and pelvis, which reduces infections
Strengthens and alleviates pain in the lower back
Lessens heaviness and soreness in the abdomen after delivery
Soothes sore nipples
Relieves weakness, tiredness, and anemia
Lifts the sagging abdominal walls and pelvic floor
Restores muscle tone
Regulates bowel movements
Reduces swelling around the anus and vagina

5 Lift your thighs and spine upward, keeping your spine and buttocks in line.

6 Your chest should not cave in, and your buttocks should not protrude.

7 Stay for 3 to 5 minutes, breathing normally.

Coming out of the pose

Reverse the process for coming back:
Place your hands on your back, bring one leg after the other back to Sarvangasana, and carefully come down.

Help

If you can't manage this asana because of weakness or anemia, you can start from Sarvangasana with a Chair (see earlier in this chapter) in order to bring your legs to Ardha Halasana with toes on a table.

Ardha Supta Konasana, with a Table

Half reclined angle pose

1st term: no
2nd term: no
3rd term: yes

1 Follow the instructions for Ardha Halasana, Toes on a Table (page 332), but spread your legs.

2 Lift your spine and thighs and keep your spine and buttocks in line.

3 Your chest should not cave in, and your buttocks should not protrude.

(For further instructions, see Chapter 3, Ardha Supta Konasana, Legs Spread, Thighs on Two Chairs, page 106.)

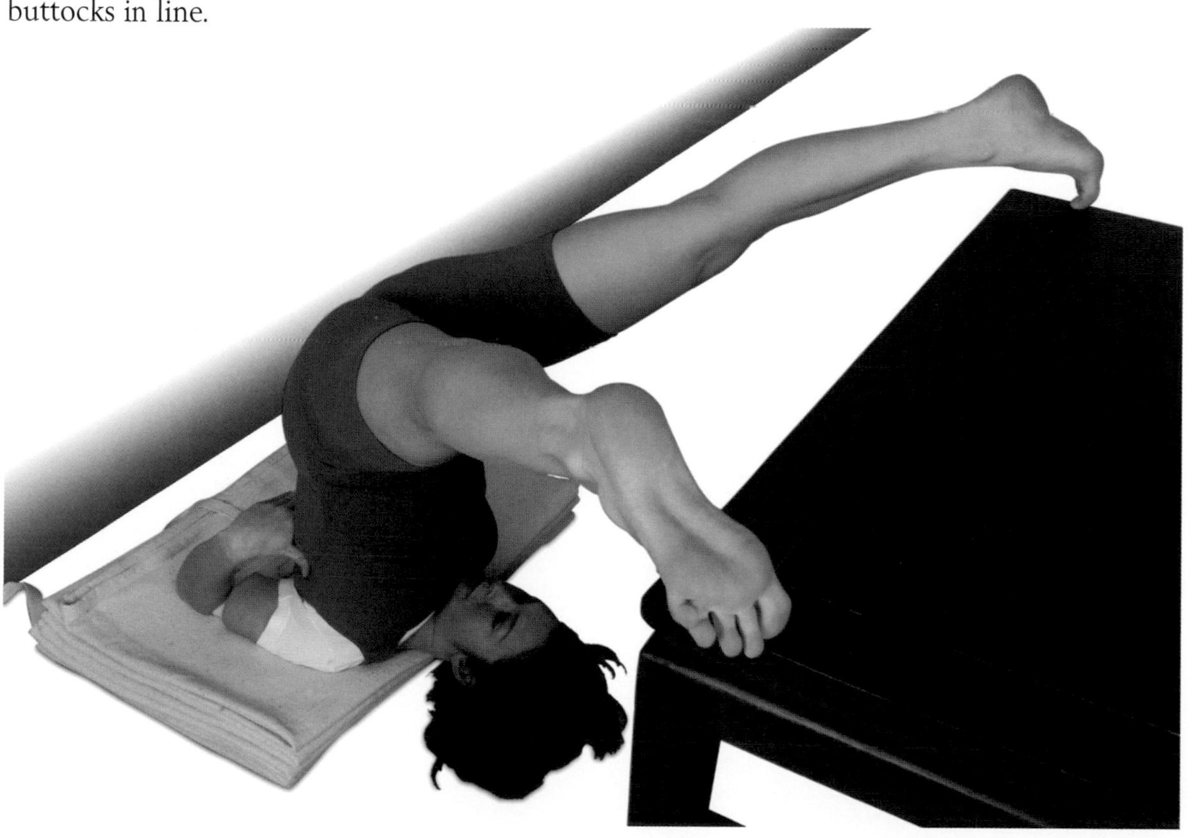

Setu Bandha Sarvangasana, on a Bench or Similar Height
Bridge formation pose

1st term: yes
2nd term: yes
3rd term: yes

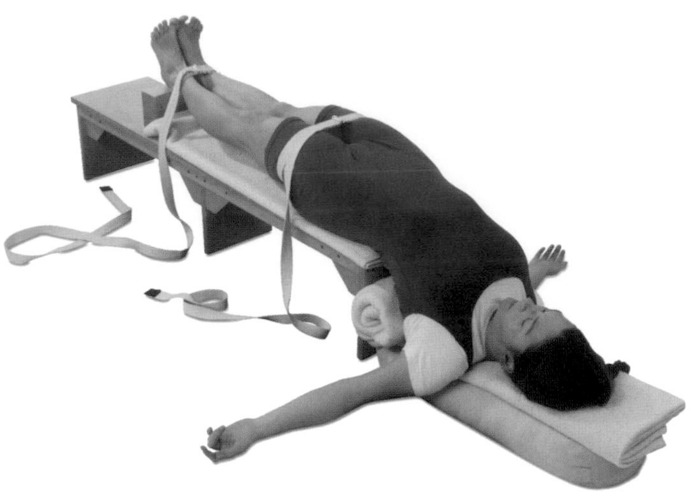

You can use belts and a block in addition to the bench.
(For further instructions, see Technique 1 for this asana, page 107.)

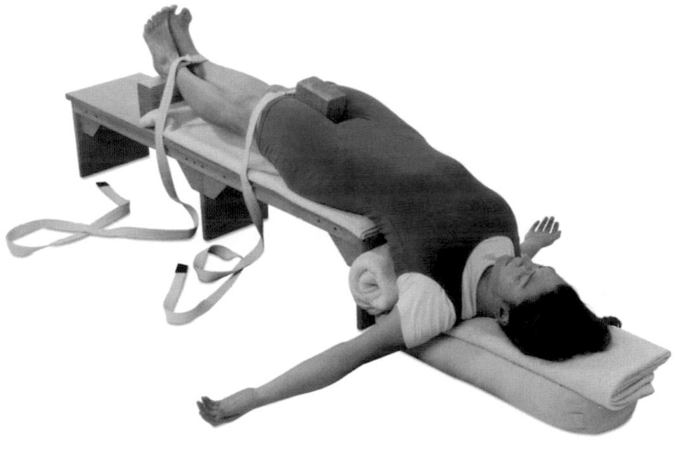

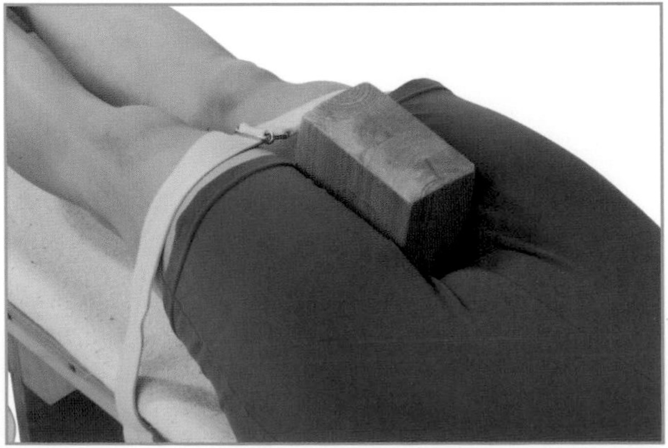

Special Instructions

For the 3rd Term

- You can practice with blocks and the wall.
- Come into and out of the pose with bent legs.
- Be aware of the alignment of your legs and keep your outer and inner knees parallel to the floor.

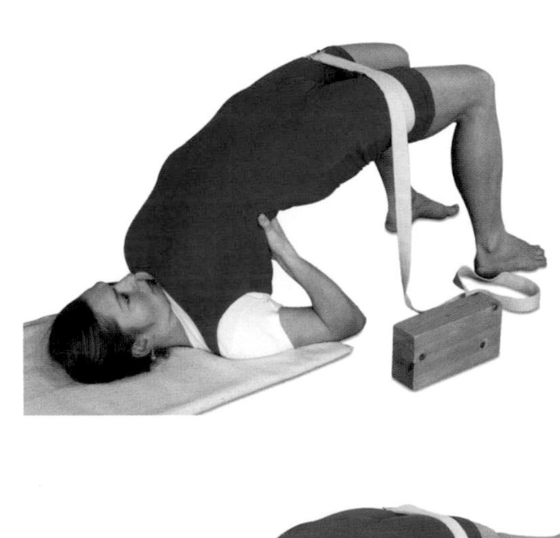

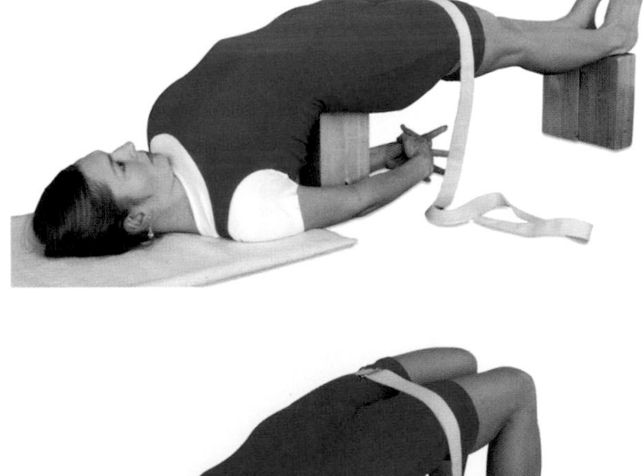

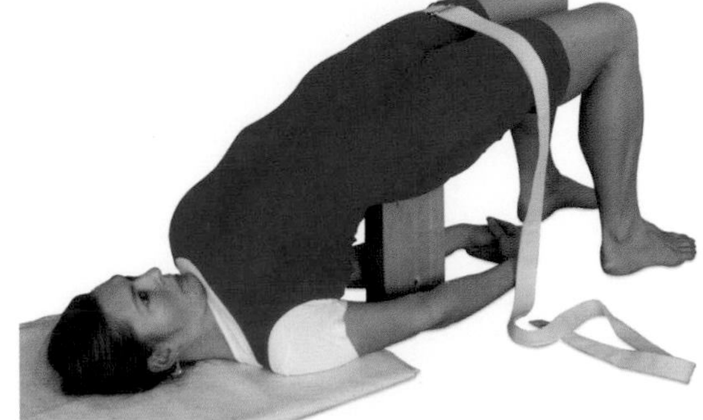

Chatushpadasana

Bridge pose

Follow the instructions given for during pregnancy, page 111.

1st term: no
2nd term: no
3rd term: yes

Benefits

See page 111

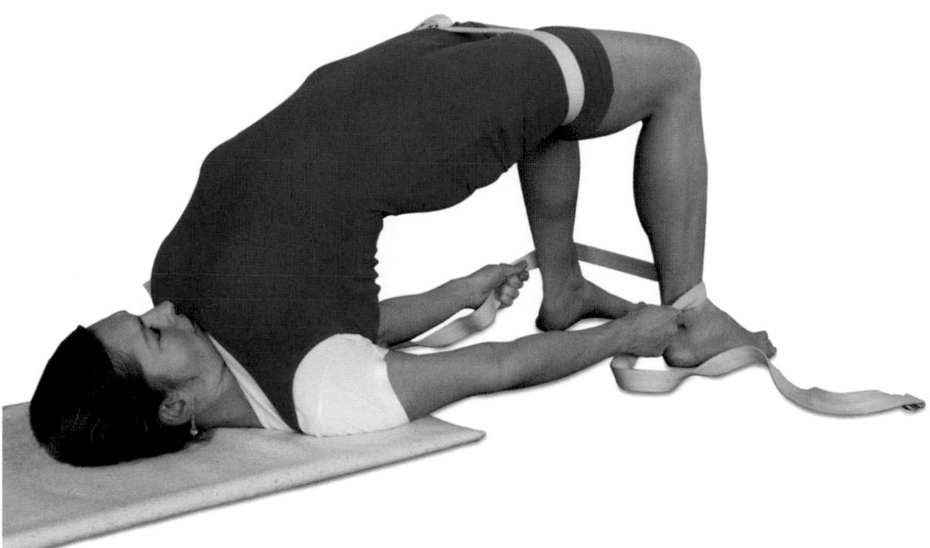

Special Instructions

- Pull from your hands, so that your shoulder blades support and open your chest and its sides.
- Using the pull of your hands and the pressing of your feet, grip and lift your spine, sacrum, and pelvis muscles.

Viparita Karani Mudra, Legs Bent on a Chair

Upward action seal pose

Follow the instructions given for during pregnancy, pages 112 – 115.

1st term: yes
2nd term: yes
3rd term: yes

Benefits

See page 113

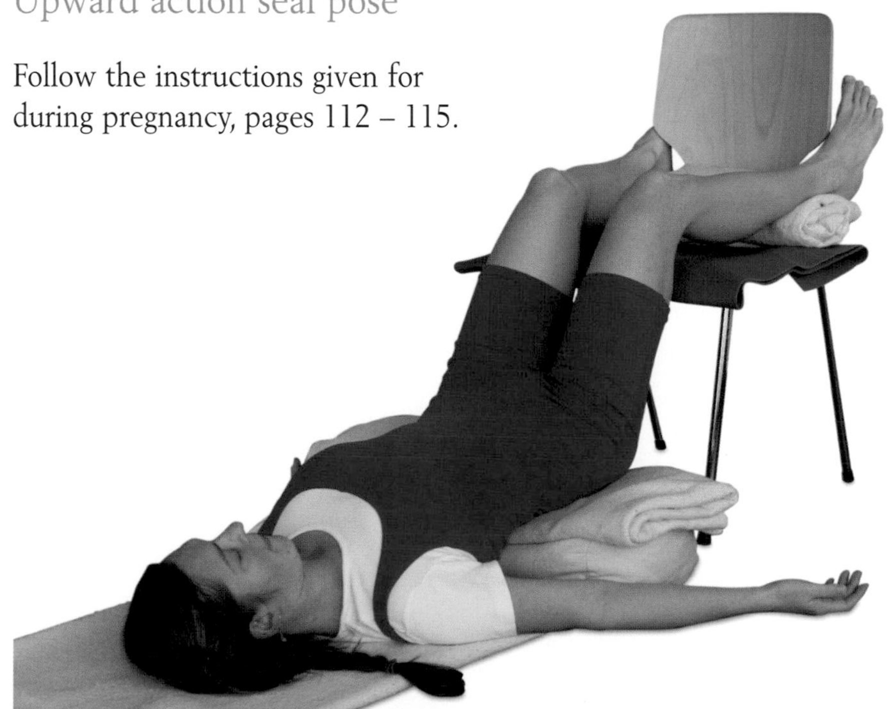

Viparita Karani Mudra
Upward action seal pose

1st term: no
2nd term: yes
3rd term: yes

For more stability we recommend using a belt for the legs.

Pages 112 – 115.

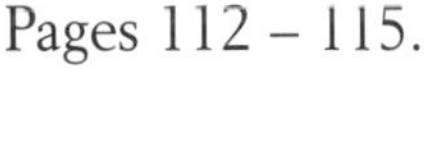

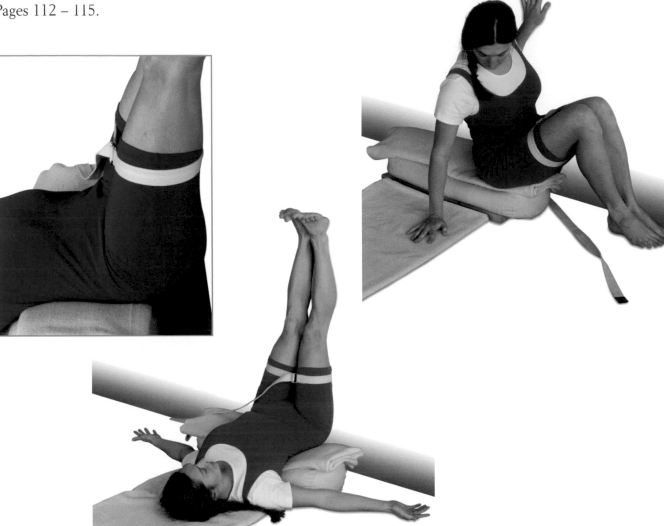

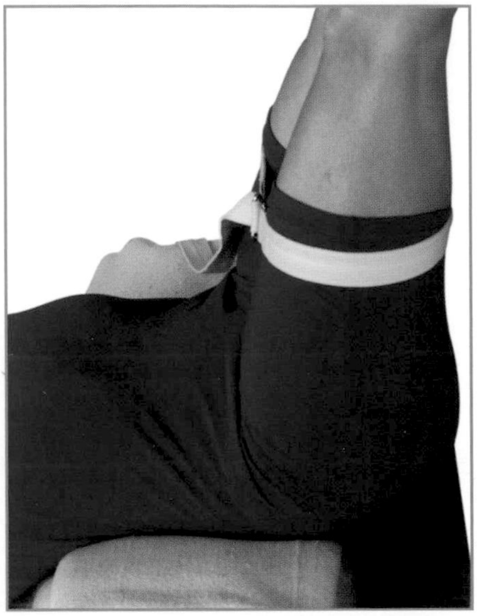

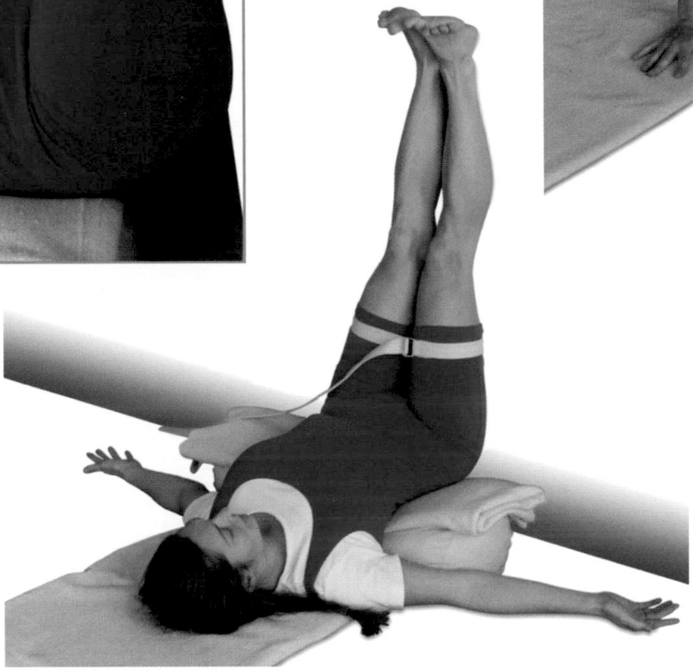

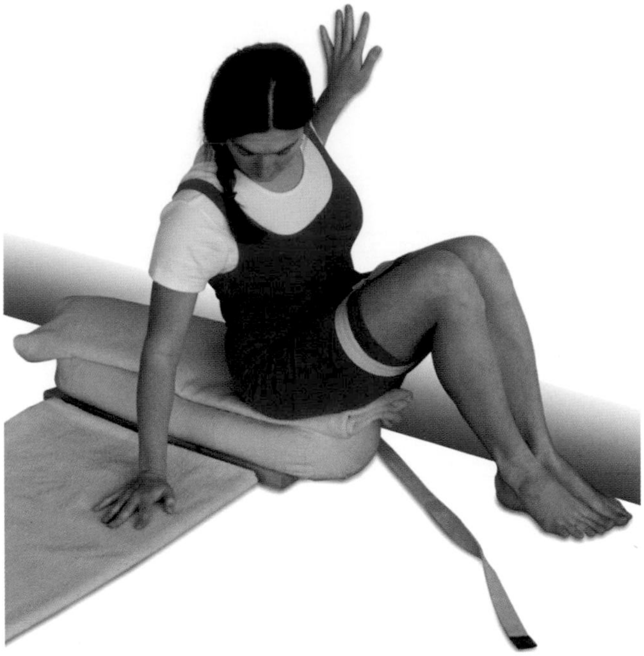

Coming out of the pose

1 Cross your legs as in Svastikasana and stay there for a few breathing cycles.

2 Push yourself away from the wall and rest your pelvis on the ground, with your legs crossed the opposite way on the bolster.

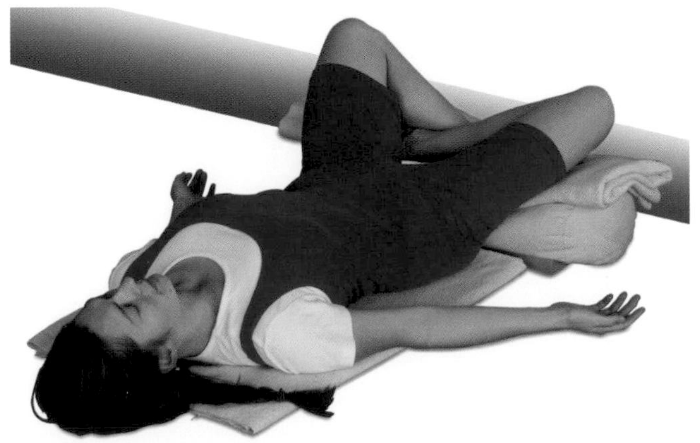

Salamba Shirshasana

Headstand pose

If you did not do Shirshasana at all before or during pregnancy, then you are a beginner as far as this asana is concerned. Don't undertake it until you've recovered fully from the strain and changes of your pregnancy. Work more with Sarvangasana and Halasana, at least for the first three months after your delivery. Afterwards, you can take up Shirshasana like any fresh student of Yoga.

If, however, you practiced Sarvangasana and Halasana regularly before or during pregnancy, then you won't have any problem balancing in Shirshasana. Your shoulder and neck muscles will have developed sufficient strength. If you are accustomed to Shirshasana and have practiced it throughout pregnancy—except perhaps for a few days towards the end—then you can do Shirshasana confidently.

With some women, hormonal imbalance after delivery causes the body to become so fragile that the muscles lose their tone, feeling loose and even painful. Breast-feeding mothers especially cannot expect the muscles to regain their strength overnight.

If this describes you, then don't assume that you should avoid Shirshasana and wait until you get your energy back. On the contrary, Shirshasana generates energy and restores the body's firmness. Together with Sarvangasana, it helps maintain your hormonal balance, which in turn rejuvenates the mind.

As always, Shirshasana should be done before Sarvangasana. This rule has not changed. However, the sequence that we recommended for pregnancy (Uttanasana, Adho Mukha Shvanasana, Maha Mudra, Shirshasana, and the reverse after Shirshasana) is not required now.

After your delivery, we recommend the following order for your practice of Shirshasana.

- Standing asanas and forward bends
- Shirshasana
- Maha Mudra
- Starting from the second term, do Sarvangasana and Halasana to bring your Yoga session to a close.

Note that Maha Mudra follows Shirshasana.

Salamba Shirshasana, in a Corner or against the Wall

Shirshasana is more than balancing on your head.
It should feel as natural as standing on your feet.

Technique for 2nd Term

1 Fold a blanket four times and place it in a corner, letting it touch both walls. Kneel on the floor as in Virasana (page 72), facing the corner.

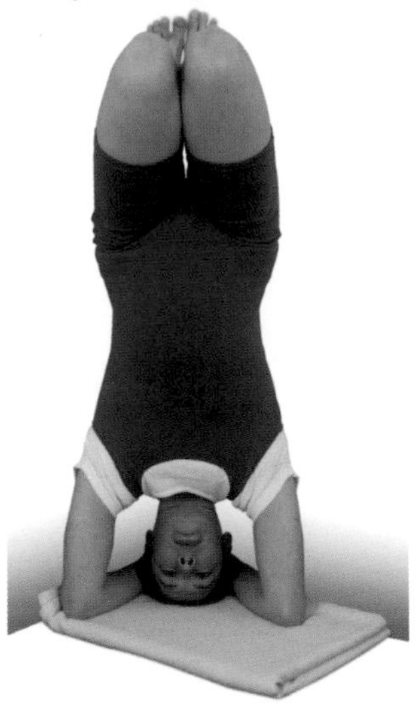

2 Interlock your fingers to the base and keep your thumbs touching, forming a semicircular cup. Place your cupped hands 2 to 3 inches away from the corner. Your little fingers and thumbs should be parallel. Keeping your hands more than 3 inches away from the corner will cause the following errors to occur in the final position:

- Your spinal column will bend and lose its extension.
- Your stomach will protrude.
- The weight of your body will bear down painfully on your elbows.
- Your face will get red and your eyes swollen and puffy.

3 Rest your forearms on the blanket, with your elbows in line. Your wrists should be upright, with the inner bone of the fore-arms touching the blanket and the outer bone directly above.

4 The distance between your elbows should be the width of your shoulders, so that your arms remain straight. If the distance is too small, there will be painful pressure on your side ribs; if it's too large, your chest won't expand and there will be pressure on your cervical (upper) spine.

5 In this position, your palms, forearms, and the space between your elbows and chest form an equilateral triangle. Don't move your elbows and forearms once you've adjusted them.

6 Raise your buttocks so that your elbows and shoulders are in line and your head is in line with your palms, and breathe normally.

7 Exhale and place the crown of your head on the blanket, so that the back of your head remains parallel to the wall and ½ inch away from your little finger. Keep your head in the cup of your hands, and don't press your head between your wrists. Your ears should be parallel to each other.

8 Exhale and raise your knees, keeping your toes on the floor. Straighten your legs and bring your feet in. Your torso should be at a right angle to the floor.

9 Keep your legs firm and pull your kneecaps in. Stay in this position for a few seconds and breathe normally.

10 Bend your knees slightly, exhale, and raise both legs with a jump (if you cannot jump, ask a helper to lift your legs). The entire action should be upward—the spine, buttocks, thighs, knees, and feet all have to be moving upward so that the weight of your body does not fall on your head and hands.

- If your spine leans slightly backward, bring it forward to keep it erect. Lift your knees so that your thighs are parallel to the floor.
- Keep your torso and buttocks in line with your head. If your buttocks drop backward, you'll topple back. If they incline forward, are loose, or are lined up with your elbows, then you'll fall forward.

11 Continue the upward motion: lift your knees to face the ceiling so that your body,

from the navel to the knees, remains erect. Your lower legs are now bent backward.

12 Tighten the muscles of your buttocks and tuck them in. Your body, from the head to the knees, should be in line. Stay in this position for a while, breathing normally.

13 Keeping your body firm from the head to the knees, raise your lower legs up to be in line with your thighs. Extend your shins and calves completely into Shirshasana.

14 Stay in this final position for 3 minutes, breathing normally (from the mid 2nd term you can slowly increase the duration). Observe the following points:

- Press your elbows and forearms down and keep your elbows firm and stationary.
- Lift your shoulders and armpits, so that your weight does not fall on your ears. Keep your armpits well opened and extended upward. Keep your shoulders well away from your wrists.
- Broaden your intercostal (rib) muscles and lift them up. To lift your breastbone and broaden your chest, tuck in your dorsal (mid) spine and shoulder blades without disturbing your head and neck. Keep the sides of your torso lifted.
- Keep the middle of your thighs and knees in line.
- Press your buttocks and thighs together and lift your inner thighs.
- Let your ankles and big toes touch each other. Straighten your feet so that they're in line with your legs and not turning in or out. Extend the bottom toes upward.

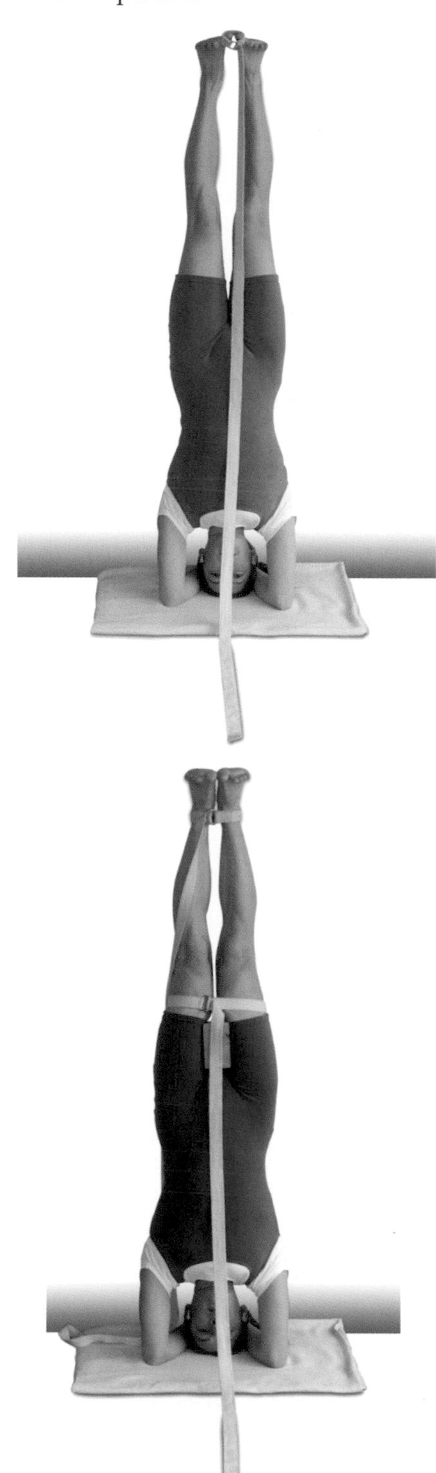

Benefits

Shirshasana's specialty is bringing about hormonal balance. In addition, it:

Elevates the depressed mind

Improves the quality of breast milk by circulating blood around the chest

Tones the breasts

Eliminates fatigue and weakness

Brings a refreshed feeling

HINT: See page 340 for an explanation on using a belt around big toes.

Coming out of the pose

1 Exhale, bend your knees, and bring your thighs parallel to the floor. Don't jolt your spine, neck, or head.

2 Rest your toes on the floor.

3 Wait in this position for 5 to 10 seconds.

4 Lift your head and unlock your fingers.

5 Begin Maha Mudra.

CHECK YOURSELF

The moment your feet are off the floor, keep your body moving upward as follows:

1. *First, your torso from the armpits to your buttocks.*
2. *Second, your groin to your knees*
3. *Last, your knees to your feet.*

Help

If you have a problem with your cervical spine, practice Shirshasana on two chairs, following the same instructions.

Caution! Do not practice Shirshasana on chairs during pregnancy. This might cause spasms and contractions of the uterus.

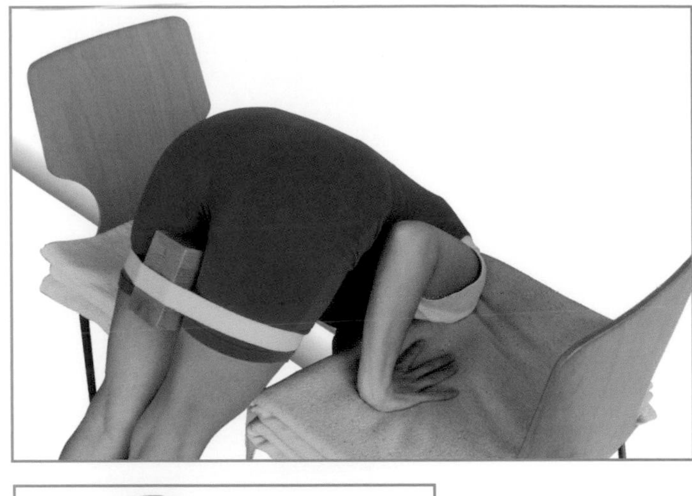

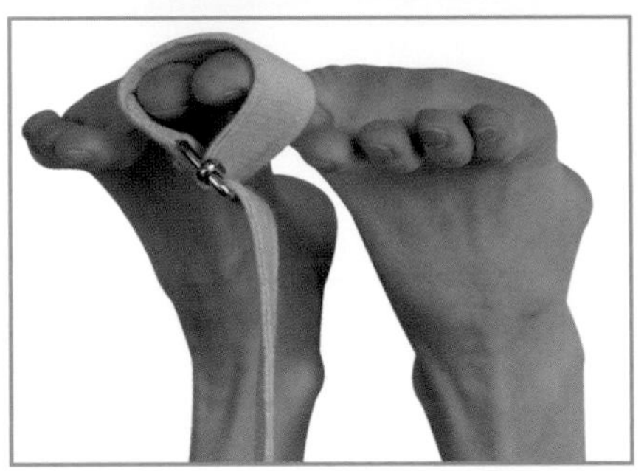

Using a block: Place a block between your legs and tie belt(s) around them to get a better grip on your thigh and pelvic muscles, to lift the inner organs, and to enjoy a rejuvenating effect on the organs and body structure.
See photos.

Using a belt for the big toes: Tie a belt around your big toes as shown. Extend the bottoms of the big toes upward towards the ceiling. This gives you a better feeling for how to grip your outer thighs and extend your inner legs. You can also do this in Sarvangasana.
See photos.

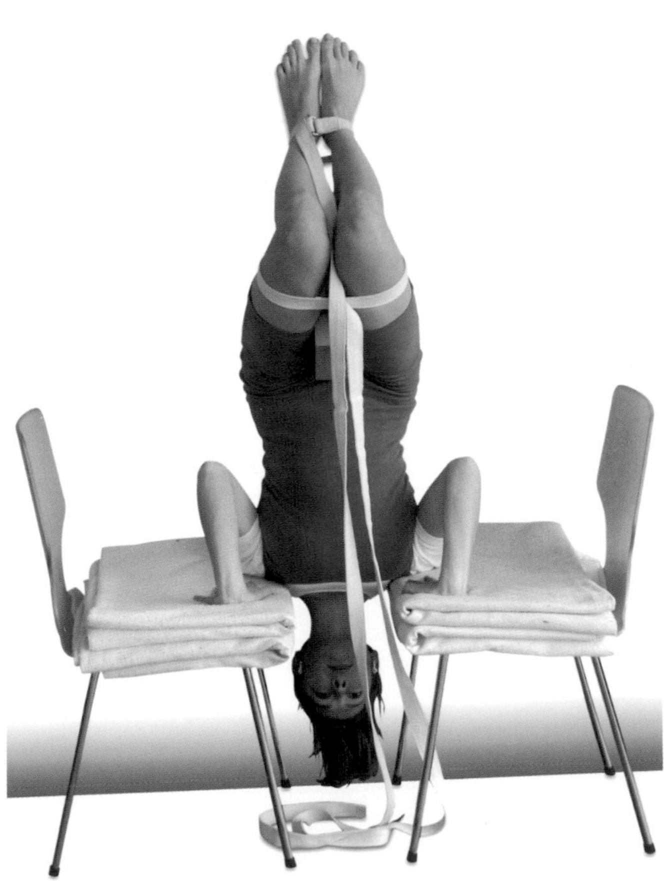

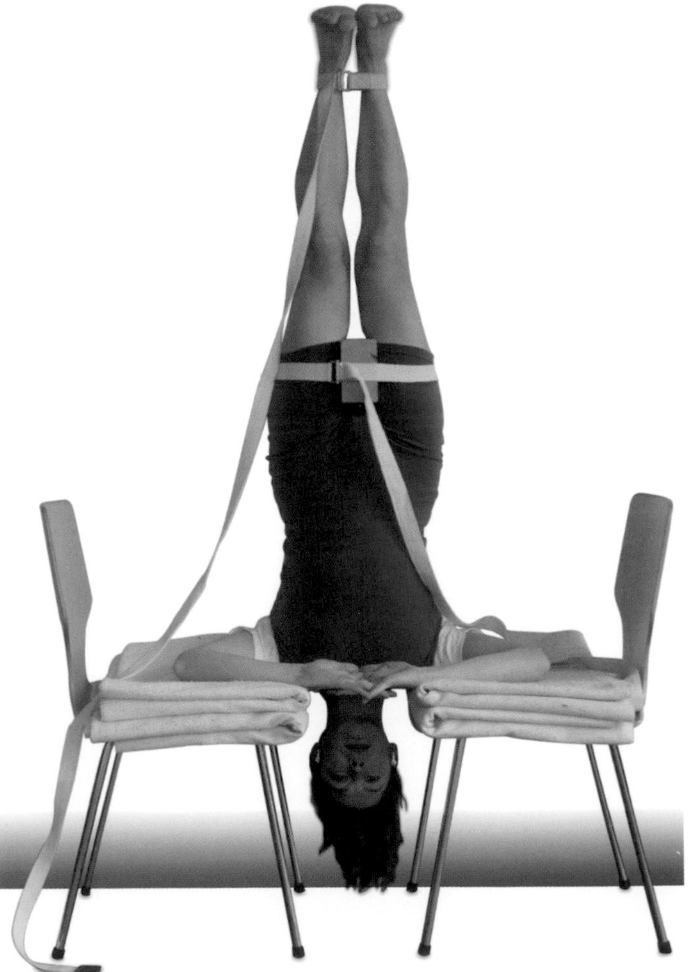

Asanas for Abdomen and Lumbar

Supta and Uttishtha Sthiti with Udara Akunchana Sthiti

After your delivery, work on your abdomen and lumbar regions becomes more comprehensive and you can add new asanas to reshape your body and build up strength and stability.

◇

Supta Padangushthasana

Reclining big toe pose

1st term: no
2nd term: yes
3rd term: yes

You can begin Supta Padangushthasana in the second term, after you've become comfortable with the less intense asanas that came earlier.

Supta Padangushthasana is a lying-down pose in which thc big toe is normally grasped with the fingers and the legs are extended in three directions. At this stage, however, we recommend the variations on the following page.

Benefits
(for Supta Padangushtasana 1 and 2)

- Eliminates stiffness of the hip joints and soothes the nerves around the hips
- Reduces fat around the waist, buttocks, thighs, and lower abdomen
- Firms the back and hip muscles
- Strengthens the abdominal organs
- Rejuvenates a sluggish digestive system

Supta Padangushthasana 1

Reclining big toe pose 1

1 Have ready a belt, and a block for the heel bone of the lower leg.

2 Lie flat on the floor. Keep your heel bone on the block, both legs together, and your knees tight. Breathe normally.

3 Inhale, bend your right knee to your chest, and loop the belt around your right foot. Grip the belt with both hands and extend your right leg upward by stretching your hamstrings (back thigh muscles).

4 Grip the end of the belt with both hands and extend it over your head.

5 Stretch your right leg up so that it's perpendicular to the floor. If possible, pull it towards your head.

6 Stay in this position for 20 to 30 seconds, breathing normally and observing the following points:

- Keep your left leg firmly pressed to the floor without bending your knee. Don't turn your left thigh out.
- Don't tilt your torso to the left.
- Press your right buttock down.
- Don't loosen your grip on the belt as you pull it over your head.

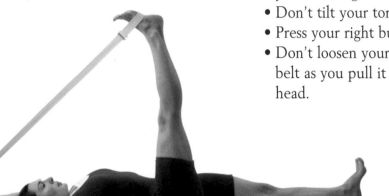

Variation with 2 Belts

For a better stretch of the pelvis and back, tie a second belt around the groin of the upper leg and the foot of the lower leg, and follow the instructions above.

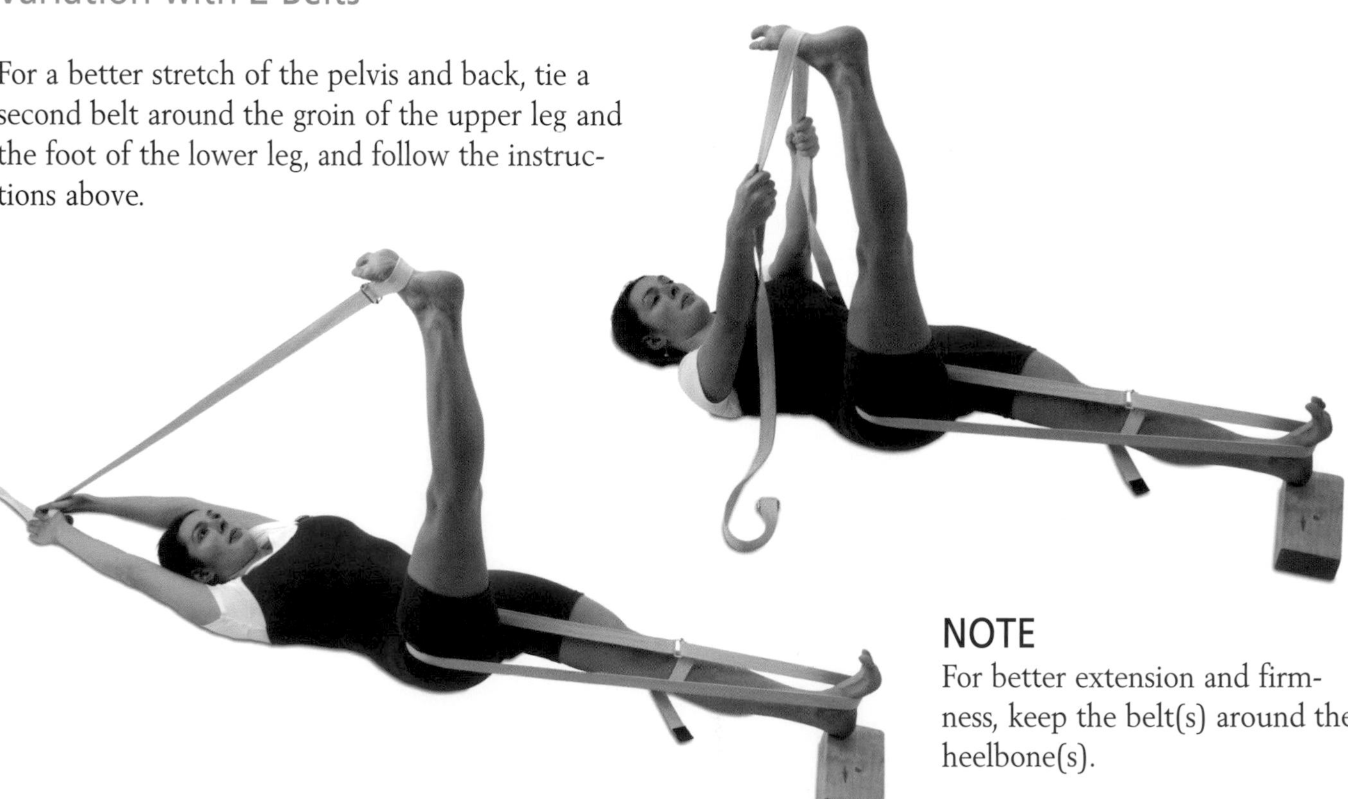

NOTE

For better extension and firmness, keep the belt(s) around the heelbone(s).

Supta Padangushthasana 2
Reclining big toe pose 2

1 Have a belt ready (and if needed, a bolster or rolled blanket).

2 Lie flat as before. Exhale and keep your left leg outstretched. Put the belt behind your head, grip it with your left hand, and pull it towards the left to the floor in line with your left shoulder.

3 Exhale and move your right leg sideways to the right until it reaches the floor or the rolled blanket. Stretch your hamstrings (back thigh muscles).

4 Stay in this position for 20 to 30 seconds, breathing normally and observing the following points:
- Bring your right foot to the level of your right shoulder.
- Don't raise the left side of your torso and your left buttock away from the floor.

CHECK YOURSELF
> *Don't loosen your grip on your foot. If you do, your knee will bend and the abdominal muscles will loosen.*

Coming out of the pose

1 Inhale and come back to Supta Padangushthasana 1.

2 Release your right foot from the belt, lower your right leg and your arms, and keep your arms by your sides.

3 Repeat the asana on the left side by raising your left leg up and proceeding as above.

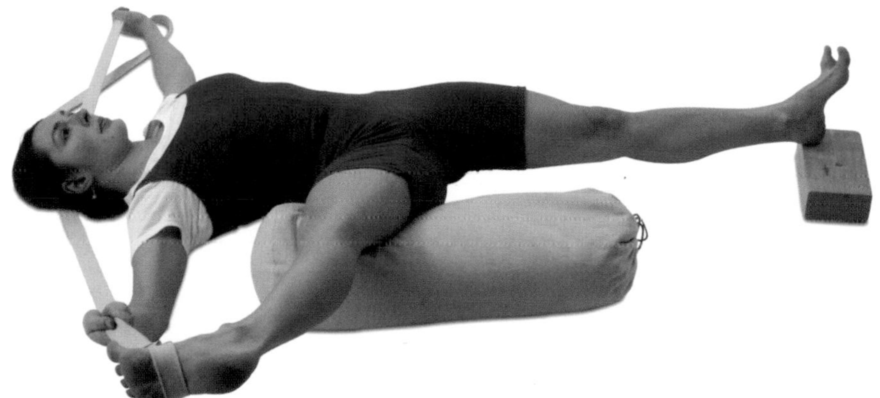

Help
- If the outstretched leg on the floor bends at the knee, keep the bottom of your left foot pressed against a wall.
- If you're having trouble pulling the raised leg towards your head, then go back to practicing the first variation (Supta Padangushthasana 1) before you proceed to this one.

Variation with 2 Belts

For a better stretch of the pelvis and back, tie a second belt around the groin of the upper leg and the foot of the lower leg and follow the instructions above.

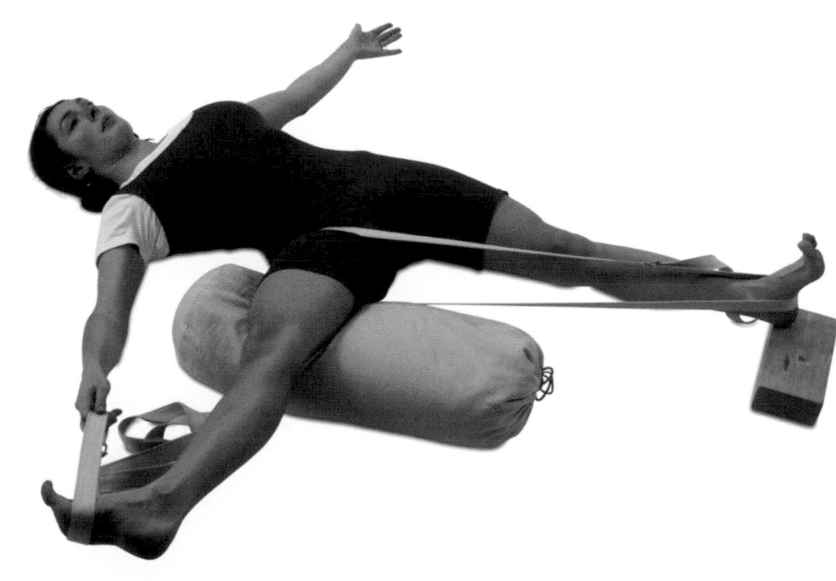

Utthita Hasta Padangushthasana 1 and 2
Extended hand to big toe poses 1 and 2

Practice this asana in the second term, after you've mastered comfortably the less intense asanas of the first term. Utthita Hasta Padangushthasana focuses on the back and the abdominal region. It helps reduce fat, firms up the back muscles, and brings back flexibility and strength to the spine.

Hasta means "hand." In this asana, you stand on one leg, extend the other leg, grip the big toe, and rest your head on your knees. It is similar to Supta Padangushthasana, but is done in a standing position so that there is freedom of movement for the spine. This is more effective in conditions such as slipped disk, backache, weakness in the hip muscles, and unequal length of the legs.

In the classic pose, Utthita Hasta Padangushthasana is done without any support. Because it's a difficult pose, however, we recommend the techniques below where you rest your outstretched leg on a table or windowsill and use a belt to get a better hold of your foot. This has more curative value.

1st term: no
2nd term: yes
3rd term: yes

Benefits
(for Utthita Hasta Padangushthasana 1 and 2)

- Reduces fat in the back and abdomen and tones them
- Relieves flatulence
- Brings flexibility and strength to the spine
- Helps eliminate backache and treat lumbago

Utthita Hasta Padangushthasana 1
Extended hand to big toe poses 1

1 Stand 2 to 3 feet away from a table or window, facing it. Take one or two breaths.

2 Exhale, bend your right knee, raise it, and place the leg on the table or windowsill so that it is parallel to the floor.

3 Loop the belt around the foot and grip both ends of the belt firmly. Stretch your right leg, keeping the foot upright. Extend both arms, catch the belt (or when you can reach farther, the windowsill) or your foot for support, and lift your torso.

4 Keep your head erect and look straight forward.

5 Keep your left leg firmly on the floor and stretch your spine from the tailbone up. Stretch both hamstrings (back thigh muscles). Stay in this position for 20 to 30 seconds, breathing normally and observing the following points:
- Don't lift your shoulders or contract your neck.
- Don't turn your right buttock out.
- Don't lean backward; keep your torso straight in an upward movement.
- Don't turn your left foot out.
- Keep your pelvic bones parallel.

6 With practice, gradually keep your right leg at a higher level. Grasp the sole of your right foot with both the hands if possible, or grip the belt more firmly. Raise your spine and extend your torso up.

7 Inhale and lower your right leg.

8 Repeat on the other side and then come back to Tadasana.

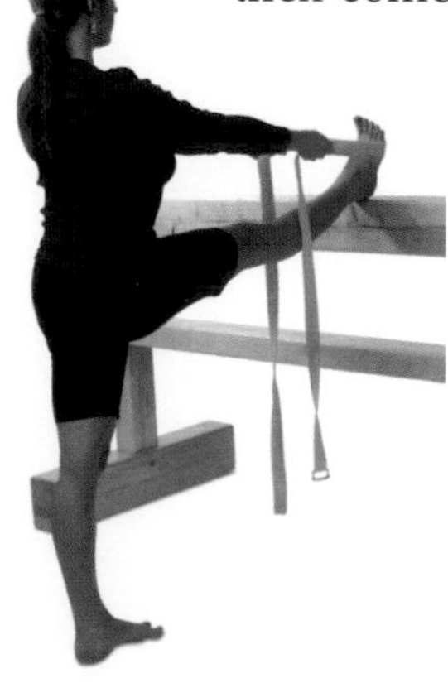

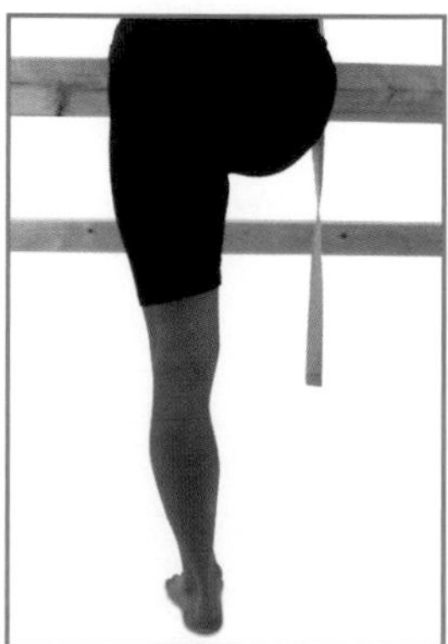

Utthita Hasta Padangushthasana 2
Extended hand to big toe poses 2

1 Turn your whole body 90° to the left. Stand 2 to 3 feet away from the table or window with your feet parallel to it. Take one or two breaths.

2 Exhale, bend your right knee, and place your right foot on the table at a right angle. Place a belt around your right foot firmly with your right hand, keep your left hand on your hip, and lift your torso.

3 With practice, increase the height and gradually rest your right foot at shoulder level.

4 Grip either your right big toe or sole with the fingers of your right hand, or grip the foot firmly with a belt, and stretch the front of your torso.

5 Stay in this position for 20 to 30 seconds, breathing normally and observing the following points:

- Don't lift your right outer buttock upward. It has a tendency to lift, which can cause backache or cramps in the thighs.
- Straighten your torso by keeping your groin firm.
- Keep your torso and buttocks in one line.
- Lift your abdominal muscles and broaden your chest.
- Don't lift your shoulders or contract your neck.

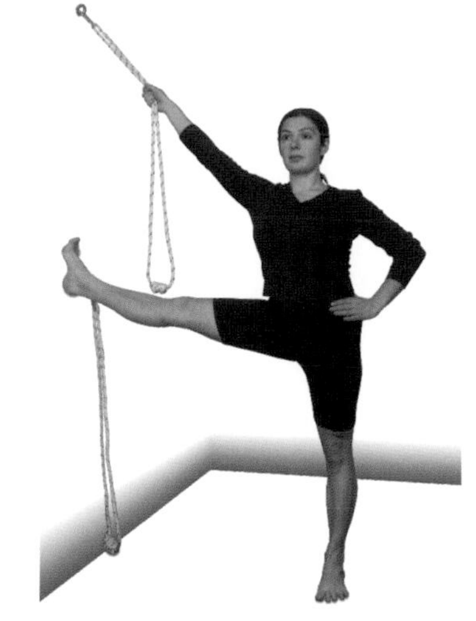

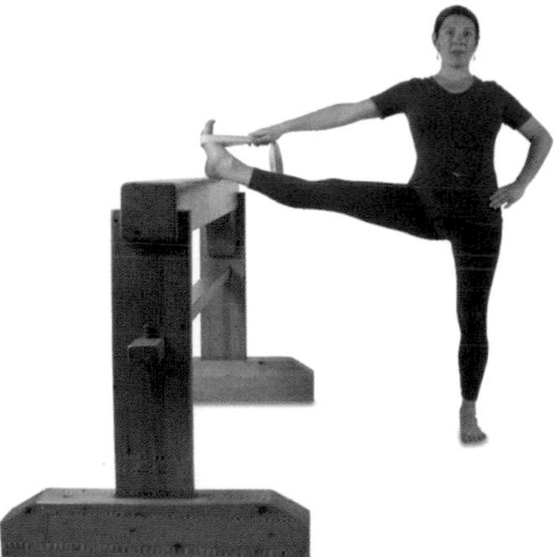

Variation with Ropes

You can use the upper and lower wall ropes for a better lift and a firmer stretch of the legs. Grip the rope behind your back as shown.

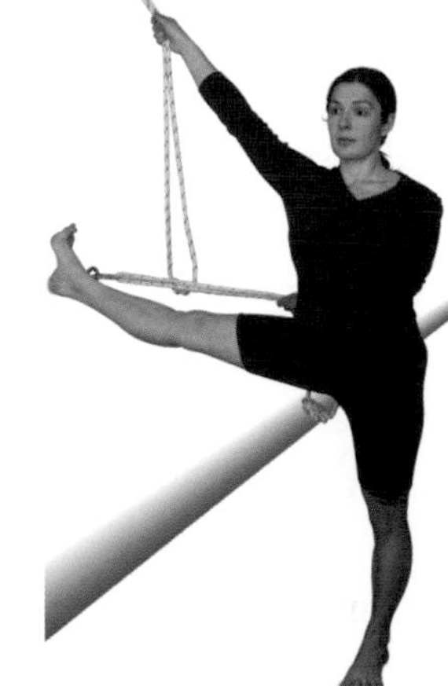

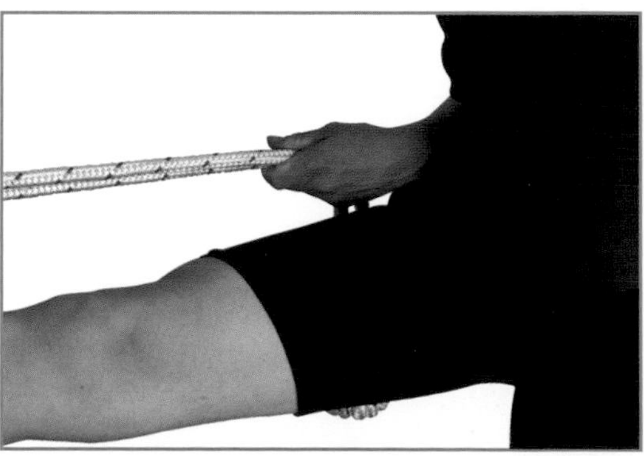

Coming out of the pose

1 Exhale, bend your right leg, and bring it down. Turn your whole body 180° and do the asana standing on your right leg and lifting the left leg up. Breathe normally.

2 Afterwards, close your feet in Tadasana.

Special Instructions

- This asana gives an intense stretch to the hamstrings (back thigh muscles), so you should place your foot onto the support very gradually. While you're learning to master the pose, raise your leg no higher than thigh level. Remember that sudden, aggressive movements can cause tearing.
- It's more important to raise your spine and keep your torso firm than to take the leg higher and higher.

Starting Abdominal Work in the Second Term

1st term: no
2nd term: yes
3rd term: yes

Yes, you want to reduce fat around your waist and abdomen. No, that does **not** mean that you should dive headlong into the practice of the asanas in this section without hesitation. Please heed the word of warning below.

Before practicing any asana that causes abdominal contraction, it is essential that you be fully trained in the asanas that come before it—the standing asanas, forward bends, and inversions. They determine whether your back and abdomen are capable of bearing the strain. Once you have concentrated on these asanas and they have provided you with the necessary strength, you can then move on to asanas for abdominal contraction, such as Navasana.

For this reason, we recommend the asanas for abdomen and lumbar only for the second term. In the beginning, you're likely to experience either abdominal pain or back pain due to weak back muscles. For relief, we will also introduce asanas to be practiced in sequence, namely Setu Bandha Sarvangasana, which removes pain that is caused by abdominal contractions, and Bharadvajasana, which eliminates back pain caused by weak muscles.

There are several ways to know if you should postpone or stop the practice of Navasana:

- If you have a menstrual disorder or displacement of the uterus, then you should not practice Navasana.
- If you don't find relief in spite of practicing Setu Bandha Sarvangasana and Bharadvajasana, then your back and abdominal muscles have not gained enough strength, and you should postpone Navasana to the third term.
- If you start bleeding or have an attack of white discharge (leukorrhea) after practicing Navasana for a week or so, then you should stop practicing it for three to four weeks, until the condition has definitely stopped.
- If you find that your breast milk production decreases, or that the quality of the milk is lower, stop Navasana.

This doesn't mean that you should stop practicing the asanas in this part of the book altogether. On the contrary, you should continue with the other asanas in the sequences. Maha Mudra and Janu Shirshasana check white discharge, Sarvangasana and Setu Bandha Sarvangasana help correct the position of the uterus, and inversions reduce bleeding.

Paripurna Navasana
Full boat pose

Paripurna means "full" or "complete," and *nava* means "boat." This asana resembles a boat with oars. The technique below is for the classic pose.

1st term: no
2nd term: yes
3rd term: yes

1 Sit in Dandasana (page 64) and extend both legs. Take one or two breaths.

2 Exhale and lean your torso slightly backward, simultaneously raising both legs off the floor.

3 Balance your whole body on your buttocks. Keep your head, torso, and legs straight; your torso should be erect and your legs firm. If your back sags, your torso will drop towards the floor. If your knees are bent, your feet will drop.

4 Raise your hands and extend them forward, parallel to the floor. Turn your palms inward, facing each other. Your shoulders and palms should be in line.

5 Remain in this position for 30 to 60 seconds, breathing normally and observing the following points:

- Keep your legs stiff and straight.
- Keep your spine firm. Your head should seem to float on your spine; if it bends forward, your neck will tighten, causing heaviness in the head. Feel as though your body is floating weightlessly like a boat.
- Look straight ahead and don't press your chin against your throat.
- Don't cave in your chest or lower your lumbar (lower) spine for the sake of balance.
- Don't touch your legs with your palms.

6 Exhale, bring your arms and legs down, and come back to Dandasana.

Benefits

- Relieves flatulence and gastric complaints
- Reduces fat
- Strengthens the abdominal and spinal muscles
- Strengthens the abdominal organs
- Tones the kidneys

Help

If you can't raise your hands after balancing on your buttocks, attempt the following actions simultaneously: reclining your torso and raising your arms and legs.

2nd Term: Using 2 Chairs

Try this variation when you first begin practicing the asana in your second term or when you still feel weak. Use one chair for your back, one for your legs, and a sticky mat in between the chairs on the floor.

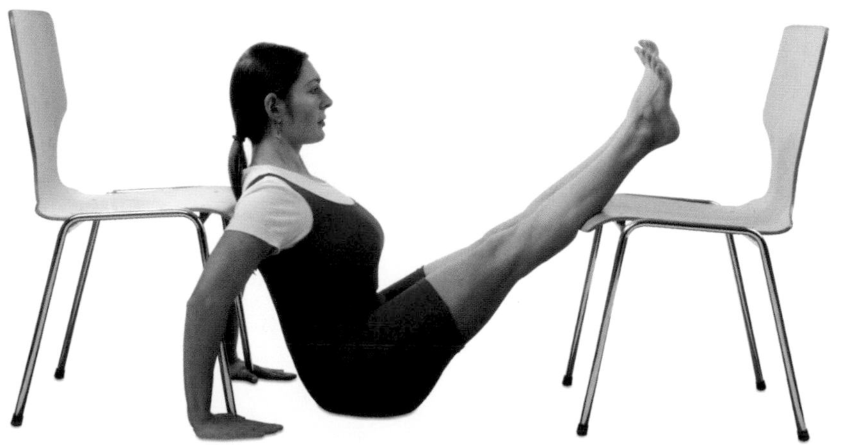

Step 1

1 Put a chair against the wall and the other 3 to 4 feet away. Have a sticky mat on the floor in front of the wall chair.

2 Sit and lean your back against the chair behind you.

3 Place your hands behind your hips on the floor, with the fingertips pointing forward.

4 Bend your knees and bring one leg after the other onto the chair in front of you.

5 Sit on your buttocks and keep your knees and feet together.

Step 2

1 Exhale and stretch your legs, keeping your legs, feet, and knees firmly together and extending your inner heels and the balls of your big toes.

If you need a rest, rest your back on the floor and your lower legs on the seat of the chair for a couple of breaths.

2 Lift your breastbone and expand your chest.

3 Stay for 1 minute, extending up to 5 minutes.

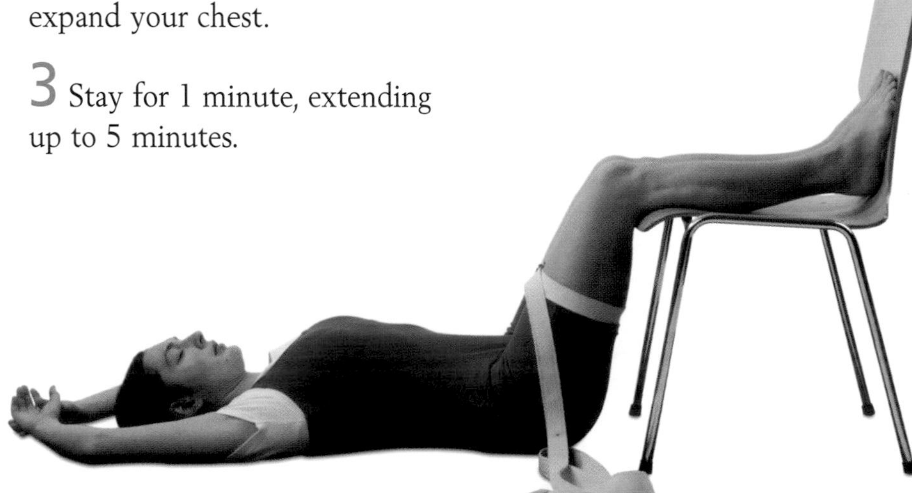

2nd Half of 2nd Term and 1st Half of 3rd term: Using 1 Chair

Grip the tops of the front legs of the chair in front of you.

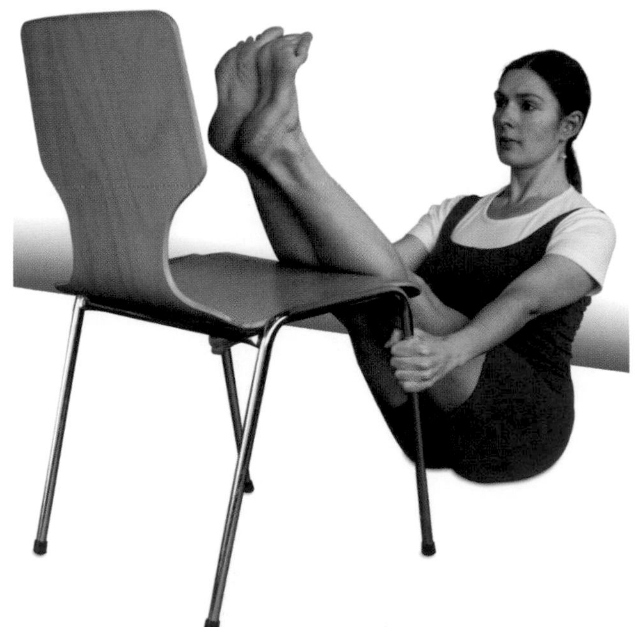

Ubhaya Padangushthasana

Both feet big toe pose

1st term: no
2nd term: no
3rd term: yes

This asana, which is a continuation of the previous one, is for the third term after your delivery and provides more lift and firmness.

Benefits

See Paripurna Navasana, page 347

Step 1

1 Begin as in the variation for Paripurna Navasana, step 1 (page 347), using two chairs and a belt.

2 Later on, when you no longer need the second chair, you can just practice with just one chair.

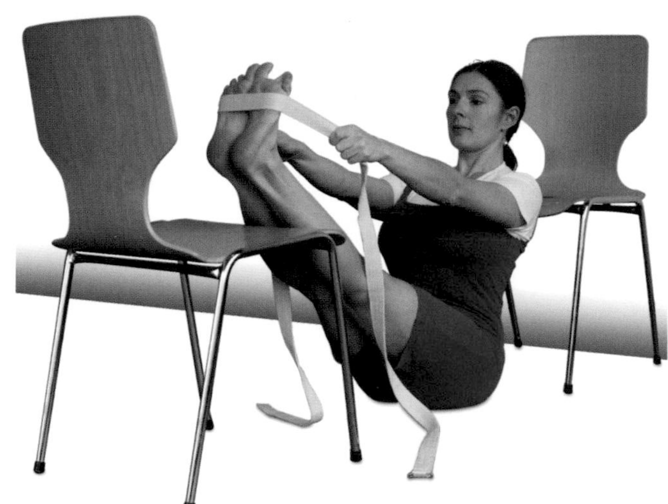

Step 2

1 Balancing on your buttock bones with bent legs and a belt around your feet, grip the belt firmly.

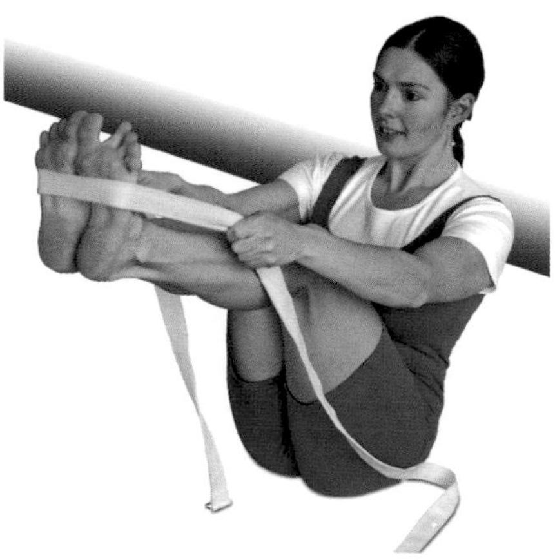

2 Extend your legs into the inner arches and pull the outer edges of your feet towards you with the belt.

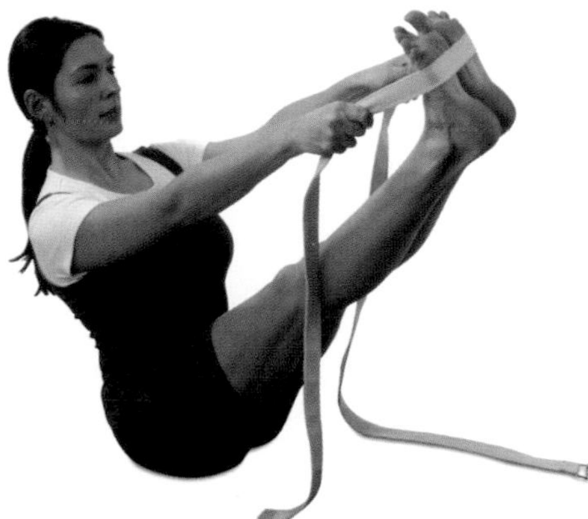

3 Lift the abdominal wall, the sides of your chest, and your breastbone by bringing your shoulder blades deep into your body.

4 Bring your chin away from your breastbone.

HINT: You can also use a block between your upper thighs.

Continuing with the Abdomen and Spine

As we recommended at the beginning of this section, the second term is the right time to take up the practice of abdominal exercises. First, a few additional cautions:

1 You may not have had any time at all for Yoga practice in the first two months after your delivery, perhaps because of a lack of help at home. If so, then don't jump right in and start practicing asanas for the second term. You must first begin with pranayama for a month and then the asanas scheduled for the first term. This holds true for any time you begin your practice of yogasanas during the first six months after delivery.

2 As long you're breast-feeding, don't attempt to do the asanas too vigorously. This can lead to fatigue, dehydration, and backache.

3 If your abdominal or lumbar (lower) back muscles are weak, then the second-term asanas will be too intensive; you should stay with the first-term asanas.

4 If you suffer from a displaced uterus, vaginal discharge (leukorrhea), weakness due to undernourishment, or poor digestion, then stay with the asanas for the first term and seek medical advice before treating these conditions through your Yoga practice.

During the second term, you'll concentrate on asanas that:

- Tone the muscles of the spine and back: Supta Padangushthasana (page 341) and Utthita Hasta Padangushthasana (page 344)
- Massage the abdominal organs: Urdhva Prasarita Padasana (page 350) and Jathara Parivartanasana (page 356)
- Bring about lateral movements of the spine: Marichyasana (pages 314 and 320) and Ardha Matsyendrasana (page 324)

These asanas also help counter flatulence, acidity, and indigestion, which are problems of middle age.

Urdhva Prasarita Padasana

Upward extended feet pose

1st term: no
2nd term: yes (3rd week)
3rd term: yes

Benefits
(for Urdhva Prasarita Padasana 1 and 2)

Tones the thigh, abdominal, and back muscles, giving you a feeling of fitness

After pregnancy, the resulting weakness of your abdominal and back muscles affects your abdominal organs as well. Common complaints include loss of appetite, urinary infection, gastritis, and flatulence. To avoid these problems, you need to tone the abdomen and back. The asanas we recommend for after your delivery accomplish this toning gradually and safely.

Supta Padangushthasana (pages 342 – 343) and Utthita Hasta Padangushthasana (pages 344 – 345), achieve several purposes. When you stretch one leg against the other, a traction effect is brought about on the spinal muscles, which helps alleviate pain in the lower back and waist. All the variations of both asanas lift the abdominal walls and massage them against the spine, lift the lower organs, and correct the position of the uterus. Practicing the asanas regularly in the first weeks of the second term brings about sufficient toning.

Only after concentrating on these poses and reaching satisfactory results should you take up more stressful poses such as Paripurna Navasana, Urdhva Prasarita Padasana, and Jathara Parivartanasana (bent legs).

Urdhva Prasarita Padasana 1
Upward extended feet pose 1

You can begin this asana in the third week of the second term. Take your time to learn it well; a learner does not become a master all at once. In this asana, you'll develop your ability to lift both legs straight up in line with your buttocks.

The buttock muscles at this stage are so stiff that it's difficult to keep the back of your buttocks down and stretch your legs at the same time; when you stretch your legs, your buttocks come up, and when your buttocks are down, your legs bend. Lack of movement in the buttocks and hamstrings (back thigh muscles) causes these problems.

The technique below for Urdhva Prasarita Padasana is an easier, intermediate pose. There are two main reasons why we recommend beginning with this version:

- It strengthens the muscles that help you keep your buttocks down and stretch your legs, and lift your legs without bending your knees.
- If you have a slipped disk, then the advanced version could aggravate your back pain.

1 Lie flat on the floor and extend your arms above your head.

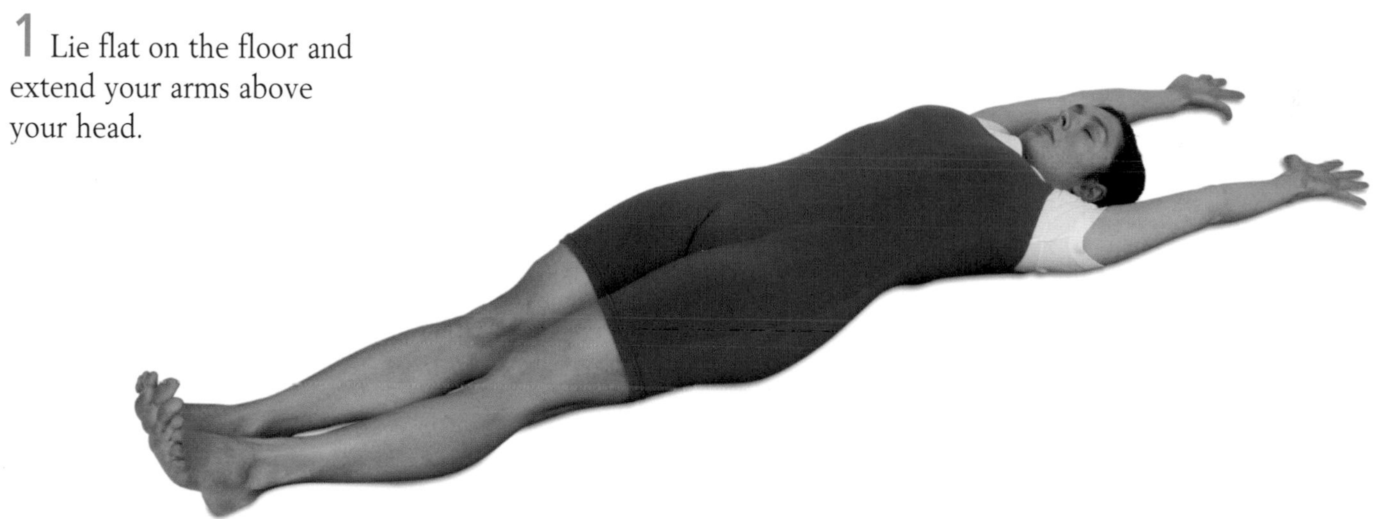

2 Bend your knees, draw them towards your stomach, and keep your heels near your buttocks. Press your knees and thighs onto your stomach. Stretch your arms further, so that your back, waist, and spine are extended.

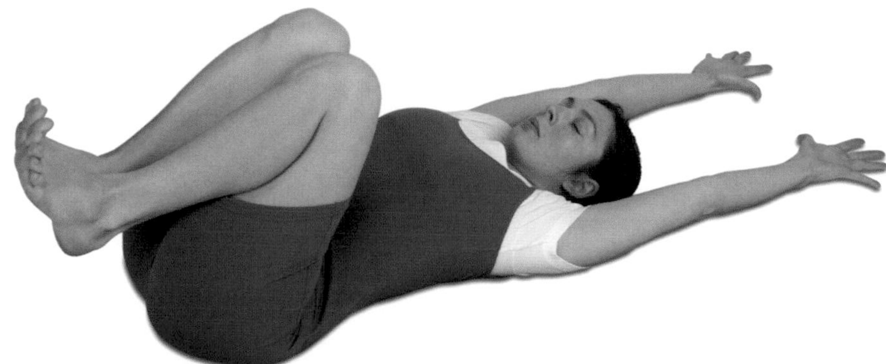

3 Encircle your legs with your arms and press your thighs down onto your stomach. Press your legs so that your back and hip muscles are pressed into the floor. This relieves weakness in the waist and legs and also backache, especially during your period.

4 Stretch your arms over your head, exhale, and raise your legs to 90°, keeping your knees straight. Remain in this position for 5 to 10 seconds, breathing normally. Gradually increase the duration.

5 Bend your knees and bring your thighs onto your stomach. Keep your arms stretched over your head.

6 If you find it difficult to keep your arms over your head, then keep them alongside your torso with the palms facing down and press them into the floor when raising your legs.

7 It's easier to lower your legs without bending your knees than to raise them, so keep your legs straight when you lower them. To raise them, however, you can bend your knees, raise them, and then straighten your legs. Once you've mastered this, then you can start raising your legs without bending your knees.

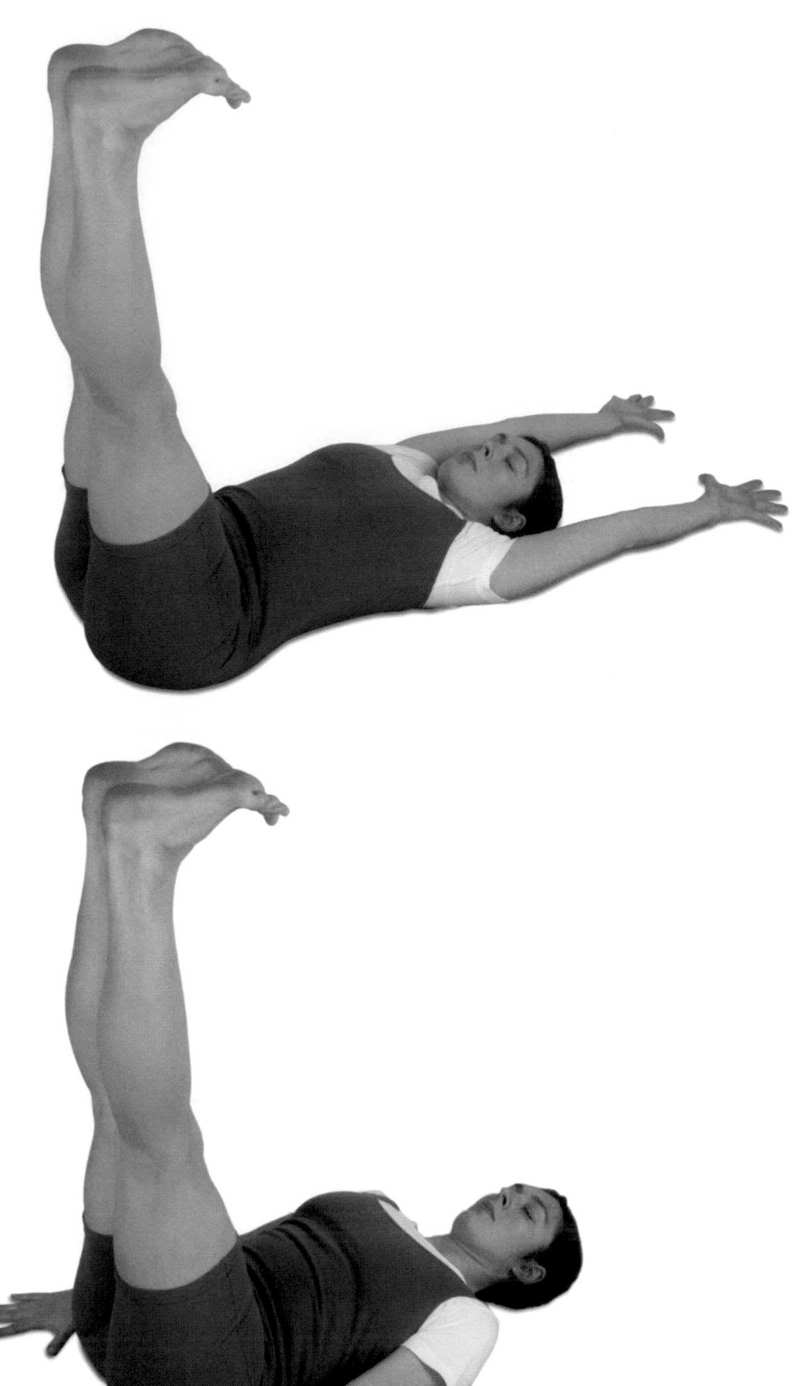

8 In the beginning, you'll experience tremors in your legs, thighs, and abdominal muscles. This is nothing to be alarmed about. At first, just do the pose once or twice and later work up to 10 to 15 times.

Variation with the Wall

If you have heavy bleeding during your period or white discharge (leukorrhea), try this pose with your legs against a wall. Your buttock bones, the back of your thighs, hamstrings, and heels should rest on the wall, forming your body into an L-shape. Your body is on the floor from head to hips, and perpendicular from buttocks to heels.

This way, your abdominal organs are supported by your spine and by the sacrum resting on the floor. With your legs resting against the wall, there is no cause for tension or pressure. Remain in this position for as long as you can.

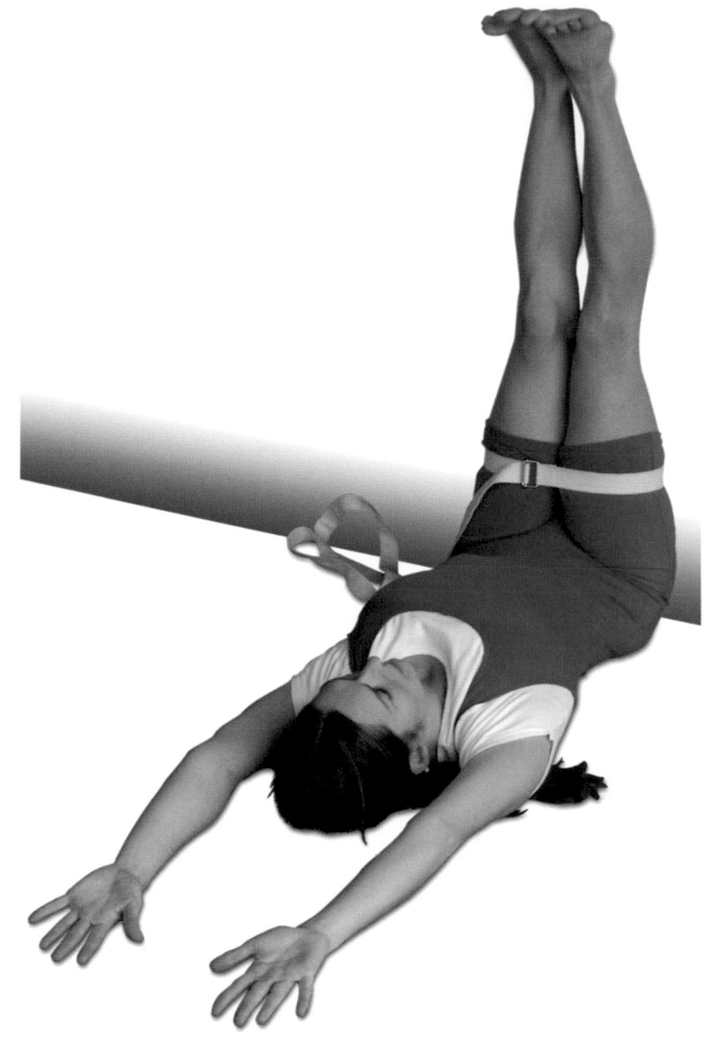

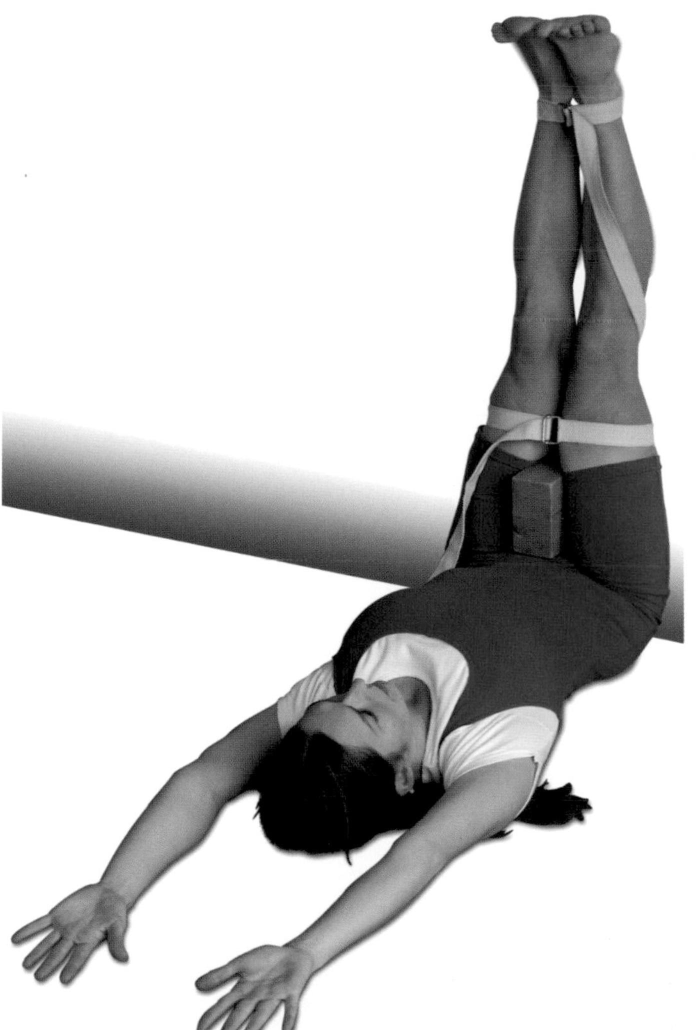

Variation with the Wall and Block

Put a block between your legs and tighten a belt around them. Grip the block firmly, which gives you a firmer grip on your leg muscles, broadens your lower back, and lifts the abdominal organs.

If you are young, strong, have given birth for the first time, feel absolutely normal, and performed this version of the asana with ease, then you can go on to the advanced technique on the next page in the third term.

Urdhva Prasarita Padasana 2, Advanced Work
Upward extended feet pose 2

Urdhva Prasarita Padasana 1 was a first step, which did not cause strain on the buttock and abdominal muscles. You can go on to the following technique in the third term when you have gained sufficient strength and muscle control.

This asana is done lying on the floor with both legs extended and stretched upward.

1 Lie flat on your back, stretch both legs, and keep your thighs, knees, ankles, and toes together and your knees tight.

2 Stretch both arms over your head with the palms facing up. Make sure that the back of your body is extending along with your arms. Take one or two breaths.

3 Exhale and raise your legs to 90°. Remain in this final position for 15 to 30 seconds, observing the following points (also in the two previous steps):
- Keep your knees tight and your legs firm.
- Extend your arms more so that the back of your torso is well stretched.
- Keep your hips and back firmly on the floor, so that the abdominal organs are massaged inside.
- Breathe normally throughout.

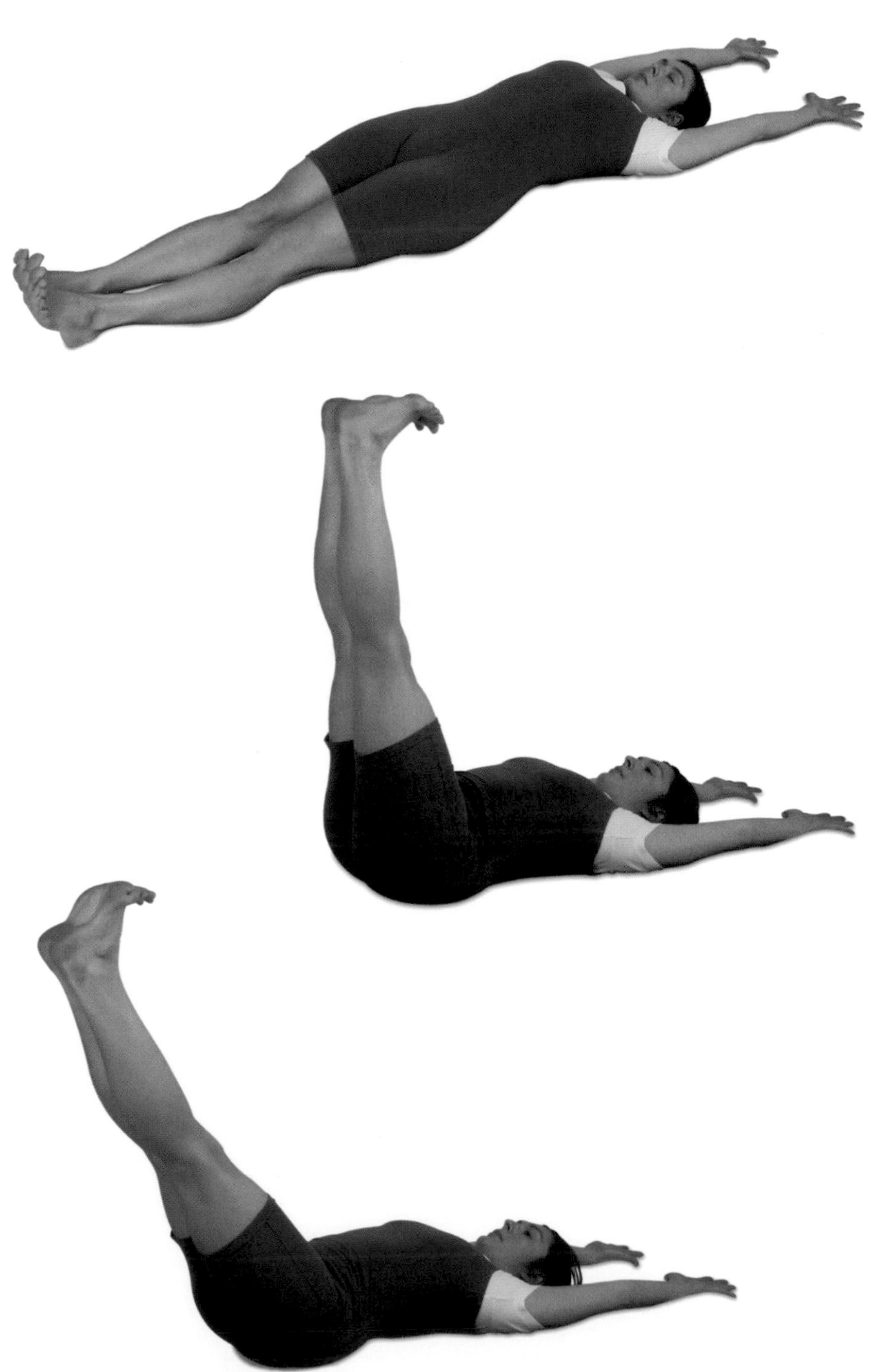

1st term: no
2nd term: no
3rd term: yes

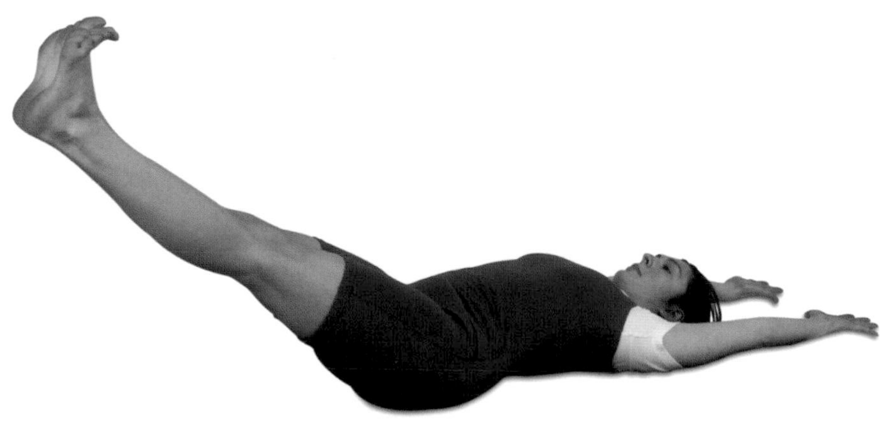

4 Exhale again and lower your legs to 60°. Stay for 5 to 10 seconds, breathing normally.

5 Exhale and lower both legs to 30°. Stay in this position for 5 to 10 seconds, breathing normally.

Coming out of the pose

1 Exhale and lower your legs slowly without bending your knees.

Try not to let your legs come down fast as a result of lack of muscle control in the lower abdomen and lower back. Pay special attention to your thighs; tighten them more, which ultimately strengthens the lower abdominal wall, and relax them after your legs have gradually reached the floor.

2 Repeat the asana 3 times for the first month of your 3rd term. Once your abdominal muscles are toned, you can repeat it 15 to 20 times.

Help

- As you learn to practice this asana, you'll experience an expected amount of tremor in the thighs and pain in the legs. If the throbbing becomes unbearable, however, you can switch to Supta Virasana, Supta Baddha Konasana, or Setu Bandha Sarvangasana. These are also good for relieving vaginal discharge (leukorrhea), abdominal cramps, and menstrual disorders.

- If you lose awareness of your breathing and hold your breath, it may cause a "catch" of your diaphragm, causing an uneasy feeling in the abdomen or chest. Practice the asanas mentioned above to relieve the feeling.

Jathara Parivartanasana, with Bent Legs
Revolved abdominal pose

Jathar means "stomach," and *parivartan* means "turning around" or "rotating." In this asana, the stomach is given an internal massage.

Because you should switch over to Jathara Parivartanasana only after you've successfully practiced Urdhva Prasarita Padasana, this asana is also in the second term, after the sixth week of the term. It's a more difficult pose than Urdhva Prasarita Padasana, since you need a strong grip on the abdomen and waist.

If you are very thin and have no tendency to put on fat, you don't need to do this asana and can stay with Urdhva Prasarita Padasana. This is particularly true if you have a weak constitution.

In the photos, you can see the asana as practiced with a block and 2 belts. This creates more space and teaches a better grip on the muscles that loosened during pregnancy.

Practice with and without the block and belts. See what the props can teach you.

Use the wall as an additional prop. At first, you can practice with your legs perpendicular to your body against the wall for:

- Better alignment of legs, buttock bones, and pelvis
- Reduced abdominal stress

1 Lie flat on your back.

2 Stretch both arms sideways in line with your shoulders, palms up. Take one or two breaths.

3 Exhale, bend your legs, and lift them together so that your upper thighs and abdomen form a right angle. Don't raise your legs straight; bend your knees. Stay in this position for some time, breathing normally.

4 Keep your knees and inner ankles firmly together and extend the soles of both feet, your inner heels, and the balls of your big toes.

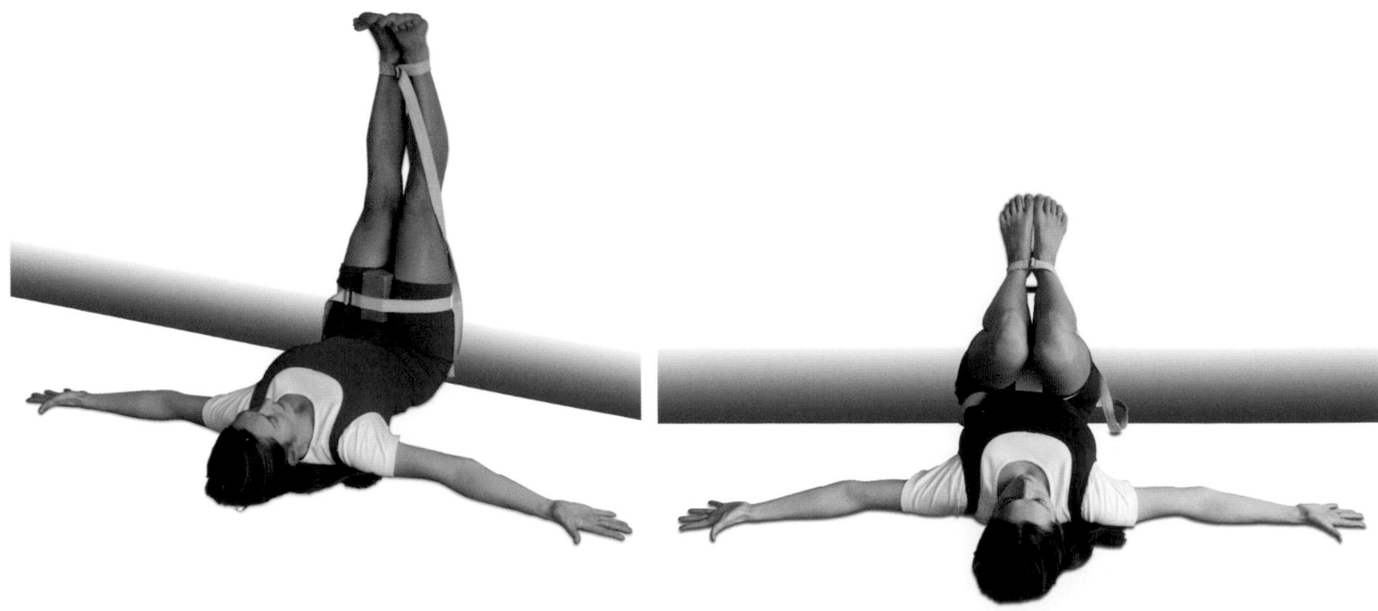

1st term: no
2nd term: yes, after 6th week of term
3rd term: yes

Benefits

See page 359

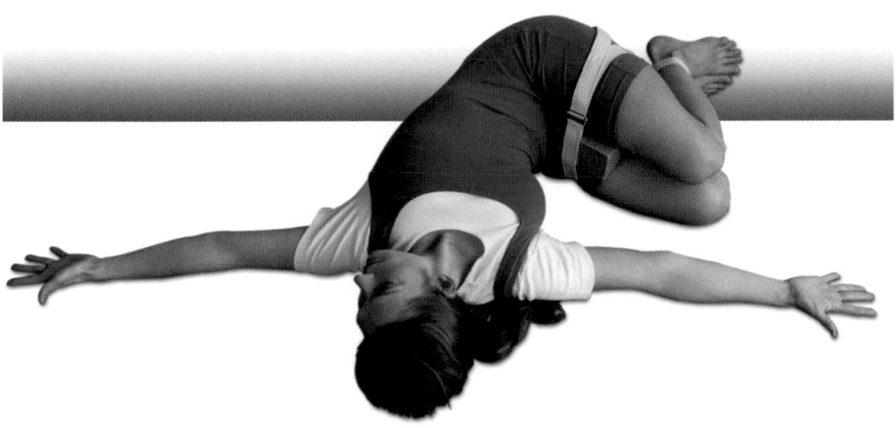

5 Exhale and slowly move your knees to the right side without dropping your feet. Keep your inner arches extended and your inner ankles and inner knees firmly together.

6 Revolve your torso, abdomen, and stomach to the left.

7 Keep the left side of your back on the floor as much as possible.

8 Stay in this position for 10 to 15 seconds, breathing normally.

9 Come back to the center and repeat on the other side.

10 As your legs move to the right, your left shoulder tends to lift off the floor. To prevent this, hold your pelvis backward and downward by holding onto a heavy piece of furniture with your left hand.

11 All these movements of the legs, whether upward or sideways, should be done very slowly without any sudden movements. The slower the movement, the better the action on the abdominal organs. If you do the pose too quickly, then only your legs benefit from the exercise.

12 In the beginning, do the asana only once. After a few weeks, you can repeat it 2 to 4 times, without lowering your legs from the perpendicular position.

Jathara Parivartanasana

In the third term, you can begin the full poses of Jathara Parivartanasana and Ardha Matsyendrasana (page 324). These two asanas are more advanced and intensive than the ones recommended for the second term. The first involves abdominal contraction, and the second, a lateral twist of the spine.

Be sure to follow the order shown below for practicing asanas like those in the third term:

1. Urdhva Prasarita Padasana (page 350) and Jathara Parivartanasana (page 356)
2. Supine poses
3. Lateral twists

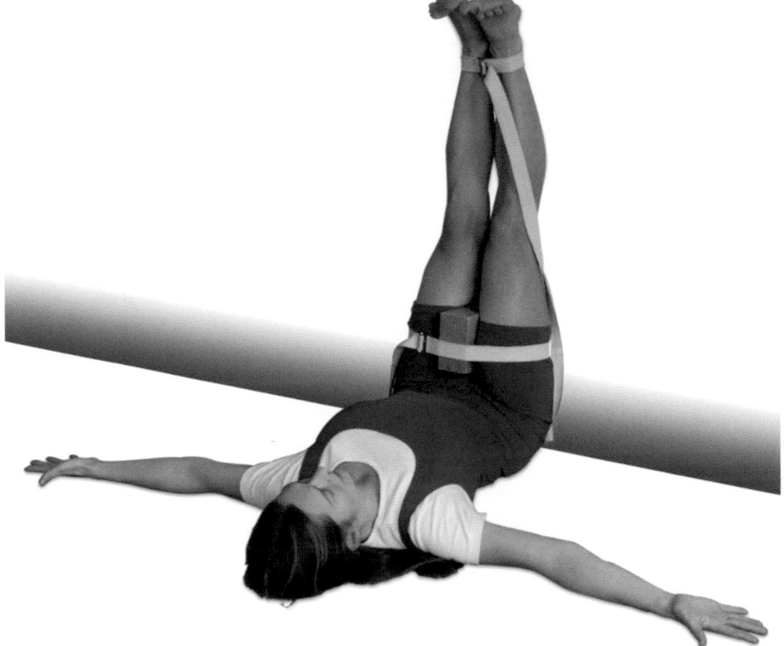

1 Lie flat on your back.

2 Stretch both arms sideways in line with your shoulders, palms up. Take one or two breaths.

3 Exhale and lift both legs together to form a right angle. Don't bend your knees. Wait in this position for some time, breathing normally.

4 Exhale and move your legs slowly sideways towards your right palm; don't let your feet touch the floor because the abdominal organs won't contract correctly. Keep your knees and thighs touching.

5 Keep the left side of your back on the floor as much as possible.

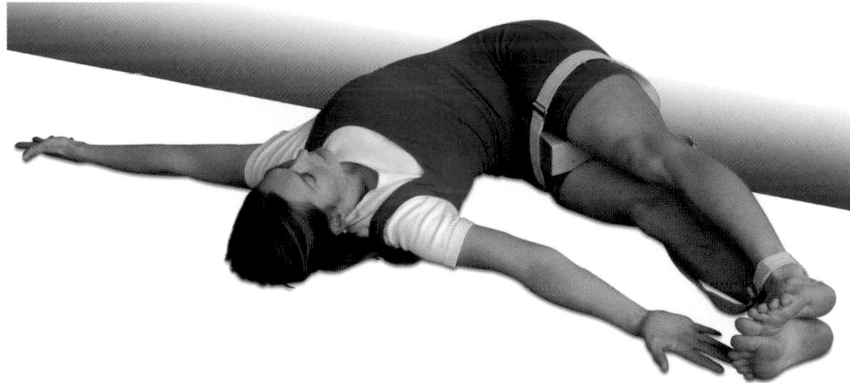

6 Stay in this position for 10 to 15 seconds, breathing normally and observing the following points:

- As your legs move to the right, revolve your torso to the left. Stretch both thighs and pull them towards your buttocks so that the left side of your back is twisted to the left.
- Turn and twist your abdomen and pelvis to the left so that the abdominal organs are tensed and exercised.
- When you move to the right, your right leg tends to lose its grip; keep it firm.
- Don't lift your right shoulder from the floor.
- Keep your feet near your palms; they tend to move away.

Coming out of the pose

1 Exhale and come back to the right-angle position by pressing your left buttock and the left side of your torso to the floor. Stay in this position for a few seconds and then repeat the pose on the left by moving your legs towards the left and revolving your abdomen to the right.

2 Stay in this position for the same length of time, breathing normally. Bring your legs to the perpendicular position and wait for a few moments. Take one or two breaths.

3 Exhale and lower both legs slowly to the floor.

4 In the beginning, do the asana only once. After a few weeks, you can repeat it 2 or 4 times, without lowering your legs from the perpendicular position.

Help

- If you can't raise your legs straight, first bend your knees and then straighten your legs.
- If you have difficulty keeping your legs together, use a belt.
- For a better overall grip on your legs, you can also try a block between your legs, a belt tied around the middle of your thighs, and/or a belt around your ankles.
- When your legs move to the right, your left shoulder tends to lift off the floor. To prevent this, hold your pelvis back and down by holding onto a heavy piece of furniture with your left hand.

1st term: no
2nd term: no
3rd term: yes

Benefits

Reduces fat

Rejuvenates sluggish liver, spleen, and pancreas

Cures gastritis

Relieves lower back pain

Strengthens the back and abdominal muscles

Special Instructions

- All these movements of the legs, whether upward or sideways, should be done very slowly without any sudden movements. The slower the movement, the better the action on the abdominal organs. If you do the pose too quickly, then only your legs gain the benefit of exercise.

- **A precaution:** Loose muscles have to be tightened, but not at the cost of causing uterine problems. Whether or not you experience cramps or other pain during Urdhva Prasarita Padasana and Jathara Parivartanasana, we recommend that you practice Supta Virasana and Supta Baddha Konasana for a minute after each of these asanas—not as counterposes (opposite movements), but as neutral poses (restful poses). These neutral poses nullify abdominal and back stress and give you release from the tremendous strain of muscular control.

Back Bends
Purva Pratana Sthiti

The backward-extending asanas we recommend here for the second and third terms are all very good for the breast-feeding mother because they open the breast area, reduce or prevent hardness of the breasts, and enhance blood circulation.

(For more information, see pages 118 – 123.)

1st term: no
2nd term: yes
3rd term: yes

Benefits

See page 122

Dvi Pada Viparita Dandasana, with a Chair
Inverted staff pose

You can also tie a belt around your upper thighs.

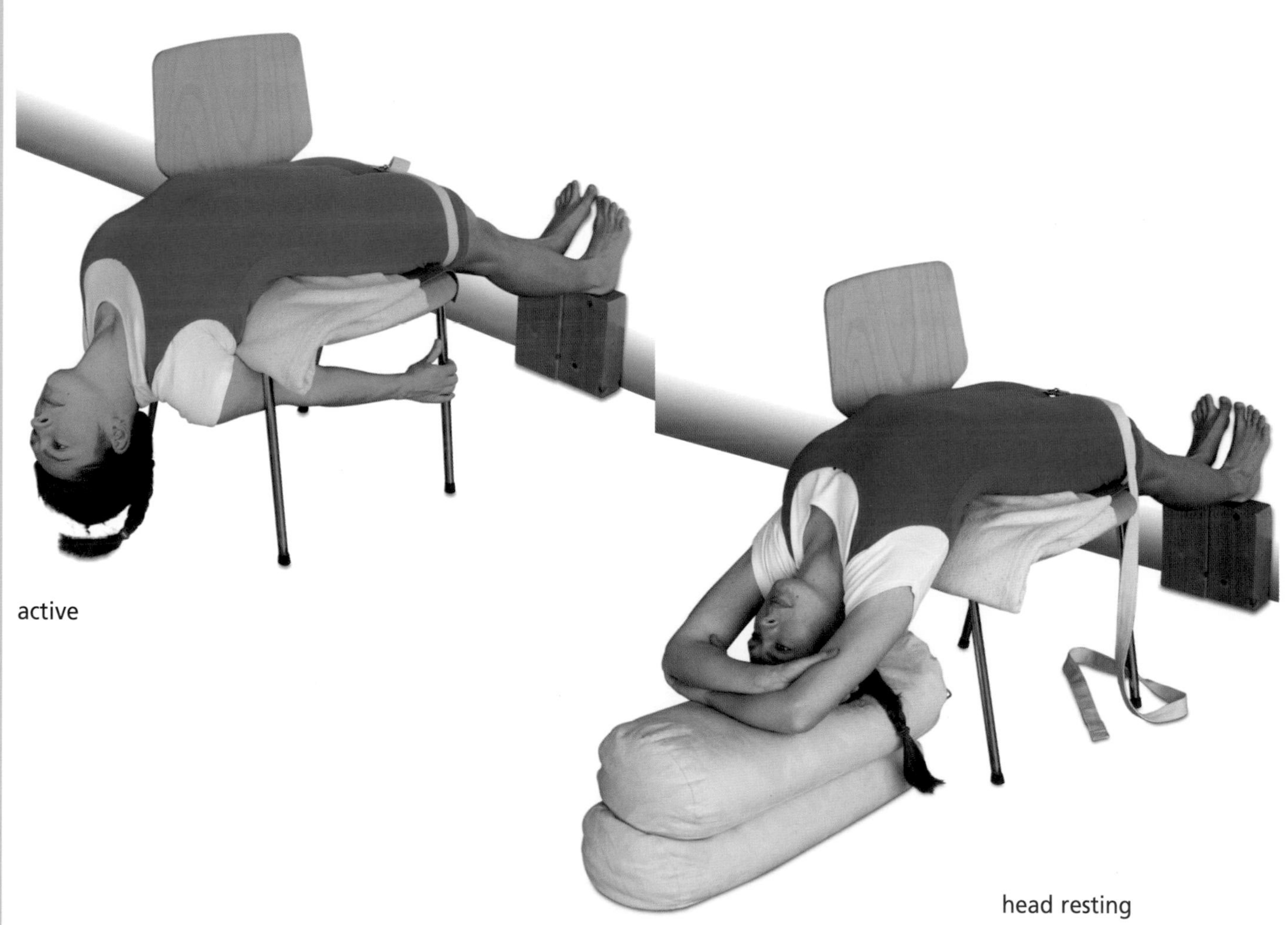

active

head resting

Dvi Pada Viparita Dandasana, with a Bench

Two-legged inverted staff pose

Use a Viparita Dandasana bench and a belt for your upper thighs.

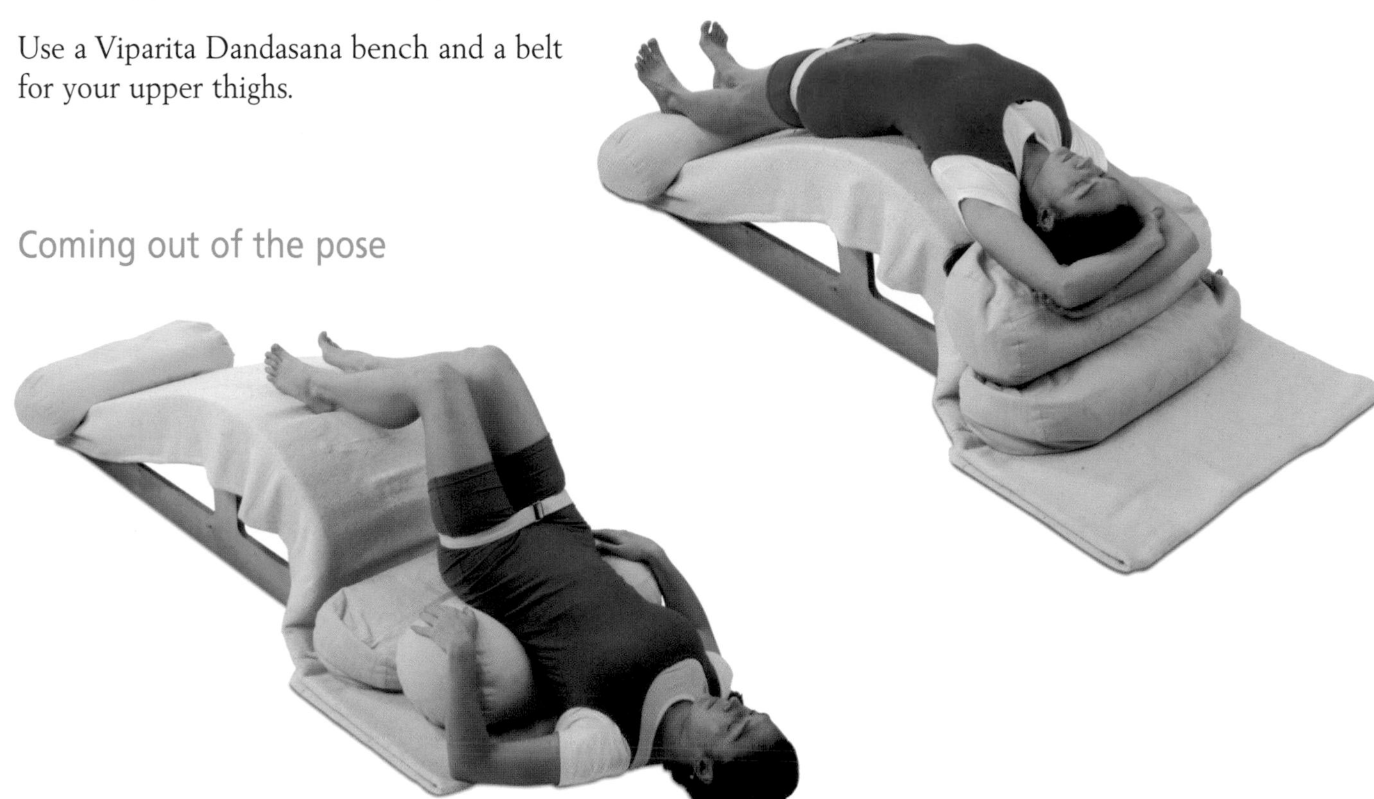

Coming out of the pose

Salamba Purvottasana, with a Chair and a Bolster

Supported eastern intense stretch pose

Use a block and a belt for your upper thighs.

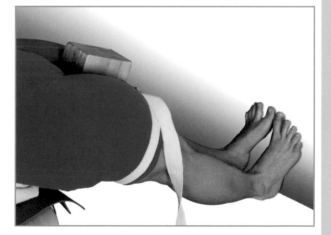

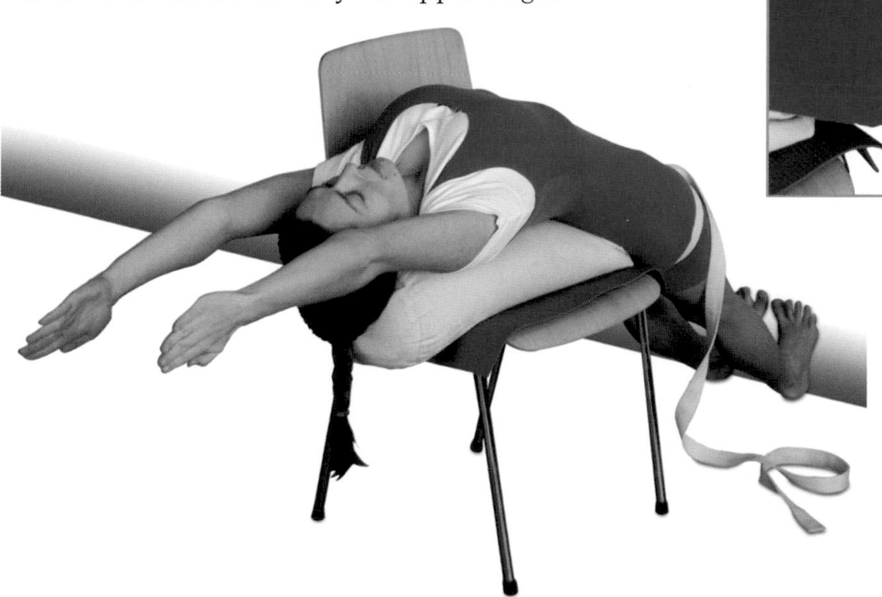

DETAILED DESCRIPTIONS OF ASANAS FOR BEGINNERS AND ADVANCED STUDENTS

Salamba Purvottasana, with a Trestle

Supported eastern intense stretch pose

For detailed instructions, see page 121.

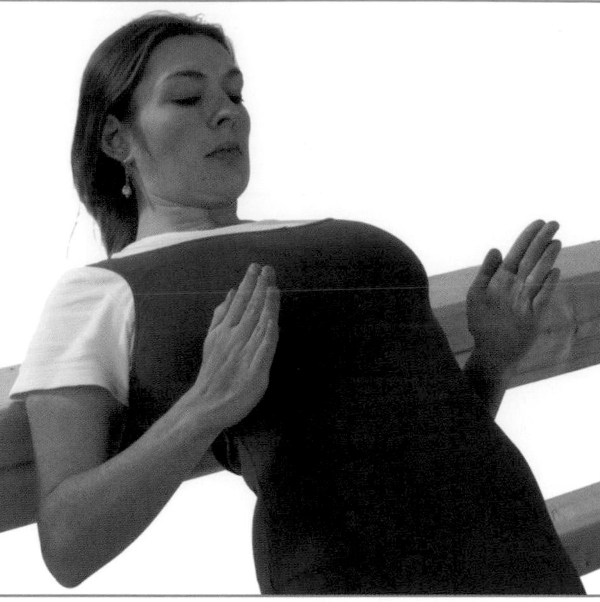

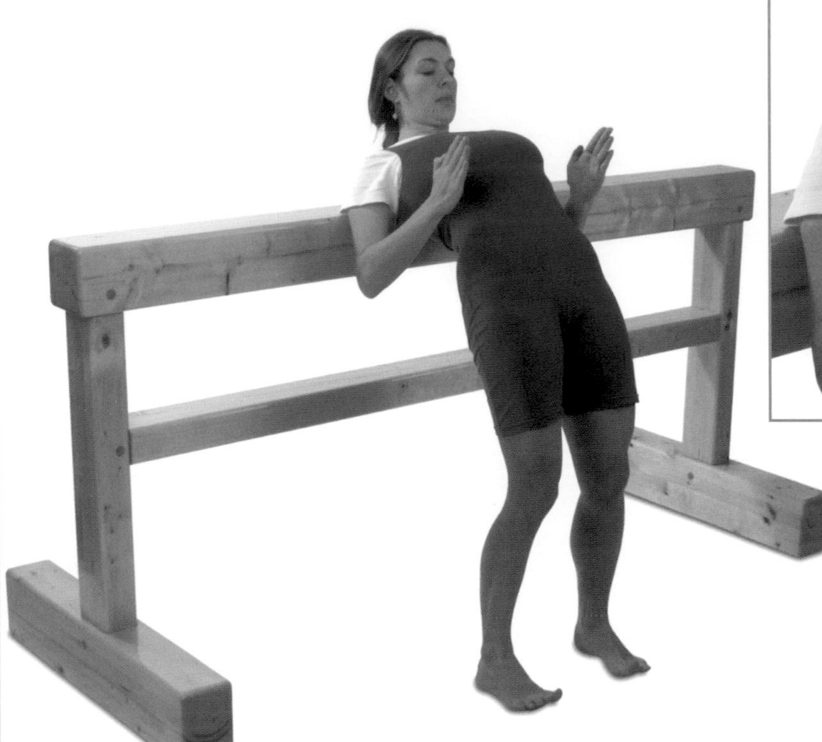

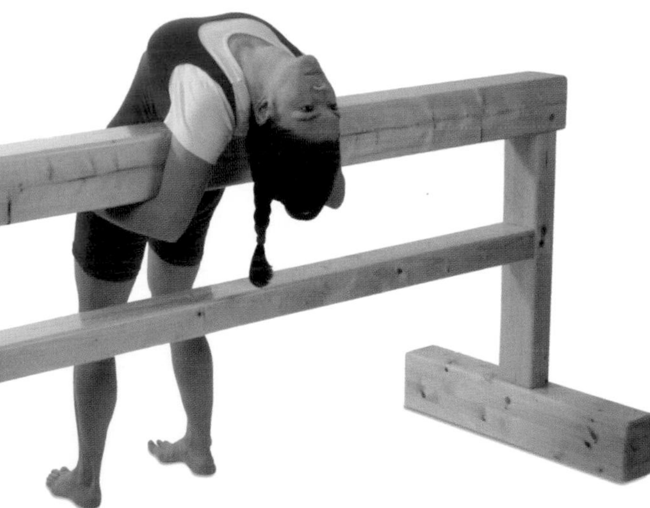

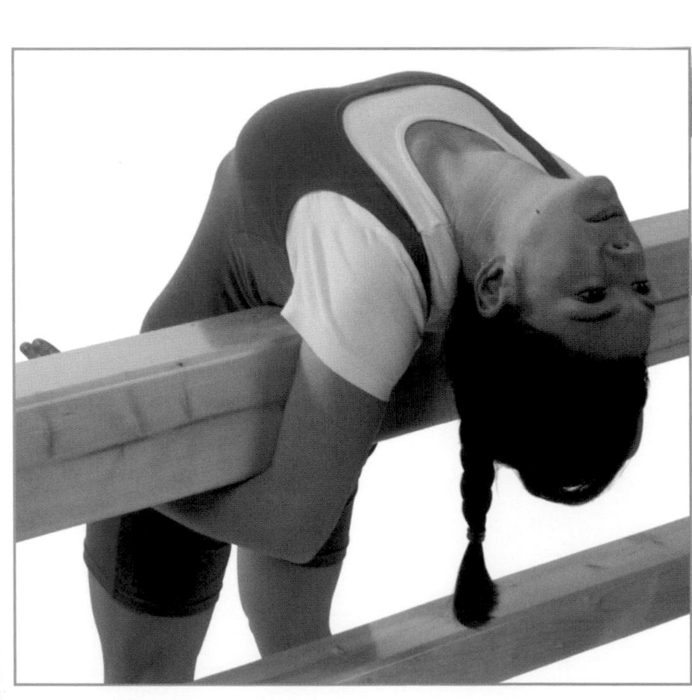

Ushtrasana, with Wall and Chair
Camel pose

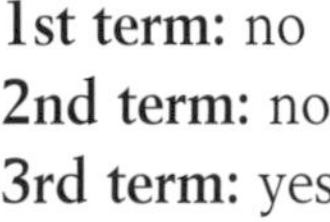

1st term: no
2nd term: no
3rd term: yes

1 Kneel in front of a wall and have a chair at your back.

2 Keep your knees and feet hip-width apart.

3 Tie a belt around your upper thighs.

4 Your shinbones are parallel, and your toes point straight back.

5 Put your hands on the chair.

6 Keep your thighs perpendicular. Your groin and pubic bone touch the wall.

7 Lengthen, extend, and lift your entire front torso.

Benefits

Gives an anti-gravitational lift to the spine, spinal muscles, and inner organs

Tones the kidneys

Relieves tension in the chest and breasts

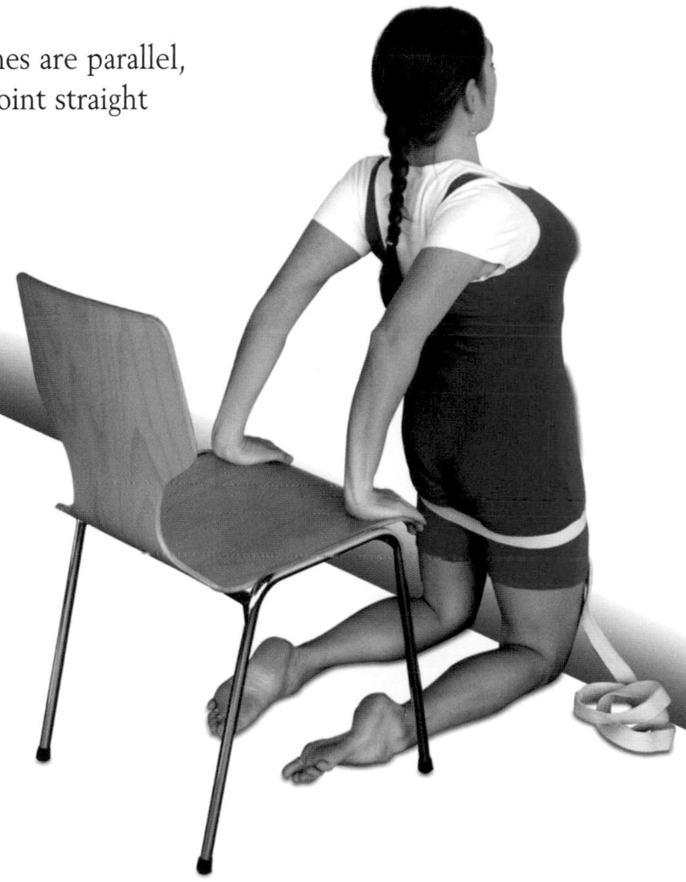

8 Tuck your buttocks in.

9 Lift your lower breastbone up and against the wall.

10 Move your dorsal (mid) spine in between your shoulder blades.

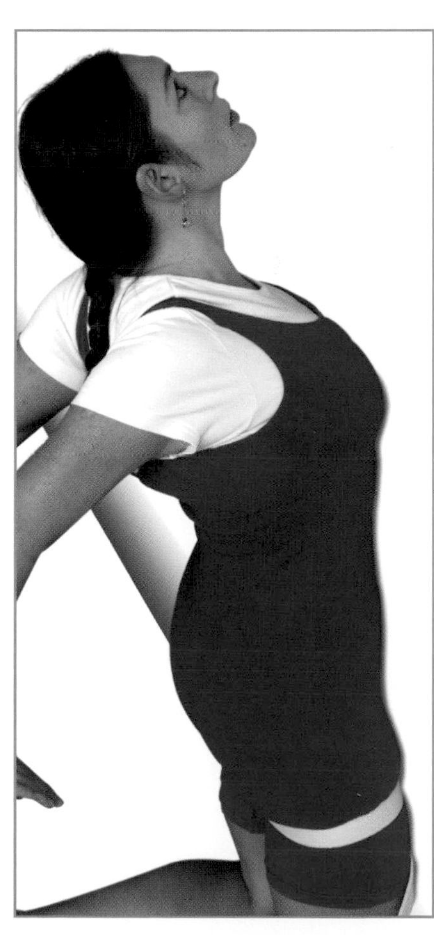

DETAILED DESCRIPTIONS OF ASANAS FOR BEGINNERS AND ADVANCED STUDENTS

11 Exhale, keep your chest well lifted, and curve your torso back.

12 Grip the front legs of the chair.

13 Pull from your hands to move your shoulder blades in and lift your chest further.

14 Keeping your neck long, bring your head back, and look behind you.

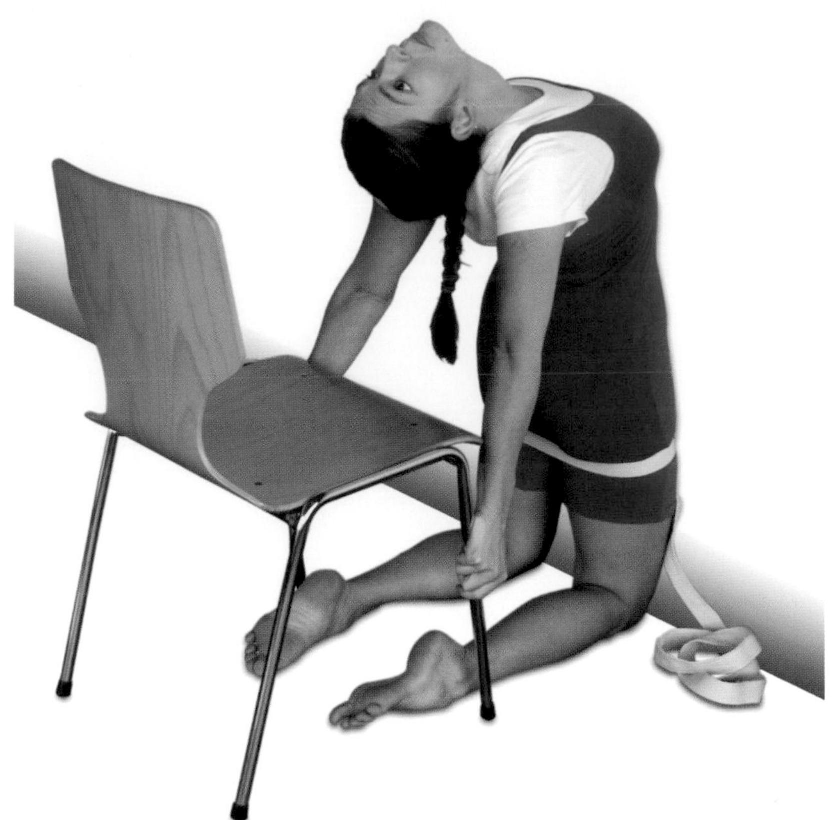

Coming out of the pose

1 Raise your head and bring your torso to the upright position by moving your hands up on the chair.

2 Sit in Virasana and put your arms up against the wall.

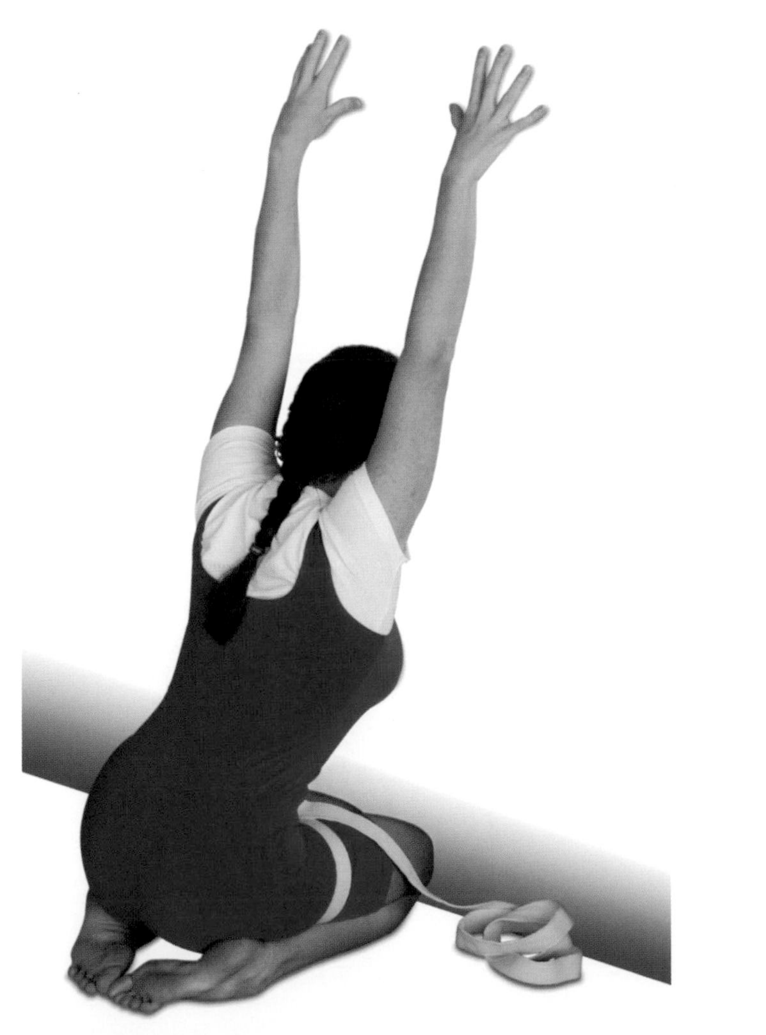

Rope Asanas
Yoga Kurunta

Ardha Uttanasana, with Ropes and Chair
Half intense forward stretch pose

1st term: no
2nd term: yes
3rd term: yes

Page 293

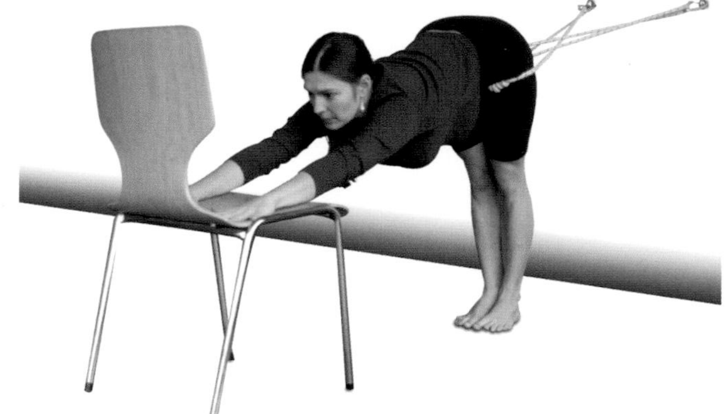

Adho Mukha Shvanasana, with Slanting Plank, Head Supported
Downward-facing dog pose

Pages 125, 214 and 299

Adho Mukha Shvanasana, with Block

1st term: no
2nd term: no
3rd term: yes

These rope asanas are ideal for the stage after delivery, when most new mothers feel loose and flabby. Using a rope, you can easily regain your sense of direction, that is, how to move and work certain muscles. With regular practice, you'll safely regain the body intelligence that tells you how and where to resist, extend, and expand.

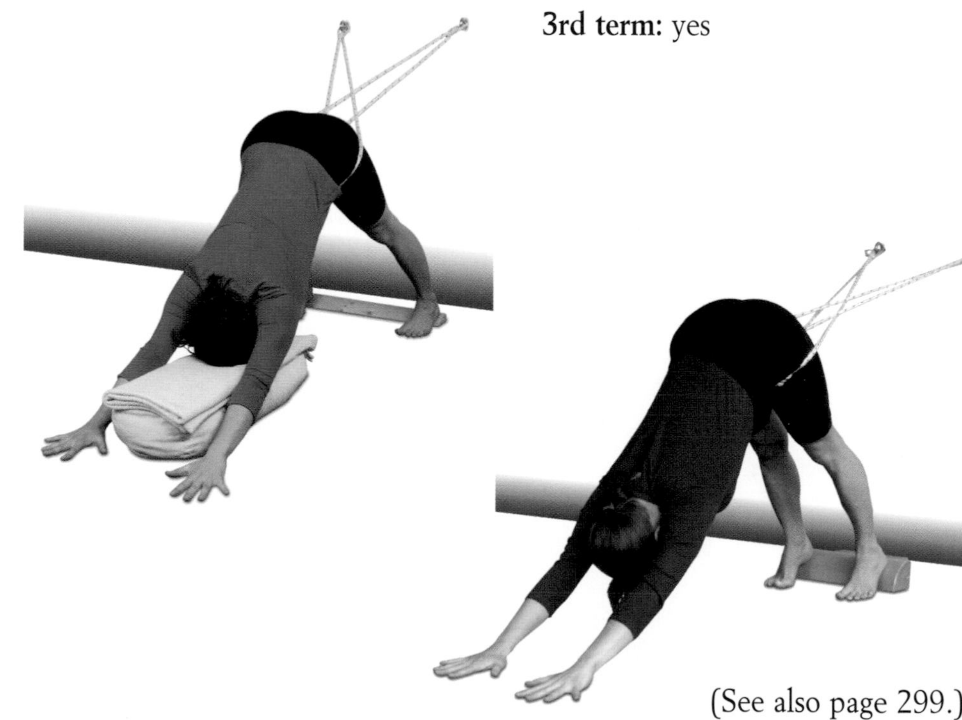

(See also page 299.)

Restorative Asanas
Vishranta Karaka Sthiti

Shavasana and Ujjayi Pranayama
Corpse pose

(For details see also pages 134 – 139 and pages 148 – 150).

During the First Month after a Normal Delivery
In the first month, you should practice only pranayama in Shavasana, which brings a balance between body and mind. Pranayama relieves fatigue and gives the body a proper rest.

It's important to take care of yourself after your delivery, not only during your pregnancy. Although you may be eager to get back in shape, you must get as much mental and physical rest as possible, even with a new baby. This is vital in the weeks after childbirth, while your uterus and other reproductive organs are gradually returning to their normal condition.

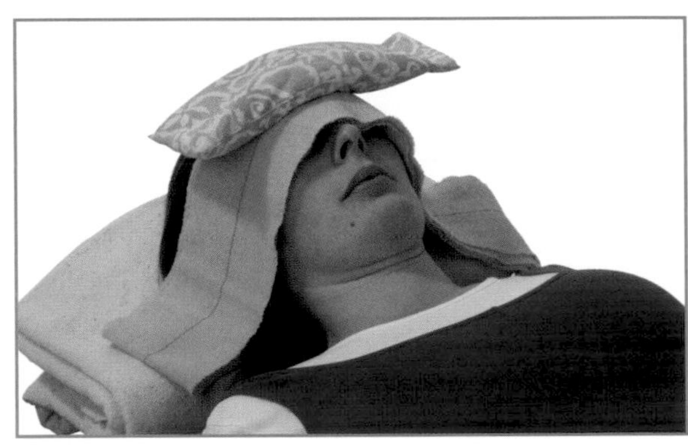

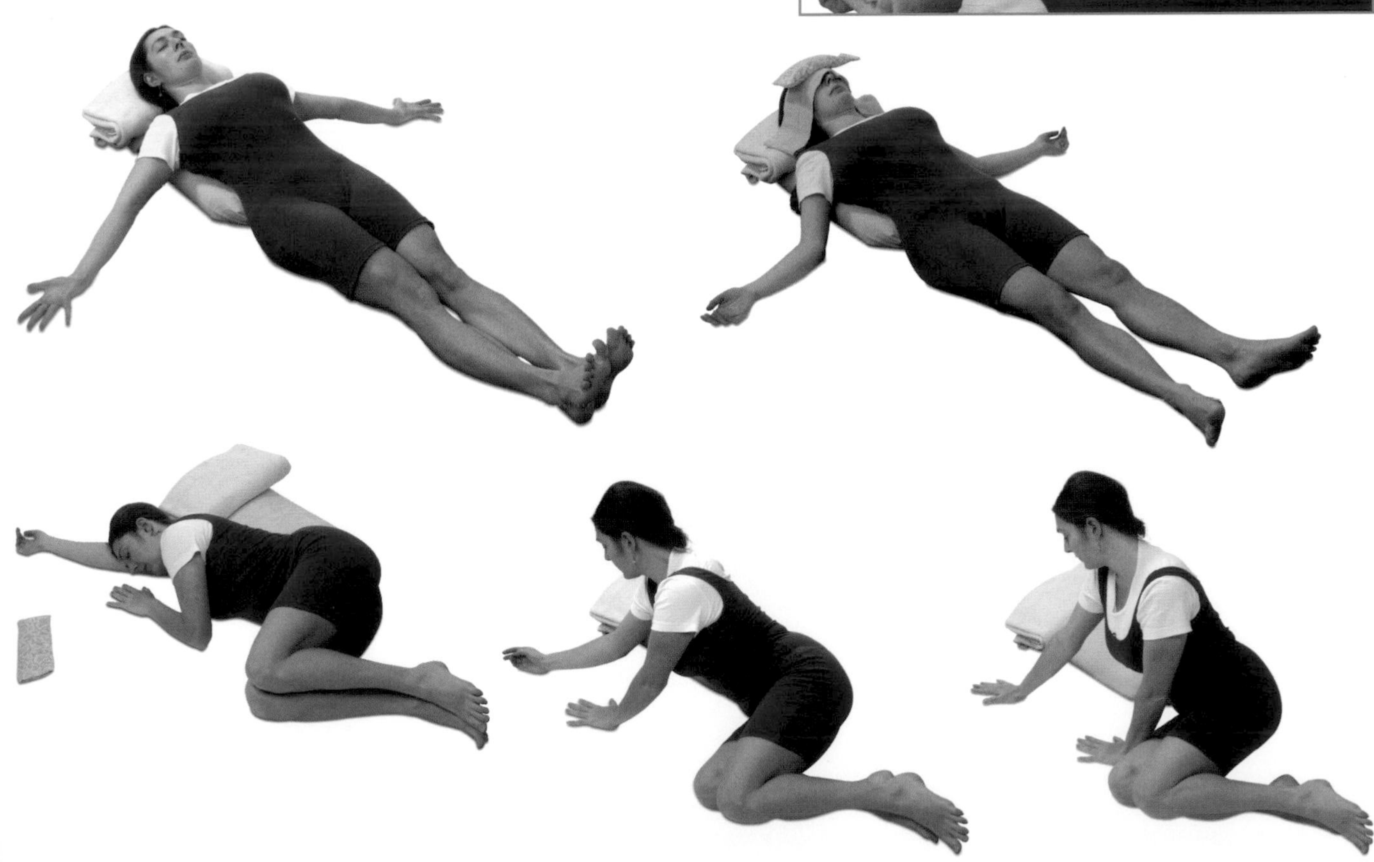

To avoid congestion and hardness of the breasts, practice asanas that open the chest, such as Setu Bandha Sarvangasana, Viparita Karani, and also Supta Baddha Konasana with the bolster crosswise, supporting the chest. Don't practice when your breasts are full; wait until after feeding.

Because it takes a lot of oxygen to make mother's milk, we recommend that you practice Shavasana and Ujjayi Pranayama 1, which increase the intake of oxygen, purify the milk, and help lactation.

General Guidelines

- Practice Shavasana often to feel rested and rejuvenated. If you suffer from back pain, use a bolster for your knees or a chair for your lower legs, as shown in Chapter 3, pages 138 – 139.
- After a cesarian section or other operation of the reproductive system, you should do Shavasana, Ujjayi Pranayama 1, and Viloma Pranayama 1 for about two months until the incision heals. After that, you can practice Salamba Sarvangasana, Setu Bandha Sarvangasana, Parvatasana, Janu Shirshasana, and Maha Mudra.

One Month after a Normal Delivery

On the following pages you can see the range of restorative asanas for all three terms after delivery. For detailed descriptions, see Chapter 3, "Restorative Asanas," page 126.

At this time, you can gradually begin practicing asanas, which will help you return to normal and maintain your health. If, and only if, the vaginal discharge after delivery (lochia) has stopped, you can resume the restorative poses:

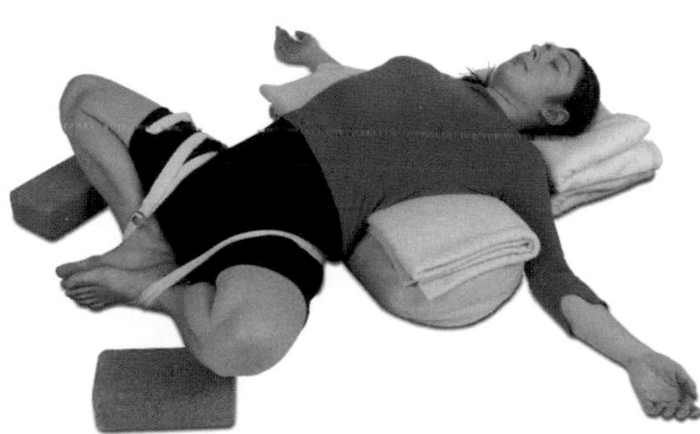

Supta Baddha Konasana (bolster crosswise, knees supported)

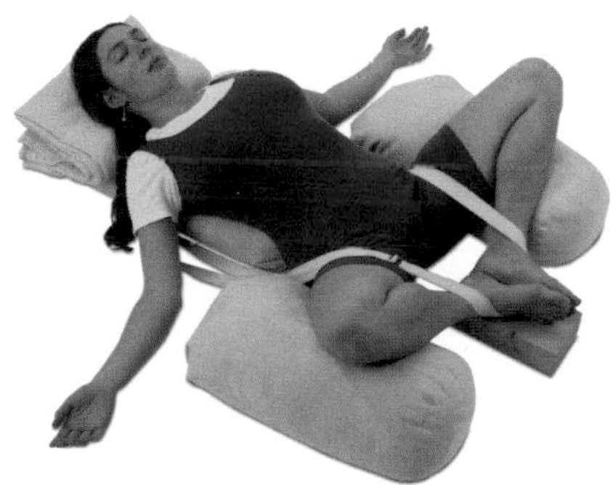

Supta Baddha Konasana (bolster lengthwise, knees supported, feet on block)

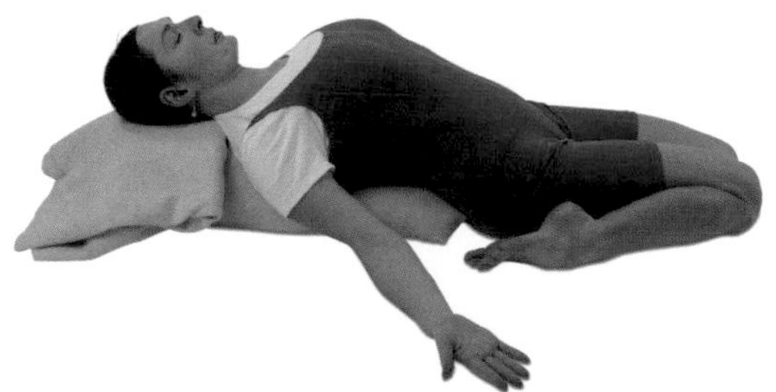

Supta Virasana (bolster/s)

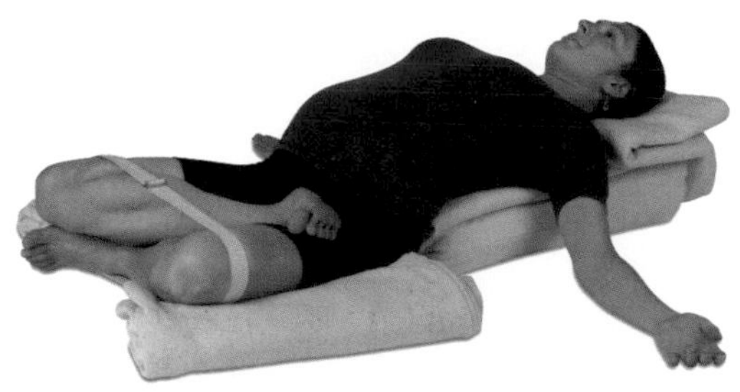

Matsyasana (bolster/s)

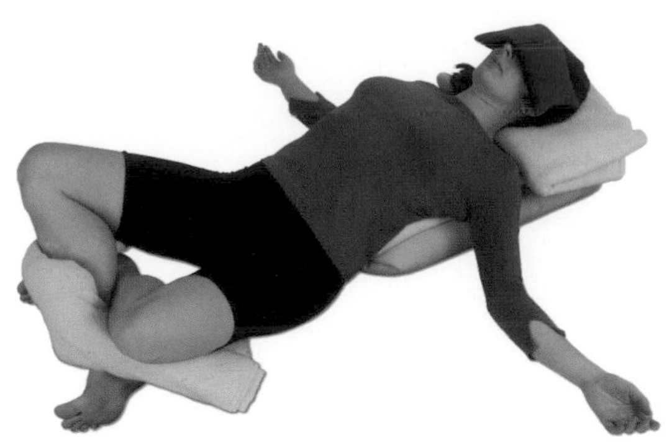

Supta Svastikasana (bolster/s)

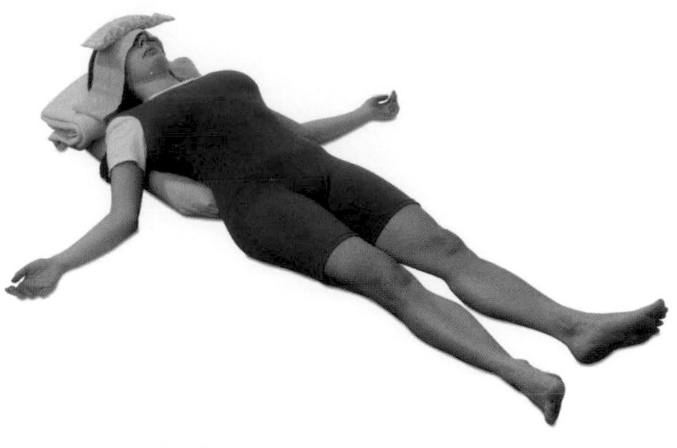

Shavasana (bolster/s)

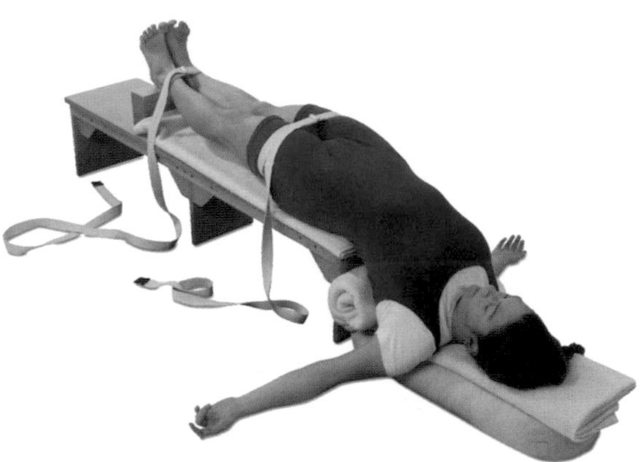

Setu Bandha Sarvangasana (bench or similar)

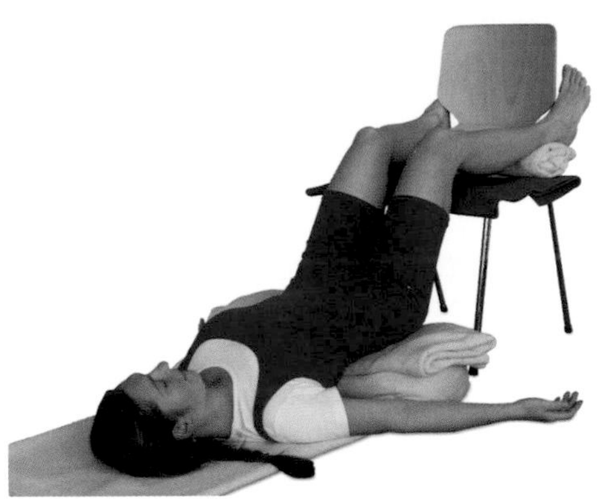

Viparita Karani (legs bent on chair in the 1st term)

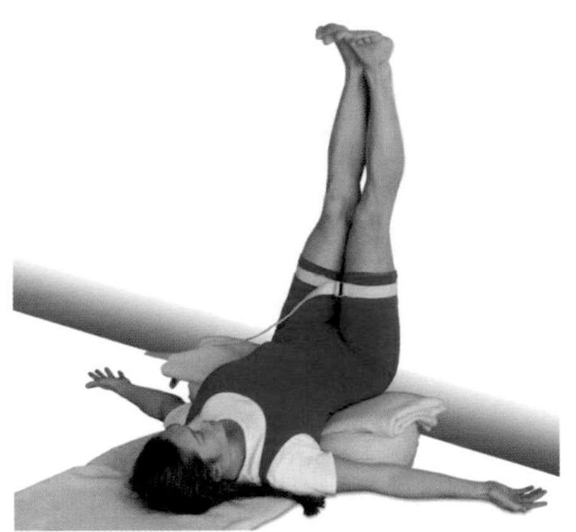

Viparita Karani (straight legs in the 2nd and 3rd terms)

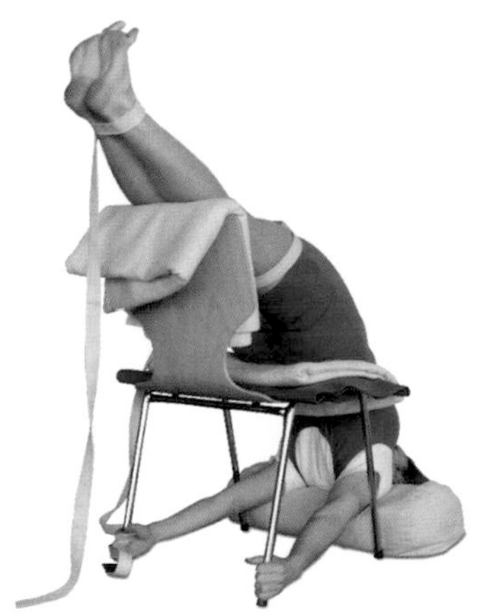

Salamba Sarvangasana (chair in 2nd and 3rd terms)

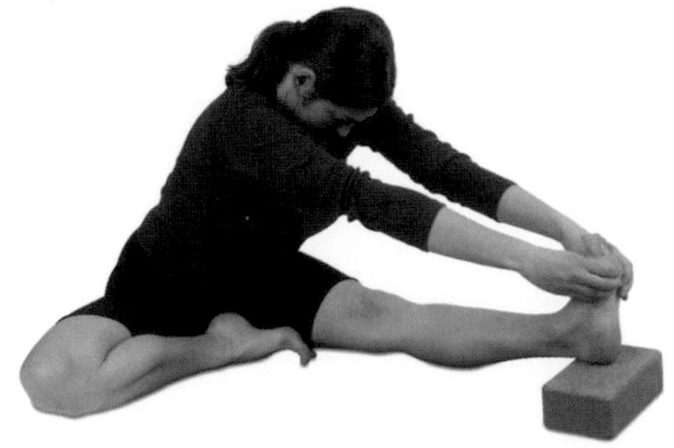

Maha Mudra (belt around foot, heel on block)

DETAILED DESCRIPTIONS OF ASANAS FOR BEGINNERS AND ADVANCED STUDENTS

Pranayama

Breathing Techniques

Ujjayi 1 and Viloma 1, Lying on a Bolster

Ocean breath 1 and interrupted 1 pose

1st term: yes
2nd term: yes
3rd term: yes

For detailed instructions, see pages 148 – 151.

After delivery, you should have mental peace, a proper diet, sufficient rest, and a relaxed body and mind. On the one hand, your body is undergoing important changes as your uterus lowers to its original position in the pelvic cavity, and on the other, you must recover your energy and health to nurse your baby. If you're agitated and annoyed, you can't provide high quality, nourishing milk.

During the first month, practicing pranayama not only provides the relaxation and renewal of energy that you need, but actually increases your oxygen intake to maximize the production and purity of your breast milk. For these purposes, we recommend that you concentrate on Shavasana and Ujjayi Pranayama.

Reminder of General Guidelines

Do a lot of Shavasana to feel energized and rejuvenated. Practicing Ujjayi in Shavasana increases your vitality and psychologically reduces your urge to "get out of the house" and overdo it. After a cesarian section or similar operation, practice Shavasana, Ujjayi Pranayama 1, and Viloma Pranayama 1 until the incision heals, about two months. Don't start any asanas less than a month after your delivery or before the vaginal discharge after delivery has stopped.

Maha Mudra

1st term: yes
2nd term: yes
3rd term: yes

For detailed instructions, see page 304.

When you practice Maha Mudra after delivery, you should lift your lower abdomen upward to lift the pelvic and other inner organs.

The special breathing technique in Maha Mudra combines pranayama with a yogasana in such a way that it rejuvenates the internal organs, the spinal muscles, and the mind.

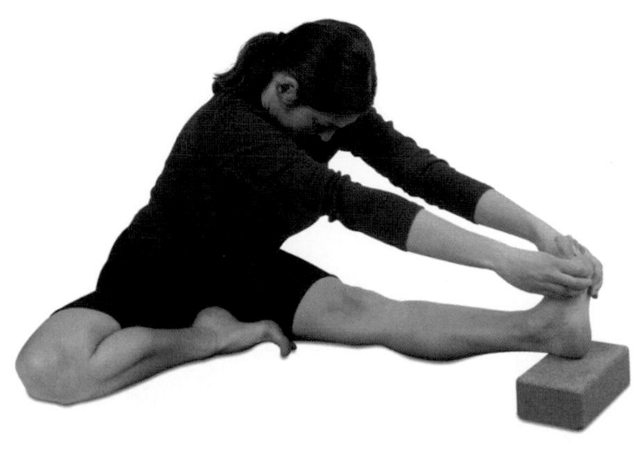

CHAPTER 9

PROBLEMS A – Z

This chapter serves as a quick reference to help you find the best asanas to relieve common problems you may experience during your pregnancy and after your delivery.

You'll see that in the "During Pregnancy" part of the book, you are usually directed to the pose as it is presented in Chapter 3, and in the "After Delivery" part, you are directed to poses that are presented in Chapter 8. In some cases, however, where the practice is the same, you are directed to Chapter 3 even after delivery. This is because the full instructions appear there.

For safety and health, please note the following *very important* guidelines for using this reference list:

- The chapter is divided into "During Pregnancy" and "After Delivery" sections; *be sure to consult only the section that applies to you.*
- The asanas are not divided into trimesters of pregnancy or terms after delivery. Please check the page given for each asana, or in the classification charts, to see whether your particular condition permits the practice of the pose. Check also whether the asana is for beginning or advanced students.
- When you go to the page listed here for each asana, we recommend that you read the entire chapter where it is found. This will complete the information you need about practicing the pose.
- The asanas are not necessarily listed in the order in which they should be practiced. If you're not sure how to work with them, we suggest you ask your Yoga teacher, or practice only the sequences as given elsewhere in the book.
- While these recommended asanas, in our experience, can help prevent or improve your condition, don't hesitate to consult your gynecologist or other physician for further medical help.

◇

During Pregnancy

Abdomen

- Heaviness: see **Heaviness**
- Muscle weakness: Parshvottanasana (Ch. 3, p. 49), Ardha Chandrasana (Ch. 3, p. 45), Dandasana (Ch. 3, p. 64)
- Pressure from the fetus: Ardha Chandrasana (Ch. 5, S. 1, p.198), Virabhadrasana 1 (Ch. 3, p. 52), Supta Baddha Konasana (Ch. 3, p. 126), Maha Mudra (Ch. 3, p. 79)
- Tightness of abdominal wall: Baddha Konasana (Ch. 3, p. 67), Supta Baddha Konasana (Ch. 3, p. 126), Upavishtha Konasana (Ch. 3, p. 70), Setu Bandha Sarvangasana (Ch. 3, p. 107)

Acidity

Sequence 5 (Ch. 3, p. 165), Prasarita Padottanasana (Ch. 3, p. 55)

Adrenal glands

Maha Mudra (Ch. 3, p. 79), Viparita Karani (Ch. 3, p. 112)

Anemia
Salamba Sarvangasana (Ch. 3, p. 102)

Ankle, sprain
Trianga Mukhaikapada Pashchimottanasana (Ch. 3, p. 89)

Anxiety
Supta Baddha Konasana (Ch. 3, p. 126), Virasana (Ch. 3, p. 72), Parvatasana from Virasana and Svastikasana (Ch. 3, p. 74), Ardha Chandrasana (Ch. 3, p. 45), Dvi Pada Viparita Dandasana (Ch. 3, p. 122), Bhujangasana with Ropes (Ch. 3, p. 119), Cross-bolsters (Ch. 3, p. 118), Chatushpadasana (Ch. 3, p. 111), Setu Banda Sarvangasana (Ch. 3, p. 107), Ujjayi Pranayama 1 and 2 (Ch. 3, p. 141), Viloma Pranayama 1 (Ch. 3, p. 151)

Appetite, lack of
Viparita Karani (Ch. 3, p. 112)

Arthritis
- Hip joint, knee, or sacroiliac joint: Utthita Parshvakonasana (Ch. 3, p. 40)
- Neck, shoulder, or elbow: Tadasana and variations (Ch. 3, p. 32)
- Wrist: Tadasana and variations (Ch. 3, p. 32), Parvatasana from Virasana and Svastikasana, (Ch. 3, p. 74)

Back pain
- Sequence 6 (Ch. 3, p. 166), Utthita Parshvakonasana (Ch. 3, p. 40), Parvatasana from Virasana and Svastikasana (Ch. 3, p. 74), Supta Svastikasana (Ch. 3, p. 131), Ardha Matsyasana (Ch. 3, p. 131), Virabhadrasana 3 (Ch. 3, p. 54), Ardha Uttanasana (Ch. 3, p. 159), Ardha Halasana (Ch. 3, p. 104)
- Upper: Tadasana and variations (Ch. 3, p. 32), Virabhadrasana 1 (Ch. 3, p. 52), Virabhadrasana 3 (Ch. 3, p. 54)

Bile
Sequence 2 (Ch. 3, p. 159), Supta Svastikasana (Ch. 3, p. 131), Ardha Matsyasana (Ch. 3, p. 131), Maha Mudra (Ch. 3, p. 79), Virabhadrasana 1 (Ch. 3, p. 52)

Bladder, incontinence, see **Urinary disorders**

Bloating, see **Flatulence**

Blood pressure, see **High blood pressure** or **Low blood pressure**

Blurred vision
Sequence 2 (Ch. 3, p. 159), Salamba Shirshasana (Ch. 3, p. 97), Viloma Pranayama 2 (Ch. 3, p. 152)

Breasts, tension
Supta Baddha Konasana (Ch. 3, p. 126), Ardha Chandrasana (Ch. 3, p. 45), Urdhva Dhanurasana with a Trestle (Ch. 3, p. 121), Shavasana (Ch. 3, p. 134)

Breath, shortness of
Sequence 5 (Ch. 3, p. 165), Utthita Parshvakonasana (Ch. 3, p. 40), Virabhadrasana 2 (Ch. 3, p. 42), Adho Mukha Shvanasana (Ch. 3, p. 62), Ardha Uttanasana (Ch. 3, p. 59), Supta Virasana (Ch. 3, p. 129, Ch. 8, p. 367), Prasarita Padottanasana (Ch. 3, p. 55), Baddha Konasana (Ch. 3, p. 67), Upavishtha Konasana (Ch. 3, p. 70), Maha Mudra (Ch. 3, p. 79), Parvatasana from Virasana and Svastikasana (Ch. 3, p. 74), Salamba Purvottanasana (Ch. 3, p. 122), Ujjayi Pranayama 1 and 2 (Ch. 3, p. 148)

Burning sensation
Baddha Konasana (Ch. 3, p. 67), Upavishtha Konasana (Ch. 3, p. 70)

Confidence, lack of, see **Anxiety**

Constipation
Sequence, 2 (Ch. 3, p. 159), Sequence for First Trimester and throughout Pregnancy (Ch. 4, p. 172), Bharadvajasana 1 (Ch. 3, p. 91)

Contractions, see **Labor Pains**

Courage, lack of, see **Anxiety**

Cramps, in calves
Tadasana with Wall and Quarter-round block (Ch. 3, p. 33), Adho Mukha Shvanasana (Ch. 3, p. 62), Virasana (Ch. 3, p. 72), Ardha Chandrasana (Ch. 3, p. 45), Salamba Shirshasana (Ch. 3, p. 97)

Depression
Adho Mukha Shvanasana (Ch. 3, p. 62), Dvi Pada Viparita Dandasana (Ch. 3, p. 122), Ardha Uttanasana (Ch. 3, p. 59), Cross-bolsters (Ch. 3, p. 118), Ardha Chandrasana (Ch. 3, p. 45), Virabhadrasana 1 (Ch. 3, p. 52), Salamba Shirshasana (Ch. 3, p. 97), Setu Bandha Sarvangasana (Ch. 3, p. 107), Chatushpadasana (Ch. 3, p. 111)

Diabetes
Sequence 4 (Ch. 3, p. 163), Adho Mukha Virasana (Ch. 3, p. 76)

Diaphragm
- Heaviness: Salamba Purvottanasana (Ch. 3, p. 126)
- Tension: Supta Baddha Konasana (Ch. 3, p. 126)

Digestion, see **Indigestion**

Discharge, vaginal, see **Leukorrhea**

Disk, slipped
Bharadvajasana 1 (Ch. 3, p. 91), Virabhadrasana 1 (Ch. 3, p. 52), Virabhadrasana 3 (Ch. 3, p. 54), Prasarita Padottanasana (Ch. 3, p. 55)

Dizziness
Sequence 2 (Ch. 3, p. 159), Parshva Janu Shirshasana: Twisting (Ch. 3, p. 95)

Edema
Sequence for First Trimester and throughout Pregnancy (Ch. 4, p. 172), Viparita Karani (Ch. 3, p. 112)

Elbow joint, stiffness
Tadasana and variations (Ch. 3, p. 32)

Endurance, lack of
Viloma Pranayama 1 (Ch. 3, p. 151)

Energy, lack of, see **Fatigue**

Fatigue
- Mental: Ardha Uttanasana (Ch. 3, p. 59), Urdhva Dhanurasana with a Trestle (Ch. 3, p. 121), Salamba Sarvangasana (Ch. 3, p. 102), Setu Bandha Sarvangasana (Ch. 3, p. 107), Restorative Asanas (Ch. 3, p. 126)
- Physical: Sequence 2 (Ch. 3, p. 159), training Sequence for First Trimester and throughout Pregnancy (Ch. 4, p. 172), Ardha Chandrasana (Ch. 3, p. 45), Ardha Uttanasana with Ropes and a Chair (Ch. 3, p. 61), Parshva Janu Shirshasana: Twisting (Ch. 3, p. 94), Chatushpadasana (Ch. 3, p. 111), Restorative Asanas (Ch. 3, p. 126), Viloma Pranayama 1 (Ch. 3, p. 151)

Feet
- Pain or heaviness: Virasana (Ch. 3, p. 72), Trianga Mukhaikapada Pashchimottanasana (Ch. 3, p. 89)
- Swollen: see Edema

Fever, persistent
Janu Shirshasana (Ch. 3, p. 82)

Flatulence
Utthita Parshvakonasana (Ch. 3, p. 40), Virabhadrasana 1 (Ch. 3, p. 52), Parvatasana from Virasana and Svastikasana (Ch. 3, p. 74), Bharadvajasana 1 (Ch. 3, p. 91), Supta Baddha Konasana (Ch. 3, p. 126), Maha Mudra (Ch. 3, p. 79), Salamba Sarvangasana (Ch. 3, p. 102), Parshva Shirshasana (Ch. 5, p. 230)

Forgetfulness
Adho Mukha Shvanasana (Ch. 3, p. 62)

Gallbladder, see **Bile**

Gas, see **Flatulence**

Gastritis
Bharadvajasana 1 (Ch. 3, p. 91), see also **Acidity**

Genital organs, irritation
Janu Shirshasana (Ch. 3, p. 82), Baddha Konasana (Ch. 3, p. 67), Upavishtha Konasana (Ch. 3, p. 70)

Genitalia, irritation, see **Genital organs, irritation**

Groin, stiffness
Upavishtha Konasana (Ch. 3, p. 70), Baddha Konasana (Ch. 3, p. 67), Trianga Mukhaikapada Pashchimottanasana (Ch. 3, p. 89)

Headache
Sequence for First Trimester and throughout Pregnancy (Ch. 4, p. 172), Adho Mukha Shvanasana (Ch. 3, p. 62)

Heartburn, see **Acidity**

Heaviness
• Sequence for First Trimester and throughout Pregnancy (Ch. 4, p. 172), Ardha Chandrasana (Ch. 3, p. 45), Setu Bandha Sarvangasana (Ch. 3, p. 107)
• Abdomen: Virabhadrasana 1 (Ch. 3, p. 52), Parshvottanasana (Ch. 3, p. 49), Prasarita Padottanasana (Ch. 3, p. 55), Janu Shirshasana (Ch. 3, p. 82), Supta Baddha Konasana (Ch. 3, p. 126), Salamba Purvottanasana (Ch. 3, p. 126), Viloma Pranayama 2 (Ch. 3, p. 152)
• Chest and upper back: Urdhva Dhanurasana with a Trestle (Ch. 3, p. 121)
• Heart: Salamba Purvottanasana (Ch. 3, p. 126), Cross-bolsters (Ch. 3, p. 118), Supta Baddha Konasana, variation with bolster crosswise (Ch. 3, p. 128)
• Lower back: Supta Svastikasana (Ch. 3, p. 131), Janu Shirshasana (Ch. 3, p. 82)
• Pelvic region: Prasarita Padottanasana (Ch. 3, p. 55), Supta Svastikasana (Ch. 3, p. 131), Trianga Mukhaikapada Pashchimottanasana (Ch. 3, p. 89)
• Uterus: Ardha Supta Konasana (Ch. 3, p. 106), Parshvottanasana (Ch. 3, p. 49), Ardha Uttanasana, with Ropes and a Chair (Ch. 3, p. 59), Ardha Uttanasana (Ch. 3, p. 61)

High blood pressure
Sequence 3 (Ch. 3, p. 161), Virasana (Ch. 3, p. 72), Adho Mukha Virasana (Ch. 3, p. 76), Ardha Uttanasana (Ch. 3, p. 59), Viloma Pranayama 2 (Ch. 3, p. 152)

Hip joint, stiffness
Virasana (Ch. 3, p. 72), Upavishtha Konasana (Ch. 3, p. 70), Baddha Konasana (Ch. 3, p. 67), Supta Padangushthasana 2 (Ch. 3, p. 115)

Indigestion
Supta Svastikasana (Ch. 3, p. 131), Ardha Matsyasana (Ch. 3, p. 131), Virabhadrasana 1 (Ch. 3, p. 52), Prasarita Padottanasana (Ch. 3, p. 55), Maha Mudra (Ch. 3, p. 79), Ardha Uttanasana (Ch. 3, p. 59)

Insomnia
Ardha Halasana (Ch. 3, p. 104)

Itching
Baddha Konasana (Ch. 3, p. 67), Supta Virasana (Ch. 3, p. 129), Supta Baddha Konasana (Ch. 3, p. 126)

In Vitro Fertilization (Ch. 2, p. 14)

Kidneys
Ardha Chandrasana (Ch. 3, p. 45), Utthita Parshvakonasana (Ch. 3, p. 40), Virabhadrasana 1 (Ch. 3, p. 52), Virabhadrasana 2 (Ch. 3, p. 42), Dandasana (Ch. 3, p. 64), Maha Mudra (Ch. 3, p. 79), Virasana (Ch. 3, p. 72), Supta Baddha Konasana (Ch. 3, p. 126), Upavishtha Konasana

(Ch. 3, p. 70), Pashchimottanasana (Ch. 3, p. 87), Chatushpadasana (Ch. 3, p. 111), Ardha Halasana (Ch. 3, p. 104), Ardha Supta Konasana (Ch. 3, p. 106), Twists (Ch. 3, p. 91), Janu Shirshasana (Ch. 3, p. 82), Viparita Karani (Ch. 3, p. 112), Shavasana (Ch. 3, p. 134)

Knees, sprains in
Trianga Mukhaikapada Pashchimottanasana (Ch. 3, p. 89)

Labor pains
Adho Mukha Virasana (Ch. 3, p. 76), Malasana, modified (Ch. 3, p. 77), Ujjayi Pranayama (Ch. 3, p. 141, Ch. 5, p. 240), Viloma Pranayama (Ch. 3, p. 141, Ch. 5, p. 240)

Legs, swelling, see **Edema**

Leukorrhea (vaginal discharge, white)
Baddha Konasana (Ch. 3, p. 67), Upavishtha Konasana (Ch. 3, p. 70), Ardha Supta Konasana (Ch. 3, p. 106), Salamba Shirshasana (Ch. 3, p. 97)

Liver, see **Bile**

Low blood pressure
Sequence 2 (Ch. 3, p. 159)

Lumbago, see **Back pain**

Lumbar area, stiff, see **Back pain**

Lung capacity, see **Breath, shortness of**

Miscarriage, disposition toward
Miscarriages and Potential Solutions (Ch. 2, pp. 22 – 24), Trianga Mukhaikapada Pashchimottanasana (Ch. 3,p. 89)

Moodiness
Adho Mukha Shvanasana (Ch. 3, p. 62), Salamba Sarvangasana with a Chair (Ch. 3, p. 102)

Morning sickness
Sequence for First Trimester and throughout Pregnancy (Ch. 4, p. 172), Virabhadrasana 2 (Ch. 3, p. 42), Parshvottanasana (Ch. 3, p. 49), Ardha Chandrasana (Ch. 3, p. 45), Virabhadrasana 1 (Ch. 3, p. 52), Prasarita Padottanasana (Ch. 3, p. 55)

Nausea
Ardha Chandrasana (Ch. 3, p. 45), Prasarita Padottanasana (Ch. 3, p. 55), Upavishtha Konasana (Ch. 3, p. 70), Maha Mudra (Ch. 3, p. 79), Twists (Ch. 3, p. 91), Viloma Pranayama 2 (Ch. 3, p. 152)

Neck pain
Tadasana and variations (Ch. 3, p. 32), Utthita Trikonasana (Ch. 3, p. 38), Twists (Ch. 3, p. 91)

Nervousness
Ardha Chandrasana (Ch. 3, p. 45), Prasarita Padottanasana (Ch. 3, p. 55), Adho Mukha Shvanasana (Ch. 3, p. 62), Viparita Karani (Ch. 3, p. 112), Salamba Purvottanasana (Ch. 3, p. 126), Cross-bolsters (Ch. 3, p. 118), Chatushpadasana (Ch. 3, p. 111), Ardha Halasana (Ch. 3, p. 104), Ardha Uttanasana with Ropes and a Chair (Ch. 3, p. 61), Salamba Sarvangasana with a Chair (Ch. 3, p. 102), Ardha Halasana (Ch. 3, p. 104), Setu Bandha Sarvangasana (Ch. 3, p. 107, Ch. 8, p. 334), Shavasana (Ch. 3, p. 134), Ujjayi Pranayama 1 and 2 (Ch. 3, p. 141), Viloma Pranayama 1 and 2 (Ch. 3, pp. 151 – 152)

Overactivity
Viloma Pranayama 2 (Ch. 3, p. 152), Salamba Shirshasana (Ch. 3, p. 97), Salamba Sarvangasana (Ch. 3, p. 102), Ardha Halasana (Ch. 3, p. 104)

Pain during contractions, see **Labor pains**

Pelvic region
- Poor blood circulation: Upavishtha Konasana (Ch. 3, p. 70), Pashchimottanasana (Ch. 3, p. 87)

• Pressure on pelvic floor (and pudendal nerve): Ardha Chandrasana (Ch. 3, p. 45)
• Tightness: Parshvottanasana (Ch. 3, p. 49), Utthita Hasta Padangushthasana 2 (Ch. 3, p. 116), Supta Padangushthasana 2 (Ch. 3, p. 115)

Perspiration, excess body heat
Janu Shirshasana (Ch. 3, p. 82), Adho Mukha Shvanasana (Ch. 3, p. 62), Ardha Halasana (Ch. 3, p. 104), Viloma Pranayama 2 (Ch. 3, p. 152)

Pituitary gland
Setu Bandha Sarvangasana (Ch. 3, p. 107)

Placenta, insufficiency
Ardha Chandrasana (Ch. 3, p. 45)

Preeclampsia, see **Toxemia**

Respiratory system, weakness of
Salamba Shirshasana (Ch. 3, p. 97), Dvi Pada Viparita Dandasana (Ch. 3, p. 122), Salamba Sarvangasana (Ch. 3, p. 102)

Rheumatism
Utthita Hasta Padangushthasana 2 (Ch. 3, p. 116), Virabhadrasana 1 (Ch. 3, p. 52), Virabhadrasana 3 (Ch. 3, p. 54), Ardha Halasana (Ch. 3, p. 104)

Sacroiliac joint, pain, see **Back pain**

Sciatica
Utthita Parshvakonasana (Ch. 3, p. 40), Supta Padangushthasana 2 (Ch. 3, p. 115), Utthita Hasta Padangushthasana 2 (Ch. 3, p. 116), Virabhadrasana 3 (Ch. 3, p. 54)

Self-confidence, lack of, see **Anxiety**

Shoulder joint, stiffness
Tadasana and variations (Ch. 3, p. 32), Virabhadrasana 1 (Ch. 3, p. 52), Virabhadrasana 3 (Ch. 3, p. 54), Twists (Ch. 3, pp. 91 – 95)

Sleeplessnes, see **Insomnia**

Spinal muscles, weakness, see **Back pain**

Spine, lower
• Stiffness and pain: see **Back pain**
• Weakness: Utthita Trikonasana (Ch. 3, p. 38), Utthita Parshvakonasana (Ch. 3, p. 40), Pashchimottanasana, Concave Back (Ch. 3, p. 87), Parshva Janu Shirshasana (Ch. 3, p. 94), Utthita Hasta Padangushthasana 2 (Ch. 3, p. 116)

Spleen
Maha Mudra (Ch. 3, p. 79), Janu Shirshasana (Ch. 3, p. 82), Supta Svastikasana (Ch. 3, p. 131), Ardha Matsyasana (Ch. 3, p. 131), Twists (Ch. 3, pp. 91 – 95)

Stiffness, see **Elbow joint, Hip joint, Shoulder joint, Sacroiliac joint, Neck pain, Back pain, Wrist, stiffness**

Stomach
• Heaviness: Supta Baddha Konasana (Ch. 3, p. 126)
• Pain: Ardha Uttanasana (Ch. 3, p. 59), Supta Svastikasana (Ch. 3, p. 131), Ardha Matsyasana (Ch. 3, p. 131), Virabhadrasana 1 (Ch. 3, p. 52)

Stress
Viloma Pranayama 1 (Ch. 3, p. 151)

Swelling, see **Edema**

Tailbone
Pain: Utthita Parshvakonasana (Ch. 3, p. 40), Virabhadrasana 2 (Ch. 3, p. 42), Ardha Chandrasana (Ch. 3, p. 45), Virabhadrasana 1 (Ch. 3, p. 52), Adho Mukha Shvanasana (Ch. 3, p. 62), Janu Shirshasana (Ch. 3, p. 82), Bhujangasana with Ropes (Ch. 3, p. 119), Dvi Pada Viparita Dandasana (Ch. 3, p. 122),

Supta Padangushthasana 2 (Ch. 3, p. 115), Ardha Parshvaika Pada Sarvangasana (Ch. 5, p. 223)

Tension
Supta Baddha Konasana (Ch. 3, p. 126), Salamba Purvottanasana (Ch. 3, p. 122), Cross-bolsters (Ch. 3, p. 118), Setu Bandha Sarvangasana (Ch. 3, p. 107), Shavasana (Ch. 3, p. 134), Viloma Pranayama 2 (Ch. 3, p. 152)

Thyroid gland
Sequence for Mental Stability (Ch. 2, p. 17), Sequence for Physical and Physiological Stability: Preparing the Ground (Ch. 2, p. 18), Supta Svastikasana (Ch. 3, p. 131), Ardha Matsyasana (Ch. 3, p. 131), Viparita Karani (Ch. 3, p. 112)

Tightness of abdominal wall, see **Abdomen**

Tiredness, see **Fatigue**

Toxemia
Sequence 3 (Ch. 3, p. 161)

Ulcers, see **Acidity** and **Gastritis**

Urinary disorders
- Sequence 2 (Ch. 3, p. 159)
- Bladder control: Trianga Mukhaikapada Pashchimottanasana (Ch. 3, p. 89), Janu Shirshasana (Ch. 3, p. 82), Maha Mudra (Ch. 3, p. 79), Twists (Ch. 3, p. 21), Salamba Sarvangasana with chair (Ch. 3, p. 102)
- Frequent urination: Baddha Konasana (Ch. 3, p. 67), Upavishtha Konasana (Ch. 3, p. 70)
- Urinary tract infection: Baddha Konasana (Ch. 3, p. 67), Twists (Ch. 3, p. 21), Ardha Halasana (Ch. 3, p. 104), Setu Bandha Sarvangasana (Ch. 3, p. 107)

Uterus
- Pain: Ardha Supta Konasana (Ch. 3, p. 106), Supta Baddha Konasana (Ch. 3, p. 126)
- Prematurely dilated cervix: Sequence 1 (Ch. 3, p. 157)
- Prolapse: Maha Mudra (Ch. 3, p. 79), Ardha Halasana (Ch. 3, p. 104)

Vagina
- Burning sensation: Supta Baddha Konasana (Ch. 3, p. 126)
- Compression of: Supta Baddha Konasana (Ch. 3, p. 126), Upavishtha Konasana (Ch. 3, p. 84)

Vaginal discharge, see **Leukorrhea**

Varicose Veins
Sequence for First Trimester and throughout Pregnancy (Ch. 4, p. 172)

Vision, see **Blurred vision**

Vomiting
Ardha Chandrasana (Ch. 3, p. 45), Maha Mudra (Ch. 3, p. 79), Viparita Karani (Ch. 3, p. 112), Salamba Shirshasana (Ch. 3, p. 97)

Water retention, see **Edema**

Weakness, see **Fatigue**

Willpower, lack of
Chatushpadasana (Ch. 3, p. 111)

Wrist, stiffness
Tadasana and variations (Ch. 3, p. 32)

After Delivery

Abdominal muscles, weak
Sequence for the 3rd term: Back to Normal (Ch. 8, p. 264), Twists (Ch. 8, p. 318), Asanas for Abdomen and Lumbar (Ch. 8, p. 341)

Abdominal and pelvic organs, weakness
Sequence for the 2nd Term: Active–Passive (Ch. 8, p. 257), Virabhadrasana 3 (Ch. 8, p. 289), Prasarita Padottanasana (Ch. 8, p. 296), Pashchimottanasana (Ch. 8, p. 308), all asanas in Ch. 8.

Adrenal glands
Maha Mudra (Ch. 8, p. 304), Viparita Karani Mudra (Ch. 8, p. 336)

Anemia
Salamba Sarvangasana (Ch. 8, p. 326)

Ankle, sprain
Trianga Mukhaikapada Pashchimottanasana (Ch. 8, p. 312)

Anxiety
Parvatasana from Svastikasana and Virasana (Ch. 8, pp. 302 – 303), Ardha Chandrasana (Ch. 8, p. 283), Dvi Pada Viparita Dandasana (Ch. 8, p. 360), Chatushpadasana (Ch. 8, p. 335), Setu Banda Sarvangasana (Ch. 8, p. 334), Ujjayi Pranayama 1 and 2 (Ch. 3, pp. 148 – 149), Viloma Pranayama 1 (Ch. 3, p. 151)

Appetite, lack of
Viparita Karani Mudra (Ch. 8, p. 336)

Arthritis
- Hip joint, knee, or sacroiliac joint: Utthita Parshvakonasana (Ch. 8, p. 282)
- Neck, shoulder, or elbow: Tadasana and variations (Ch. 8, p. 274)
- Wrist: Tadasana and variations (Ch. 8, p. 274), Parvatasana from Svastikasana and Virasana (Ch. 8, pp. 302 – 303)

Back pain
- Utthita Trikonasana (Ch. 3, p. 38), Utthita Parshvakonasana (Ch. 8, p. 282), Ardha Chandrasana (Ch. 8, p. 283), Parvatasana from Svastikasana and Virasana (Ch. 8, pp. 302 – 303), Supta Padangushthasana 2 (Ch. 8, p. 343), Utthita Hasta Padangushthasana 2 (Ch. 8, p. 345), Supta Svastikasana (Ch. 3, p. 131), Ardha Matsyasana (Ch. 3, p. 131), Virabhadrasana 3 (Ch. 8, p. 289), Twists (Ch. 8, p. 318), Ardha Uttanasana (Ch.8, p. 292), Pashchimottanasana (Ch. 8, p. 308)
- Upper back: Tadasana and variations (Ch. 8, p. 274), Parivritta Trikonasana (Ch. 8, p. 290), Virabhadrasana 1 (Ch. 3, p. 52), Virabhadrasana 3 (Ch. 8, p. 289), Bharadvajasana (Ch. 8, p. 319)

Bile
Supta Svastikasana (Ch. 3, p. 131), Ardha Matsyasana (Ch. 3, p. 131), Maha Mudra (Ch. 8, p. 304), Virabhadrasana 1 (Ch. 3, p. 52), Janu Shirshasana (Ch. 8, p. 306), Pashchimottanasana (Ch. 8, p. 308), Twists (Ch. 8, p. 318), Jathara Parivartanasana (Ch. 8, p. 356)

Bladder
- Enlarged: Twists (Ch. 8, p. 318)
- Incontinence: see **Urinary disorders**

Bloating, see **Flatulence**

Blood pressure, see **High blood pressure** and **Low blood pressure**

Blurred vision
Salamba Shirshasana (Ch. 8, p. 338), Viloma Pranayama 2 (Ch. 3, p. 152)

Breast glands, underdeveloped
Dvi Pada Viparita Dandasana (Ch. 8, p. 360)

Breast milk, low quantity
Shavasana (Ch. 3, p. 134), Ujjayi Pranayama 1

and 2 (Ch. 3, pp. 148 – 149), Salamba Shirshasana (Ch. 8, p. 337), Salamba Sarvangasana (Ch. 8, p. 338)

Breasts
- Hardness: Back bends (Ch. 8, p. 360), Setu Bandha Sarvangasana (Ch. 8, p. 334), Viparita Karani Mudra (Ch. 8, p. 336), Restorative Asanas (Ch. 3, p.126)
- Heaviness (when breasts are full): Supta Baddha Konasana (Ch. 3, p. 126), Shavasana (Ch. 3, p. 134), Ujjayi Pranayama 1 (Ch. 3, p. 148)
- Congestion: Supta Baddha Konasana (Ch. 3, p. 126), Shavasana (Ch. 3, p. 134), Ujjayi Pranayama 1 (Ch. 3, p. 148)

Cesarean section
Sequences for Terms 1 – 3, After a Cesarian Section (Ch. 7, p. 251)

Congestion, breasts, see **Breasts**

Confidence, lack of, see **Anxiety**

Courage, lack of, see **Anxiety**

Cramps, abdominal
Supta Padangushthasana 1 and 2 (Ch. 8, pp. 342 – 343), Utthita Hasta Padangushthasana 1 and 2 (Ch. 8, p. 344), Paripurna Navasana (Ch. 8, p. 347), Urdhva Prasarita Padasana 1 (Ch. 8, p. 351) Restorative Asanas (Ch. 8, p. 366)

Depression, see **Postpartum depression**

Digestion, see **Indigestion**

Discharge, vaginal, see **Leukorrhea** or **Lochia**

Disk, slipped
Bharadvajasana, sitting on a chair (Ch. 8, p. 319), Utthita Marichyasana (Ch. 8, p. 323)

Endurance, lack of
Viloma Pranayama 1 (Ch. 3, p. 151)

Energy, low, see **Fatigue**

Fatigue
- After delivery: Sequence for the 1st term: Passive - Active (Ch. 8, p. 255), Restorative Asanas (Ch. 8, p. 366)
- Depression, with: Ardha Chandrasana (Ch. 8, p. 283), Uttanasana (Ch. 8, p. 294), Adho Mukha Shvanasana (Ch. 8, p. 299), Setu Bandha Sarvangasana (Ch. 8, p. 334)
- Mental: Ardha Uttanasana (Ch. 8, p. 292), Restorative Asanas (Ch. 8, p. 366)
- Physical: Parvatasana from Svastikasana and Virasana (Ch. 8, pp. 302 – 303), Ardha Chandrasana (Ch. 8, p. 283), Adho Mukha Shvanasana (Ch. 8, p. 299), Chatushpadasana (Ch. 8, p. 335), Urdhva Dhanurasana with a Trestle (Ch. 8, p. 362), Salamba Shirshasana (Ch. 8, p. 338), Salamba Sarvangasana with a Chair (Ch. 8, p. 329), Twists (Ch. 8, p. 318), Restorative Asanas (Ch. 3, p. 126), Ujjayi Pranayama 1 and 2 (Ch. 3, pp. 148 – 149), Viloma Pranayama 1 (Ch. 3, p. 151)

Fever, persistent
Janu Shirshasana (Ch. 8, p. 306)

Flabbiness
Rope Asanas (Ch. 8, p. 365)

Flatulence
Utthita Parshvakonasana (Ch. 8, p. 282), Virabhadrasana 1 (Ch. 3, p. 52), Parvatasana from Svastikasana and Virasana (Ch. 8, pp. 302 – 303), Twists (Ch. 8, p. 318), Supta Baddha Konasana (Ch. 3, p. 126), Maha Mudra (Ch. 8, p. 304), Salamba Shirshasana (Ch. 8, p. 338), Salamba Sarvangasana (Ch. 8, p. 329)

Forgetfulness
Adho Mukha Shvanasana (Ch. 8, p. 299)

Gallbladder, see **Bile**

Genital organs, irritation
Janu Shirshasana (Ch. 8, p. 306), Baddha

Konasana (Ch. 8, p. 234), Upavishtha Konasana (Ch. 8, p. 316)

Genitalia, irritation see **Genital organs**

Headache
Adho Mukha Shvanasana (Ch. 8, p. 299), Setu Bandha Sarvangasana (Ch. 8, p. 334)

Heaviness
• Abdomen: Virabhadrasana 1 (Ch. 3, p. 52), Parshvottanasana (Ch. 8, p. 285), Prasarita Padottanasana (Ch. 8, p. 296), Janu Shirshasana (Ch. 8, p. 306), Supta Baddha Konasana (Ch. 3, p. 126), Dvi Pada Viparita Dandasana (Ch. 8, p. 360), Viloma Pranayama 2 (Ch. 3, p. 152)
• Body: Ardha Chandrasana (Ch. 8, p. 283), Salamba Shirshasana (Ch. 8, p. 338), Salamba Sarvangasana with a Chair (Ch. 8, p. 329), Setu Bandha Sarvangasana (Ch. 8, p. 334)
• Breasts (when breasts are full): see **Breasts**
• Chest and upper back: Urdhva Dhanurasana with a Trestle (Ch. 8, p. 362)
• Heart: Urdhva Dhanurasana with a Trestle (Ch. 8, p. 362), Supta Baddha Konasana, Bolster Crosswise (Ch. 3, p. 128)
• Lower back: Parvatasana from Svastikasana and Virasana (Ch. 8, p. 303), Janu Shirsasana (Ch. 8, p. 306)
• Pelvic region: Prasarita Padottanasana (Ch. 8, p. 296), Parvatasana from Svastikasana and Virasana (Ch. 8, pp. 302 – 303), Trianga Mukhaikapada Pashchimottanasana (Ch. 8, p. 312), Maha Mudra (Ch. 8, p. 304)
• Uterus: Ardha Supta Konasana (Ch. 8, p. 333), Parshvottanasana (Ch. 8, p. 285), Ardha Uttanasana (Ch. 8, p. 292)

Hernia
Twists (Ch. 8, p. 318)

High blood pressure
Parshvottanasana (Ch. 8, p. 285), Prasarita Padottanasana (Ch. 8, p. 296), Adho Mukha Shvanasana (Ch. 8, p. 299), Ardha Uttanasana (Ch. 8, p. 292), Parvatasana in Virasana (Ch. 8, p. 303), Forward Bends (Ch. 8, p. 304), Supta Baddha Konasana (Ch. 3, p. 126), Viloma Pranayama 2 (Ch. 3, p. 152)

Indigestion
Virabhadrasana 2 (Ch. 8, p. 284), Prasarita Padottanasana (Ch. 8, p. 296), Ardha Uttanasana (Ch. 8, p. 292), Uttanasana (Ch. 8, p. 294), Maha Mudra (Ch. 8, p. 304)

Insomnia
Ardha Halasana (Ch. 8, p. 332)

Knees, sprains
Trianga Mukhaikapada Pashchimottanasana (Ch. 8, p. 312)

Leukorrhea (vaginal discharge, white)
Begin only from the end of the 2nd term: Setu Bandha Sarvangasana (Ch. 8, p. 334), Supta Padangushthasana 1 and 2 (Ch. 8, pp. 342 – 343), Utthita Hasta Padangushthasana 1 and 2 (Ch. 8, p. 344), Paripurna Navasana (Ch. 8, p. 347), Urdhva Prasarita Padasana 1 (Ch. 8, p. 351)

Liver, see **Bile**

Lochia (discharge, until 4 to 6 weeks after delivery)
"Resuming Your Yoga Practice" (Ch. 7, p. 249)

Low blood pressure
Parvatasana from Svastikasana and Virasana (Ch. 8, pp. 302 – 303), Twists (Ch. 8, p. 318), Salamba Shirshasana (Ch. 8, p. 338), Setu Bandha Sarvangasana (Ch. 8, p. 334), Viparita Karani Mudra (Ch. 8, p. 336)

Lumbago
Utthita Hasta Padangushthasana 2 (Ch. 3, p. 345), Twists (Ch. 8, p. 318)

Lumbar area, stiff, see **Back pain**

Menstrual cycle, irregular
Sequence for the 1st Term (Ch. 8, p. 255), Sequence for the 2nd Term, During Your Period (Ch. 8, p. 257), Sequence for the 3rd Term, During Your Period (Ch. 8, p. 263)

Moodiness
Adho Mukha Shvanasana (Ch. 8, p. 299), Salamba Sarvangasana with a Chair (Ch. 8, p. 329)

Muscles, weakness, see **Abdominal muscles** and **Back pain**

Neck pain
Tadasana and variations (Ch. 8, p. 274), Utthita Trikonasana (Ch. 3, p. 38), Twists (Ch. 8, p. 318)

Nervousness
Ardha Uttanasana (Ch. 8, p. 365), Chatushpadasana (Ch. 8, p. 335), Salamba Sarvangasana with a Chair (Ch. 8, p. 329), Setu Bandha Sarvangasana (Ch. 8, p. 334), Ardha Halasana (Ch. 8, p. 332), Ardha Chandrasana (Ch. 8, p. 283), Prasarita Padottanasana (Ch. 8, p. 296), Adho Mukha Shvanasana (Ch. 8, p. 299), Uttanasana (Ch. 8, p. 293), Viparita Karani Mudra (Ch. 8, p. 336), Shavasana (Ch. 3, p. 134), Ujjayi Pranayama 1 and 2 (Ch. 3, pp. 148 – 149), Viloma Pranayama 1 and 2 (Ch. 3, pp. 151 – 152)

Organs, see **Abdominal and pelvic organs**

Overactivity
• 1st term after delivery: Supta Baddha Konasana (Ch. 3, p. 126), Shavasana (Ch. 3, p. 134), Ujjayi Pranayama 1 and 2 (in Shavasana), (Ch. 3, p. 141)
• 2nd term onward: Salamba Shirshasana (Ch. 8, p. 338), Salamba Sarvangasana (Ch. 8, p. 326), Ardha Halasana (Ch. 8, p. 332), Shavasana (Ch. 3, p. 134), Viloma Pranayama 2 (Ch. 3, p. 152)

Oxygen, lack of
Ujjayi Pranayama 1 and 2 (Ch. 3, pp. 148 – 149)

Perspiration (excess body heat)
Ardha Uttansana (Ch. 8, p. 292), Adho Mukha Shvanasana, with Slanting Plank, Head Supported (Ch. 8, p. 299), Ardha Halasana (Ch. 8, p. 332), Janu Shirshasana (Ch. 8, p. 306), Viloma Pranayama 2 (Ch. 3, p. 152)

Pituitary gland
Setu Bandha Sarvangasana (Ch. 8, p. 334)

Postpartum depression
Sequence for the 1st Term: Passive–Active (Ch. 8, p. 255)

Prolapse, uterus
Maha Mudra (Ch. 8, p. 304), Ardha Halasana (Ch. 8, p. 332), Ardha Supta Konasana (Ch. 8, p. 333), Ardha Uttanasana (Ch. 8, p. 365), Parshvottanasana (Ch. 8, p. 285), see also **Abdominal and pelvic organs, weakness**

Reproductive organs, weakness
Parivritta Trikonasana (Ch. 8, p. 290), Virabhadrasana 2 (Ch. 8, p. 284), Virabhadrasana 3 (Ch. 8, p. 289)

Rheumatism
Utthita Hasta Padangushthasana 2 (Ch. 8, p. 345), Parivritta Trikonasana (Ch. 8, p. 290), Virabhadrasana 2 (Ch. 8, p. 284), Virabhadrasana 3 (Ch. 8, p. 289), Ardha Halasana (Ch. 8, p. 332)

Sacroiliac joint
• Pain: see **Back pain**
• Stiffness: Prasarita Padottanasana (Ch. 8, p. 296)

Sciatica
Utthita Parshvakonasana (Ch. 8, p. 282), Supta Padangushthasana 2 (Ch. 8, p. 343), Utthita Hasta Padangushthasana 2 (Ch. 8, p. 345), Virabhadrasana 3 (Ch. 8, p. 289)

Self-confidence, lack of, see **Anxiety**

Shoulder joint, stiffness
Tadasana and variations (Ch. 8, p. 274), Parivritta Trikonasana (Ch. 8, p. 290), Virabhadrasana 1

(Ch. 8, p. 288), Virabhadrasana 3 (Ch. 8, p. 289), Twists (Ch. 8, p. 318)

Sleep disorders, see **Insomnia**

Sleeplessness, see **Insomnia**

Spine, lower
- Stiffness and pain: see **Back pain**
- Weakness: Utthita Trikonasana (Ch. 8, p. 281), Utthita Parshvakonasana (Ch. 8, p. 282), Pashchimottanasana (Ch. 8, p. 308), Parshva Shirshasana (Ch. 7, p. 230), Utthita Hasta Padangushthasana 2 (Ch. 8, p. 345)

Spleen
Maha Mudra (Ch. 8, p. 304), Janu Shirshasana (Ch. 8, p. 306), Supta Svastikasana (Ch. 3, p. 131), Ardha Matsyasana (Ch. 3, p. 131), Twists (Ch. 8, p. 318), Jathara Parivartanasana (Ch. 8, p. 356)

Stiffness, see **Shoulder joint, Sacroiliac joint, Neck pain, Back pain, Wrist**

Stomach
- Heavy feeling: Supta Baddha Konasana (Ch. 3, p. 126)
- Pain: Ardha Uttanasana (Ch. 8, p. 292), Supta Svastikasana (Ch. 3, p. 131), Ardha Matsyasana (Ch. 3, p. 131), Virabhadrasana 2 (Ch. 8, p. 284)

Tailbone
Pain: Utthita Parshvakonasana (Ch. 8, p. 282), Ardha Chandrasana (Ch. 8, p. 283), Virabhadrasana 2 (Ch. 8, p. 284), Virabhadrasana 3 (Ch. 8, p. 289), Adho Mukha Shvanasana (Ch. 8, p. 299), Janu Shirshasana (Ch. 8, p. 306), Dvi Pada Viparita Dandasana, with a Bench (Ch. 8, p. 360), Supta Padangushthasana 2 (Ch. 8, p. 343)

Tension
Supta Baddha Konasana (Ch. 3, p. 126), Setu Bandha Sarvangasana (Ch. 8, p. 334), Shavasana (Ch. 3, p. 134), Viloma Pranayama 2 (Ch. 3, p. 152)

Thyroid gland
Sequence for Mental Stability (Ch. 2, p. 17), Sequence for Physical and Physiological Stability: Preparing the Ground (Ch. 2, p. 18), Supta Svastikasana (Ch. 3, p. 131), Ardha Matsyasana (Ch. 3, p. 131), Viparita Karani (Ch. 3, p. 112)

Tiredness, see **Fatigue**

Urinary disorders
- Stress incontinence: Trianga Mukhaikapada Pashchimottanasana (Ch. 8, p. 312), Janu Shirshasana (Ch. 8, p. 306), Maha Mudra (Ch. 8, p. 304), Twists (Ch. 8, p. 318), Salamba Sarvangasana (Ch. 8, p. 326), see also **Abdominal and pelvic organs, weakness**
- Urinary tract infection: Baddha Konasana (Ch. 3, p. 67), Supta Baddha Konasana (Ch. 3, p. 126), Twists (Ch. 8, p. 318), Ardha Halasana (Ch. 8, p. 332), Setu Bandha Sarvangasana (Ch. 8, p. 334)

Uterus
- Aid in involution and regeneration: Sequences in Chapter 7 and Chapter 8
- Pain: Ardha Supta Konasana (Ch. 8, p. 333), Supta Baddha Konasana (Ch. 3, p. 126)
- Prolapse: see **Prolapse, uterus**

Vagina, burning sensation
Supta Baddha Konasana (Ch. 3, p. 126)

Vaginal discharge, see **Leukorrhea** or **Lochia**

Vision, see **Blurred vision**

Willpower, lack of
Chatushpadasana (Ch. 8, p. 335)

Wrist, stiffness
Tadasana and variations (Ch. 8, p. 274), Supta Baddha Konasana (Ch. 3, p. 126)

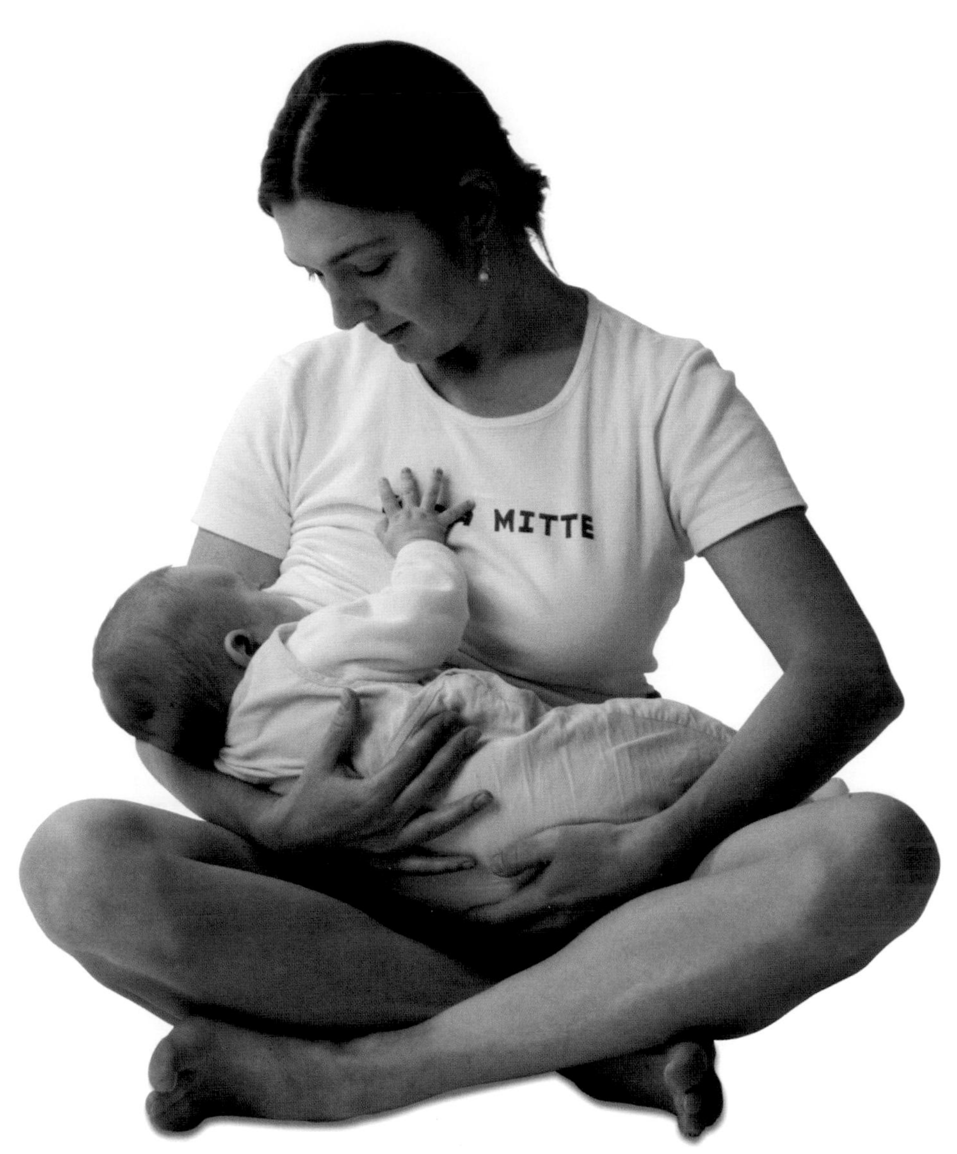
MITTE

PART IV
Miscellaneous

CHAPTER 1

ANATOMY, PHYSIOLOGY, AND PROCREATION

This chapter explains the anatomy of the female pelvis, specifically the bones and joints, and the position and characteristics of the pelvic organs, pelvic floor, and perineum. Pregnancy is like a journey full of surprises. Especially while doing Yoga, you will gain a new awareness of your body. This chapter provides you with a source of more information about the structures that are mentioned in the description of asana work throughout the book.

This chapter also contains further explanation of the menstrual cycle, to enhance your understanding of the cyclic changes in your body and the need to adjust your Yoga practice accordingly. This is especially important after delivery, so your body can slowly recover and return to a healthy and fertile monthly rhythm.

We have outlined the development of the fetus from fertilization through birth: implantation of the embryo in the uterus, development of the organs, formation of umbilical cord and placenta, and other milestones. This information, while interesting in itself, is included in order to help sharpen your awareness of your baby and why and how Yoga practice should be adjusted according to the stage of your pregnancy.

Changes in your body during pregnancy sometimes lead to various conditions that may cause discomfort or pain; for these, Yoga offers profound relief. Throughout this chapter, you'll find boxes called Helpful Yogasanas, which refer you to relevant asanas in the book. In addition to these, we suggest that you consult the chapter "Problems A – Z," where you'll find more recommended poses.

Yoga helps to prepare you for delivery and can be a good friend to guide you through childbirth and the time afterward. That's why this chapter deals with the stages of labor and the changes in your body after delivery.

At the end of the chapter, we give you a glimpse of the philosophies of motherhood and procreation from the perspective of the ancient Ayurvedic texts.

The Female Pelvis

Bones and Joints

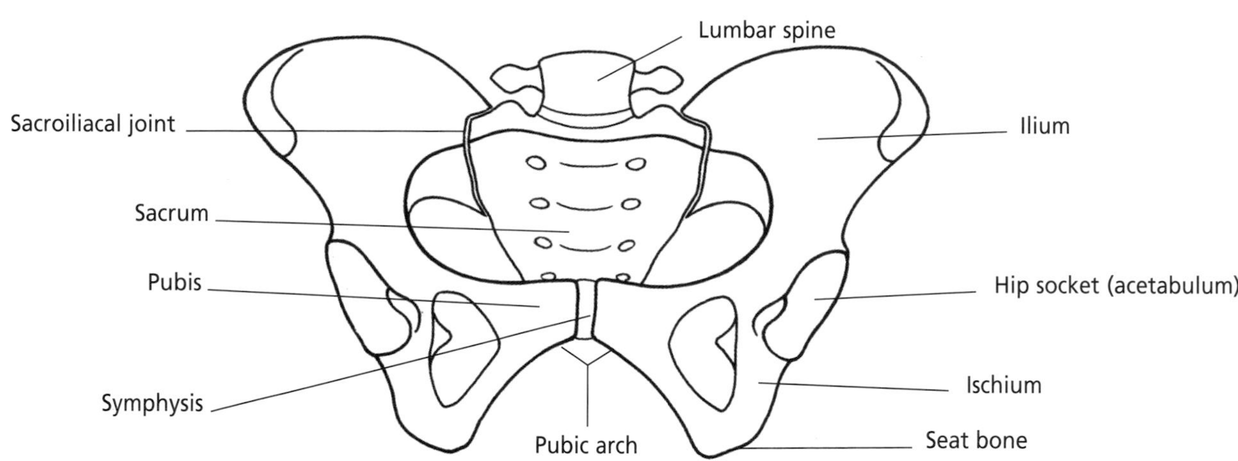

Fig. 1: Anterior (frontal) view of the pelvis, according to Rohen.

The human pelvis is a basin-shaped ring, which, in the upright position, bears the weight of the body and the abdominal organs and transfers this burden by way of the hip joints to the legs. The pelvic bones also form a protective ring around the pelvic organs without obstructing their outlets.

The pelvic interior serves as a bony birth canal and has different diameters at different levels (planes), to which the baby's head has to adjust during birth. (This is discussed in the section "Delivery" further on in this chapter.) The female pelvis is shorter and broader than the male's, which results in a greater distance between the hip joints. A woman's legs also have a different shape in the standing position from a man's. Because of the greater distance between her hip joints, the relation between hip joints and knees suggests an X-shape (valgus type), whereas in men the position is more of an O-shape (varus type).

The bony ring of the pelvis consists of the two large hipbones, the sacrum, and the coccyx (tailbone).

Each hipbone consists of three bone segments, which intersect in a firm junction located in the center of a cavity that forms the hip socket (acetabulum). The three bone segments are called the ilium, ischium, and pubis. The ilium is shaped like a flat shovel or scoop. Both ilia together, acting like two cupped hands, support the weight of the abdominal organs against gravitational pull from below. The space they create is called the greater pelvis. The pubis, ischium, and sacrum form the lesser pelvis.

The pubic bones articulate, or connect to form a joint, at the mons pubis (the area covered by pubic hair) to form the pubic symphysis. Strong ligaments tighten this joint, which is the frontal closing of the pelvic ring. The ischium is the lowest part of the hipbone. It is also called the seat bone or buttock bone because it has a prominent tuberosity (bulge), which can be distinctly felt on both sides when you are sitting upright. At the level of the lesser pelvis, the hipbone has a natural opening (foramen), located between the pubis and ischium, which is closed by a membrane and attached muscles.

The sacrum is the hardest bone of the body. It consists of five fused vertebrae, which you can see by its shape. The sacrum articulates with the coccyx, or tailbone, which is made up of small, connected, sometimes fused bones composing a rudimentary tail, which is an evolutionary remnant. The coccyx can move slightly. During birth, it can be forced backwards by the baby's head, thus permitting an enlargement of the pelvic outlet.

The spine is stably embedded in the pelvis by way of the wedge-formed sacrum, which articulates with the hipbones in the form of two sacroiliac joints (joints where the sacrum and ilium meet).

These joints are firmly connected by strong ligaments, which also allow the sacrum to move slightly back and forth within the pelvis. Any blockage of this limited, but important, movement of the sacroiliac joints causes back pain. When there is no obstruction, the hipbones and the sacrum slip easily past each other, such as when you bend your torso from a standing position. During pregnancy, the ligaments stabilizing the pelvis loosen. Therefore, the forward pull of the abdomen can cause pressure on the sacroiliac joint and result in pain.

The hip joint consists of the head of the femur (thigh bone) and the acetabulum (hip socket). In order to permit stable, erect standing and walking, the acetabulum is positioned sideways in the pelvic ring and is tilted so that it partially forms a roof over the head of the femur.

It is important that the head of the femur is well contained in its socket for healthy development of the hip joint during childhood and afterwards. That is why newborn babies are given an ultrasound to check whether the acetabulum is sufficiently covering the femur. If not, the hip joint can be realigned with the help of broad or straddle bandaging.

Yogasanas create freedom and flexibility in the hip joint, and also help to keep the two bone partners of the joint firmly connected, which helps to prevent arthrosis.

The pelvic organs are located within the pelvic cavity. The pelvic cavity and the abdominal cavity are separated by the peritoneum (transparent membrane that lines the abdominal cavity). The position of the pelvic organs is referred to as subperitoneal (under the peritoneum), and that of the abdominal organs as intraperitoneal (within the peritoneum). Behind the abdominal cavity lies the retroperitoneal (behind the peritoneum) cavity, which contains the kidneys, ureters (ducts that carry urine from the kidneys to the bladder), abdominal aorta, and inferior vena cava (vein that returns blood to the heart).

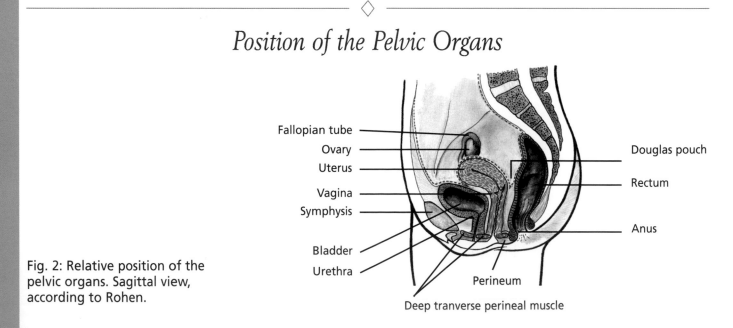

Position of the Pelvic Organs

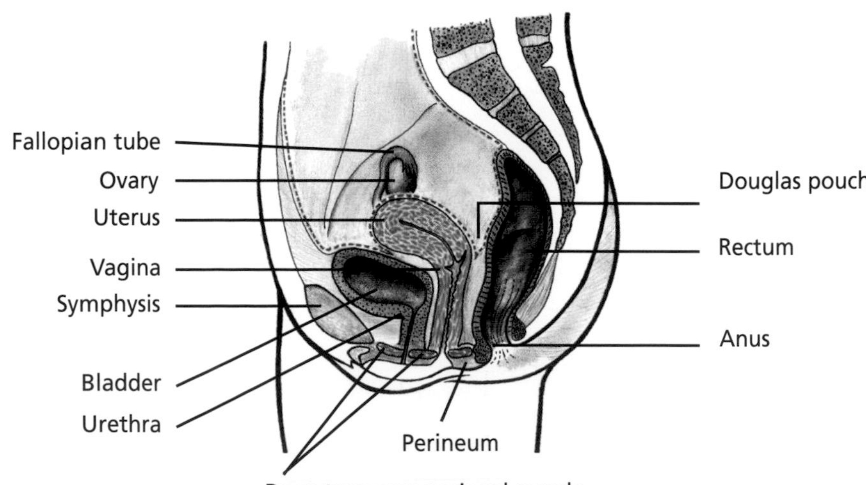

Fig. 2: Relative position of the pelvic organs. Sagittal view, according to Rohen.

The bladder lies directly behind the symphysis. If the bladder is full, it rises higher than the mons pubis and can then be felt between the symphysis (the midline cartilaginous joint uniting the superior rami of the left and right pubic bones) and the navel.

The uterus lies behind and rises above the top of the bladder. It is physiologically bent forwards (anteversion) in relation to the body axis, and bent still more forwards (anteflexion) on its own axis. This plays an important role during pregnancy in allowing it to stretch out in the right direction towards the abdominal cavity. If the uterus is tilted backwards (retroflexion), its growth is, in rare instances, impeded by the sacrum.

The rectum lies behind the uterus. It is the part of the large intestine that is close to the anus. The rectum begins in the abdominal cavity, but its lowest part is found in the pelvic cavity. There is a small space between the uterus and the rectum, which is called the Douglas pouch. This gap is the lowest point of the abdominal cavity and is lined with peritoneum. The roof of the uterus and the bladder are also covered by the peritoneum. When the uterus enlarges during pregnancy, it pushes the peritoneum and the abdominal organs upward and it also creates pressure on the neighboring bladder and the rectum.

Description of the Pelvic Organs

All hollow organs of the body consist of similar layers: an inside mucous membrane, a middle layer of smooth muscle (which enables peristalsis), in some cases a layer of connective tissue, and an outer membrane.

Bladder

In the mucous membrane of the bladder, the cells have a cylindrical structure. The smooth muscle of the bladder has a special function. Its fibers are arranged like a scissor lattice and meet at the neck of the bladder, where they form the inner closing muscle (internal sphincter). A quantity of approximately 5 – 14 fluid ounces of urine causes the urge to urinate. The smooth muscle of the bladder wall contracts during urination to push the urine out. This contraction, together with the arrangement of the muscle fibers, causes the involuntary inner closing muscle of the bladder to open like a funnel. This is followed by the relaxation of the outer closing muscle, which can allow the urine to flow or can voluntarily hold it back. This external sphincter is part of the pelvic floor muscles.

Physiological Changes in Pregnancy

During the first trimester, there is an increased urge to urinate. The uterus, which is still situated entirely within the pelvis, has already increased in size and is pressing on the neighboring bladder. In the second trimester, the uterus rises towards the abdomen, thereby relieving the pressure on the bladder. In the last trimester, the much-enlarged uterus again presses on the bladder, so that even small quantities of urine create the urge to urinate. It also becomes more difficult to hold the urine when you cough or sneeze.

Urinary Tract Infections

The vesical trigone is a triangular structure on the bladder floor. The ureters, which are ducts that carry urine from the kidneys to the bladder, open in the upper corners on each side. The urethra originates from its lower corner. In women the urethra is just over an inch long and runs vertically to the pelvic floor.

Thus bacteria from the external genital area and the neighboring anal area can migrate into the bladder and cause cystitis. To prevent such infections, **it is important to drink adequately. Regular urination rinses the bladder from the inside.**

During pregnancy, the hormone that prevents contractions, progesterone, also relaxes the smooth muscle of the urinary tract. There is a tendency towards stagnation of the urine in the ureters, which increases the danger of ascending urinary tract infection that can also affect the kidneys. Therefore, it is especially important to drink enough during pregnancy.

Helpful Yogasanas

We recommend suptas and the twisting asanas allowed during pregnancy. These stimulate the flow of urine and improve blood circulation in the kidneys.

Uterus

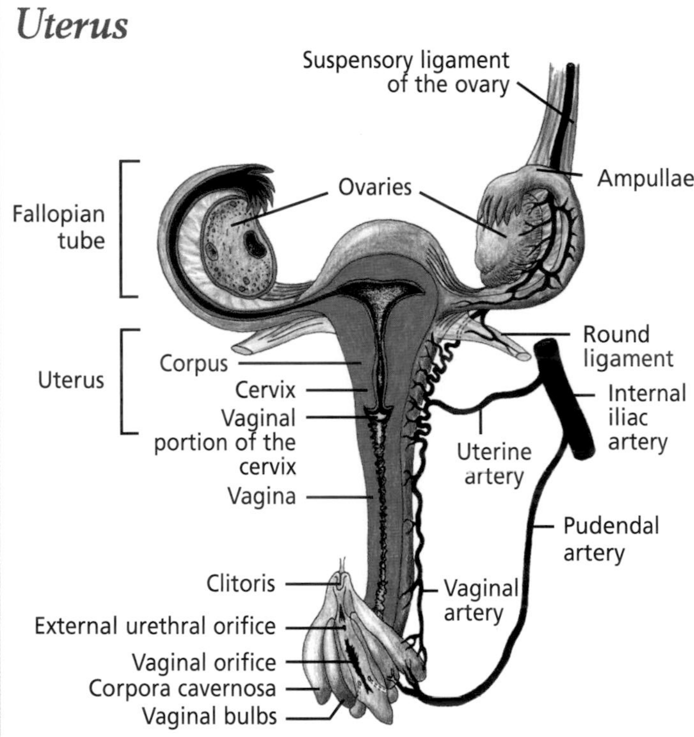

Fig. 3: Ovaries and development of follicles, uterus, and vagina, according to Rohen.

The uterus is a pear-shaped, hollow organ that is approximately three inches long and weighs approximately three and one-half ounces. During pregnancy, its weight can reach as much as three and one-third pounds. It is divided into the cervix and corpus (main part of the uterus). The cervix is the lower, narrow part that protrudes downward into the vagina. The part of the cervix visible from the vagina is called the vaginal portion, where you find the uterine orifice. In women who have not yet given birth, this orifice looks like a little dimple. After birth it becomes somewhat wider and rounder.

The fallopian tubes extend like two little arms from the upper poles of the uterus on each side. At their ends are the ampullae (part of the tube that is dilated like a flask) and the ovaries.

The uterus has the typical wall layers of a hollow organ, but they are used for very special purposes. The mucous membrane of the uterus, or endometrium, undergoes cyclical changes regulated by various hormones. In the first phase of the 28-day menstrual cycle (proliferation phase), the membrane becomes thicker and stores nutrients. Ovulation in the middle of the cycle is followed by the transformation phase (secretion phase), during which the membrane begins to show glandular changes and loosening. At the end of the cycle, the majority of the membrane, called the lamina functionalis (functional layer), is usually discarded except for the lamina basalis (layer near the base). This results in menstrual bleeding. If fertilization takes place, the membrane remains intact and no menstruation occurs.

The muscle layer of the uterus, or myometrium, has various functions. During pregnancy, when it provides the growing fetus with sufficient space, the individual muscle cells become much enlarged. New cells are formed only to a minimal extent. The muscles are also used during birth to expel the child. Similarly to the muscle fibers of the bladder, these muscles are arranged in a scissor lattice fashion, so that they can exert pressure on the uterine cavity during birth.

There are fewer muscle fibers on the transition to the cervix, because these areas dilate rather than contract during labor. After birth, the muscle fibers of the uterus facilitate the expulsion of the placenta and, through contractions, stop any bleeding and help the uterus return to its normal size.

Ligaments of the Uterus

The muscle layer is connected to a layer of connective tissue, the parametrium, which is part of a complex positioning and support apparatus for the uterus. Two broad ligaments connect the sides of the uterus to the lateral wall of the pelvis. Together with the uterus, the broad ligaments form a kind of partition wall across the pelvic cavity that separates the bladder and the rectum. The broad ligaments also enclose the fallopian tubes, the ovaries and their suspensory ligaments, and the blood vessels and nerves of the uterus.

The uterus also has other ligaments, which are reinforced by smooth muscle fibers connected with the smooth muscles of the uterine wall. These help to fasten the uterus towards the front, sides, and back of the pelvis.

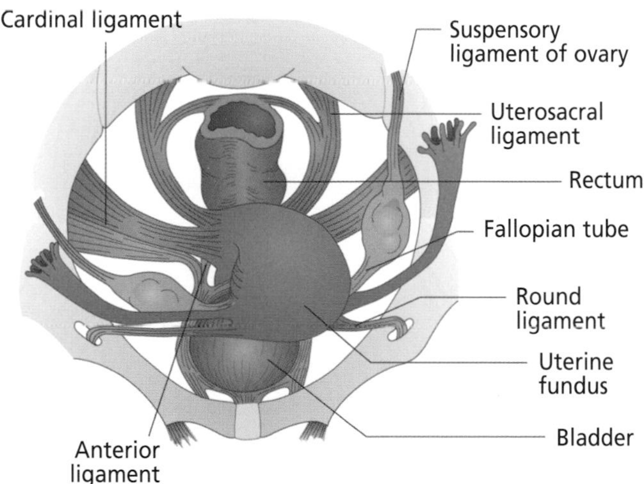

Fig. 4: Ligamentous connections of the pelvic organs. View from the upper pelvis, according to Pfleiderer, Breckwoldt, and Martius.

The cardinal ligaments, found at the sides of the uterus, are part of the base of the broad ligaments and help to attach the uterus to the pelvic wall. Toward the front, the uterus is fastened by a more muscular, anterior ligament that runs around either side of the bladder to the mons pubis. Towards the back, a ligament runs around the colon to the inner surface of the sacrum (uterosacral ligament).

The round ligaments are two ligaments that follow a unique route from the corner of the uterus from which the fallopian tubes extend, through the inguinal canal (that runs through the groin), into the connective tissue of the labia majora (see "External Genitals," page 390). These ligaments hold the uterus in its forward-tilted position. When the uterus becomes larger, these "reins" hold a heavy weight. Pregnant women sometimes feel a pulling in the labia or in the groin due to the increased pressure on the round ligaments.

Helpful Yogasanas

During pregnancy, there is a loosening of all ligament structures of the uterus. Therefore, it is very important to retighten these ligaments after birth to regain their original form. In the inverted positions of Yoga, the ligaments no longer have to support the weight of the organs, since the gravitational effect is reversed. There is a relaxation of the ligaments. In combination with a certain amount of leg and pelvic floor work in these positions, the ligaments are toned and tightened, and they regain their former elasticity.

Ovaries *(Fig. 3, page 388)*

The ovaries and fallopian tubes are located behind the peritoneum. They are supported by the suspensory ligament of the ovary, which encloses the nutritive vessels of the ovaries. The ovary consists of an outer (cortical) layer and the inner (medullary) substance. Before birth, there is a pool of several million egg cells present in the cortical layer. Each egg cell is surrounded by a wreath of nutrient cells. This unit of egg cell and nutrient cells is called a follicle. The number of follicles declines with age.

Until puberty, the follicles remain inactive in the ovary. By means of a complex hormonal interplay guided by the brain (hypothalamus and hypophysis) during puberty, cyclical hormonal changes develop (Fig. 7, page 393). Every month a cohort of follicles starts to grow, and usually one of them fully ripens and becomes competent to ovulate. The egg that is ready to be fertilized is discharged and transported by way of the fallopian tube in the direction of the uterus. The follicular tissue remaining after the discharge of the egg is transformed into the corpus luteum (yellow mass of tissue). Both the follicular tissue and, after discharge of the egg, the corpus luteum produce hormones in this cycle. Special cells of the follicle produce estrogen, and the corpus luteum secretes progesterone.

Vagina

The vagina is a tubular cavity consisting of smooth muscle cells and many elastic fibers. This structure gives the vagina the elasticity required for the baby's head to pass through during delivery.

At the transition from the outer opening of the cervix, the vagina forms a pouch called the vaginal fornix. This is a recess at the vault of the vagina formed by the protrusion of the cervix into the vagina. The vagina itself possesses two lengthwise, vein-filled folds or lips, which are the internal erectile tissue of the woman. One of these lies in direct proximity to the urethra.

The vagina is lined with a mucous membrane which is lubricated by a process called transudation. During pregnancy, it is normal to have increased vaginal discharge (leukorrhea), which is usually clear and odorless. The vagina has special bacteria, among which are Döderlein bacilli. These bacteria liquefy cells shed by the vaginal mucous membrane and transform their sugar content into lactic acid, which results in an acidic pH value. This acidic environment protects the vagina against infections.

External Genitals (Vulva)

The vagina opens into the vaginal orifice, which has at its upper edge the exit of the urethra. The vaginal orifice is cushioned with paired masses of erectile tissue (vaginal bulbs), which join just above the external urethral orifice.

The vaginal orifice, which is lubricated by the secretion of glands, is delineated by the labia minora and majora. The labia minora unite at an upper pole, where the clitoris is located. The clitoris has the largest concentration of nerve endings in the female body and is also surrounded by another paired mass of erectile tissue (corpora cavernosa), which are attached close to the pubic bones (Fig. 3, page 388).

Pelvic Floor

The muscular structure of the pelvic floor can be divided into three layers. The first, outermost layer is closely connected to the external genitals and erectile tissue. The vaginal orifice and its erectile tissue are encircled by the bulbospongiosus muscle, which encloses the vaginal orifice. This muscle is interbraided with the external anal sphincter, the muscle that closes the external anal orifice, in a figure-eight shape.

At each side of the pubic bones are two muscles, called ischiocavernous muscles, which directly surround the erectile tissue of the clitoris (corpora cavernosa). The two branches of the pubic bones are cross-connected by the superficial transverse perineal muscle. In Fig. 5, you can see that the ischiocavernous muscles and the superficial transverse perineal muscle form a triangular frame at the frontal exit of the pelvis.

This frame is closely attached to the deep transverse perineal muscle, which spans the frontal part of the pelvic outlet horizontally, like a triangular sheet. This is the second layer of muscle, called the urogenital diaphragm.

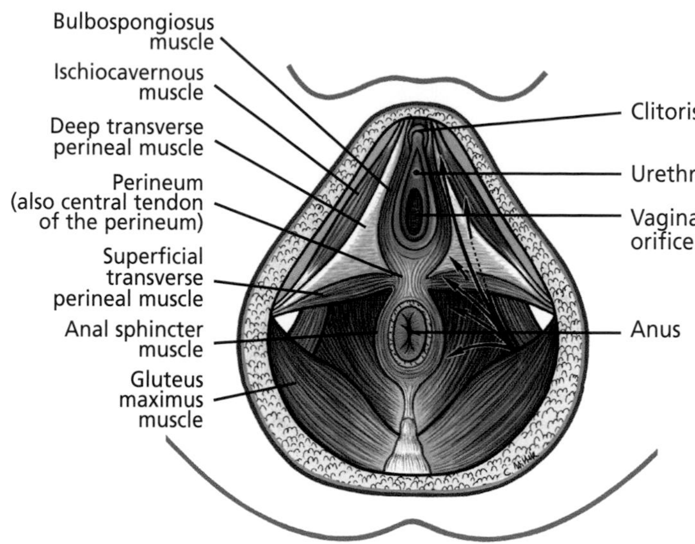

Fig. 5: The pelvic floor muscles, observed from the bottom, according to Rohen.

The third layer consists of the deeper pelvic floor muscle structure, called the pelvic diaphragm. It is mainly formed by the levator ani muscle. This funnel-shaped, broad layer of muscle is suspended like a hammock and fills the important function of preventing the pelvic organs from sagging under the pressure of the abdominal cavity. It rises from the sides of the lesser pelvis and from the fascial (connective tissue) ring of the internal obturator muscle.

In the front, the levator ani muscle rises from the back surface of the pubic bone, but behind the symphysis it leaves a gap for the urethra and vagina. It runs towards and around the rectum like a sling. Its fibers enter the side of the rectum and are capable of lifting the back wall of the rectum above the column of excrement during defecation. The muscle also extends into the sphincter muscle and plays an important role in voluntary fecal continence.

The levator ani muscle also extends into the back wall of the vagina. Women can use this muscle voluntarily to contract the vagina. The muscle protects the vagina and the uterus from sagging. Posteriorly, the muscle is connected to the sacrum and coccyx by the strong anococcygeal ligament and the coccygeal muscle.

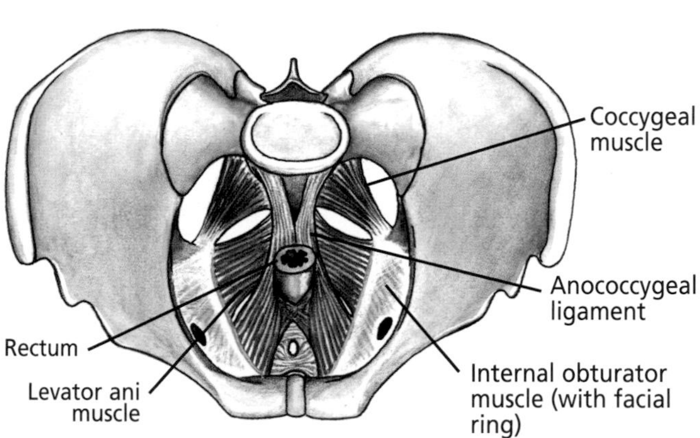

Fig. 6: Levator ani muscle observed from the above, according to Rohen.

Perineum

The area of the pelvic floor between the vagina and the anus is called the perineum. The perineum has a strong, tendon-reinforced point that connects the external anal sphincter and the bulbospongiosus muscle in an 8-shaped manner (Fig. 5). This "central tendon of the perineum" is an important hub, connecting fibers of the superficial pelvic floor muscles with those of the deeper pelvic floor (pelvic diaphragm). It is also connected with the smooth muscles of the posterior vaginal wall.

Helpful Yogasanas

The central tendon of the perineum plays an important role in Yoga. In the Maha Mudra ("great seal") exercise, this anatomical point is drawn inside the body. By means of this exercise, the entire pelvic floor and the inner organs can be lifted.

Episiotomy

During birth, the pelvic floor must widen in order to allow the baby's head to emerge. The perineum is subjected to tension, and it must be protected by the hand of the birth assistant.

An episiotomy may be performed when it is necessary to ease the exit of the baby's head through the muscle structure of the pelvic floor, or if the perineum has been stretched too far and threatens to tear. An episiotomy entails cutting into the bulbospongiosus muscle. This muscle surrounds the vaginal outlet and is part of the 8-shaped muscle loop that is bound by way of the central tendon of the perineum with the external anal sphincter. The incision is performed in a way that permits full healing of the muscle fibers and avoids damage to the external anal sphincter muscle. Because of the minimized circulation in the stretched perineum, an episiotomy performed at the right moment is not painful for many women, and is in fact a relief. Sometimes an episiotomy is an emergency measure, such as when the tense perineum has delayed the birth too long and the baby becomes distressed. Thorough oiling of the perineum before and during birth keeps the perineum supple, which can reduce the need for an incision.

Helpful Yogasanas

During birth, the muscles of the pelvic floor, which surround the vaginal outlet, must widen and relax to an extreme degree. Even during pregnancy they must tolerate considerable stress, because together with the ligaments, they carry the weight of the baby and the uterus.

In the *prenatal* Yoga exercises, the first task is the widening of the muscle structure of the pelvic floor by spreading the legs. The outward rotation of the hips is of special significance, since the levator ani muscle rises from the fascial (connective tissue) ring of the internal obturator muscle, which belongs to the deep outward rotators of the pelvic muscle structure. Due to the close connection of these two muscles, outward rotation can widen the pelvic floor.

In the *postnatal* Yoga program, when the emphasis is on regaining form, the pelvic floor is toned to support and lift the pelvic organs again. The pelvic floor is suspended between the pubis, the ileum, the sacrum, and the coccyx. Realigning the pelvis by working on these points can achieve better distribution of body weight, which can then be better transferred to the legs. This entails using all the muscles bordering on the pelvis (hip, leg, abdominal, and pelvic). The coccyx and sacrum are pulled into the body and lowered, and the pubic bone and lower abdominal muscles are elevated. This alone tones the pelvic floor muscles and supports the pelvic organs.

This work also creates alignment from head to toe. Stretching these body points and aligning them to one another integrates the pelvis into the body, so that the entire inner body is lengthened and aligned into an erect position. This is reinforced by the use of inverted positions such as headstands and shoulderstands, in which the ligaments of the uterus and the muscles of the pelvic floor are pulled inside with the help of inverted gravitational force.

The Menstrual Cycle

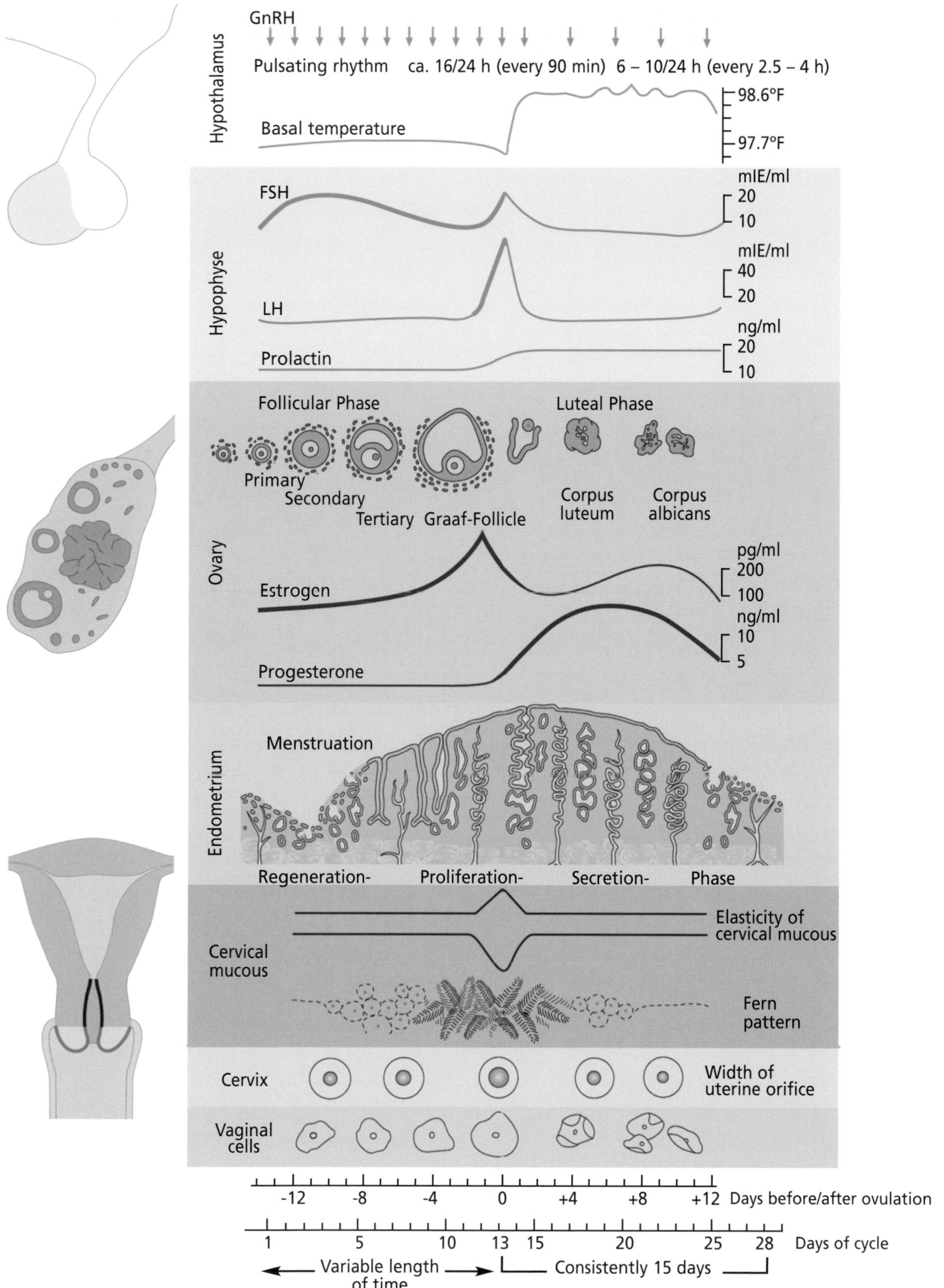

Fig. 7: The cycle-dependent changes in the female organism, according to Pfleiderer, Breckwoldt, and Martius.

Follicular Phase

Before birth, a female is equipped with a pool of several million egg cells. The cells are inactive until the woman becomes sexually mature. By puberty, this pool has declined to approximately 500,000 egg cells, of which approximately 500 ripen during the woman's period of fertility. Hormonal changes during puberty result in the establishment of an approximately 28-day cycle.

In a pulsating manner, the hypothalamus secretes the hormone GnRH (gonadotropin releasing hormone). This hormone gives the impulse to the pituitary gland (hypophysis) to release FSH (follicle stimulating hormone). FSH stimulates the reproductive cells in the ovary.

An egg cell in the ovary is surrounded by protective cells, which provide its nourishment. The unit of egg cell and protective cell is called a primary follicle. FSH causes the growth of a cohort of primary follicles, which in later stages of ripening are called secondary and tertiary follicles. The larger follicles secrete the hormone estrogen. The fully ripened form is a fluid-filled bubble or blister known as a Graaf follicle. It secretes the hormone inhibin, which suppresses the growth of less competent follicles by suppressing FSH. This dominant follicle continues growing, forms a bulge near the surface of the ovary, and soon becomes competent to ovulate.

Under the influence of estrogen in this first phase of the female cycle, the body prepares itself for possible conception and implantation of the fertilized cell. The mucous membrane of the uterus thickens to approximately four-tenths of an inch and stores a supply of sugar and nutrients (proliferation phase). The cervix widens. The mucous plug, which seals the neck of the uterus, is loosened and liquified. The mucous threads line up in parallel formation. When they crystallize, they have a characteristic "fern pattern." This formation of the mucous threads permits easier entry for the sperm.

In the vagina, with the help of estrogen, there is a proliferation of well-nourished cells, which are shed. The Döderlein bacilli liquify these shed cells and metabolize their sugar to lactic acid. Thus, in the first half of the cycle, the vagina is well moistened and its environment is acidic.

Further effects of estrogen on the female body include:

- Favorable influence on the mineral content of bone
- Thick hair growth, strong and well-nourished tissue
- Positive change in mood
- Stimulation of the parasympathetic (calming) nervous system
- Protection against arteriosclerosis by widening of the arteries and reduction of the cholesterol level
- Low basal temperature (early morning: 97.7° F)

Ovulation

Due to increasing estrogen and low FSH levels in the middle of the cycle, the pituitary gland releases the ovulation-inducing hormone LH (luteinizing hormone). On average, by the 14th day, the Graaf follicle has reached the cortical layer and arches its wall outwards. LH tears the skin of the ovary, and the egg cell is expelled from the follicle bubble. The funnel of the fallopian tube places itself close enough to pick up the egg cell and propels it by movement of tiny glistening hairs towards the uterus. The egg cell requires approximately four to five days to find its way through the fallopian tube. Following ovulation, the sperm cells have about 12 hours to fertilize the egg. The usual fertilization site is the fallopian tube.

Luteal Phase

After ovulation, the follicular tissue remaining in the ovary is transformed into the corpus luteum, which forms the hormone progesterone.

Progesterone steers the second half of the female cycle. In this phase, the mucous membrane of the uterus is prepared for the implantation of a fertilized egg. The built-up mucous membrane is loosened, also with glandular changes, and the many small arteries shorten into spirals (secretion phase).

Progesterone, which is extremely important in preserving the pregnancy throughout its course, narrows the cervix. The mucous threads form a network to produce a viscous and impermeable cervical plug. The mucous membrane of the vagina is dry and only a few folded cells are formed. The acidic pH protection is weakened.

Further effects of progesterone on the female body include:

- Proliferation of mammary glands, and tenderness or heaviness of the breasts
- Increase of the basal temperature (early morning: 98.6 to 99.5° F)
- Depressed mood
- Influence on the sympathetic nervous system in preparation for pregnancy

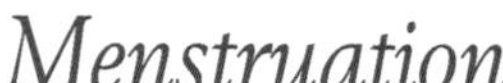

Menstruation

If the egg is not fertilized, the hormone production of the corpus luteum is usually exhausted after 14 days. When the hormone is depleted, the mucous membrane of the uterus is shed from the basal membrane, and menstruation ensues. The changes in the mucous membrane brought about by progesterone are also necessary for it to be separated and shed.

Helpful Yogasanas

During menstruation, practice only the sequences for that period. Inverted poses are not suitable, because they disturb the blood flow. We recommend that you follow the guidelines and sequences for the phases before and after ovulation to promote a healthy menstrual cycle (see *Part I, Chapter 2, "Preparing for Pregnancy"*). After delivery, your body needs to recover and to return to a normal menstrual cycle. For this purpose, we have adapted the Yoga program for after delivery into three terms and recommended different Yoga sequences during your period for each (see *Chapter 8, "Sequences for After Delivery"*).

CHAPTER 1

Development of the Embryo

Fertilization

During sexual intercourse, semen is ejaculated into the posterior vaginal vault. The seminal fluid consists of sperm cells produced in the testicles and the secretion of the prostate and seminal glands. The secretion of these glands is alkaline and neutralizes the acidity of the vagina, so that the sperm become mobile. It also contains fructose, a source of energy for sperm mobility. Each ejaculation contains about 300 million sperm cells. The sperm cell consists of head, neck, connective piece, and tail. The connective piece and the tail are significant for the sperm's mobility. In the head section there is a cell nucleus with the genetic information. Several million sperm cells penetrate through the liquified mucous of the cervix. Some atypical sperm or insufficiently mobile ones may be filtered out at this barrier. The neck of the uterus stores sperm cells for three to four days and releases them little by little. They continue their ascent into the uterine cavity and finally reach the fallopian tubes. If a sperm cell comes into contact with an egg cell in the fallopian tubes, enzymes help it to penetrate the outer layer of the egg. After fertilization, the outer layer of the egg becomes impermeable to other sperm cells. Fertilization occurs by a melting together of the egg cell and the sperm cell. Each one has only half a set of chromosomes (containing information of inherited traits). Thus, maternal and paternal genetic information are combined in a single cell. The sex of the fetus is determined by which sex chromosome is in the fertilizing sperm cell. If it is an X chromosome, then the child will be female. If it is a Y chromosome, the child will be male.

If the egg gets fertilized, no menstruation occurs. The fertilized egg very soon starts producing the hormone beta-HCG (human chorion gonadotropin), which preserves the corpus luteum and the endometrium during the first stage of pregnancy. Beta-HCG can be detected by commercially available pregnancy tests on the very first day of the missed period. For the pregnancy to progress, preservation of the corpus luteum during the first trimester is important. Later, the placenta takes over the production and secretion of progesterone.

Implantation

It takes about five to six days for the fertilized egg cell to make its way through the fallopian tube. During this time it divides five times, finally reaching the uterus at the 32-cell stage. It then acquires the form of a blastocyst, a sphere of cells with a fluid-filled cavity. This consists of two parts: the inner cell mass, which adheres to the wall of the cavity and is responsible for the actual formation of the embryo (embryoblast), and an outer layer of cells that later forms the supportive, nutritive tissue like the embryonic part of the placenta and amniotic membranes (trophoblast).

The blastocyst usually implants at the top of the uterus near the exits of the fallopian tubes. The trophoblast forms enzymes that dissolve the mucous membrane of the uterus, gradually embedding itself firmly into the uterine wall. The dissolved cell material serves as nutrients for gestation. The tissue of the trophoblast sends hair-like projections (villi) into the mucous membrane of the uterus. The maternal blood flows into little pools around the villi of the embryo, so that a metabolic exchange can take place. Later this system forms a multibranched system of villi and maternal blood pools, called the placenta.

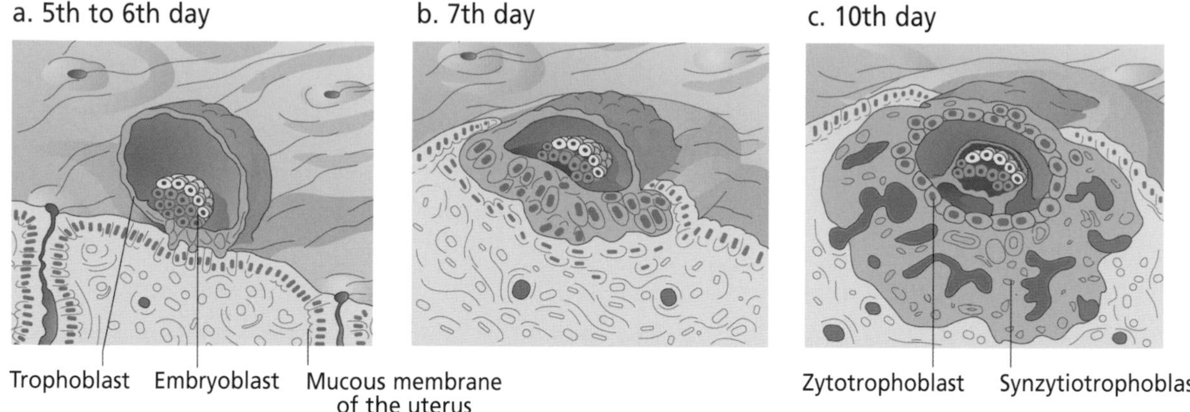

Fig. 8: Implantation, according to Pfleiderer, Breckwoldt, and Martius.

Organogenesis

By the first week of pregnancy, the embryonic system has already become differentiated. Within the embryonic knot, the amniotic cavity forms. This becomes larger during the course of the pregnancy and surrounds the embryo. The amniotic cavity's outer membrane (amnion) is lined with cells from the trophoblast. These cells form the amniotic fluid.

The embryonic system differentiates into two layers, the outer ectoderm and the inner endoderm. In week three, a third layer, mesoderm, is formed between them. The three layers form the germinal disk. This is the beginning of organogenesis, where specific tissues, organs, and systems become differentiated to create the basic human body structure. The formation of the organs takes place during weeks four to eight of pregnancy (see box).

The earliest organ to begin functioning is the heart. Then other systems, such as the circulatory, digestive, urogenital, and nervous systems, begin to take shape. The neural tube begins to develop, which forms the central nervous system (brain and spinal cord).

At this stage, sensory placodes (platelike, thickened areas) will form specific components of the ear, nose, and eyes. Limb buds start to grow.

Ectoderm: epithelium of the skin, nervous system, epithelium of the sensory organs, and pituitary gland
Mesoderm: connective tissue, muscles, bones and joints, heart, blood and lymph nodes, gonads, brain, spleen, and blood cells
Endoderm: stomach and intestinal tract, lung and respiratory tract, liver, pancreas, urinary tract, thymus, and larynx

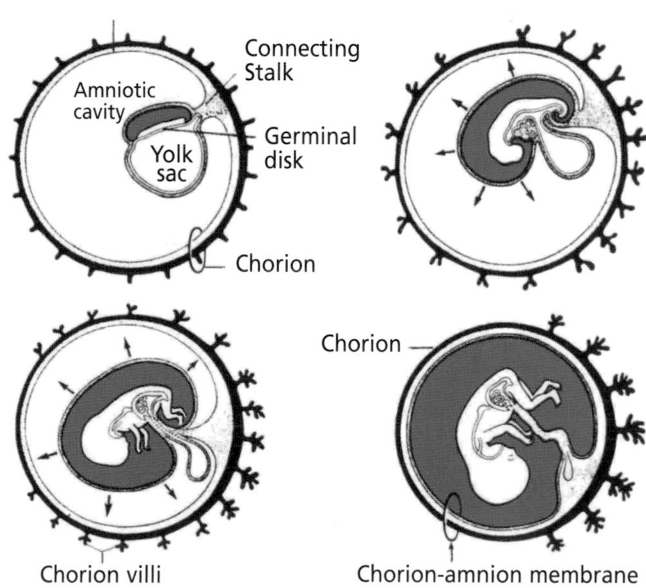

Fig. 9: Development of the Amniotic Cavity

Brandis/Schönberger, *Anatomie und Physiologie*, 9th edition 1999 © Elsevier GmbH, Urban & Schwarzenberg

Formation of the Umbilical Cord

A yolk sac helps to nourish the fetus during early pregnancy (Fig. 9 & 10, page 397 and below). By the end of week three, the embryo is attached to the placenta with a connecting stalk. Within this stalk are the beginnings of the early circulatory system, out of which by the end of week five the umbilical cord is formed.

The umbilical cord serves as the lifeline between the fetus and the placenta. Two arteries transport waste from the fetus back to the placenta, where it is transferred to the mother's blood and disposed of by way of her kidneys. One umbilical vein transports blood enriched with oxygen and nutrients to the fetus. The umbilical cord is surrounded by a gelatinous tissue (jelly of Warthon) to prevent the vessels from tangling and being clamped off. Due to further enlargement of the amniotic cavity, the amnion adheres firmly to the chorion (membrane formed by the trophoblast) (see Fig. 10).

◇

Amniotic Fluid

Amniotic fluid provides a medium for mobility and shock absorption for the fetus. It is formed and reabsorbed by way of the amnion and the vessels of the umbilical cord. The amniotic fluid increases and decreases as the fetus swallows it and excretes it again in the form of primitive urine. It helps in the development of the fetus's lungs.

At week 20 of pregnancy, there are approximately 17 fluid ounces of amniotic fluid. At week 38, there are approximately 50 fluid ounces. The fetus is protected from the amnionic fluid by a water-repellent protective film.

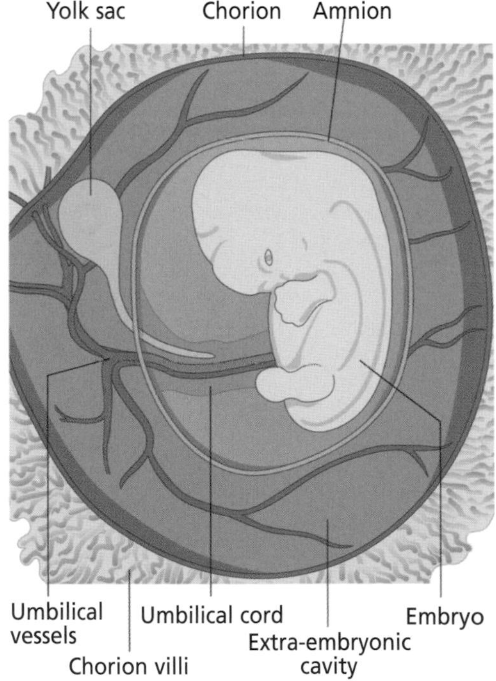

Fig. 10 - (a): Embryo in week five of pregnancy, according to Pfleiderer, Breckwoldt, and Martius.

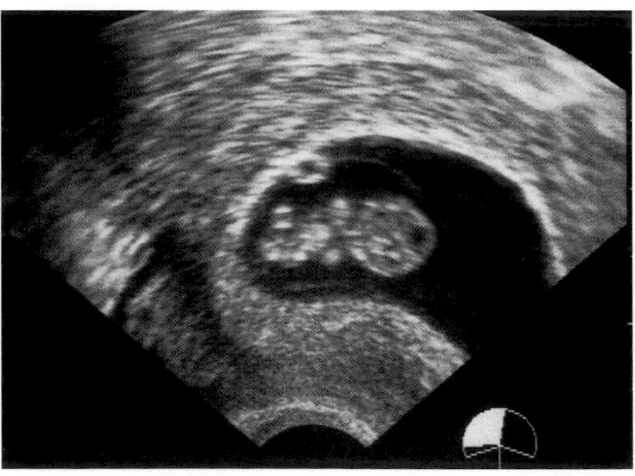

Fig. 10 - (b): Embryo in week nine of pregnancy, according to Pfleiderer, Breckwoldt, and Martius.

Placenta

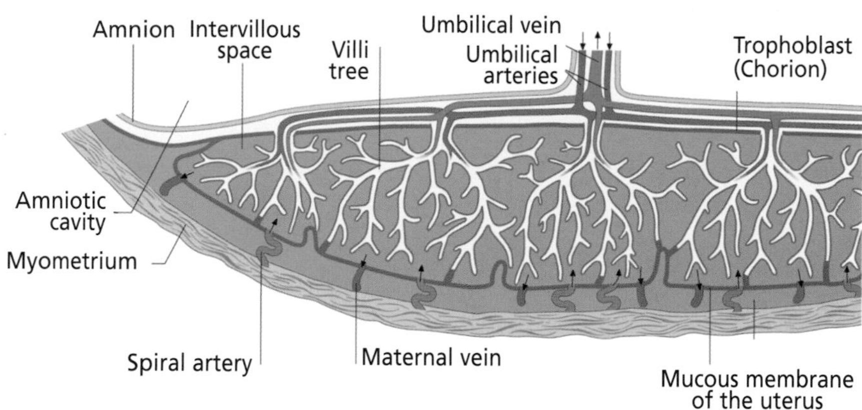

Fig. 11: The placenta, according to Pfleiderer, Breckwoldt, and Martius.

The villi of the fetus form little tree-like branches that permeate the mucous membrane of the uterus. The placenta is approximately six to eight inches long and almost one inch thick. On the maternal side, the blood of the spiral arteries of the uterine mucous membrane flows in little pools, into which the villi trees penetrate. By way of membranes, the oxygen-rich blood of the mother can enrich the fetus's blood, which contains less oxygen. The hemoglobin of the fetus has a different structure than adult hemoglobin and can absorb oxygen more easily. Aside from the free diffusion of oxygen, nutrients and antibodies are transported for the immune protection of the fetus. Only the existing immune protection of the mother can be passed on. If the mother develops an acute infection during pregnancy, the newly formed antibodies are not transferred to the fetus. For this reason, vaccinations are recommended to prospective mothers before conception.

Fetal Circulation

In the circulatory system of the adult, there is the pulmonary circulation, in which blood from the right side of the heart is directed to the lungs for oxygen enrichment. The enriched blood is then sent to the left side of the heart and pumped from there into the systemic circulation. It flows past the intestines, liver, and spleen, and then returns, detoxicated and nutrient-enriched, but low in oxygen, to the right side of the heart.

In the fetus's circulatory system, the opposite occurs. The oxygen-enriched blood flows through the umbilical cord vein into the inferior vena cava (large vein that returns blood to the heart) of the fetus and to the right side of the heart. By way of a short-circuit connection (ductus venosus), it bypasses the liver and lungs, which are not yet developed, and is pumped directly into the main circulatory system.

For this purpose, there is an open connection between the right and left side of the heart (foramen ovale). However, some blood also passes from the right side of the heart in the direction of the lesser circulation. In order to bypass the lung, a further short cut (ductus arteriosus) carries blood from the pulmonary artery directly to the aorta. An umbilical artery runs back to the placenta from both femoral arteries.

After birth, with the first breaths the baby takes, the fetal circulation changes and the short cuts begin to shrivel and close off.

Milestones of the Fetus's Development

Month 1

Fertilization and implantation in the lining of the uterus occur. The mother misses her menstrual cycle and may feel morning sickness (sometimes throughout the first trimester). The fundamental development of organs, brain, and spinal cord starts. The first organ to function is the heart (from week three). Arm and leg buds and sensory placodes (from which sensory organs will develop) appear, and muscles begin forming. The embryo is one-quarter inch long (10,000 times larger than the fertilized egg).

Month 2

By the end of the second month, most organs are established. The lung system is forming. Muscles work together, and the fetus begins to move. The skeleton is formed. Fingers and toes are defined, and the fetus has permanent fingerprints. Its eyelids are forming, and the ears develop. In week eight, the embryonic period ends, and the fetal period begins.

Month 3

The face is well formed. The fetus can suck its thumb and kick, and its fingers can make grasping movements. It can hear the mother's voice. Lung and brain growth are nearly complete. The eyelids remain closed, although they can open. The fetus is about three inches long. By week 12, the uterus has grown to the point where its upper edge (fundus) can be palpated or felt above the pubic plate.

Months 4 – 6

The mother has her first perception of the fetus's movements. The sex of the fetus can be identified by ultrasound (with great certainty by week 20). Its heartbeat can be heard with a stethoscope. The mother can feel her baby's hiccups. This is the time of rapid growth. The fetus weighs about one pound and is about one foot long (at five months). Downy hair covers the body, and the delicate skin is protected by a waxy substance. The fetus practices breathing by inhaling amniotic fluid into its developing lungs. Fingernails and toenails are present. The fetus produces feces (meconium) in the intestinal tract. By week 24 the upper edge of the uterus can be felt near the navel.

Months 7 – 9

The lungs continue to mature. Fat deposits make the thin, wrinkled skin smoother. By eight months, movements like kicks are visible from the outside. At week 36, the upper edge of the uterus has risen as high as the rib cage. By week 40, the upper edge of the uterus has lowered to four-fifths of an inch under the rib cage due to the entry of the fetus's head into the birth canal. At end of the ninth month, the fetus weighs about seven and one-half pounds and is about 19 to 20 inches long.

Physiological Changes during Pregnancy

As your body gradually adjusts to the new situation of being pregnant, many changes occur. Especially at the beginning, but sometimes throughout your pregnancy, you might feel morning sickness, dizziness, weakness, tiredness, or heaviness.

Helpful Yogasanas

Please refer to Chapter 3, "Sequences for Common Problems in Pregnancy," pages 159 – 160, Sequence 2 for dizziness, fatigue, and headache. And to Chapter 4, "Sequence for 1st trimester and throughout Pregnancy," pages 172 – 174.

Hormonal Changes

- HCG (human chorion gonadotropin) is formed by the fetus for maintenance of the corpus luteum. The hormone can be detected from the fourth day of pregnancy, even on the first day of the missed period.
- Progesterone is produced first by the corpus luteum, and from the second month of pregnancy, by the placenta. It has the following functions: maintaining pregnancy, preventing labor, producing milk, and developing the mammary glands.
- Estrogen is produced in the suprarenal glands of the mother and the fetus, and in the placenta. It has the following functions: growth and softening of the mother's tissues (uterus, ligaments, pelvic floor, and cervical dilation during labor). It also causes fluid retention.
- HPL (human placenta lactogen) is formed in the placenta and has an effect on the catabolic metabolism of the mother. It decreases her own consumption of blood sugar to ensure a good supply for the fetus. It increases the breakdown of fat in the mother and provides energy to the fetus between the mother's meals. (This metabolism is also regulated by the hormones cortisone and estrogen.)
- Cortisone suppresses immunity in the mother to prevent a possible rejection of the fetus. It helps the fetus's lungs mature.

◇

Heart and Circulatory System

- Adjustments in blood circulation ensure proper circulation in the placenta and as a result, in the fetus. Approximately 27 fluid ounces of blood per minute flow through the placenta.
- The mother's heart increases in size and beats faster, up to approximately 100 beats per minute.
- The leg veins widen and store more blood, so the circulating blood volume decreases. This activates the kidney hormones that cause the retention of salt and water. The water retained amounts to approximately eight quarts, of which one and one-half quarts are in the blood vessels. Because of this, the circulating blood volume then increases by 30-40%. Standing for long periods can put increased pressure on the leg veins and cause water retention in the lower legs and feet (peripheral edema).
- Pressure is increased in the inferior vena cava (large vein that returns blood to the heart) because it is partially compressed by the growing size of the uterus.

Helpful Yogasanas

Supine and inverted poses in particular can decrease edema of the legs, because they improve the draining of the retained fluid (lymph fluid) from the limbs. At the same time, they are done in a way that opens the rib cage and facilitates breathing. They improve the blood flow from the periphery to the trunk, so the blood flow to the vital organs of the mother and the fetus is also improved.

Pathological Conditions of the Circulatory System

Supine Hypotensive Syndrome

The name of this condition means low blood pressure when lying on your back. In this position, the inferior vena cava (large vein that returns blood to the heart) is clamped off by the weight of the fetus, thus preventing the blood from flowing back to the heart. This can lead to severe low blood pressure, which is signaled by nausea, dizziness, and cold sweats, and can eventually lead to fainting and shock. Since the inferior vena cava is on your right side, it is very important to immediately place the pregnant woman on her left side!

Helpful Yogasanas

See the variations of Shavasana in Chapter 3, "Instructions and Benefits."
In all the supine positions during your pregnancy, your torso is elevated by bolsters to create more space and improve the flow of blood back to the heart. If you still feel uncomfortable in these positions (especially in the last trimester), you should either increase the height of the support below your back or turn onto your side.

Preeclampsia or Toxemia

Preeclampsia is characterized by high blood pressure, increased excretion of protein in the urine, and edema (accumulation of fluid in the body). The condition can also lead to eclampsia (in which convulsive seizures appear). Preeclampsia usually develops in the third trimester of pregnancy. It is more frequent among women giving birth for the first time and those who are either pregnant with twins or more, at risk for high blood pressure, diabetic, or suffering from a kidney disorder.

Helpful Yogasanas

If you have high blood pressure, or develop high blood pressure during your pregnancy, please refer to Chapter 3, "Sequences for Common Problems in Pregnancy," Sequence 3 for high blood pressure, pages 161 – 162. Be sure to have frequent gynecological check-ups as well.

Other Changes

- Kidneys: Increase in the filtration rate due to increased circulation.
- Urinary tract: The ureters may become compressed, impeding the flow of urine. Progesterone limits the peristalsis of the ureters, which causes the urine to stagnate in the urinary tract for a longer time. This increases the risk of infection and the formation of kidney stones.
- Gastrointestinal tract: Peristalsis becomes weaker, and there is a tendency to become constipated.
- Esophagus: The abdominal organs are pushed in the direction of the diaphragm, thus causing a backflow of stomach acid into the esophagus (heartburn).
- Gall bladder: The emptying of the gallbladder into the small intestines is lessened, due to the effect of progesterone. This increases the risk of gallstones.
- Carbohydrate metabolism: Blood sugar levels can rise because of the increased demands of the fetus. About two to five percent of women develop diabetes during pregnancy. The diabetic metabolic state usually improves after giving birth. However, blood sugar readings must be carefully monitored to avoid complications, and the doctor must decide whether a dietary restriction during pregnancy is sufficient. Women who were diabetic prior to pregnancy also experience a change in their glucose metabolism during

Helpful Yogasanas

The changes in the mother's digestive tract are caused by the fetus, which is crowding her abdominal organs and exerting pressure on her diaphragm, and also by the progesterone in her body. As a pregnancy-supporting hormone, it limits contractions during pregnancy. It also, however, limits the peristalsis of all the smooth muscles of the digestive tract.
Yoga asanas can help with difficulties such as heartburn and constipation and also prevent the formation of gallstones or stagnation of urine in the ureters. Supine positions or twists are helpful because of their stimulating effect on the entire digestive tract.
See also Chapter 3, "Sequences for Common Problems in Pregnancy," Sequence 4 for diabetes, pages 163 – 164, and Sequence 5 for tension, heartburn, and shortness of breath, pages 165 – 167.

pregnancy. In this case, it is absolutely necessary to watch the blood sugar readings and carefully adjust the need for insulin medication.

- Fat metabolism: In early pregnancy, the woman's body builds up fatty tissue. Later on, fat is increasingly burned, resulting in elevated cholesterol and triglyceride levels.
- Lungs: Breathing becomes fast and shallow due to the pressure of the fetus on the diaphragm.
- Blood count: The fetus's metabolism requires iron. This increased demand can result in iron deficiency anemia in the mother, and often an increase in the white cell count.
- Blood clotting: The liver produces more clotting factors, thus increasing the risk of a thromboembolism (the blockage of a blood vessel by a blood clot).
- Thyroid gland: The increased demand for iodine can cause iodine deficiency and goiter formation in the mother.
- Skin and hair: Pigment cells are stimulated, thus hyperpigmentation often occurs on parts of the face exposed to sun light. There is often the formation of a dark line between the navel and the mons pubis.

Changes in the Body in Preparation for Birth

Due to the estrogen-induced relaxation of the ligaments and muscles, there is often increased tension in the pelvic ring and pain in the iliosacral joint. Many women complain of pain of the labia majora, which is caused by the pressure on the round ligament. Because the abdomen is pulling away from the spine, backache can occur. The formation of mammary glands can cause tension in the breasts.

Helpful Yogasanas

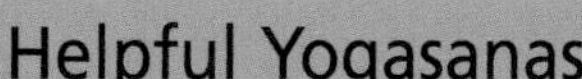

Please refer to Chapter 4, "Sequence for Third Trimester, Preparing for Delivery," pages 187 – 188.

Asanas can also be helpful in the case of back or pelvic pains by relieving the pressure on the sacrum and the lower back. Please refer to Chapter 3, "Sequences for Common Problems in Pregnancy," Sequence 6 for back pain, pages 166 – 167.

Psychological Effects

Every woman experiences her pregnancy in an individual way. The following are some frequently reported feelings:

First trimester – ambivalence, lack of bonding with the fetus, fear of losing the baby

Second trimester – a pronounced feeling of well-being, increased connection to the fetus because the first movements are felt and its growth can be seen in ultrasound pictures

Third trimester – fears and anxiety regarding any of the following: becoming a mother, the birth, the health of the fetus and one's own health, the process of separation from the fetus

Helpful Yogasanas

We recommend asanas that help to create mental and psychological stability, especially the practice of pranayama.

ANATOMY, PHYSIOLOGY, AND PROCREATION

Delivery

According to Naegele's Rule, the due date for a 40-week pregnancy (from the first day of the last menstrual cycle) can be calculated according to the following formula:
1st day of your last period – 3 months + 7 days + 1 year
The rule effectively states that a pregnancy should last approximately 40 weeks (280 days) from the last menstrual cycle. Giving birth before week 37 of pregnancy is termed premature; post-term is a birth exceeding 42 weeks of pregnancy.

During pregnancy, Braxton-Hicks contractions may occur. Because they are not capable of inducing birth, they are also known as false labor.

Labor is divided into the following three stages:

Stage 1

In the first stage, contractions induce the dilation of the cervix at a rate of approximately four- to eight-tenths of an inch per hour, up to the maximum dilation of four inches. For women who have already given birth, the first stage is often shorter than for those giving birth for the first time.

How, exactly, do the contractions cause the dilation of the cervix? Before the birth, there are hormonal changes. The progesterone level is reduced, which increases the contractions induced by the hormone oxytocin. The contractions stimulate the smooth muscles of the uterus. In the cervix, there are more elastic fibers than muscles. When the uterus contracts, the baby's head is already pressing into the cervix. The cervix itself does not contract, but widens and dilates. This process can be compared to pulling on a turtleneck pullover.

The effacement, or thinning, of the cervix is induced by hormones as well. Estrogen softens and loosens the tissue. Prostaglandin widens the vessels and causes cells to release enzymes that further soften the tissues of the cervix.

When the mucous plug that has closed the uterine orifice during the entire pregnancy dislodges, some bleeding may occur due to the tearing of small blood vessels. It may occur during the first stage or even before the onset of labor.

The rupture of the amniotic membranes, or the water breaking, can occur at various points. They may rupture early during the period of dilation or even before onset of labor, which is called premature rupture of the membranes. This can indicate or cause the induction of labor. If a child is born together with intact membranes, it is called late rupture of the membranes.

Stage 2

Once the cervix is fully dilated, the second stage of labor can begin. The contractions are more frequent, and the baby's head has entered the birth canal.

The bony part of the birth canal is a firm passageway that the baby's head (its largest and hardest structure) must penetrate first. The bony part of the birth canal consists of the pelvic inlet, the mid-pelvic plane, and the pelvic outlet. Each of these has a different shape, so the baby must change position in order to pass through them.

The pelvic inlet is horizontally oval. It runs from the upper surface of the sacrum (sacral promontory) to the upper edge of the symphysis. Since the human head is a lengthwise oval, the baby's head has to turn sideways when it enters the pelvic inlet. By this time, the baby's body is usually lying with its lengthwise axis in the lengthwise axis of the mother, commonly turning its back towards the left side.

The mid-pelvic plane is round and runs from the bottom edge of the symphysis to the tip of the sacrum. In order to enter this part of the bony pelvis, the baby turns with the back of its head downward. The back of the baby's head (occiput) turns forward toward the pubic bone, and the baby's chin is thus bent onto its chest.

The pelvic outlet is a lengthwise oval, limited by the pubic arch, ischium, and coccyx. As a rule, first the back of the baby's head, then the top, and then the face pass through the pelvic outlet. The mother's tailbone (coccyx) is pushed backward by the baby's head; this dilates the pelvic outlet so the baby can pass through.

The bony birth canal leads into the soft birth canal, which is made up of the lower segment of the uterus, the cervix, the vagina, and the muscular pelvic floor. When the baby's head enters the middle pelvic area, the muscular part of the soft birth canal forms a bulge that is pushed outwards by the pressure of the baby's head. At this point, you can already see the fontanel (back of the baby's head) through the vagina. The anus widens under the pressure. The baby's head then presses onto the muscular pelvic floor, which has to give way to allow the baby to pass through. This pressure on the pelvic floor increases the contractions, and there is a strong urge to push. At this stage, it is advantageous for the mother to close her larynx (not to cry out) and actively squeeze, and push, as during defecation. This also soothes the perception of labor pains.
When the pelvic floor muscle is stretched outward during delivery, the birth assistant protects the perineum with her hand. Sometimes, however, the pelvic floor presents an obstacle that delays the delivery. If the mother or child becomes distressed and the child cannot be born promptly, an episiotomy can shorten the soft birth canal and speed up delivery. If the baby's head does not emerge, other means may be used (such as forceps or vacuum extraction).

Once the baby's head has emerged, the birth assistant turns the baby to the side. By means of a gentle pull downward, first the shoulder facing the front emerges. With a gentle pull upward, the other shoulder emerges, followed by the rest of the body.

Immediately after birth the baby's face is cleaned so that he or she can breathe. Then the baby is dried off and given a health examination. Now the newborn can be laid on the mother's chest.
The time for cutting the umbilical cord may vary. The umbilical cord is clamped off at each end and then cut off between the two clamps. The remainder of the umbilical cord, which is left on the child, eventually dries and falls off.

Stage 3

After the baby is born and the umbilical cord has been cut, the afterbirth is delivered. It consists of the placenta and the maternal part of the umbilical cord. The placenta becomes dislodged during postpartum labor, so a slight tug on the umbilical cord will allow the birth assistant to pull the placenta out through the vagina.

This stage is important for blood coagulation and for the uterus's return to its proper shape.

Helpful Yogasanas

In preparation for birth, asanas are used to widen the hips and the pelvic floor. It is important for the pregnant woman to learn straight positioning of the pelvis, so she will gain an instinctive and confident sense of the direction in which to exert pressure during the bearing-down phase.
The poses promote patience and confidence in one's own body and inner relaxation. This includes pranayama, which encourage deep breathing into the pelvic floor. Deep breathing relaxes the muscles during and after labor and helps with breathing through the pain. This also includes active breathing directed towards the child. Other pranayama help with recovery between painful contractions, so that the mother can gather strength and relax (see Chapter 4, "Sequence for Third Trimester, Preparing for Delivery, pages 187 – 188").

Cesarean Section

Situations when a cesarean section is clearly indicated include:

- Cord prolapse: when the umbilical cord descends into the vagina to lie in front of the baby
- Placental presentation: when the placenta lies across the cervix before or during labor
- Severe preeclampsia

Situations when a cesarean section may be indicated include:

- A breech or transverse position that can make a vaginal delivery impossible
- Fetal distress
- Diseases of the mother (such as infections)
- Multiple births (twins or more)

After Delivery

Position of the Uterus

Position of the Uterus

The uterus gradually regains its shape. Directly after the afterbirth is pushed out, the top of the uterus (fundus) is located between the ischium and the navel. On the first day after birth, it is one finger's width below the navel. By the tenth day, it is at the upper edge of the ischium.

Lochia

Lochia is a bloody discharge, similar to menstruation, which occurs for four to six weeks after birth as a result of the postpartum healing process. There is a progressive change in its color: Immediately after birth, it is most bloody. It then becomes rust brown, then yellowish, and finally quite clear and watery.

The discharge is infectious, and it is advisable to change sanitary napkins and wash your hands frequently, especially before breast-feeding. Cleaning the genital area is best done with pure water. Lukewarm chamomile solution may also be used, but no soap, in order to maintain the protective acidic milieu of the vagina.

Hormonal Adjustment

Directly after birth, there is a withdrawal of all hormones produced by the placenta. This may cause a significant change in the mother's moods on the second or third day postpartum. Depression and mood swings are completely normal and occur in many women. They are usually self-limiting, and end when the hormones return to a balanced state.

Breast-Feeding

Hormonal changes during pregnancy lead to the development of the mammary glands. After birth, the hormone prolactin regulates the formation of breast milk. Breast milk secretion is assisted by the hormone oxytocin through the suckling reflex of the baby. This hormone also induces contractions of the uterus, so breast-feeding helps the uterus regain its shape.

The increased prolactin level suppresses the other hormones of the menstrual cycle, so that fertility may be limited for about 30 weeks postpartum. However, you should not rely solely on this for birth control purposes.

The mother's milk is produced according to the requirements of the newborn. In the first two or three days, the baby receives a unique pre-milk fluid, called colostrum, which is highly nutritious and rich in antibodies. In the following two weeks, the mother's milk becomes particularly rich in fat. After this period, normal breast milk is produced. The mother's milk contains an assortment of nutrients, important trace elements, and vitamins that are appropriate for the baby's metabolism and for his or her immune system. It is very good for the development of healthy intestinal bacteria and can help prevent the formation of allergies in early years.

Full nursing (meaning breast milk only) is recommended for at least six months before introducing solid food. The midwife usually gives instructions and assistance in breast-feeding. It is important that the nipple is taken properly into the baby's mouth and that the baby can breathe. To prevent minor injuries to the breast, the baby has to latch on correctly. Both breasts should be offered to the baby and emptied. The breasts should be kept dry and clean in order to prevent infections. Nursing is important for mother-child bonding, so the mother and baby should not be disturbed. (See also Part IV, Chapter 3, "Ayurvedic Recipes and Health Tips.")

Procreation from the Ayurvedic Point of View

The ancient Ayurvedic texts, mainly *Vagbhata Samhita* (circa 7th century), *Sushruta Samhita* (circa 1,500–1,000 BC), and *Charaka Samhita* (circa 1,000 BC), described conception, pregnancy, and birth in detail.

The formation of the embryo takes place as the *atman* (individual soul), impelled by the afflictions of its own past actions (*klesha-karma*), enters the union of pure (not impaired by *doshas*) *shukra* (semen) and *shonita* (egg cell). This union of *atman*, *shonita*, and *shukra* takes place in the uterus (*garbhashaya*) and gives rise to the formation of an embryo (*garbha*) in a predetermined manner, like the fire that originates from two pieces of wood rubbed together. (2/1)

Just as the rays of the sun passing through a lens and converging on a piece of paper are not seen—although suddenly the piece of paper catches fire—the *atman* enters the womb, and suddenly life activity is felt. (2/2)

Like molten metal that takes the shape of the mold into which it is poured, the *atman* takes on different shapes and conditions of birth according to its actions in former lives. According to the *Samkhya* and Yoga philosophy, good actions cause good things in the new life, and bad actions cause bad conditions (principle of similarity and dissimilarity = *samyama* and *vaishesika vedanta*). (2/3)

"The accumulated imprints of past lives, rooted in afflictions, will be experienced in present and future lives. As long as the root of actions exists, it will give rise to class of birth, span of life, and experiences. According to our good, bad, or mixed actions, the quality of our life, its span, and the nature of birth are experienced as being pleasant or painful." (2/15)

Conception

Just as the lotus closes at the end of the day, so also the *yoni* (female reproductive organs) close after the *ritu kala* (the period suitable for conception); thereafter the woman will not be receptive to *shukra* (semen). (2/4)

The immediate signs of conception are:

- A sense of contentment
- A sense of heaviness and throbbing in the lower abdomen and vaginal tract
- Cessation of flow of semen after copulation
- Cessation of menstruation
- Throbbing in the heart
- Stupor, thirst, fatigue, and goose bumps (2/5)

Development of the Embryo (Five Elements)

The signs of early pregnancy (second month) are:

- Cessation of menstruation
- Fatigue, urge to do nothing, yawning
- Heaviness in the body
- Fainting
- Vomiting (early morning nausea), watery sensation in the mouth, heartburn
- Various kinds of cravings, especially for sour-tasting food
- Development of the breasts, darkening of the nipples, sometimes a little lactation
- Edema (fluid accumulation) of the feet
- A dark line under the navel

The embryo grows gradually in the womb, nourished by the essence of the food of the mother.

According to the *Charaka Samhita*, different organs can be derived from the mother, the father, and the soul. The text says in the third chapter of the second volume according to the translation of R. K. Sharma Bhagwan Dash:

"The fetus is produced from the mother. Without the mother, there is no possibility of conception and birth of viviparous creatures. We shall thereafter describe those organs which are derived from the maternal source (from the ovum) and which are formed because of the existence of the mother. They are skin, blood, flesh, fat, umbilicus, heart, lung, liver, spleen, kidneys, bladder, rectum, stomach, colon, upper and lower part of the anus, small intestines, mesentery and omentum.

"The fetus is produced from the father. Without the father, there is no possibility of conception and birth of viviparous creatures. We shall thereafter describe those organs which are derived from the paternal source (from the sperm) and which are formed because of the existence of the father. They are hair of the head, hair of the face, small hairs of the body, nails, teeth, bones, veins, ligaments, arteries, and semen. These organs are derived from the paternal source.

"The fetus is also produced out of the soul. The *jivatman* [soul inside the animal body] is the same as *garbhatman* [soul in the fetus]. This is known as embodied or animated soul. The soul is eternal. It does not get afflicted by diseases. It does not undergo the process of aging. It does not succumb to death. It does not undergo diminution. It cannot be penetrated. It cannot be cut. It cannot be made or get irritated. It is invisible. It is without beginning or end, and it is unchangeable."

Patanjali describes the soul as an entity separate from the body, mind, and intelligence. It is latent and exists everywhere. It is the very essence of the core of one's being. It has no actual location in the body but exists everywhere.

Charaka Samhita describes further: "By entering into the uterus, it gets combined with the sperm and the ovum and thereby reproduces itself in the form of a fetus. Thus the fetus takes the designation of the soul. Factors derived from the *atman* [soul] are: taking birth in different wombs, life span, self-realization, mind, senses, to take things in and excrete things from the body, stimulation and substance of sense organs, characteristic shape, voice and complexion of the individual, desire for happiness and sorrow, liking or disliking, consciousness, courage, intellect, memory, egoism, and efforts."

The development of the embryo is regulated by the causative and subtle *mahabhutas* (five elements) and the entry of *atman* (soul). (2/6)

The five elements are *akasha* (element of space), *vayu* (element of air), *tejas* (element of fire), *apa* (element of water), and *prithvi* (element of earth). As *shukra* (semen) and *shonita* (ovum) both are elemental, *jivatman* (soul inside the animal body) unites with these elements.

Charaka Samhita, Vol 2, IV:8 states that the soul first unites with the element of space before uniting with the other elements. This is compared to the creation of space by God after the deluge. As God, the indestructible one, equipped with the mind, created space first and then the other elements whose attributes are successively more and more manifest, so does the soul, desirous of creating another body, first unite with the element of space and then with the other four elements. All these actions take place in a very short time.

The five elements (*panchamahabhutas*) and their actions are:
1. *Akasha* (space)
The element of space is important in creating the hollowness or space of the organs. It helps the development of the ear regarding the sense of sound, and the development of all rhythms, rhythmic actions, and sounds in the body such as breathing and heartbeat. Lightness, subtlety, and distinction are derived from this element.

2. *Vayu* (air)
The element of air is important in structuring and formatting the body, creating the channels and ways of transportation of the tissues, and creating the principle of movement. It helps develop the sense of touch and the sense organ that corresponds to touch, which is the skin. Roughness and impulsion refer to this element.

3. *Tejas* (fire)
Like blowing into hot glass to give it shape, the fire and air elements work together to shape the structure of the body. They create the inner hollowness of all organs. Fire is also the element that creates the principle of transformation in the body; it develops different *agnis* (fires) that can digest and transform. The heat of the body refers to the element of fire. Fire creates brightness, the sense of sight, and the corresponding sense organ, the eye.

4. *Apa* (water)
This element makes all liquid parts of the body (*kledah*), controlled by drinking, sweating, and urination. It forms the tissue of plasma (*rasa*) and creates the sense of taste and its corresponding sense organ, the tongue. Coldness, softness, unctuousness, and stickiness are derived from this element.

5. *Prithvi* (earth)
This element creates the principle of mass of the body. It creates heavy tissues like muscles (*mamsa*) and bones (*asthi*). It develops the sense of smell and its corresponding sense organ, the nose. Heaviness, hardness, and steadiness are derived from this element.

When accompanied by all five elements, the soul takes the form of an embryo. During the first month of gestation, it takes the form of jelly, because of the intimate mixture of the five elements. These develop in the subsequent months into the seven tissue elements of the body, which are *rasa* (plasma), *rakta* (blood), *mamsa* (muscle), *meda* (fat), *asthi* (bones), *majja* (bone marrow), and *shukra* (semen).

The *dhatus* (seven tissues of the body) are built up in steps, one on top of the other. If we take food, some of it gets transformed into energy for the body, some gets excreted, and some gets assimilated into the first tissue of the body, which is *rasa* (plasma). Rasa gets transformed into the next body tissue, which is *rakta* (blood). Then come muscle (*mamsa*), fat (*meda*), bones (*asthi*), bone marrow (*majja*), and the reproductive cells (*shukra* and *shonita*). For each of these steps, the Ayurveda knows different digestive fires (*agni*).

In order to maintain good health, the *doshas* (active principles of the body) have to be balanced, so that their functions of preserving, transforming, and excreting are well balanced, and so that no waste products (*ama*) remain in the body. When the last *dhatu* is built (*shukra* and *shonita*), it gets transformed into the essence of life (*ojas*). *Ojas* is the very core of the energy of life and exists in a very small quantity in the body. The quantity and quality of *ojas* depends on the functioning of the metabolism.

Month by Month

During the first month, the embryo has no particular form, and its organs are both manifest and latent. (*Charaka Samhita, Vol 2, IV:9*)

By the second month, the embryo has formed into a shape with some firmness—somewhat round (*pinda*) in a male child and more oval (*peshi*) in a female child (2/7). During this month, the mother may show the signs of pregnancy mentioned earlier. If she has cravings for certain things, she should have them in small quantities; it is said that denying her cravings could lead to abnormalities in the fetus. (2/8)

In the third month, the five parts of the body become manifest: the head, two legs, two arms, and all the minor parts. Simultaneously with the formation of the head, the knowledge of pleasure and pain comes into existence. (2/9) The umbilical cord is formed, which is said to make a connection between the heart of the mother and the heart of the fetus, so that the fetus can express its desires through the heart of the mother. The fetus derives nourishment like a cornfield does from an aqueduct. (2/10)

In the fourth month, all parts become clearly formed. The fetus becomes stabilized, and the mother experiences excessive heaviness in the body as a result.

In the fifth month, the *cetana* (consciousness) enters. *Cetana* can also be translated as liveliness of the fetus, which is due to more activity of the *atman* (soul) of the child. The blood and the muscles of the child develop, and it is said that the mother loses weight as the child grows.

In the sixth month, the tendons, nails, skin, hair, strength, and color develop, and the child gains weight. In comparison to the other months, there is a marked increase in the strength and complexion of the fetus during this month, so the mother loses considerable strength and complexion herself.

In the seventh month, the fetus is well developed and nourished. The *doshas* of the mother, being pushed up by the fetus towards her heart, can cause itching and burning in the palms and soles of the feet, heartburn, and pregnancy striae (stretch marks). (2/11) There is an overall development of the fetus during this month, causing the mother to become deficient in all aspects of her health.

In the eighth month, *ojas* travels from the child to the mother and from the mother to the child. Both become fatigued or contented respectively. Ojas is an essence of he body responsible for strength and is essential for life. It is said to be present in the heart, and its loss leads to death. Its presence in the mother and the fetus produces strength and contentment; its absence leads to fatigue and anxiety. If the child is born in this month, when the ojas travels between mother and child, it is said to be very dangerous for one or the other because of the absence of ojas. (2/12)

In the ninth month, the child is ready to be born. It is recommended that the mother often have ghee (a clarified butter used in Indian cooking, page 417) and an outer application of oil (abhyanga, page 417), as well as a rolled cloth dipped in oil applied to the vagina, to ease the delivery.

The Doshas

The five elements build up three active principles of the body, called *tridosha*. The word *dosha* means "able to disturb." Doshas, once they are impaired, can disturb the health of the body. A person with balanced doshas enjoys good health. From birth, we have a certain constitution, mostly with one or two dominating doshas. But the activity of the doshas can be diminished or aggravated, as everything we do, sense, think, eat, or drink has certain qualities (*gunas*) or tastes (*rasas*) that increase or decrease the doshas. The constitution of the embryo depends on that of both parents and on all the influences the mother undergoes during her pregnancy.

The three doshas are:

The ***kapha dosha*** comes from the elements of earth and water. Its main function is to build up and preserve the body. Its main seat is in the head and thoracic region, as well as the upper gastrointestinal tract from the mouth cavity to the stomach.

This dosha is strong in winter and early spring, in the early morning after sunrise. It is dominant in childhood and youth, when the body and the personality are developing. It is very important especially for conception, as it preserves a good quality of the reproductive organs and is dominant in early pregnancy.

According to Ayurveda, things similar to *kapha* can increase the kapha dosha, and opposite things can decrease it. Qualities that increase kapha are: heavy, solid, slimy, cold, slow, oily, moist, stable, and soft. Qualities that decrease kapha are: light, liquid, rough, hot, fast, dry, mobile, and hard. Tastes that increase kapha are: sweet, sour, and salty. Tastes that decrease kapha are: hot, astringent, and bitter.

People who have a predominance of kapha dosha in their constitution have a certain outer appearance. They have a rather heavy body with big bones, good muscles, and stable joints. They gain weight easily, their skin is moist and cool, and their veins are not visible. They have full hair and white eyeballs.

The temperament of people with kapha constitution is calm, friendly, and forgiving. They make friendships slowly, but once they have decided, they are steadfast. They do their duty quietly and methodically, and have a good memory.

Signs and diseases of increased/impaired kapha include diseases of the respiratory tract and the head. The person feels heavy and tired. If the kapha dosha becomes impaired, it decreases the digestive power (*agni*), which leads to the assimilation of waste products (*ama*). People gain weight and experience heaviness and stiffness in their limbs. They feel hungry even after eating and have a watery sensation in the mouth.

The ***pitta dosha*** comes from the element of fire. Its main function is the principle of transformation and digestion (by *agnis*, which are special digestive fires).

The main seat of pitta dosha in the body is the region around the navel and the small intestines. It is strong in summer, at high noon, when the sun is at its peak. The pitta dosha gets stronger in the middle period of life, when people create their own existence and career.

In pregnancy, the pitta dosha gets stronger up to the third trimester.

Qualities that increase pitta are: hot, light, odorous, watery, slightly oily, and flowing. Qualities that decrease pitta are: cold, heavy, odorless, rough, and stable. Tastes that increase pitta are: hot (pungent), sour, and salty. Tastes that decrease pitta are: sweet, bitter, and astringent.

People with a predominance of pitta dosha have an attractive appearance, shiny skin, and are always warm and soft. They cannot tolerate missing a meal and can digest everything without gaining weight. Their hair gets gray very early. They have good eyesight and shining eyes, but sometimes yellowish or red eyeballs.

People with pitta constitution like to be the center of attention; they can entertain and lead a group. They often lose their temper if they don't control themselves. They work quickly and accurately. They have a good capacity for understanding and getting a point, as pitta dosha transforms and also assimilates.

The signs and diseases of impaired pitta include heartburn, inflammation, diarrhea, excessive thirst or hunger, itching and burning, and sleeplessness.

The ***vata dosha*** comes from the elements of air and ether. Its main function in the body is the principle of transport and movement. Its main seat is in the area below the navel, colon, and rectum. Vata is enhanced in autumn and winter, in the evening and before dawn. It is strong later in life.

In pregnancy, the vata dosha increases towards birth and is very high after delivery.

Qualities that increase vata are: dry, light, rough, minute, moving, and fast. Qualities that decrease vata are: oily, moist, heavy, slimy, gross, stable, and slow. Tastes that increase vata are: bitter, astringent, and pungent. Tastes that decrease vata are: sweet, sour, and salty.

People with vata constitution have a light body structure and difficulty gaining weight. They have dry skin that wrinkles early and visible veins. Their skin is cool, and they always feel cold. The vata element is responsible for excretion and the withdrawal of water from the feces in the colon. Since the vata dosha has a drying capacity and decreases moisture and oiliness in the body, vata-dominated people tend to suffer from constipation and meteorism (gas). People of this constitution have thin hair and early hair loss. Their eyes are deep in the eye socket and sometimes surrounded by dark rings. Their eye color is often brown.

The vata dosha is responsible for all the movements in the body, including the movement of the limbs, the circulation of the blood in the vessels, and the transmission of nerve impulses. Therefore it is also responsible for sensing and pain. The element makes all rhythmic actions in the body, such as breathing and the heartbeat.

The vata dosha is fast moving and controls the speed of thoughts. People of this constitution think very quickly, sometimes so much so that they cannot finish their thoughts. Often they don't finish one job because they already have so many ideas for the next one. They like to talk, and they get to know many people without having deep relationships.

The signs and diseases of increased vata are: constipation and meteorism (gas), agitation and restlessness, pain, arthritis, a lot of talking with little meaning, weight loss, sleeplessness, shivering, and tremor.

Special Note

After birth, due to labor pains and the hollow space in the body after delivery, the vata element greatly increases. This can lead to vata disorders. The mother should therefore use oil on her body, especially around the waist, and should eat foods that are oily and sweet. Lack of rest, stress, and strain can impair vata, leading to the signs and symptoms mentioned above.

The Delivery

The following signs indicate the approach of the delivery:

1. Exhaustion of the limbs and general tiredness
2. Drooping of the eyes and facial skin
3. Soft abdomen
4. Feeling in the chest as if a knot is being untied
5. Feeling that something is coming down from the pelvis
6. Heaviness in the lower part of the body
7. Pain in the groin, thighs, waist, pelvis, bladder, sides of the chest and back, and pulsation and pain in the cervix
8. Onset of discharge from the vaginal tract
9. Increased urination
10. Loss of appetite and watery sensation in the mouth (2/13)

Afterwards, true labor pains start, which are associated with the excretion of amniotic fluid. A bed should be prepared on the ground and covered with soft material, and the mother should be asked to sit on it.

Female attendants should remain all around the mother and soothe her with comforting words. The attendants should have certain qualities: they should have had their own experience in giving birth, and be affectionate, constantly attached to the mother, well mannered, resourceful, naturally disposed to love, free from grief, tolerant of hardship, and able to give courage.

If delivery does not take place in spite of severe labor pains, the sages are of the view that the pregnant woman should not strain herself, but can be allowed to walk around. At intervals, the mother should be anointed with warm oil at her waist, sides of the chest, back, and thighs, and these places should be gently massaged. This brings the fetus downward.

When the mother feels that the fetus has gotten separated from her heart, entered into the lower abdomen, and approached the perineum, and when the frequency of labor pain has increased and the fetus has turned and come downward, then the physician should have her lie on a bed especially prepared for this purpose. The mother should be asked to push to facilitate the delivery, but her attendants should instruct her not to push in the absence of labor pains.

Pushing in the absence of labor pains does not serve any useful purpose. On the contrary, it causes morbidity and deformity in the fetus and produces conditions like shortness of breath, cough, consumption, and enlargement of the spleen.

On the other hand, the mother should push when she does feel a contraction. Just as it is difficult and dangerous to suppress a natural urge such as sneezing or belching, the mother should never fail to push when she feels the urge to do so.

The mother should listen to the instructions. She should apply pressure slowly in the beginning and gradually increase it. As she pushes, the attendants should thank her enthusiastically for her efforts and let her know that she has delivered the child. This gives her relief and joy and helps her regain her vitality.

Immediately after delivery, she should be examined to ascertain whether the placenta has come out. If not, the following measures should be taken: One of the female attendants should press the mother's abdomen with her right hand from above the umbilical region downward, with the left hand supporting her back. Other methods to expel the placenta are also described in the *Charaka Samhita*; they all help to create a downward movement of *vayu* (vata dosha) in the abdomen, which results in the expulsion of the placenta as well as gas, urine, and stool. These may cause an obstruction inside the abdomen, preventing the placenta from coming out.

The child should be cleaned and cleared of the vernix caseosa (pasty covering that protects the fetus), and his or her breathing passage should be cleared. The umbilical cord should be separated by cutting and ligature.

The *Vagbhata Samhita* describes a mantra for immediately after birth. A sound should be made at the child's right ear by hitting two stones together, and the following should be recited:

"You have been born from every organ of the body and the hrdaya (heart, mind).
You are myself in the form of a child.
May you live for a hundred years, may you attain long life, let the stars, the quarters, nights, and days protect you."

CHAPTER 2

AYURVEDIC RECIPES AND HEALTH TIPS - DURING PREGNANCY

The Ideal Diet

To understand the necessity for balanced, or *sattvic*, nutrition when you're pregnant, it helps to first understand the hormonal changes that take place in the blood once you've conceived. The dominating hormone in pregnancy is progesterone, which is secreted to prevent labor contractions from beginning before they are due. It also affects the peristalsis of the uterus, colon, and other internal organs. *(See also Part IV, Chapter 1, "Anatomy, Physiology, and Procreation".)*

This is why many pregnant women experience constipation, bloating, and hard stools. Passing hard stools can put pressure on the veins and cause hemorrhoids, swelling of the legs, and varicose veins.

Consequently, you should avoid eating dry food such as bread (beyond a moderate amount), day-old leftovers, frozen food, dried pulses (peas, beans, lentils, etc.), and cabbage.

Restrict how much coffee and black tea you drink, because these dehydrate. Have instead green tea, fennel tea, and hot or warm water instead of cold drinks.

If you eat heavy proteins such as black lentils or cheese, you should eat them for lunch to ensure full digestion before bedtime.

◇

Foods to Avoid

- Laxative foods, which can cause spasms of the uterus: aloe vera, angelica, papaya, pineapple, asafetida, beans, saffron, rhubarb, nutmeg, citrus, fenugreek, chebulic myrobalan
- Hot and spicy dishes cooked with chilies and lots of garlic and onions
- Acidic or oily foods: meat, white sugar, sweeteners, vinegar, and sour fruits

Healthy Foods

Foods you should eat include alkaline foods like vegetables, green leaves, juicy fruits, cereals, and homemade bread made from organic whole or German wheat.

The following are recommended foods that balance the *agni*, the fire of digestion:

Grains

Organic whole wheat, German wheat, oats, basmati rice, millet, barley, mung beans, pasta made from organic whole or German wheat or millet, and homemade bread from organic whole or German wheat or millet

Fruit

Ripe, juicy, sweet fruit (can be slightly cooked for easier digestion), including apples, pears, apricots, plums, and pomegranates. (Grapes and cherries, though sweet, can cause bloating.)

Cooked Vegetables

Carrots, celery, onion, Chinese cabbage, zucchini, tomatoes (ripe), beet root, cucumbers, sprouts, potatoes (in moderation), sweet potatoes, green beans, cassava, mushrooms, plenty of green herbs and green leaves, and asparagus

Note

Nightshades such as paprika, eggplant, potatoes, pumpkin, and zucchini can cause bloating. Find out how to prepare them with warming spices like black pepper and cumin.

Nuts and Seeds

Roast these without fat in a pan: almonds, sesame seeds, pumpkin seeds, coconut, macadamia nuts, pine nuts, and walnuts

Fats

Sesame oil, olive oil, pumpkin seed oil, mustard oil, and ghee (a clarified butter used in Indian cooking; for recipe see page 417)

Herbs

- Ginger, coriander, black pepper, celery seeds, fennel seeds, cumin seeds, mustard seeds, anis, cinnamon, Ayurvedic masalas (spice mixtures), and rock salt
- Small amounts of: turmeric, saffron, and cardamom
- Instead of salt, try to use herbs like parsley, basil, rosemary, thyme, and American raspberry.

Milk Products

- Fresh cow's milk (1 cup per day), buttermilk, ghee, fresh goat cheese, fresh sheep cheese, and cream
- Don't mix milk products with fruit. This causes a curdling of the milk product, which forms a kind of cheese in the acidic stomach environment that is heavy to digest and can even cause joint problems.

Nonlactic Proteins

Soy milk, tofu, and miso soup (from barley or soy)

Beverages

Have 2 to 3 quarts of hot water a day and follow this procedure:

- Boil the water for 10 minutes and pour half of it into a thermos bottle.
- Boil the rest of the water for 5 more minutes with 3 slices of fresh or dried ginger and 1 teaspoon of celery seeds and add it to the water in the thermos. (You can also try 1 teaspoon of fennel instead.) These ingredients warm the stomach, improve digestion, and reduce gas formation.

Sugar

Jaggery (unrefined brown sugar), cane sugar, and honey

"Let him, with an attentive mind, first taste that which has a sweet flavor, he may take salt and sour things in the middle course and finish with those

which are pungent (and bitter), etc. The man who commences his meal with fluids, then partakes of solid food and finishes with fluid again, will ever be strong and healthy."
(Vishnu Purana III, 11:87–88)

Suggested Daily Menu

Breakfast - **Porridge**

Instructions

1. Boil 2 cups of water with 1/2 teaspoon ghee (clarified butter).
2. Stirring constantly, add 1/2 pound oats, German wheat, or organic whole wheat.
3. Bring to a boil.
4. Add 2 teaspoons raisins (or dried figs or apricots) and 1 teaspoon ground coconut or dried almonds.
5. Serve with honey and if you like, cinnamon.

Alternative: Toast and Honey
Toast made from fresh, homemade bread with ghee and honey

How to Make Ghee

1. Heat 1 pound of fresh, pure biological butter (with no additives) in a large pan or pot on a very low flame (don't use soured butter or butter from sweet cream).
2. After 15 to 20 minutes, the protein will settle on the bottom of the pan and start to thicken. The butter will smell like fresh popcorn.
3. As soon as the butter stops bubbling, take it off the fire, let it rest for 5 minutes, and filter the clarified butter into a ceramic pot.
4. You can keep the clarified butter for 2 to 3 months outside the refrigerator.

Snack - Fruit or fruit juice

Lunch - **Kichadi with Buttermilk Curry Sauce**

You can have this dish, which cleans and supports the bodily systems, 1 to 2 times a week.

Ingredients

1 to 2 tablespoons finely chopped ginger

3 tablespoons ghee

1/2 teaspoon cumin seeds

1/2 teaspoon fennel seeds

1 teaspoon coriander

3 or 4 curry leaves*

1 tablespoon finely chopped onion

1/2 teaspoon freshly ground black pepper

1 cup split mung beans

1 1/2 cups basmati rice

1 pound asparagus (If not available, use green leaves such as spinach or silver beet)

1/2 teaspoon sea salt

1 1/2 quarts fresh water

1/2 teaspoon cumin powder

Instructions

1. Wash the beans and the rice thoroughly and soak them in the water for 1 hour in 2 tablespoons of ghee.
2. Fry the cumin seeds, coriander, and fennel seeds over a low flame until the seeds are brown.
3. Add the curry leaves* and the onion.
4. Fry over a low flame until the onions are transparent.
5. Drain the beans and the rice and add them together with the water and the black pepper. Cook for 1 hour.
6. While the kichadi is cooking, cut the asparagus into 1-inch pieces.
7. Cook it in 2 cups of boiling water for 5 to 10 minutes.
8. Add the asparagus, 1 tablespoon of ghee, the salt, and the cumin powder to the kichadi.

Serve with:

Buttermilk Curry Sauce

Ingredients

1 1/2 cups buttermilk

1/2 cup water

1/2 teaspoon black pepper

1/2 teaspoon dried powdered ginger

4 to 6 crunched curry leaves*

Instructions

1. Mix the buttermilk and the water, pepper, ginger, and curry leaves.
2. Simmer on a low flame, stirring constantly, for 10 minutes.

Snack - Fruit or fruit juice

---

* Curry leaves, Murrayaa koenigii (not to be confused with curry powder) are small, pointed leaves native to tropical Asia, southern India and Sri Lanka. They have a strong aroma somewhat similar to citrus and anise.

Dinner - **Soup with toast**

Basic Soup Recipe

Ingredients

2 tablespoons sesame oil

1 teaspoon mustard seeds

½ teaspoon turmeric powder

2 teaspoon chopped onion

Any vegetables recommended for pregnancy (earlier in this chapter)

½ cup barley or rice (optional)

1 quart water

Salt and fresh herbs to taste

Instructions

1. Heat the oil in a wok.
2. Add the mustard seeds and fry them until the seeds pop up.
3. Add the onion and fry it on a low flame until transparent.
4. Add the turmeric powder and stir well.
5. Add the vegetables. If you want to make the soup thicker, add the barley or rice.
6. Stir well over a low flame for 5 to 10 minutes.
7. Add the water, stir, and cook for another 10 to 20 minutes.
8. Depending on the vegetables you use, add salt and fresh herbs to taste.

HINTS:

> Assimilating iron: Adding a tablespoon of lemon juice to the vegetables as they cook will improve your assimilation of vegetable iron.

> Counteracting dryness: Increase your consumption of ghee and good oils to alleviate vata problems like hard stools, bloating, disturbed sleep, and dry skin.

> Improving sleep: Before going to bed, warm ½ cup of milk (or soy milk) and add a teaspoon of ghee. This provides good sleep, cools your body, and supports the digestive system. Try also oiling the soles of your feet and your ankles with almond oil or sandalwood oil.

Oil Massage during Pregnancy

In India, massage is a must for pregnant women. To maximize your body's immune system, increase the elasticity of your skin and its sublayers, and strengthen your veins, oil your body daily with a good massage oil or simple almond oil. If you have a problem with varicose veins, oil your legs from your feet upward and don't rub the skin.

After oiling, wait for 20 to 30 minutes and then take a warm bath or shower.
(For more information on massaging, see Chapter 3, "Oil Massage after Delivery, page 426.")

In the Last Trimester

Oil the perineum, outer part of the vagina, and anus with St. John's wort oil. Prepare your nipples for breast-feeding by massaging them with a soft brush. Afterwards, oil them and the rest of your body with sesame or almond oil.

Chapter 3

Ayurvedic Recipes and Health Tips - After Delivery

40 Days of Uninterrupted Union

According to Ayurveda, mother and child should stay together, withdrawn from the outside world, for a full 40 days (six weeks) after delivery. There are several reasons for this:

- The mother can recover without having to bother about her work and household chores.
- The child is sheltered in the presence of its mother. Children who are kept in such a quiet atmosphere for the first six weeks have been found to be much more balanced than others, according to the *vaidyas* (experienced Ayurvedic doctors).
- The mother needs rest so that the process of breast-feeding will start smoothly and mother and child can get into a rhythm. The mother can breast-feed "on demand," that is, whenever the baby wants.

For the first nine days, the breast milk is very fatty and contains a high percentage of antibodies. It is mature only from the tenth day, and from then on, is fully adapted to the needs of the child.

According to medical studies, 400 ounces of oxygen are needed for one ounce of maternal milk. This is why we recommend that you:
Lie down in Shavasana at least twice a day for 15 to 20 minutes, and practice Ujjayi deep breathing in Shavasana.

Perform Supta Baddha Konasana with the bolster both crosswise and lengthwise.

The relaxation and higher intake of oxygen "purify" the milk and thus increase its quality. At the same time, tension in the breasts is reduced.

For the first ten days after delivery, you should eat hot cereal in order to calm down the vata state. Add as much ghee as you like. During pregnancy, pitta is dominant, whereas after delivery, vata is dominant.

Ayurvedic Recipes for Breast-Feeding

These recipes give you strength and enhance the quality of your breast milk.

Drink for after the morning and evening meals
(You can purchase these ingredients in a health food store.)

Mix thoroughly:
1 teaspoon Ashwagandha (available in Ayurvedic or Indian groceries
2 teaspoons Shatavari (Indian asparagus)
1 teaspoon licorice

Drink this mixture with half a cup of boiled milk.

Lunch

A kichadi recipe for the health of the reproductive system

Ingredients

1/2 teaspoon saffron

3 tablespoons ghee

1/2 teaspoon cumin seeds

1/2 teaspoon fenugreek seeds

3 or 4 curry leaves (page 418)

1 tablespoon finely chopped onion

1/8 teaspoon asafetida

1 cup split mung beans

1 1/2 cups basmati rice

1 pound asparagus (if not available, use green leaves such as spinach or silver beet)

1 teaspoon sea salt

1 1/2 quarts water

1/2 teaspoon cumin powder

Instructions

1. Fry the saffron.
2. Add 2 tablespoons ghee, the cumin, and the fenugreek seeds.
3. Fry over a low flame until the cumin seeds are brown.
4. Add the curry leaves, the onion, and the asafetida. Fry over a low flame until the onions are transparent.
5. Add the beans, rice, water, and salt, and cook for 1 hour.
6. While the kichadi is cooking, cut the asparagus into 1-inch pieces and cook it in 2 cups of boiling water for 5 to 10 minutes.
7. Add the asparagus, 1 tablespoon of ghee, and the cumin powder to the kichadi.

Serve with:
Buttermilk Curry Sauce
page 418

Dinner

You can have this rice dish every day, or whenever it is convenient to cook.

Ingredients

1 cup rice

3 tablespoons fenugreek seeds

1/2 teaspoon cumin seeds

1/2 teaspoon celery seeds

1/2 teaspoon coriander powder

1 tablespoon finely chopped onions

1 tablespoon ghee

3 cups water

Salt

Instructions

1. Cook the rice in the water and the spices for 30 minutes.
2. Fry the onions in the ghee until they are light brown.
3. Add the onion ghee to the rice and salt to taste.
4. Stir well.

Serve with steamed vegetables.

CHAPTER 3

The Ideal Diet

Foods to Avoid

When you're breast-feeding, you should stay away from:

- Dried pulses (peas, beans, lentils, etc.), with the exception of mung beans and soy beans
- Cabbage, with the exception of Chinese cabbage
- Hot and spicy dishes cooked with chilies and lots of garlic and onions
- Acidic or oily foods: meat, sugar, sweeteners, vinegar, and sour fruits

These might cause bloating, not only for you, but also for the baby.

Avoid eating dry food such as bread (beyond a moderate amount), day-old leftovers, and frozen food.

Restrict how much coffee and black tea you drink, because these dehydrate. Have instead green tea, fenugreek tea, and hot or warm water instead of cold drinks.

If you eat heavy proteins such as black lentils or cheese, you should eat them for lunch to ensure full digestion before bedtime.

Healthy Foods

Foods you should eat include alkaline foods like vegetables, green leaves, juicy fruits, cereals, and homemade bread made from organic whole wheat.

The following foods are recommended because they:

1. Balance the fire of digestion, the agni
2. Alleviate the vata state
3. Promote lactation

Grains

Organic whole wheat, oats, basmati rice, millet, barley, mung beans, *urid dhal* (Indian black lentil soup), pasta made from organic whole wheat or millet, and homemade bread from organic whole wheat or millet.

Fruit

Ripe, juicy, sweet fruit (can be slightly steamed for easier digestion), including apples, pears, apricots, plums, pomegranates, dates, figs, limes, sweet oranges, papaya, and peaches. (Grapes and cherries, though sweet, can cause bloating. Dried fruit can increase vata, as well.)

Cooked Vegetables

Carrots, celery, onion, Chinese cabbage, zucchini, tomatoes (ripe), beet root, cucumbers, sprouts, potatoes (in moderation), sweet potatoes, spinach, mangold (a kind of beet), green beans, cassava, mushrooms, asparagus, plenty of green herbs and green leaves. (If the baby's stool turns green, cut green leaves from your diet.)

Note

Nightshades such as paprika, eggplant, potatoes, pumpkin, and zucchini can cause bloating. Find out how to prepare them with ghee and spices that warm the stomach, such as ginger, nutmeg, black pepper, and cumin seeds, to enhance digestibility.

Nuts and Seeds

Roast these without fat in a pan: almonds, sesame seeds, pumpkin seeds, coconut, macadamia nuts, pine nuts, and walnuts.

Fats

Sesame oil, olive oil, pumpkin seed oil, mustard oil, sunflower seed oil, and ghee

Herbs

Ginger, cardamom, black pepper, nutmeg, celery seeds, fennel, cumin, mustard seeds, turmeric, anis, cinnamon, cloves, Ayurvedic masalas (spice mixtures), rock salt, fenugreek, turmeric, saffron, coriander leaves, rosemary, and basil

Milk Products

- Fresh cow's milk (1 cup per day), buttermilk, ghee, fresh goat cheese, fresh sheep cheese, fenugreek cheese, and cream
- Don't mix milk products with fruit. This causes a curdling of the milk product, which forms a kind of cheese in the acidic stomach environment that is heavy to digest and can even cause joint problems.

Nonlactic Proteins

Soy milk, tofu, and miso soup (from barley or soy)

Beverages

Have 2 to 3 quarts of hot water a day and follow this procedure:
Boil the water for 10 minutes and pour half of it into a thermos bottle.
Boil the rest of the water for 5 more minutes with 3 slices of fresh or dried ginger and 1 teaspoon of celery seeds. (You can also try 1 teaspoon of fenugreek instead of these ingredients.) Ginger warms the stomach, celery seeds prevent bloating, and fenugreek improves the condition of the body.

Sugar

Jaggery (unrefined brown sugar), cane sugar, and honey

CHAPTER 3

Oil Massage after Delivery

Starting with the fourth day after delivery and for forty days thereafter (or longer, if possible), you and your baby must receive *abhyanga*, a "loving hands" oil massage, as regularly as nourishment. Although many women today feel that they can't afford to "take off" forty days, your physical and mental health will suffer if you don't. You especially need the cleansing effect of massage, since the yogasanas you can do during this time are limited to Shavasana, Supta Baddha Konasana, and pranayama.

Massage helps you relax and helps your system reorganize itself after the physical and mental strain of delivery. It also helps your body, especially the musculature of the stomach region, return to its prepregnancy state.

More Good Reasons for Oil Massage

Preventing arthritis: Pregnancy and breast-feeding can make your joints more susceptible to arthritis. Massage helps with this problem.

Averting depression: These feelings can be caused by hormonal changes after delivery and by changes in a new mother's situation at home. Studies conducted in Great Britain estimated that more than 50 percent of new mothers suffer from depression.

Dr. Elizabeth Young, a gynecologist at Homerton University Hospital in London, recommends abhyanga, Ayurvedic oil massage, to mothers who have just given birth. The entire body is gently massaged with warm sesame oil or almond oil, with the main emphasis on the head, forehead, back, and lower abdomen. Dr. Young found that women who received the massages were clearly less nervous, exhausted, and depressive.

Regeneration: Oil massage supports the uterus in quickly returning to its normal state. The expanded tissue of the pelvic and abdominal areas recovers faster, and pain in the back and lower abdomen is reduced.

◇

Abhyanga Techniques

The technique below is for both mother and child.

You can massage yourself, if necessary, although you'll need help for your upper back. If there is no such help available, just do as much as you can.

After you have enjoyed an oil massage, you or the baby's father can also massage the baby. For both of you, be sure to warm the oil first.

The Ayurveda recommends starting to massage the baby six days after birth. You can do the massage, which strengthens and develops the muscles and bones, at bath time.

For the first months, gently oil the head first, followed by the front of the body: torso, arms, and legs, and then the same in the back, following the direction of the growth of the body hair. Babies enjoy being massaged, and also seem to sleep more deeply and have a stronger immune system if they are regularly massaged.

Before starting the massage, oil the anus and wash your hands.

1. Head

Begin with the head, using your fingers and fingertips. Massage the following areas in circular movements from the inside to the outside:

- The crown of the head, clockwise
- The left and right side of the neck, from bottom to top
- The sides of the throat, from bottom to top (where the hair starts)
- The forehead, from the center down to the temples
- The temples, from top to bottom, down to the cheeks
- The cheeks: from the outer cheeks towards the nose, from the nose down to the lips, the corners of the lips down to the chin, and the lower cheeks towards the ears
- The ears, from bottom to top and from outside to inside
- Back to the forehead
- Repeat 7 times

2. Front torso

Massage with flat hands in 14 circular movements, clockwise.

- The navel, with small circular movements
- Slowly widen the movements, until they reach the pubic plate, the sides of the torso, the floating ribs, and the area below the breast.
- The left breast, with your flat right hand, in 7 circular movements from inside to outside, starting in the area around the breast and becoming more narrow
- Repeat for the right breast, with your flat left hand

3. Armpits, shoulders, arms, and hands

Armpits

- The left armpit, with your flat right hand, in 7 circular movements from inside to outside, starting in the center of the armpit and becoming wider
- Repeat for the right armpit, with your flat left hand

Shoulders

- The left shoulder, with your flat right hand, one stroke from the breastbone towards the shoulder and then 7 circular movements on the shoulder
- Repeat 3 times
- Repeat for the right shoulder, with your flat left hand

Arms and hands

- Start at the left shoulder, with the side of your right index finger, 1 circular movement around the shoulder and then 7 long strokes alternating 1 on the inside and 1 on the outside of the upper arm, down towards the elbow
- The elbow joint, with your thumb, 7 circular movements alternating on the inside and the outside
- The lower arm, with your thumb, 7 long strokes alternating 1 on the inside and 1 on the outside, towards the wrist
- The wrist, with your thumb, 7 circular movements alternating on the inside and the outside
- From the wrist towards the fingertips and beyond the fingertips, with your thumb or palm, 7 circular movements, and then, with your fingers and thumbs, long strokes
- Repeat for the right arm with your left hand

4. Sides of the waist

With flat hands and your fingers pointing forward, 7 circular movements from back to front, and 7 circular movements from front to back, extending the circular movements up to the floating ribs and down to the pelvic rim.

5. Hips and legs

Hips

- With flat hands and your fingers pointing forward, 7 circular movements from back to front, and 7 circular movements from front to back
- With the last movement, extend your hands (with the thumbs spread apart) down to the upper thighs

Legs

- For each leg, with both hands, 7 long strokes on the front, the inside, the outside, and the back of the thighs down to the knee
- The knee, mainly with both thumbs, in 7 circular movements on the front, the inside, the outside, and the back
- With both hands, again 7 long strokes on the front, the inside, the outside, and the calf down to the ankle
- Mainly with your fingers and thumbs, 7 circular movements on the front, the inside, and the outside
- For the foot, apply the same technique as for the hands: 7 circular movements on the sole and then 7 long strokes from the ankle to the tips of the toes.

6. Back torso

- Ask a friend to help you by doing the following, with flat hands in circular movements
- Starting on the sacrum (spine just above the tail-bone), with one or both hands, 7 circular movements, clockwise
- With both hands, movements from inside out:
  - Lower back, 7 circular movements
  - Towards the back of the waist, 7 circular movements upward
  - Middle back, 7 circular movements
  - Sides of the torso, 7 circular movements
  - Upper back, 7 circular movements
  - Shoulder blades, 7 circular movements
  - Shoulders, 7 circular movements
- With both hands:
  - Top to bottom down to the lower back, 7 long strokes
  - Back of the shoulders and the back of the arms towards the hands, 7 long strokes

7. Sacrum, buttocks, legs, and feet

- Your friend can help you with this as well, using circular movements:
- Starting on the sacrum, with one hand, 7 circular movements, clockwise
- With both hands, movements from inside out:
  - Buttocks and hips, 7 circular movements
  - Back of the left leg towards the back of the knee, 7 strokes
  - Back of the knees, 7 circular movements
  - Lower leg towards the ankle, 7 strokes
  - Ankle, 7 circular movements
  - Sole, 7 circular movements
  - From heel to toes, 7 strokes
- Repeat for the right leg.
- Finish the back with flat hands, from buttocks to toes, 7 strokes

USEFUL LINKS AND ADDRESSES

B. K. S. Iyengar website : www.bksiyengar.com

USA

Iyengar Yoga Association of the United States
3940 Laurel Canyon Blvd #947
Studio City , CA 91604, USA
1 800 889-YOGA
www.iynaus.org

Iyengar Yoga Association of Greater New York
150 West 22nd Street, 11th floor
New York, NY 10011, USA
212-691-YOGA (9642)
212.255.1773 fax
Info@iyengarnyc.org
www.iyengarnyc.org

BKS Iyengar Yoga Center of Las Vegas
6342 W Sahara Ave ,
Las Vegas , Nevada – 89146, USA
702.222.9642
iyasn@iynaus.org
www.iyclv.com

BKS Iyengar Yoga Studio of Dallas
5539 Dyer Street ,
Dallas , Texas – 75206, USA
214.365.9642
marj1@airmail.net
www.dallasiyengaryoga.com

The Yoga Center of Nashville
2822 Columbine Place ,
Nashville , Tennessee - 37204-3104, USA
615.383.0785
jcampbell@yogacenternashville.com
www.yogacenternashville.com

BKS Iyengar Yoga Studio of Tucson
3400 E Speedway Suite 200,
Rancho Center, Tucson, Arizona – 85716, USA
520.743.7142
iyengartucson@msn.com

BKS Iyengar Yoga Studio of Philadelphia
2200 Ben Franklin Pkwy, South Bldg, Lower Level,
Philadelphia, Pennsylvania – 19130, USA
215.568.1961
mariang102@aol.com
www.philayoga.com

Iyengar Yoga Center of Boulder
2299 Pearl Street ,
Boulder , Colorado – 80302, USA
brenda@iyengaryoga.org
www.philayoga.com

Iyengar Yoga Center of Denver
770 S Broadway ,
Denver , Colorado – 80209, USA
303.316.8466
iycd@earthlink.net
www.iyengaryogacenter.com

Iyengar Yoga Institute of Los Angeles
8233 W Third Street ,
Los Angeles , California – 90048, USA
213.399.9877
yogarth@comcast.net
www.iyogala.org

BKS Iyengar Yoga Centers of San Diego
4704 East Mountain View Dr ,
San Diego , California – 92116, USA
619.226.2202
info@sandiegoyoga.com
www.sandiegoyoga.com

Iyengar Yoga Institute of San Francisco
2404 27th Avenue ,
San Francisco , California – 94116, USA
415.753.0909
www.iyisf.org

BKS Iyengar Yoga Institute of Champaign-Urbana
407 W Springfiled ,
Urbana , Illinois – 61801, USA
217.344.9642
info@yoga-cu.com
www.yoga-cu.com

BKS Iyengar Yoga Center Minneapolis
2736 Lyndale Ave S.,
Minneapolis, Minnesota – 55408, USA
612.872.8708
iyengaryogampls@yahoo.com
www.iyengaryogampls.com

Iyengar Yoga in Harvard Square
154 Mt Auburn St ,
Cambridge, Massachusetts – 02138, USA
617.661.7370
Eleanor@yoga.com

Iyengar Yoga in West Roxbury
Emmanuel Church,
Boston , Massachusetts – 02132, USA
617.323.4289
laureen@yogaclasses.net

CANADA

Iyengar Yoga Association of Canada
infoNOSPAM@iyengaryogacanada.com
www.iyengaryogacanada.ca

Centre de Yoga Iyengar de Montréal
917, avenue du Mont-Royal est
Montréal, Québec H2J 1X3, Canada
514 528-8288
www.iyengaryogamontreal.com

Iyengar Yoga center of Victoria
202 - 919 Fort Street,
Victoria, B.C., V8V 3K3, Canada
250-386-YOGA (9642)
iyoga@telus.net
www.iyengaryogacanada.ca

Iyengar Yoga Center Ottawa
784 Bronson Avenue
Ottawa, Ontario K1S 4G4, Canada
(613) 761-7888
iyoga@canada.com
www.iyoga.ca

Glossary of Sanskrit Terms

The terms below appear in an adapted Sanskrit, i.e., in an English transliteration of the Sanskrit words, throughout the book. These Sanskrit terms are used all over the world and provide a common linguistic basis among practitioners of Yoga. Translations, however, although useful, can only approximate the original meaning.

Adho - downward

Angushtha - big toe

Ardha - half

Asana - pose

Ayurveda - knowledge of long life, formed from *ayur* (long life) and *veda* (knowledge)

Baddha - bound, caught

Bandha - bondage, formation, construction

Bharadvaja - the name of a sage

Chandra - moon

Chitta - composed of mind, intellect, and ego

Danda - Stick

Dhanu - bow

Dosha - one of three active principles of the body according to Ayurveda, namely *vata*, *pitta*, and *kapha*

Dvi - two

Eka - one

Hala - plough

Hasta - hand

Jala - net

Janu - knee

Jathara - stomach

Kapha - one of the three *doshas*; the earth and water principle, the static and stabilizing energy

Kona - angle

Mantra - a word or words that are compressed, concise, and powerful in meaning

Marichi - grandfather of the Sun God (*Surya*)

Matsya - fish

Mudra - seal, closing, control

Nava - boat

Pada - foot

Padma - lotus

Paripurna - complete

Parivartana - turning round, rotating

Parivritta - twisted

Parshva - side, flank, lateral

Parvata - mountain

Pashchima - west, the back of the body

Pitta - one of the three *doshas*; the fire principle, responsible for digestion and transformation

Prakriti - in *Amkhya* philosophy, original matter in its unmanifested form, also constitution, the nature of an individual that remains throughout life

Prana - breath, vital force

Prasarita - spread apart

Salamba - with support

Sarvanga - entire body

Shavasana - motionless like a corpse

Setu - bridge

Shirsha - head

Supta - sleeping pose, supine

Shvana - dog

Tada - steady, erect like a mountain

Tri - three

Triang - three parts (foot, knees, and buttocks)

Ujjayi - formed from *ud* (upwards, superior in rank, expanding, blowing, indicating a sense of power) and *jaya* (victory, conquest)

Upavishta - seated, sitting

Urdhva - above

Ushtra - camel

Uttana - lying on back, intense stretch

Utthita - extended

Vata - one of the three *doshas*; ether and wind principle, the dynamic force

Viloma - against the hair, against the natural order of things, formed from *vi* (negation) and *loma* (hair)

Viparita - opposite, reverse or inverted

Vira - brave, a hero

Virabhadra - a warrior

Vrksha - tree

Index

C

D

E

V

W

Y

References

Chapter 1

1/1 Translation from B. K. S. Iyengar, *Light on Yoga* (Schocken; Revised edition, 1995).

1/2 *Charaka Samhita*
Chowkhamba Sanskrit Series Office
Varanasi, 1997

1/3 *Hatha Yoga Pradipika*
by Svatmarama
Adyar Library, Madras, India, 1972

1/4 Parts of Chapter 1 were taken from Geeta S. Iyengar, *Gem for Women*, Allied Publishers Private Ltd, 1983.

Chapter 2

The following references refer to the *Vagbhata, Ashtanga Hrudaya*, Vol. 1, Section 2, Chapter 1: Garbhavakranti Sharira/Embryology, following the translation by Prof. K. R. Srikatha Murthy:

2/1 Sloka 1
2/2 Sloka 3
2/3 Sloka 4
2/4 Sloka 21b – 22a
2/5 Sloka 35b – 36
2/6 Sloka 2
2/7 Sloka 49b – 50a
2/8 Sloka 50 – 54a
2/9 Sloka 54b – 55
2/10 Sloka 56
2/11 Sloka 57
2/12 Sloka 62 – 63
2/13 Sloka 74b – 76
2/14 and 2/15 B. K. S. Iyengar, *Light on the Yoga Sutras of Patanjali*, Harper Collins Publishers, 1993, London

Chapter 3

3/1 *Samkhya*
2nd Indian Edition, 1979
Oriental Books Reprint Corporation, New Delhi

Chapter 5

5/1 *Hatha Yoga Pradipika*
by Svatmarama
Adyar Library, Madras, India, 1972

ACKNOWLEDGEMENTS

Over the past few years, many individuals have contributed to the making of this book and have helped in one way or another to give it its present form. We feel deep gratitude towards all of them and at the same time, we offer our apologies for not being able to mention each and every one by name.

It is the depth and brilliance of B. K. S. Iyengar's teaching and his profound insights into the benefits and effectiveness of yogic (asana and pranayama) practice during and after pregnancy that inspired us initially to make this knowledge available to a larger audience. We are forever grateful for the many fruitful discussions we had with him concerning the contents of the book, which helped us gain clarity about the needs of women in relation to Yoga practice throughout pregnancy and especially after delivery.

We also thank Prof. Dilip Gadgil, an experienced, well-known lecturer and Ayurvedic medical doctor at Tilak Maharashtra Vidyapeeth, an Ayurvedic university in Poona, for reviewing the chapter on Ayurveda.

As the illustrative photos are an integral part of the book, meant to convey a maximum of information in combination with the text, we are grateful to our photographer Dominik Ketz for his excellent craftsmanship and for being there for us whenever we needed to take pictures over the last four years.

Part of the charm of the photos is the fact that we were able to work with the same model during all phases of pregnancy. Special thanks therefore to our good friend G. Fraunhofer for her willingness and patience to have herself photographed during two pregnancies and the time after delivery between the two pregnancies.

We would also like to thank Gabi Doron from the Iyengar Yoga Center, Neve Tzedek, Tel-Aviv, and Horst Binski from the Iyengar Yoga Institut Rhein-Ahr, Cologne, for their special support and help.

Geeta S. Iyengar, Rita Keller, and Kerstin Khattab